A PRACTICE OF CARDIAC PACING

Third Edition

A PRACTICE OF CARDIAC PACING

Third Edition

by

Seymour Furman, MD, FACS, FACC

Attending Cardiothoracic Surgeon
Montefiore Medical Center
Professor of Surgery
Professor of Medicine
Albert Einstein College of Medicine of Yeshiva University
Bronx, New York

David L. Hayes, MD

Consultant, Division of Cardiovascular Diseases
and Internal Medicine
Director, Cardiac Pacing Services
Mayo Clinic and Mayo Foundation
Associate Professor of Medicine
Mayo Medical School
Rochester, Minnesota

David R. Holmes, Jr., MD

Consultant, Division of Cardiovascular Diseases
and Internal Medicine
Mayo Clinic and Mayo Foundation
Professor of Medicine
Mayo Medical School
Rochester, Minnesota

Futura Publishing
Company, Inc.
Armonk, New York

Library of Congress Cataloging-in-Publication Data

Furman, Seymour.
    A practice of cardiac pacing / by Seymour Furman, David L. Hayes,
David R. Homes, Jr.—3rd ed.
          p.   cm.
    Includes bibliographical references and index.
    ISBN 0-87993-538-3
    1. Cardiac pacing.   I. Hayes, David L.   II. Holmes, David R.,
1945–   . III. Title.
    [DNLM: 1. Cardiac Pacing, Artificial—methods.   2. Pacemaker,
Artificial.   WG 168 F986p 1993]
RC684.P3F867   1993
617.4′12059—dc20
DNLM/DLC
for Library of Congress   92-48502
                                                                      CIP

Copyright 1993
Futura Publishing Company, Inc.

Published by
Futura Publishing Company, Inc.
135 Bedford Road
Armonk, New York 10504

L.C. No.: 92-48502
ISBN No.: 0-87993-538-3

Every effort has been made to ensure that the information in this book is as
up to date and accurate as possible at the time of publication. However, due
to the constant developments in medicine, neither the author, nor the editor,
nor the publisher can accept any legal or any other responsibility for any
errors or omissions that may occur.

Printed in the United States of America

FOREWORD

A rich literature about cardiac pacing exists in the major world languages. Many books have been published, almost all multiauthored and, indeed, with the editor only one of many authors. The book that presents either a single point of view or one with only the viewpoints of several contributor-authors is uncommon. This book, now in its third edition, is an attempt at such a limited perspective of the evolving field of cardiac pacing within the rapidly developing discipline of electrical stimulation of the heart. Indeed, electrical cardiac stimulation for arrhythmia control is a field barely a quarter of a century old. In the first edition implantable cardioversion and defibrillation, one of the major areas of such stimulation, received only the most cursory mention. By the second edition a chapter had been included that has now been rewritten and enlarged. Additional chapters on rate modulation and the variety and intricacy of dual-chamber function have also been added with overall substantial enlargement of the effort. While something may be lost limiting the number of authors, a great deal is gained by a personal approach from two large practices of cardiac stimulation, Montefiore Medical Center and the Mayo clinic. This book is intended to be a readable and accessible tutorial, responsive to the needs of the less experienced worker and valuable even to the more experienced. For those goals we hope it will be a useful contribution to the cardiac stimulation literature.

The volume is extensively illustrated with many ECGs, x-rays, and diagrams of the operation of pacing modes. The bibliography focuses on those references that seem most necessary rather than attempting to be exhaustive. The text is intended to be a practical exposition of how pacemakers work with emphasis as well on basic science related to the electrophysiology of cardiac stimulation. An understanding of how pacemakers work, and what telemetric, radiological, and electrocardiographic findings are associated with normal and abnormal function is intended. These analyses should delineate anomalous and normal function and help to clarify the complexity of modern cardiac pacing and implantable defibrillator therapy. We attempt not only to delineate the anomalous and normal functions but also to integrate the diagnostic capabilities of modern cardiac pacemaker systems into daily practice. We have also emphasized the utility of modern dual-chamber and rate modulated pacemakers and the variety of timing systems, atrial and ventricular based, that now make up cardiac pacing. In all we have emphasized modern, basic, and practical single- and dual-chamber pacing and the associated complications, the individual indications for each, and the operational differences among hardware.

Much has transpired in the seven years since the first edition. The dual-chamber approach is now a mainstay of cardiac pacing in the United States and rate modulated pacing, especially single chamber, is widely used around the world. The use of the implantable cardioverter defibrillator (ICD) for management of ventricular arrhythmias is increasing progressively and rapidly and has gone from an innovative approach to a mainstay of management of malignant ventricular arrhythmias. This is reflected in a large chapter, newly written, about the implanted cardioverter defibrillator. Much information has been added to this edition. Each chapter has been revised to some degree and several chapters have been extensively revised. The volume is larger than the first or second editions. We hope that the reader will find that we have succeeded in the attempt to provide a sense of the practice of cardiac pacing and implanted defibrillation and will consider the volume as providing an experienced "consultant" when one is needed.

The authors want to thank Shari Gardner for her support of the writing process and Joanne Lama whose assistance in preparing all three editions has been integral to its completion and above and beyond the call of duty.

CONTENTS

PART I.

BASIC CONSIDERATIONS

Chapter 1

INDICATIONS FOR PERMANENT PACING

David L. Hayes

The precise criteria for the implantation of a permanent pacemaker vary from institution to institution. Some conduction disturbances generally are accepted to be definite indications for permanent pacing, and for some others, there is general agreement that permanent pacing is not necessary. In a number of conduction disturbances, the need for permanent pacing is debatable but pacing is probably necessary and depends on the clinical circumstances. Because of changes in diagnosis and therapy, the absolute indications for permanent pacing are constantly evolving. Difficulties arise when an attempt is made to list rigid indications for implanted pacemaker insertion.

Before concluding that permanent pacing is in the best interest of the patient, the physician must carefully and thoughtfully analyze the patient. This analysis should include the general medical status, as well as the specifics of the cardiac rhythm disturbance. Although at one time permanent pacemakers were used solely for the treatment of atrioventricular (AV) block, pacing is appropriate for the control of any symptomatic bradyarrhythmia. Recent advances in pacemaker technology also have increased the indications for dual-chamber pacemakers. Pacemakers with antitachycardia capabilities have extended pacer treatment to include complex bradyarrhythmias and tachyarrhythmias. Controversy still exists over the implantation of pacemakers for bifascicular and trifascicular block, for new-onset bundle branch block in acute myocardial infarction, and for treatment of patients with bradycardia-related low cardiac output syndromes including, chronic congestive heart failure and others.

GUIDELINES FOR PACEMAKER IMPLANTATION AND REIMBURSEMENT

Guidelines for implantation of cardiac pacemakers have been established by a task force formed jointly by the American College of Cardiology and the American Heart Association. The first set of guidelines was published in 1984. A revised set of guidelines was published in 1991. Although there are occasional cases that cannot be categorized according to the ACC/AHA guidelines they are, for the most part, all-encompassing and have been widely endorsed.

In addition, Medicare has established approved and nonapproved indications for the justification of permanent pacing. Most third-party payers also follow the Medicare guidelines. If a clinical decision is made that permanent pacing is indicated and the indication does not fit within the approved Medicare guidelines, then it is advisable when dealing with non-Medicare patients, to seek preapproval from the third-party payer. For Medicare patients, depending upon state regulations, preapproval may not be possible. If no preapproval practice exists in a given state, then it is best to proceed with permanent pacing when it is believed to be clinically indicated. In addition, all symptoms, objective evidence of a rhythm disturbance, and the logic by which it is felt that permanent pacing is indicated should be thoroughly documented in the patient's records. If the pacemaker implant is challenged by the Medicare system, all of this information will be useful to avoid denial of payment.

Hospitals are reimbursed for pacemaker-related procedures by diagnosis-related groups (DRGs). The four pacing DRGs do not give specific indications for pacing but simply provide the diagnosis-related group for both initial and replacement procedures. The pacing DRGs currently are defined as follows:

115. Permanent pacemaker implant with primary diagnosis of acute myocardial infarction, heart failure or shock.
116. Permanent pacemaker implant without primary diagnosis of acute myocardial infarction, heart failure, or shock.
117. Pacemaker revision in all cases except those in which the pulse generator is the only component being replaced.
118. Pacemaker pulse generator replacement only.

Combinations of procedures also are considered. A pacing procedure that is coupled with another cardiovascular surgical procedure is placed in the DRG with the heavier weight. For example, a patient simultaneously requiring a prosthetic heart valve and an initial implant of a pacemaker would be in the DRG of the prosthetic heart valve. The hospital would receive the reimbursement rate associated with the DRG category of the prosthetic heart valve only.

Although some indications for permanent pacing are relatively certain or unambiguous, others require considerable expertise and judgment. It is easiest to consider indications for pacemaker implantation in three specific groups. Following is the definition for each of the 3 Groups and a list of indications that corresponds to that category. Subsequently, specific conduction system disturbances are discussed individually.

Group 1

Group 1 includes conditions in which implantation of a cardiac pacemaker is considered acceptable and necessary, provided that the conditions are chronic and recurrent and not due to transient causes, such as acute myocardial infarction, drug interaction, and electrolyte imbalance. If the rhythm disturbance is chronic or recurrent, a single episode of a symptom such as syncope, presyncope, or seizure is adequate to establish medical necessity.

1. Acquired complete AV block. Potential symptoms include: syncope, seizure, congestive heart failure, dizziness, confusion, and limited exercise tolerance. However, asymptomatic acquired complete AV block is a generally accepted indication for pacing (Figures 1 and 2).
2. Congenital complete heart block with severe bradycardia, significant physiological deficit, or significant symptoms due to the bradycardia.

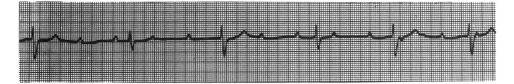

Figure 1. Complete heart block is characterized by dissociation between atrial and ventricular activity. The atrial rate approximates 95 bpm while the ventricular rate is about 35 bpm. While antegrade conduction seems entirely lost, the fifth ventricular complex is followed by a retrograde P wave, indicating retained retrograde conduction, a circumstance which occurs in about 10% of fixed antegrade complete AV block.

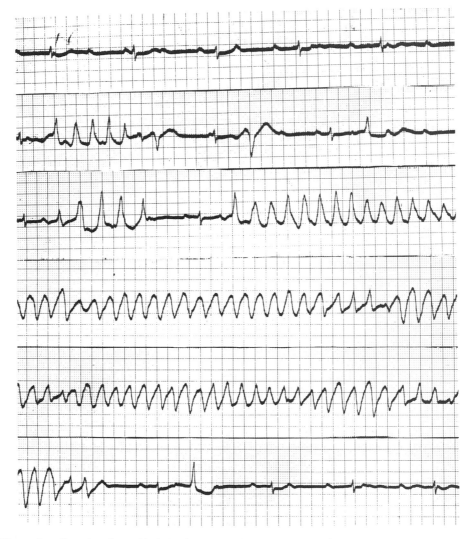

Figure 2. Complete heart block is characterized by dissociation between atrial and ventricular activity. Several ventricular foci may exist. Symptoms of circulatory arrest follow ventricular asystole, or as in this case, ventricular tachycardia, monomorphic or polymorphic.

3. Symptomatic Mobitz II AV block (Figure 3).
4. Symptomatic Mobitz I second-degree AV block with symptoms related to hemodynamic instability (Figure 4).
5. Symptomatic sinus bradycardia (syncope, seizures, congestive heart failure) or substantial sinus bradycardia (heart rate of <40 bpm) associated with dizziness or confusion (Figure 5). The guidelines state that the correlation between symptoms and bradycardia must be documented or the symptoms must be clearly attributed to the bradycardia rather than to some other cause.
6. A less distinct group of patients with sinus bradycardia of lesser severity (heart rate >40 bpm) and dizziness or confusion. Again, correlation between symptoms and bradycardia must be documented in the patient.
7. Symptomatic sinus bradycardia that is the consequence of long-term required drug treatment for which there is no acceptable alternative.
8. Sinus node dysfunction and symptomatic bradycardia with or without tachyarrhythmias or AV block. This category includes tachycardia-bradycardia syndrome, sinoatrial block, and sinus arrest.
9. Sinus node dysfunction with or without symptoms when there are potentially life-threatening ventricular arrhythmias or tachycardia secondary to bradycardia.
10. Bradycardia associated with significant symptoms and with supraventricular tachycardia and high-degree AV block unresponsive to appropriate pharmacological management. Included here are patients with carotid sinus hypersensitivity and syncope due to bradycardia who do not respond to prophylactic medical measures.

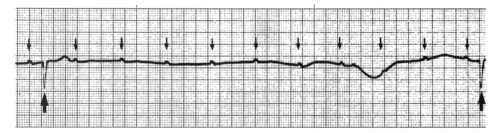

Figure 3. *High-grade AV block in which there is sporadic failure to conduct from atrium through AV node. In this example the first and last P waves appear to result in ventricular depolarization with a PR interval of approximately 220 ms. However, between QRS complexes there are 9 P waves that are not conducted through the AV node and result in a 7.4-second period of ventricular asystole.*

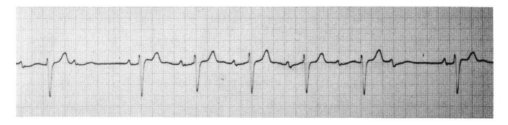

Figure 4. *Wenckebach AV block (Mobitz I) conduction defect allows progressive prolongation of the PR interval until a P wave is blocked. The cycle then recurs.*

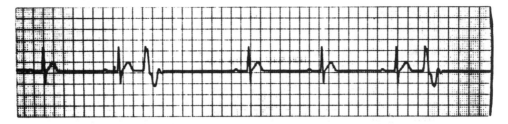

Figure 5. *Sinus bradycardia occurs at a rate of 39 bpm. The patient was symptomatic at this rate.*

Group 2

Group 2 includes conditions in which use of a cardiac pacemaker may be found acceptable or necessary, provided the medical history and prognosis of the patient can be documented and there is evidence that pacemaker implantation will assist in overall management.

1. Congenital complete heart block with less severe bradycardia.
2. Bifascicular or trifascicular block accompanied by syncope that is attributed to transient complete heart block after other plausible causes of syncope have been reasonably excluded.
3. Prophylactic pacemaker use after recovery from acute myocardial infarction during which there is transient, complete, or Mobitz II second-degree AV block.
4. Asymptomatic Mobitz II second-degree AV block.
5. Symptomatic sinus bradycardia (heart rate <45 bpm) that is a consequence of long-term necessary drug treatment for which there is no acceptable alternative.
6. Overdrive pacing in patients with recurrent and refractory ventricular tachycardia (overdrive pacing) to prevent ventricular tachycardia.

Group 3

Group 3 includes conditions that are considered unsupported by adequate evidence to benefit from permanent pacing and, therefore, generally should not be considered appropriate uses for pacemakers in the absence of indications noted in group 1 and group 2.

1. Syncope of undetermined cause. This requires vigorous investigation, including ambulatory monitoring, neurological evaluation, and electrophysiological testing (including tilt-table testing), in selected patients. (If the history strongly suggests that the syncope is of cardiogenic etiology, cardiac pacing may be considered. In such cases, the patient must understand that permanent pacing may not alleviate the symptoms since no correlation between symptoms and rhythm has been documented. When possible, preapproval for pacemaker implantation should be sought from the patient's insurance provider.)
2. Sinus bradycardia without significant symptoms.
3. Sinoatrial block or sinus arrest without significant symptoms.

4. Prolonged RR intervals with atrial fibrillation or other causes of transient ventricular pause.
5. Bradycardia during sleep.
6. Right bundle branch block with left axis deviation without syncope or other symptoms of intermittent AV block.
7. Asymptomatic second-degree Mobitz I (Wenckebach) AV block (Figure 4).
8. First-degree AV block. (There are case reports of pacing for first-degree AV block when the PR interval is so long that there is effective loss of AV synchrony with hemodynamic compromise.)

Categories of conduction disturbances to be considered individually include: acquired AV block, AV block occurring with myocardial infarction, bifascicular and trifascicular block (chronic), sinus node dysfunction, and carotid hypersensitivity. Antitachycardia pacing is discussed in Chapter 13.

AV Block

AV block is the impairment of conduction of a cardiac impulse from the atrium to the ventricles. It can occur at different levels, depending on whether it is proximal to the AV node, at the level of the AV node, or at the level of the His-Purkinje conduction system.

Electrocardiographically, AV block has been divided into first-, second-, and third-degree (complete) heart block (Table I). First-degree heart block is a prolonged PR interval without failure of ventricular conduction. The normal PR interval is defined electrocardiographically as a range of 120–200 ms. First-degree AV block is usually secondary to a delay of impulse conduction through the AV node or the atrium. It is a nonspecific finding and not an indication for pacing (Figure 6).

Table I
Atrioventricular Block

Degree	Pacemaker Necessary	Pacemaker Probably Necessary	Pacemaker Not Necessary
Third	Symptomatic congenital complete heart block Acquired symptomatic complete heart block Atrial fibrillation with complete heart block Acquired asymptomatic complete heart block		
Second	Symptomatic type I Symptomatic type II	Asymptomatic type II Asymptomatic type I at intra-His or infra-His levels	Asymptomatic type I at supra-His (AV nodal) level
First			Asymptomatic or symptomatic

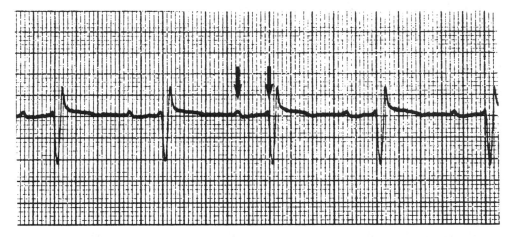

Figure 6. *First-degree AV block in which there is, by definition, prolongation of the PR interval greater than 200 ms. This conduction disturbance is benign and does not require treatment. PR interval in this illustration is noted by the arrows and measures approximately 300 ms.*

Second-degree heart block (Figures 3, 4, 7, 8) occurs when an atrial impulse that should be conducted to the ventricle is not. The nonconducted P waves may be intermittent or frequent, at regular or irregular intervals, and preceded by fixed or lengthening PR intervals. A distinguishing feature is that conducted P waves relate to the QRS complex in a recurrent pattern and are not random. Second-degree AV block has been classified into type I and type II Mobitz block. Typical type I second-degree AV block (Wenckebach block, Mobitz I) is characterized by progressive PR prolongation culminating in a nonconducted P wave (Figure 4). In type II second-degree AV block (Mobitz II), the PR interval remains constant before the blocked P wave (Figure 3). The AV block is intermittent and generally repetitive and may result in several nonconducted P waves in a row. Mobitz I and II are applied to the two types of block, whereas "Wenckebach block" refers to Mobitz I block only.

Separating second-degree AV block into type I and type II is important and, in most cases, can be done by ECG. Type II second-degree AV block often

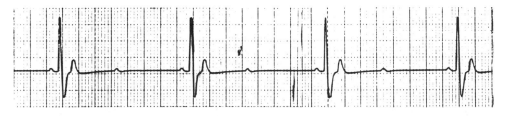

Figure 7. *AV block, 2:1, in which the QRS complex appears narrow. When the conduction ratio remains in a 2:1 pattern, it is impossible to tell from the ECG exactly where in the AV node the conduction disturbance occurs. A narrow QRS complex suggests that the conduction defect is "intra-His" as opposed to "infra-His," which would result more commonly in a wide QRS complex.*

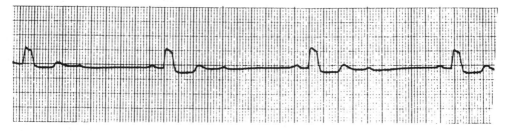

Figure 8. *AV block, 2:1, with a left intraventricular conduction delay. This pattern is suggestive of an infra-His conduction defect.*

precedes the development of higher grades of AV block, whereas type I second-degree AV block is usually a less severe conduction disturbance and does not consistently progress to more advanced forms of AV block. Type I AV block with a normal QRS complex usually takes place at the level of the AV node proximal to the His bundle.

AV block that is 2:1 may be type I or type II second-degree AV block. If the QRS complex is narrow, the block is more likely to be type I, that is, located in the AV node, and one should search for transition of the 2:1 block to 3:2 block, during which time the PR interval lengthens in the second cardiac cycle (Figure

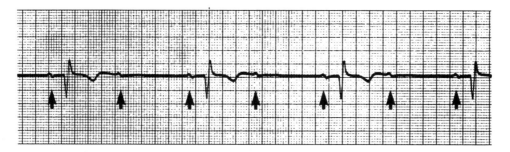

Figure 9A. *2:1 AV block. It is unclear if the conduction defect is intra-His or infra-His.*

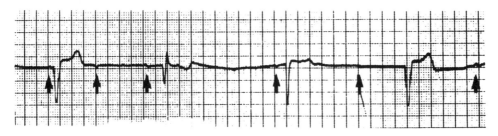

Figure 9B. *Subsequent electrocardiographic recording of the same patient shows intermittent complete heart block with junctional escape beats. (Arrows denote P waves.)*

7). If the QRS complex is wide (Figures 8 and 9), the level of block is more likely to be distal to the His bundle. The escape focus then is usually less reliable. If pre-existing bundle branch block is present, the block may be located either in the AV node or in the His-Purkinje system.

AV block may occur simultaneously at two or more levels of the conduction system. This occurrence makes the distinction between type I and type II second-degree block difficult.

Third-degree (complete) AV block implies that there is no conduction of the atrial impulses to the ventricle. It is important to separate this from AV dissociation. In AV dissociation, a subsidiary pacemaker, usually junctional, is more rapid than the underlying sinus rate. This contrasts with third-degree AV block in which the atrial rate is faster and there is no AV nodal conduction.

Third-degree (complete) AV block may be congenital or acquired. In the congenital form of complete heart block, there is anatomical discontinuity in the conduction pathway. Although for many years patients with this disorder were left untreated (if no associated congenital anomaly existed) and seemingly did well with their ventricular escape rates, controversy now exists about whether these patients should receive permanent pacing. Hemodynamic as well as arrhythmic consequences must be considered. VVI pacing would offer little benefit to such patients but DDD or VDD pacing would restore both atrioventricular synchrony and rate responsiveness. Symptomatic patients with congenital heart block should be paced. The ultimate fate of congenital complete heart block over the course of a lifetime remains to be determined.

Acquired complete heart block most commonly occurs due to aging with or without calcification of the conduction system or secondary to ischemic disease, i.e., previous myocardial infarction with damage extending to involve the conduction system. Complete heart block can also be related to a number of systemic illnesses, many of which have been described as single case reports. Iatrogenic causes of complete heart block also exist. Postoperative complete heart block has been the most common iatrogenic etiology in the past. However, AV nodal ablation for the definitive treatment of supraventricular tachyarrhythmias has become an increasingly more common acquired cause of complete heart block. Table II lists categories of causes of acquired atrio-ventricular block.

Acquired complete heart block can be either intermittent or fixed. Patients with abnormalities of AV conduction may be asymptomatic or experience severe symptoms related to profound bradycardia or ventricular arrhythmias. Decisions on the need for a pacemaker in the patient with impaired AV conduction, whether complete heart block or second-degree AV block, are influenced by a number of factors, most important of which is the presence or absence of symptoms that may be directly attributed to the arrhythmia. It has been well documented that patients with complete heart block and syncope have improved survival with permanent pacing.

Atrial fibrillation with a slow ventricular response should be considered as AV block, although it often is mistakenly categorized as sinus node dysfunction. These patients should be paced if symptoms occur (Figures 10 and 11).

Table II
Causes of Acquired Atrioventricular Block

Idiopathic (Senescent) AV Block
Coronary Artery Disease
Calcific Valvular Disease
Postoperative/Traumatic
AV Node Ablation
Therapeutic Radiation of the Chest
Infectious
  Syphilis
  Diphtheria
  Chagas' disease
  Tuberculosis
  Toxoplasmosis
  Lyme disease*
  Viral myocarditis (Epstein-Barr, Varicella, etc.)
  Infective endocarditis
Collagen-Vascular
  Rheumatoid arthritis
  Scleroderma
  Dermatomyositis
  Ankylosing spondylitis
  Polyarteritis nodosa
  Systemic lupus erythematosus
  Marfan's syndrome
Infiltrative
  Sarcoidosis
  Amyloidosis
  Hemochromatosis
  Malignancy (lymphomatous or solid tumor)
Neuromuscular
  Progressive external ophthalmoplegia-Kearns-Sayre syndrome
  Myotonic muscular dystrophy
  Peroneal muscular atrophy–Charcot Marie Tooth disease
  Scapuloperoneal syndrome
  Limb-girdle dystrophy
Drug Effect
  Digoxin
  Beta blockers
  Calcium-blocking agents
  Amiodarone
  Procainamide
  1C Agents: propafenone, encainide, flecainide

* See Chapter 7, Temporary Cardiac Pacing.

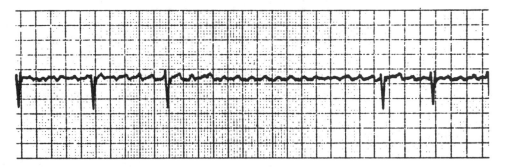

Figure 10. *Atrial fibrillation with a slow ventricular response and a single period of asystole of approximately 3-seconds duration.*

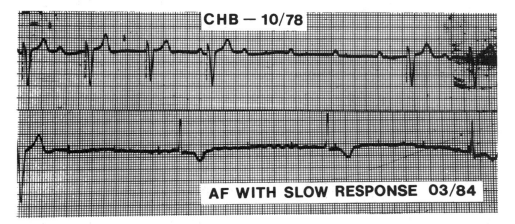

Figure 11. *Upper panel demonstrates an electrocardiographic recording of complete heart block. Lower panel demonstrates atrial fibrillation with a slow ventricular response in the same patient recorded several years later. Atrial fibrillation with a slow regular ventricular response is best categorized as complete heart block.*

Permanent Pacing After Acute Myocardial Infarction

Patients with myocardial infarction may experience a variety of conduction disturbances largely related to the site of the infarction and the coronary artery involved. Rigid classification is difficult because of the variations in coronary circulation (Table III).

Inferior Myocardial Infarction

Patients with an inferior myocardial infarction may have a variety of conduction disturbances. Supraventricular arrhythmias associated with an inferior myocardial infarction include (1) sinus bradycardia, (2) sinus arrest, (3) atrial fibrillation, and (4) atrial flutter.

AV nodal conduction disturbances may also occur, including first-degree

Table III
Permanent Pacing After Acute Myocardial Infarction

Pacemaker Necessary	Pacemaker Probably Necessary	Pacemaker Not Necessary
Persistent complete heart block	New bundle branch block with transient complete heart block	First-degree AV block
Persistent type II second-degree AV block	Newly acquired bifascicular bundle branch block	Asymptomatic type I second-degree AV block
Persistent symptomatic bradyarrhythmias		Pre-existing right or left bundle branch block
		New unifascicular block
		Asymptomatic sinus bradycardia

AV block, Mobitz I (Wenckebach) AV block, and in a minority of patients, higher grades of AV block (Mobitz II and complete heart block) will develop. Patients require temporary pacing if they are hemodynamically unstable. Few have persistent high-grade AV block or sinus node dysfunction that requires permanent pacing.

Anterior Myocardial Infarction

Anterior myocardial infarctions are more likely to be accompanied by intraventricular conduction defects or AV block (or both). Temporary pacing will be required for (1) new-onset bifascicular block, (2) bilateral bundle branch block, (3) intermittent complete heart block, and (4) persistent complete heart block.

Permanent pacing in patients with intraventricular conduction defects is predicated on the potential for development of complete heart block. In patients with newly acquired bifascicular block or transient or persistent trifascicular block, permanent pacing will most likely be required.

The long-term prognosis in survivors of acute myocardial infarction who have had AV block is related primarily to the extent of myocardial injury rather than to the AV block per se. Patients with acute myocardial infarction and intraventricular conduction defect (with the exception of isolated left anterior hemiblock) have unfavorable short- and long-term prognoses and an increased incidence of sudden death.

It should be stressed that the requirement for temporary pacing in the setting of acute myocardial infarction does not constitute an indication for permanent pacing. Indications for temporary pacing are presented in Chapter 7.

Chronic Bifascicular and Trifascicular Block

Permanent pacing in patients with conduction disturbances of two or more fascicles of the ventricular conduction system depends on assessment of the risk of development of complete AV block, either transient or permanent. A high mortality and a significant incidence of sudden death are known to be associated with bifascicular or trifascicular block and syncope, which, without pacing, commonly lead to complete heart block. Thus, defining the cause of syncope in patients with bifascicular and trifascicular block is important for documenting whether intermittent complete heart block is present. If this is documented, permanent pacemaker implantation should be performed. However, the incidence of progression of bifascicular block to complete heart block is low. Furthermore, no clinical or laboratory variables have proved valuable or definitive in identifying patients at a high risk of death from future bradyarrhythmias due to progression of the conduction disease. Specific controversy has arisen about patients with right bundle branch block and left anterior hemiblock. Although these patients have increased cardiovascular mortality, conduction abnormalities and bradycardia are not the cause of death in a sufficiently high proportion to warrant routine prophylactic pacing.

Measurement of the H-V interval (a measure of conduction of the His-Purkinje system) at times helps in identifying patients at higher risk for developing symptomatic high-grade AV block. In patients with a markedly prolonged H-V interval, prophylactic pacing may be indicated because of an increased incidence of developing symptomatic bradycardia. The degree of H-V interval lengthening necessary to justify prophylactic pacemaker placement is controversial. Some have advocated pacing for an H-V interval of >100 ms and others have considered pacing for an H-V interval of >70 ms, especially if the patient is to be placed on cardioactive drugs that have the potential to further impair the conduction system. For other patients with normal or a less prolonged H-V interval, electrophysiological testing does not reliably distinguish high-risk from low-risk groups. The clinical usefulness of routine electrophysiological studies is not established in patients with bifascicular block. Therefore, such studies in asymptomatic patients with bifascicular block usually are not necessary (Table IV).

Table IV
Chronic Bifascicular and Trifascicular Block

Pacemaker Necessary	Pacemaker Probably Necessary	Pacemaker Not Necessary
Symptomatic patients with fascicular block and significantly prolonged H-V interval by electrophysiological study	Patients with syncope and bifascicular or trifascicular block with other etiologies of syncope excluded	Asymptomatic fascicular block without AV block
Symptomatic patients with block distal to His at atrial paced rates of <100–120	Pacing-induced block distal to His at atrial paced rates of <130 bpm	Asymptomatic fascicular block and first-degree AV block
Symptomatic patients with bifascicular block and intermittent type II second-degree AV block or third-degree AV block	Asymptomatic patients with fascicular block and intermittent type II second-degree or third-degree AV block	

Sinus Node Dysfunction

Sinus node dysfunction, sick sinus syndrome, and tachycardia-bradycardia syndrome include a variety of cardiac arrhythmias that have been classified in several ways. Sinoatrial disturbances included are: (1) sinus bradycardia (Figure 5); (2) sinus arrest (Figure 12); (3) sinoatrial block; and (4) paroxysmal supraventricular tachycardias alternating with periods of bradycardia or asystole (Figure 13).

The definition of bradycardia varies, but it is generally agreed that it denotes rates of <40 bpm during waking hours. There is disagreement about the absolute cycle length of an asystolic period that should require pacing. Sinus pauses of

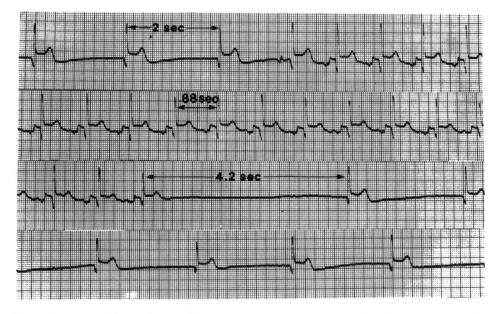

Figure 12. *A continuous electrocardiographic tracing from a patient with tachycardia-bradycardia syndrome shows sinus rhythm with sudden prolonged junctional escapes of up to 4.2 seconds.*

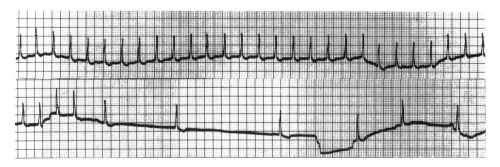

Figure 13. *Tachycardia-bradycardia syndrome with an episode of PSVT followed by an episode of bradycardia.*

Table V
Sinus Node Dysfunction

Pacemaker Necessary	*Pacemaker Probably Necessary*	*Pacemaker Not Necessary*
Symptomatic bradycardia	Symptomatic patients with sinus node dysfunction with documented rates of <40 bpm without a clear-cut association between significant symptoms and the bradycardia	Asymptomatic sinus node dysfunction
Symptomatic sinus bradycardia due to long-term drug therapy of a type and dose for which there is no accepted alternative		

3 seconds or sustained symptomatic sinus rates below 40 bpm in the awake patient are indications for permanent pacing. Sinus bradycardia during sleep in an otherwise asymptomatic patient should not be considered an indication for pacing. Because of the uncertainty of the definition of bradycardia and the duration of sinus pauses that requires treatment, it is important to take the patient's clinical condition into consideration, including age, associated disease, medications, and symptoms.

In sinus node dysfunction, correlation of symptoms with the specific arrhythmia is essential. Patients who have episodes of both tachycardia and bradycardia and are asymptomatic require no therapy. Others become symptomatic when treated for tachycardia because the treatment produces symptomatic bradycardia. Treatment for tachycardia may, therefore, require permanent antibradycardia pacing (Table V).

Neurally Mediated Syncope

There are several types of neurally mediated syncope, some of which may be an indication for permanent pacing. The terminology used for the various disorders is unnecessarily confusing. Disorders include asymptomatic carotid sinus hypersensitivity, carotid sinus syndrome, benign vasovagal syncope, and malignant vasovagal syncope.

Understanding the physiology involved is crucial to understanding the clinical manifestations. The carotid sinus reflex is the physiological response to pressure exerted on the carotid sinus. Stimulation results in activation of baroreceptors within the wall of the carotid sinus. Vagal efferents then result in cardiac slowing. Although this reflex is physiological, some persons have an exaggerated or even pathological response. This reflex has two components, a cardioinhibitory response and a vasodepressor response. A cardioinhibitory response results from increased parasympathetic tone and may be manifested by any or all of the following: sinus bradycardia (Figure 14), PR prolongation, and advanced AV block. The vasodepressor response is due to decreased sympathetic activity and secondary hypotension. While pure cardioinhibitory or pure vasodepressor responses may occur, it is most common to observe a mixed response.

The definitions of normal and abnormal responses are somewhat arbitrary. Ventricular asystole of 3 seconds or a substantial decrease in blood pressure, i.e., 30 to 50 mm Hg (or both) is abnormal (Table VI). An abnormal response to carotid sinus massage occurs in 25% to 30% of patients over 50 years of age. Men are affected approximately twice as frequently as women, and the right carotid sinus usually is more sensitive than the left. Although most of these patients are asymptomatic during carotid sinus massage and have no clinical history of syncope, others may have had recurrent syncope. Patients with syncope may have a typical history related to a tight collar or neck extension but more commonly have not identified any definite provocative maneuvers. If carotid sinus massage reproduces the patient's symptoms and is associated with significant cardioinhibition or vasodepression, then a diagnosis of carotid sinus syndrome can be made and treatment could be initiated. If carotid sinus massage is positive but does not reproduce the patient's symptoms, then a hypersensitive carotid reflex has been demonstrated but may not be of clinical significance and other etiologies for syncope should be investigated. However, if carotid sinus massage is negative then tilt-testing may be indicated.

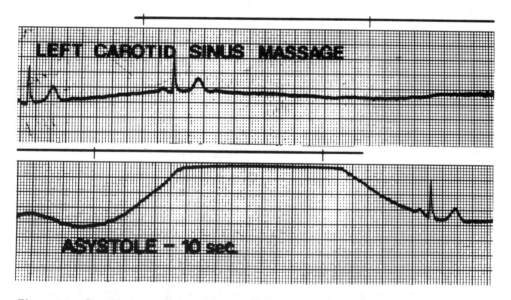

Figure 14. *Carotid sinus massage often is effective in demonstrating the basis of syncope or dizziness. Gentle massage of the carotid sinus, at the bifurcation of the common carotid artery, may produce AV block or, in this instance, prolonged sinus arrest without junctional escape. This level of sensitivity is associated with symptoms that pacing relieves.*

Table VI
Neurally Mediated Syncope

Pacemaker Necessary	*Pacemaker Probably Necessary*	*Pacemaker Not Necessary*
Patients with recurrent syncope associated with clear spontaneous events provoked by carotid sinus stimulation in whom carotid sinus massage induces asystole of >3 seconds	Patients with recurrent syncope without clear, provocative events who have a positive response to carotid sinus massage Symptomatic patients in whom tilt-table testing provokes a symptomatic bradycardia	Asymptomatic patients with a positive response to carotid sinus massage but without overt syncope who have only vague symptoms, i.e., dizziness or lightheadedness

Tilt-testing can provide the physiological environment to reproduce malignant vasovagal syncope. With head-up tilt, susceptible patients will have decreased venous return and subsequent decrease in left ventricular filling that may result in efferent vagal discharge. Stimulation of baroreceptors and adrenergic discharge may also result in efferent vagal discharge. Vasodilatation and hypotension as well as cardiac slowing may result from efferent vagal discharge. It is important to document whether the predominant cause of symptoms are cardioinhibitory or vasodepressor in origin because therapy will differ. Tilt-table testing often is helpful in determining the predominant cause (Figure 15). In the patient with significant cardioinhibition, permanent pacing is appropriate and should eliminate most, if not all, of the patient's symptoms. In the patient with pure vasodepression, however, other measures, i.e., drugs and compressive stockings, would be the treatment of choice. In the patient with a mixed response, but with a significant vasodepressor response, dual-chamber permanent pacing with the capability of hysteresis has been shown to help blunt the vasodepressor-related symptoms. In this situation the pacemaker would be programmed to a hysteresis rate that would allow the patient to remain in normal sinus rhythm the majority of the time, i.e., 40 to 50 ppm, and a pacing rate of 80 to 100 ppm. Therefore, when an episode of cardioinhibition and vasodepression occurs, as the patient's intrinsic heart rate slows to less than the hysteresis rate, the pacemaker would begin pacing at the programmed rate of 80 to 100 ppm. Ideally, to allow restoration of the patient's intrinsic rhythm, the pacemaker should be capable of search hysteresis whereby the pacemaker will intermittently, at programmed intervals, suspend pacing to determine if the patient's intrinsic rate is once again greater than the hysteresis rate.

Benign vasovagal syncope or a "simple faint" usually does not require therapy. Associated rhythms usually are prolonged sinus arrest without nodal or ventricular escape and may be associated with dramatic symptoms, including syncope, often undiagnosed for very prolonged periods (Figure 16). Syncope has been reported during many activities such as swallowing, coitus, cough, micturition, and respiration (Figure 17). Pacemaker implantation may be an effective means of preventing syncope, but there is some controversy as to whether these patients should receive permanent pacing. The argument against pacing is that such vagally mediated events usually do not result in significant reduction in mortality. However, the situations during which the events occur, i.e., operating a motor vehicle or heavy machinery, may predispose the patient or bystanders to danger.

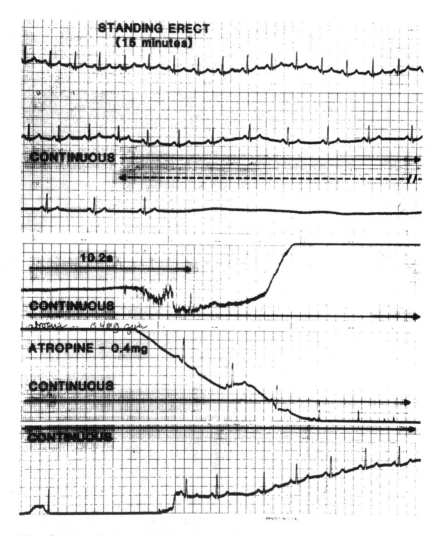

Figure 15.   *Continuous electrocardiographic recording during a tilt-table test. The upper panel shows sinus rhythm with some slowing in the second panel. In the third panel, sinus arrest occurs and persists until atropine is administered and the patient is placed supine.*

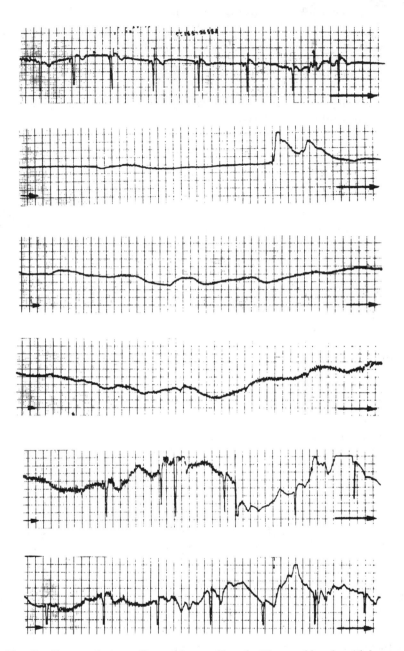

Figure 16. *Continuous electrocardiographic recording of a 55-year-old male with hypervagotonia with greater than 30 seconds of asystole. The patient recovers with sinus bradycardia in the fifth panel.*

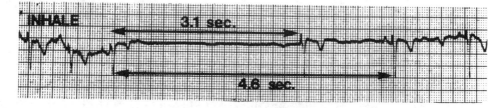

Figure 17. *Respiration can cause sinus arrest as it does in this 21-year-old woman. A modest depth of respiration causes 3.1 seconds of sinus arrest with asystole and 4.6 seconds of sinus bradycardia before resuming a normal atrial rate.*

SELECTION OF THE APPROPRIATE PACING MODE

Once it has been established that a conduction disorder exists that warrants permanent pacing, it then is necessary to determine the appropriate pacemaker. In selecting the ideal pacing mode, the patient's overall physical condition, associated medical problems, exercise capacity, and chronotropic response to exercise must be considered along with the underlying rhythm disturbance. Table VII describes clinical applications of various pacing modes in three classifications: conduction disorders for which a given pacing mode is indicated, conduction disorders for which a given pacing mode is controversial, and conduction disorders for which a given pacing mode is contraindicated. Algorithms for determining the appropriate pacing mode for patients with sinus node disease and AV node disease are shown in Figures 18 and 19, respectively.

VVI pacing remains the most commonly used pacing mode. Although VVI pacing will protect the patient from lethal bradycardias, it has significant limitations such as pacemaker syndrome.

The earliest indication for cardiac pacing was high-grade or complete heart block with recurrent Stokes-Adams attacks. In patients with this disorder, establishing a stable ventricular rhythm was lifesaving and prevented catastrophic asystole. This fact alone overshadowed the observation that although ventricular pacing improved cardiac output and/or patients' symptoms, it did not re-establish normal function. In addition, some patients with intermittent heart block experienced symptomatic hemodynamic deterioration with ventricular pacing. Adverse hemodynamics that are associated with a normally functioning pacing system resulting in overt symptoms or limiting the patients' ability to achieve optimal functional status is referred to as pacemaker syndrome. (See Chapter 5, Hemodynamics of Cardiac Pacing.) Pacemaker syndrome initially was recognized with ventricular (VVI) pacing. However, pacemaker syndrome may occur anytime there is AV dissociation. It has also been described with AAI and DDI pacing modes.

AAI pacing is appropriate for patients with sinus node dysfunction but is used infrequently in the United States. The obvious disadvantage of atrial pacing is lack of ventricular support should AV block occur. If the patient with sinus node dysfunction is assessed carefully for the presence of AV node disease at the time of pacemaker implant, the occurrence of clinically significant AV nodal

Table VII
Indications for Various Pacing Modes

Mode	Generally Agreed Upon Indications	Controversial Indications	Contraindicated
VVI	Atrial fibrillation with symptomatic bradycardia in the CC* patient	Symptomatic bradycardia in the patient with associated terminal illness or other medical conditions from which recovery is not anticipated and pacing is life-sustaining only	Patients with known pacemaker syndrome or hemodynamic deterioration with ventricular pacing at the time of implant CI† patient who will benefit from rate response Patients with hemodynamic need for dual-chamber pacing
VVIR	Fixed atrial arrhythmias (atrial fibrillation or flutter) with symptomatic bradycardia in the CI† patient	As for VVI	As for VVI
AAI	Symptomatic bradycardia as a result of sinus node dysfunction in the otherwise CC* patient and when AV conduction can be proven normal		Sinus node dysfunction with associated AV block either demonstrated spontaneously or during preimplant testing When adequate atrial sensing cannot be attained
AAIR	Symptomatic bradycardia as a result of sinus node dysfunction in the CI† patient and when AV conduction can be proven normal		As for AAI
DVI[1]			
VDD[2]	Congenital AV block AV block when sinus node function can be proven normal		Sinus node dysfunction AV block when accompanied by sinus node dysfunction When adequate atrial sensing cannot be attained AV block when accompanied by paroxysmal supraventricular tachycardias
VDDR[3]			

(*continued*)

Table VII   (Continued)

Mode	Generally Agreed Upon Indications	Controversial Indications	Contraindicated
DDI	AV block and sinus node dysfunction in the presence of significant PSVT in the CC* patient Need for dual-chamber pacing in the presence of significant PSVT in the CC* patient	Sinus node dysfunction in the absence of AV block in the presence of significant PSVT in the CC* patient	Chronotropic incompetence in the patient with a demonstrated need or improvement with rate responsiveness
DDIR	AV block and sinus node dysfunction in the CI† patient in the presence of significant PSVT Other need for dual-chamber pacing, i.e., hemodynamic need, in the presence of significant paroxysmal supraventricular tachycardias in the CI† patient	Sinus node dysfunction without AV block in the CI† patient in the presence of significant PSVT	
DDD	AV block and sinus node dysfunction in the CC* patient Need for AV synchrony, i.e., to maximize cardiac output, active patients Previous pacemaker syndrome	For any rhythm disturbance when atrial sensing and capture is possible, i.e., with the exception of atrial fibrillation or flutter, for the potential purpose of minimizing future atrial fibrillation and improved morbidity and survival For the suppression of tachyarrhythmias by overdrive suppression	Presence of chronic atrial fibrillation, atrial flutter, giant inexcitable atrium or other frequent paroxysmal supraventricular tachyarrhythmias When adequate atrial sensing cannot be attained
DDDR	AV block and sinus node dysfunction in the CI† patient	As for DDD	As for DDD

[1] DVI as a stand-alone pacing mode, i.e., a pacemaker capable of DVI as the only dual-chamber mode of operation, is obsolete. All primary uses of this mode should be considered individually.

[2] VDD as a stand-alone pacing mode, i.e., a pacemaker capable of VDD as the only dual-chamber mode of operation, currently is used primarily as a single-lead VDD system. If a dual-lead system is implanted, then the capability of DDD pacing is desirable.

[3] VDDR is a misnomer by the current NBG code for pacing modes. The "R" in this context generally would indicate the capability of dual-chamber sensor-driven pacing. However, VDD by definition excludes atrial pacing. The designation of VDDR is being used by manufacturers as a device that operates in a P-synchronous mode except when sensor-driven during which time pacing may be VVIR or DDDR depending upon the specific device.

* CC = chronotropically competent; † CI = chronotropically incompetent.

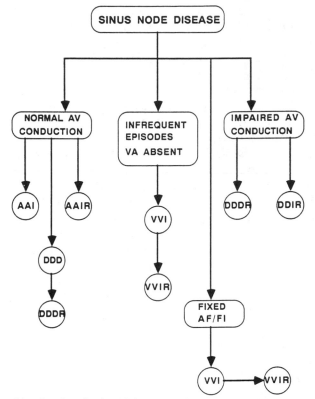

Figure 18. *Algorithm for the selection of the appropriate pacing mode in patients with sinus node disease.*

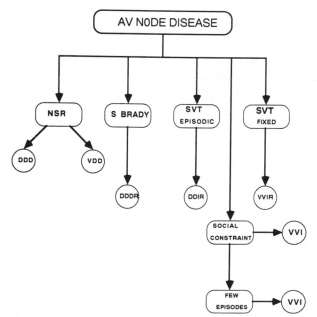

Figure 19. *Algorithm for the selection of the appropriate pacing mode in patients with AV node disease.*

disease is very low, i.e., <2% per year. Assessment prior to use of an AAI system should include incremental atrial pacing at the time of pacemaker implant. Although criteria vary among institutions and implanting physicians, the adult patient should be capable of 1 to 1 AV nodal conduction to rates of 120 to 140 bpm.

DVI pacemakers were at one time implanted in a large number of patients often with a very satisfactory outcome. However, DVI pacing is limited by the absence of atrial sensing which prevents the restoration of rate responsiveness in the chronotropically competent patient. In addition, lack of atrial sensing may lead to competitive atrial pacing and initiation of atrial rhythm disturbances. For these reasons, DVI pacing rarely is selected as the mode of choice at the time of implant. It is a programmable option in most DDD pacemakers and may be used in the patient with a DDD pacemaker who develops atrial failure to sense.

The competitive atrial pacing seen with DVI pacing can be avoided by using the DDI pacing mode. In this pacing mode there is atrial sensing and pacing but the pacemaker is incapable of tracking intrinsic atrial activity. Therefore, there is only a single rate programmed, and the paced ventricular rate will never exceed the programmed rate. This mode may be advantageous in the patient with paroxysmal supraventricular tachycardias that could result in rapid ventricular pacing if the patient were programmed to the DDD mode.

VDD pacing is appropriate for the patient with normal sinus node function and conduction disease of the AV node. Dual-chamber (2 lead) VDD pacing systems have largely been supplanted by DDD pacemakers. However, VDD as the preimplant pacing mode of choice is gaining new acceptance with the introduction of a single-lead VDD pacing system. (In this system atrial sensing is accomplished from "floating" sensing electrodes on the atrial portion of the ventricular pacing lead).

The DDD pacing system combines the functions of ventricular, atrial, AV sequential, and atrial synchronous. Pacing and sensing occur in both atrium and ventricle. The atrium is stimulated if sinus bradycardia exists. Both atrium and ventricle are stimulated if bradycardia exists independently in both chambers; if heart block exists with normal sinus function, the ventricle will be paced in synchrony with the atrium, and if sinus rhythm exists, the pacemaker will be totally inhibited. Therefore, there are four different rhythms that can be seen as a result of normal pacemaker function: (1) normal sinus rhythm; (2) atrial pacing; (3) AV sequential pacing; and (4) P-synchronous pacing. The DDD pacing mode is most successful for patients with normal sinus node function and AV block. DDD pacing is considered by some to be the mode of choice in carotid sinus hypersensitivity with symptomatic cardioinhibition.

DDD pacing is not the "universal" pacing mode it was first purported to represent. It was apparent from the outset that DDD or P-synchronous pacing had definite limitations in some patients. P-synchronous pacing is not possible in the presence of chronic atrial fibrillation or in patients with a paralyzed or nonexcitable atrium. A limitation not well appreciated until more recently is chronotropic incompetence—the inability to appropriately increase the atrial rate with exercise. In the chronotropically incompetent patient, DDD pacing is suboptimal because rate responsiveness will not be restored.

Indications For Rate Adaptive Pacemakers

Current indications for rate adaptive pacemakers are also listed in Table VII. VVIR pacing, like VVI, is contraindicated if ventricular pacing results in retrograde (VA) conduction and/or a fall in blood pressure. VVIR pacing should not be used as an excuse to forego attempts at placing an atrial lead in a patient who is undergoing pacemaker implantation and has normal sinus node function and would benefit from rate adaptive pacing. If the sinus node is intact, P-synchronous pacing should still be considered the optimal rate adaptive parameter and utilized when possible.

AAIR pacing can be considered in the patient with sinus node dysfunction and normal AV node function as this mode will restore rate responsiveness and maintain AV synchrony. If AAIR pacing is contemplated, normal AV node conduction must first be determined as previously discussed for AAI pacing.

The ideal patient for DDDR pacing is one with combined sinus nodal and AV nodal dysfunction in whom DDDR pacing would restore rate responsiveness and AV synchrony. In a patient with paroxysmal atrial rhythm disturbances, programming the pacemaker to the DDIR mode will allow rate modulation and AV synchrony but not allow tracking of any rapid pathological atrial rhythms (DVIR may be used when DDIR is not available, but DVIR is less useful since atrial competition can occur).

POTENTIAL HEMODYNAMIC INDICATIONS FOR PERMANENT PACING IN THE ABSENCE OF SYMPTOMATIC BRADYCARDIA

There are three conditions where controversy exists as to whether permanent pacing should be considered for the possible hemodynamic advantage that it may confer even in the absence of symptomatic bradycardia.

The first of these is paroxysmal atrial fibrillation. As previously discussed there have been multiple retrospective studies showing lowered morbidity and mortality in DDD or AAI paced patients versus VVI pacing. The improvement is due to a lower incidence of atrial fibrillation, congestive heart failure, thromboembolic phenomena, and death. Some, but not all, investigators have found that paroxysmal atrial fibrillation is alleviated when patients are paced in the AAI or DDD mode. The hypothetical extension of this data has been that pacing should be considered a therapeutic option in the patient with paroxysmal atrial fibrillation to "stabilize" the atrial rhythm. At this point, the data is inconclusive, it is not accepted practice and further studies are needed.

Pacing patients with dilated cardiomyopathy for potential hemodynamic gain also has been advocated. Literature supporting this indication for permanent pacing is very limited, and the existing information fails to demonstrate the mechanism by which hemodynamic improvement might occur. Treatment options in dilated cardiomyopathy are limited and any new, potential therapy is given much attention. Nonetheless, this indication for permanent pacing is not accepted practice and again, additional studies are necessary to substantiate potential benefit.

Permanent pacing for patients with hypertrophic obstructive cardiomyopathy (HOCM) is less controversial. Multiple investigators have shown reduction in left ventricular outflow gradient and symptoms in patients with HOCM with dual-chamber pacing. Presumably the hemodynamic improvement occurs because of the paced alteration of ventricular depolarization. That is, the septum is depolarized later than it would be during intrinsic conduction and septal motion may even be paradoxical, thus preventing some of the left ventricular outflow tract collapse that translates to a lower gradient. If pacing is eventually accepted as an equal therapeutic option to drugs and surgery, it would likely be preferred by many patients since it avoids the possibility of dependence on drugs and their side effects and obviates the need for a large, albeit often successful, surgical procedure. It should be emphasized that ventricular (VVI) pacing should not be used in HOCM. Although ventricular pacing would still alter ventricular depolarization, the hypertrophic ventricle is noncompliant and loss of AV synchrony may result in severe clinical deterioration.

BIBLIOGRAPHY

Abi-Samra F, Maloney JD, Fouad-Tarazi FM, et al: The usefulness of head-up tilt testing and hemodynamic investigations in the work-up of syncope of unknown origin. PACE 1988; 11:1201–1214.

Almquist A, Goldenerg IF, Milstein S, et al: Provocation of bradycardia and hypotension by isoproterenol and upright posture in patients with unexplained syncope. N Engl J Med 1989; 320:346–351.

Breivik K, Ohm OJ: Improved quality of life from pacemaker treatment in the very aged. In FP Gomez: Cardiac Pacing: Electrophysiology, Tachyarrhythmias. Mount Kisco, NY, Futura Media Services, 1985; 1207–1211.

Brignole M, Menozzi C, Lolli G, et al: Pacing for carotid sinus syndrome and sick sinus syndrome. PACE 1990; 13 (12 pt 2):2071–2075.

Brignole M, Sartore B, Barra M, et al: Ventricular and dualchamber pacing for treatment of carotid sinus syndrome. PACE 1989; 12:582–590.

Bru P, Levy S, Metge M, et al: Remote occurrence of high degree heart block following failure of transcatheter AV junctional ablation: Incidence and clinical significance. PACE 1987; 10:937–942.

Campbell RW: Chronic Mobitz type I second degree atrioventricular block. Has its importance been underestimated? Br Heart J 1985; 53:585–586.

Col JJ, Weinberg SL: The incidence and mortality of intraventricular conduction defects in acute myocardial infarction. Am J Cardiol 1972; 29:344–350.

Dewey RC, Capeless MA, Levy AM: Use of ambulatory electrocardiographic monitoring to identify high-risk patients with congenital complete heart block. N Engl J Med 1987; 316:835–839.

Dhingra RC, Denes P, Wu D, et al: The significance of second degree atrioventricular block and bundle branch block: Observations regarding site and type of block. Circulation 1974; 49:638–646.

Domenighetti G, Perret C: Intraventricular conduction disturbances in acute myocardial infarction: Short- and long-term prognosis. Eur J Cardiol 1980; 11:51–59.

Donoso E, Adler LN, Friedberg CK: Unusual forms of second-degree atrioventricular block, including Mobitz type II block, associated with the Morgagni-Adams-Stokes syndrome. Am Heart J 1964; 67:150–157.

Dreifus LS, Gillette PC, Fisch C, et al: ACC/AHA Task Force Report: Guidelines for implantation of cardiac pacemakers and antiarrhythmia devices. J Am Coll Cardiol 1991; 18:1–13.

Dubois C, Pierard LA, Smeets JP, et al: Long term prognostic significance of atrioventricular block in inferior acute myocardial infarction. Eur Heart J 1989; 10:816–820.

Fisch GR, Zipes D, Fisch C: Bundle branch block and sudden death. Prog Cardiovasc Dis 1980; 23:187–224.

Fitzpatrick A, Theodorakis G, Ahmed R, et al: Dual chamber pacing aborts vasovagal syncope induced by head-up 60° tilt. PACE 1991; 14:13–19.

Frye RL, Collins JJ, DeSanctis RW, et al: Guidelines for permanent cardiac pacemaker implantation, May 1984. A Report of the Joint American College of Cardiology/American Heart Association Task Force on Assessment of Cardiovascular Procedures(Subcommittee on Pacemaker Implantation). J Am Coll Cardiol 1984; 4:434–442.

Gammage M, Schofield S, Rankin I, et al: Benefit of single setting rate responsive ventricular pacing compared with fixed rate demand pacing in elderly patients. PACE 1991; 14:174–180.

Ginks WR, Sutton R, Oh W, Leatham A, et al: Long-term prognosis after acute anterior infarction with atrioventricular block. Br Heart J 1977; 39:186–189.

Hatano K, Kato R, Hayashi H, et al: Usefulness of rate responsive atrial pacing in patients with sick sinus syndrome. PACE 1989; 12:16–24.

Hayes DL, Holmes DR, Jr: Atrial pacing: A viable pacing mode for the 1980s? Clin Prog Pacing Electrophysiol 1984; 2:339–348.

Hindman MC, Wagner GS, JoRo M, et al: The clinical significance of bundle branch block complicating acute myocardial infarction. 2. Indications for temporary and permanent pacemaker insertion. Circulation 1978; 58:689–699.

Hochleitner M, Hortnagl H, Ng CK, et al: Usefulness of physiologic dual-chamber pacing in drug-resistant idiopathic dilated cardiomyopathy. Am J Cardiol 1990; 66:198–202.

Johnston FA, Robinson JF, Fyfe T: Exercise testing in the diagnosis of sick sinus syndrome in the elderly: Implications for treatment. PACE 1987; 10:831–838.

Kallryd A, Kruse I, Ryden L: Atrial inhibited pacing in the sick sinus node syndrome: Clinical value and the demand for rate responsiveness. PACE 1989; 12:954–961.

Kappenberger L, Jeanrenaud X, Vogt P, et al: Pacemaker treatment of hypertrophic obstructive cardiomyopathy (HOCM): Acute and long term efficacy. (abstract) PACE 1991; 14(4 Pt II):668.

Kerr CR, Tyers GF, Vorderbrugge S: Atrial pacing: Efficacy and safety. PACE 1989; 12 (7 Pt I):1049–1054.

Kolettis TM, Miller HC, Boon NA: Atrial pacing: Who do we paceand what do we expect? Experiences with 100 atrial pacemakers. PACE 1990; 13:625–630.

Kugler JD, Danford DA: Pacemakers in children: An update. Am Heart J 1989; 113:665–679.

Lamas GA, Dawley D, Splaine K, et al: Documented symptomaticbradycardia and symptom relief in patients receiving permanent pacemakers: An evaluation of the Joint ACC/AHA pacing guidelines. PACE 1988; 11:1098–1104.

Lamas GA, Muller JE, Turi ZG, et al: A simplified method to predict occurrence of complete heart block during acute myocardial infarction. Am J Cardiol 1986; 57:1213–1219.

Mavric Z, Zaputovic L, Matana A, et al: Prognostic significance of complete atrioventricular block in patients with and without right ventricular involvement. Am Heart J 1990; 119:823–828.

McDonald KM, Maurer B: Permanent pacing as treatment for hypertrophic cardiomyopathy. Am J Cardiol 1991; 68:108–110.

McElroy P, Janicki JS, Weber KT: Physiologic correlates of the heart rate response to upright isotonic exercise: Relevance to rate responsive pacing. J Am Coll Cardiol 1988; 11:94–99.

Mymin D, Mathewson FAL, Tate RB, et al: The natural history of primary first-degree atrioventricular heart block. N Engl J Med 1986; 315:1183–1187.

Nicod P, Gilpin E, Dittrich H, et al: Long-term outcome in patients with inferior myocardial infarction and complete atrioventricular block. J Am Coll Cardiol 1988; 12: 589–594.

Ritter WS, Atkins J, Blomqvist CG, et al: Permanent pacing in patients with transient trifascicular block during acute myocardial infarction. Am J Cardiol 1976; 38:205–208.

Rosenfeld LE: Bradyarrhythmias, abnormalities of conduction, and indications for pacing in acute myocardial infarction. Cardiol Clin 1988; 6:49–61.

Rosenqvist M, Brandt J, Schuller H: Long-term pacing in sinus node disease: Effects of stimulation mode on cardiovascular morbidity and mortality. Am Heart J 1988; 116: 16–22.

Ryden L: Atrial inhibited pacing—An underused mode of cardiac stimulation. PACE 1988; 11:1375–1379.

Schmidinger H, Probst P, Schneider B, et al: Subsidiary pacemaker function in complete heart block after His-bundle ablation. Circulation 1988; 78:893–898.

Shaw DB, Kekwick CA, Veal D, et al: Survival in second-degree atrioventricular block. Br Heart J 1985; 53:587–593.

Sholler GF, Walsh EP: Congenital complete heart block in patients without anatomic cardiac defects. Am Heart J 1989; 118:1193–1198.

Strasberg B, Amat-Y-Leon F, Dhingra RC, et al: Natural history of chronic second-degree atrioventricular nodal block. Circulation 1981; 63:1043–1049.

Sutton R: Pacing in patients with carotid sinus and vasovagal syndrome. PACE 1989; 12(Part 2):1260–1263.

Sutton R, Bourgeois I: Clinical presentation of conduction defects and indications for pacing. In R Sutton, I Bourgeois (eds.): The Foundations of Cardiac Pacing, Pt. I: An illustrated guide to basic pacing. Mount Kisco, NY, Futura Publishing Co, 1991, pp 137–148.

Vardas PE, Fitzpatrick A, Ingram A, et al: Natural history of sinus node chronotropy in paced patients. PACE 1991; 14:155–160.

Chapter 2

BASIC CONCEPTS

Seymour Furman

BASIC ELECTRICITY

Understanding some of the basic concepts of electrical theory is important in dealing with cardiac pacing issues. It allows the understanding and calculation of pulse generator output, pulse generator longevity, and the consequences of lead insulation disruption and conductor fracture.

OHM'S LAW

Ohm's law is a basic law of electricity and should be understood by anyone involved in electrical work and in cardiac stimulation. Electricity is a flow of electrons in a conductor. The force that drives the electron flow is the **electromotive force (E)** and is measured in **volts (V)**. The flow of **current (I)** is measured in **amperes (A)** and the **resistance (R)** to that flow is measured in Ohms (O). Each of the factors is commonly measured in much smaller factors than a full volt, ampere, or ohm when dealing with biological systems and pacemaker level outputs. One thousandth ($\frac{1}{1000}$) of a volt or an ampere is a milliampere or millivolt (mA or mV) and one millionth ($\frac{1}{1,000,000}$) is a microampere or microvolt. The formula for Ohm's law is $I = E/R$. It can be solved for each of the three factors, thus $E = IR$ and $R = E/I$. Energy is measured in joules and is the product of volts, current, and time: **ENERGY = EIt**. It too can be calculated in small amounts for pacemaker work, i.e., microjoules, or in much larger quantities, i.e., joules when dealing with defibrillators. The output of an implantable cardioverter defibrillator (ICD) shock is, therefore 10,000 times as great as a single pacemaker stimulus.

When a battery causes the potential difference to produce current flow through a conductor, the flow occurs from a point of higher potential difference to one of lower potential difference, just as a flow of water would be from a higher level to a lower level. The flow of a current of electrons is always through a resistance, whether low, such as conductive wire, or relatively high, such as a pacemaker system lead. That resistance will cause the fall of the entire electromotive force across the resistance. If there is more than one resistance in series, connected end to end, the fall in voltage across each resistance will be proportional to the amount of resistance it represents of the total. For example, if there are two resistances in series and one is 10 ohms and the other 40 ohms, the total will be 50 ohms. The voltage drop across the lesser resistance will be

20% (one fifth) of the total and the voltage drop across the greater resistance will be 80% (four fifths) of the total.

If the resistances are parallel, the total resistance will be less than each individually, i.e., the product of the resistances divided by their sum. A group of parallel resistances can be analogous to a short circuit and is seen when an insulation defect occurs. If a lead resistance is 500 ohms and an insulation defect adjacent to the connector has a resistance of 10 ohms, the flow of current will be proportional to the two parallel resistances and the net resistance of the circuit will be 9.8 ohms. Some 50 times the current will flow via the insulation defect "short circuit" than via the remainder of the lead. If the output voltage of the system were 5.0 V and the lead resistance 500 ohms, the output would have been 10 mA. At a total resistance of 9.8 ohms (i.e., with the parallel insulation defect) the current flow will be 510 mA. While internal pulse generator resistance will limit the total flow well below that level, it will be far above the normal level and drain the power supply rapidly (Figure 1).

Measurement of the resistance of a lead system is very useful to determine the nature of a malfunction. Most normal lead systems have a resistance of 400–

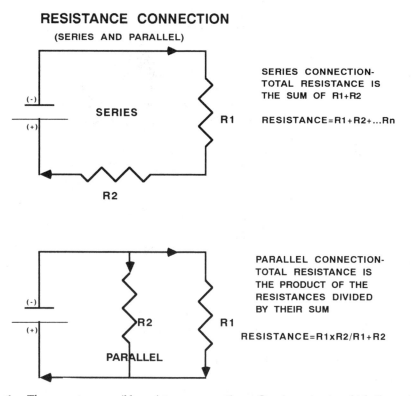

RESISTANCE CONNECTION

(SERIES AND PARALLEL)

SERIES

R1

R2

SERIES CONNECTION-
TOTAL RESISTANCE IS
THE SUM OF R1+R2

RESISTANCE=R1+R2+...Rn

R2

R1

PARALLEL

PARALLEL CONNECTION-
TOTAL RESISTANCE IS
THE PRODUCT OF THE
RESISTANCES DIVIDED
BY THEIR SUM

RESISTANCE=R1xR2/R1+R2

Figure 1. *There are two possible resistance connections. One is **series** in which the resistances are additive. The beginning of one resistance is connected to the end of another. A lead fracture is an example of a series resistance. As the resistance is high, little current flows. The second is **parallel** in which the resistances are all connected to the same point. The net resistance is the product of the resistances divided by their sum. The resulting resistance is low and a great deal of current flows. Insulation disruption is an example of a parallel resistance.*

600 ohms (some designs are somewhat higher or lower). Normal pulse generator output is based on the assumption that the lead resistance will be in this range. If the resistance is higher, less current will flow and if it is lower, more current will flow. If the current flow is too low, the heart will not be stimulated adequately. If it is too high, the pulse generator battery will be drained prematurely.

The power supply from the battery can be in series or in parallel. When two cells comprise the battery they are usually connected end to end (i.e., series) so that the total output voltage is added. Two 2.8 V lithium iodine cells, connected in series provide an output of 5.6 V. This is not usually done. A single lithium iodine cell is used, and if higher voltages are desired (as they are), a voltage transformer is used. When mercury zinc cells powered pulse generators, series connections of 4 cells (each 1.35 V) to provide 5.4 V or 5 cells to provide 6.75 V were routine (Figure 2).

The electrical output of a pulse generator may be constant current or constant voltage though the term "constant" must be understood in context. Each is "constant" within a range rather than infinitely. The output load through

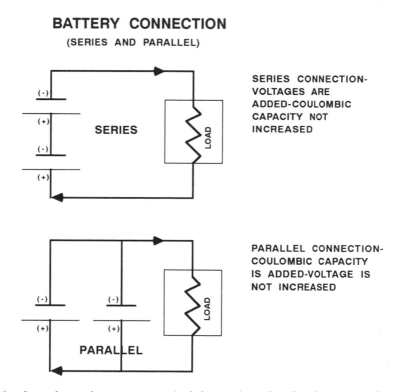

BATTERY CONNECTION

(SERIES AND PARALLEL)

Figure 2. *In modern pulse generators a single battery is used so that the output voltage from the power source is that of a single cell. In the instance of the lithium iodine cell, the output is 2.8 V, sufficient to operate the circuit. A higher output is obtained with a voltage transformer. If two cells are connected into the circuit they may be in* **series**, *in which the negative terminal of one is connected to the positive of the second. The voltage is then additive, but the overall capacity is that of a single cell. Alternatively, the cells may be connected in* **parallel**, *in which case the capacity of the cells is additive, but the voltage is that of a single cell.*

which the pulse generator discharges is the lead electrode system, and the output of the generator is designed to accommodate the nominal resistance of that system, which is 510 Ohms. In a constant current system the internal resistance of the circuit is large compared to the load, which is the resistance through which the pulse generator discharges itself. In a pacing system the load is the lead system. Changes in the lead resistance will have relatively little effect on overall resistance and therefore on the output current. Such circuits are commonly used for temporary cardiac pacing where lead connections and the leads used are far more variable in electrical characteristics than for implanted pacemakers. No implanted constant current pulse generators are now manufactured. A constant voltage output pulse generator has a lower internal resistance so that the load (lead) resistance is a larger part of the total output resistance and therefore changes in resistance will have a larger effect on current flow through the load (Figure 3).

The consequences are that an increase in load resistance will promptly reduce the current flow and a decrease in load resistance will increase the current flow. Changes are according to Ohm's law (Voltage = current × resistance). All implantable pulse generators are constant voltage and are therefore sensitive

CONSTANT CURRENT & VOLTAGE

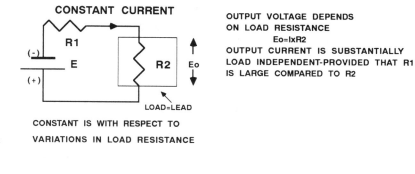

CONSTANT CURRENT

R1

(−)

E

R2   Eo

(+)

LOAD=LEAD

OUTPUT VOLTAGE DEPENDS ON LOAD RESISTANCE
$Eo = I \times R2$
OUTPUT CURRENT IS SUBSTANTIALLY LOAD INDEPENDENT-PROVIDED THAT R1 IS LARGE COMPARED TO R2

CONSTANT IS WITH RESPECT TO VARIATIONS IN LOAD RESISTANCE

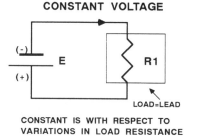

CONSTANT VOLTAGE

(−)

E

R1

(+)

LOAD=LEAD

OUTPUT CURRENT DEPENDS ON LOAD RESISTANCE
$I = E/R$
OUTPUT CURRENT IS LOAD DEPENDENT

CONSTANT IS WITH RESPECT TO VARIATIONS IN LOAD RESISTANCE

Figure 3.   *The terms constant current and constant voltage output depend on whether the resistance within the pulse generator is high or low compared to the lead resistance (load). If the additional resistance, represented by the lead, connector, etc. is small compared to the internal resistance, then the output current will vary little with changes in resistance.* **The circuit will be constant current.** *If the additional resistance, represented by the lead, connector, etc., is large compared to the internal resistance, the output current will vary widely with changes in resistance. The circuit will be* **constant voltage.**

to changes in load. For example, a polarity programmable pulse generator, i.e., one in which a bipolar lead is placed but that can be programmed to unipolar or bipolar output will have higher resistance in the bipolar mode and a lower output current. If the lead insulation has become defective, the resistance will drop, the voltage will remain constant, and the current output will increase. A practical effect is that in the presence of insulation failure with a short circuit of current and low resistance, the pulse generator battery is drained rapidly and even a relatively new generator (in place during exploration for insulation failure) should be replaced.

PACEMAKER OUTPUT

A pacemaker output circuit can be readily understood by a hydraulic comparison. In those terms the significance of high output or low output and the significance of high-impedance or low-impedance leads or the effect of single- or dual-chamber pacing can all be understood.

The hydraulic comparison is traditional in understanding electrical circuits. Flow of water is readily compared to flow of current, and the various impedances to flow can be equally compared. Many persons have difficulty comprehending electrical terms but have an intuitive understanding of hydraulic events (Figure 4).

The five major factors are energy, voltage, current, charge. and impedance. They can be redefined as:

Voltage—The force moving the current. This is analogous to the height of the reservoir above the point of delivery of the current flow.

Current—The actual continuing volume of flow of electricity or of water.

Charge—The quantity of electricity or of water that has flowed. Because of the measurement of volume and the duration of flow, the charge is given in volume multiplied by time, i.e., Watt-hours or more commonly in Coulombs, which are amperes (the quantity) multiplied by time.

Energy—This is the result of multiplying the electromotive force (voltage) by the charge (the current multiplied by the time of flow).

Impedance—This is the numerical sum of all of the resistances to the flow (either of water or of electricity). The calculation may be very complex, especially in a biological system, but in the simplest form, once a number has been selected as being reasonably accurate, calculation of the derived functions can be accomplished. Battery capacity is given in voltage (electromotive force) and in a capacity of current delivery. The voltage is a result of the chemistry of the battery and cannot be modified once a specific chemistry is selected. The capacity of the cell to deliver current is given by the amount it will deliver for the time it will deliver. Consequently batteries will be identified by voltage and by ampere hours, i.e., current × time. A small lithium iodine battery may have an output of 2.8 V and a capacity of 0.8 ampere hours, while a larger battery will have a voltage of 2.8 V and 3.0 ampere hours. The actual longevity of a pulse generator with either battery implanted will depend on how rapidly the battery is drained as well as the capacity of the battery. Because voltage is a function of battery

PACEMAKER CIRCUIT

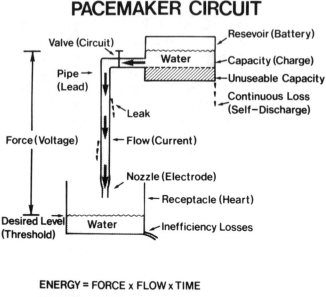

ENERGY = FORCE x FLOW x TIME

CHARGE = CURRENT x TIME (of Flow)

CURRENT = QUANTITY OF FLOW

VOLT = FORCE OF FLOW

Figure 4. *In this diagram the battery is the reservoir of fluid above the point of delivery. The height above the point of delivery (the nozzle) is the force with which the fluid is delivered. The size of the nozzle presents a resistance to flow and the valve in the circuit represents all of the other increases or decreases in resistance to current flow. In the reservoir (i.e., the battery) water above the egress pipe is wholly usable, some below the pipe is not usable, and because the reservoir is incompletely sealed there is some continuing loss, even if no water flows. The flow therefore depends on the resistance to flow, the height of the reservoir above the nozzle, the duration and rate of flow, and the usable capacity of the reservoir.*

chemistry it declines slowly until the current is almost completely drained. In effect it is the charge and not the voltage that is the consumable component. The longevity of the pacemaker can be calculated from the knowledge of the battery capacity and the rate of drain caused by the sensing circuit efficiency, pacing circuit efficiency, and the factors under the control of the operator of a programmable pacemaker, which are the:

1. pacemaker rate;
2. programmed output voltage;
3. programmed pulse duration;
4. percent of time pacing.

The current output of a pacemaker can be calculated by the output, voltage and by the impulse duration. Consequently, output can be given as energy —

Formula 1.   Energy = volts × current × time;
or
volts × current × pulse duration;
or
Formula 2.   As current only;
or
Formula 3.   As charge, i.e., current × time.

The current that will flow is a function of the resistance of the circuit to current flow and the voltage that is applied.

Generally, Ohm's law will be applicable, i.e.:

Formula 4.   Voltage = current × resistance.

This formula may be solved for any of the three functions, i.e.

Formula 4a.   Current = voltage/resistance;

Formula 4b.   Resistance = voltage/current.

It is best to calculate and give pacemaker output in charge as this (see above) is the consumable component. Giving output in energy is less meaningful because of the shape of the strength-duration curve. The pulse duration at which output occurs must always be known to appreciate its effectiveness.

THRESHOLD OF CARDIAC STIMULATION

Comprehension of the threshold of cardiac stimulation is basic to pulse generator and electrode design. The programming of and the setting of the minimum output, which will (1) accommodate threshold; (2) set an adequate safety factor; and (3) allow maximum pulse generator longevity, is based on the comprehension of the factors concerning the long-term stability of threshold and specifically the strength-duration curve of stimulation. A variety of electrode factors are involved and each must be considered.

I. Myocardial Factors
   A. Fibrosis or local infarction increases threshold;
   B. Endocardial thickening increases threshold;
   C. Drugs, the effect is variable;
   D. Electrolyte balance, the effect is variable.
II. Lead and Electrode Factors
   A. Electrode maturity—i.e., duration of the electrode in position;
   B. Distance of the electrode from sensitive tissue—the effect of which is the same as I-1 and 2;
   C. Unipolar or bipolar electrode—i.e., anodal size;
   D. Electrode surface area and shape;
   E. Electrode material;
   F. Lead insulation;
   G. Solid and porous electrodes;
   H. Steroid leads
   I. Lead fixation;
   J. Anodal or cathodal stimulation;

I. Myocardial Factors

A. Fibrosis or Local Infarction

Neither fibrous nor infarcted tissue is sensitive to stimulation. The nearest viable tissue will be stimulated if its threshold is reached. Extensive fibrosis or infarction about an electrode increases the size of the "virtual" electrode, which is the surface area of the encasement of such tissue about an electrode. As threshold is directly related to "virtual" electrode size, the larger the fibrotic area, the higher the threshold (Figure 5).

B. Endocardial Thickening

This separates the electrode from the stimulatable tissue as does fibrosis. The greater the distance between the stimulating electrode surface and the responsive tissue, the higher the threshold and the poorer the sensed electrogram.

C/D. Drugs/Electrolyte Balance

Changes in electrolyte concentration affect stimulation threshold. Administration of potassium (chloride) in Ringer's solution reduces threshold by as much as 20%–40% consistently but briefly, while potassium in combination with insulin increases threshold by 17%–30%, also briefly. Hypertonic (3%) sodium

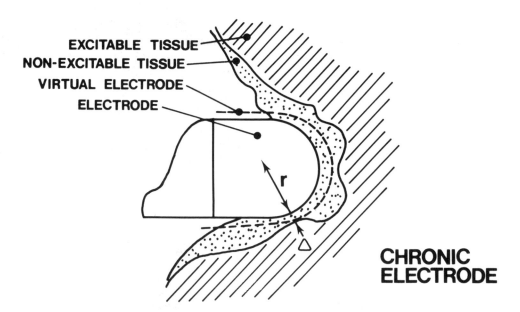

Figure 5.   *Each electrode is surrounded by an insensitive layer of fibrous tissue. As the interface of the fibrous layer with adjacent stimulatable tissue is where stimulation actually occurs, the surface area of the "virtual" electrode is that which determines the chronic stable stimulation factors. The size of the fibrous layer may be decreased by porous electrode and local steroids.*

chloride increases the blood sodium concentration and threshold by 50%–60%, while calcium gluconate has a slight lowering effect. An increase in pO_2 has little effect, a slight decrease of pO_2 increases threshold, and marked hypoxia reduces threshold. An increase in pCO_2 increases threshold and a decrease has little effect. The glucocorticoids (methylprednisone, dexamethasone, prednisone) and epinephrine and ephedrine decrease threshold. Isoproterenol, aldactone, propranolol, verapamil, quinidine, ajmaline, and flecainide all increase threshold. Digitalis, morphine, lidocaine, and procainamide, administered in the usual therapeutic dose range, have little effect. Still, drug administration has little significant or sustained effect on threshold. Only flecainide need be considered as a cause for threshold increase during cardiac pacing. None is an effective means of long-term threshold reduction. Even where a pronounced immediate effect occurs, continued drug administration is accompanied by a gradual return to the pretreatment baseline over several hours. The major problem that can occur is the acute loss of pacing during severe electrolyte imbalance. The best method of management is prompt restoration of electrolyte balance.

II. Lead and Electrode Factors

A. Electrode Maturity

The duration of the electrode in situ affects the threshold in two ways. Early after implant the threshold of stimulation increases, i.e., more energy is required, probably because of a nonstimulatable reactive layer about the electrode. This evolution may be affected by the use of local steroids incorporated in an electrode for slow local dissemination. Early threshold increase is reduced and may be useful in avoiding the need for electrode revision. The chronic threshold of a steroid-eluting lead is about the same as a similar nonsteroid electrode. As the reactive layer becomes smaller, because of decreasing edema, the threshold decreases. The threshold peak usually is reached within the first month after implant, although occasional patients will evolve over a longer period, uncommonly as long as 6 months and rarely even longer (Figure 6).

B. Distance of Electrode from Sensitive Tissue

Once an electrode is in position, threshold evolves over a matter of days; but longer term evolution may occur. The peak evolution (in a nonsteroid electrode) may commonly represent a charge threshold increase of 3–5 times over that at implant and is largely determined by separation of the electrode from sensitive tissue by fibrous tissue and/or local reaction. Such an increase is sufficiently small so that it will not be noted if pacer output is at conventional levels. Threshold may, in as much as 5%–10% of the cases, rise to 10 times that at implant. In more than 90% of such instances, threshold will return within weeks or more slowly, possibly over 6 months, to the usual 1–3 times threshold at implant. Even where threshold has evolved to 10 times that at implant, continued increase is very unusual and rare, but it can occur. The typical pattern is

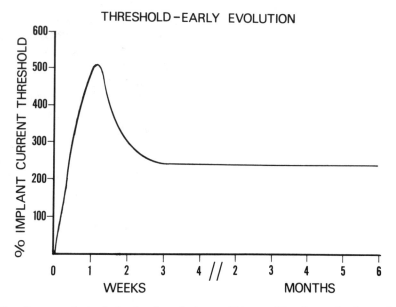

Figure 6. *Once an electrode is placed against or within sensitive tissue, local reaction causes enlargement of its surface area as the virtual electrode is formed. As chronicity is reached, the virtual electrode is smaller than early after implant and threshold decreases. The height and duration of the threshold increase are highly variable.*

for return toward a lower threshold even if that level is higher than is customary (Figure 7).

Once stability has been reached it is, for all practical purposes, permanent. About 20% of chronically implanted leads will develop a slow progressive threshold increase that will not exceed the output capability of a conventional pulse generator in less than a decade. An equal number will have a drifting, but progressive decline. About 60% will remain broadly stable, increasing or decreasing about a mean with variation caused by medication, food intake, electrolyte balance, activity, or sleep (Figure 8).

C. Unipolar or Bipolar Electrode

A unipolar electrode is the stimulating surface of a single insulated conductor (the lead) with a proximal connector to the pulse generator and the electrode in contact with sensitive tissue. The cardiac stimulator is always the cathode (negative) terminal of the pulse generator, the second is always the anode (positive) terminal. The second pole of the system is remote from the heart, usually part of the pulse generator case. It is in the subcutaneous tissue where the circuit is completed. Since the pulse generator case in the unipolar system is electrically active it may sense the adjacent pectoral or other somatic muscle to cause electromyographic interference and stimulate that muscle.

The bipolar electrode consists of two stimulating surfaces in contact with the heart. Both may be identical as they are for a myocardial implant where two

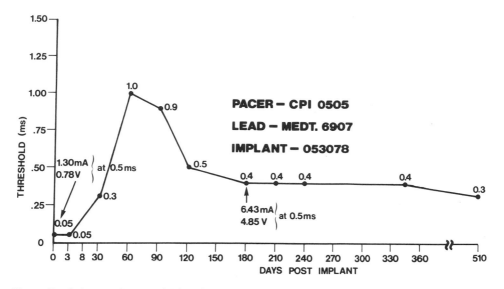

Figure 7. *Infrequently a very high and prolonged threshold evolution will occur. Such an evolution may return to a normal threshold chronically or the threshold may be high and stable. If evolution ends with a chronic threshold within the output capability of a conventional pacemaker, the utilization of a high output from the output programmable pulse generator will have been very valuable.*

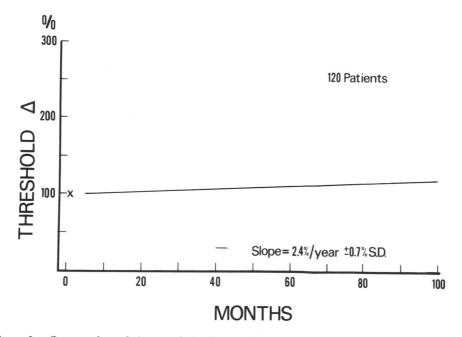

Figure 8. *Once an electrode is properly in place, prolonged and even indefinite stability of threshold can be anticipated. Progressive increase in threshold may occur, but at so slow a rate as to be practically meaningless. In this instance, 120 patients were analyzed and compared to the first threshold after implant. The rate of increase was 2.4% per year.*

electrodes are implanted to comprise the bipolar electrode. The bipolar endo-cardial lead has a stimulating tip (the cathodal electrode and a ring proximally), the anode. Depending on the model, separation between the two will be 2–3 cm. The tip should stimulate the heart while the ring should not. Modern cathodal electrodes are 8–10 mm^2 in surface area, the ring (designed to have a high stimulating threshold and, preferably, be incapable of stimulating the heart) is 40–50 mm^2 in surface area.

Bipolar Lead Construction.   Unipolar endocardial leads have been constructed of a coil encased by insulating material since 1965. This coil has been progressively reinforced by progression from a monofilar to multifilar conductor, i.e., multiple wires comprising one coil. Guidance of the lead is achieved by placing a flexible guide wire inside the coil to lend shape and direction to the lead. Prior to that a twisted flat wire without a lumen was used. That lead was positioned in the heart by its introduction into the venous system and movement of the patient until the lead was floated into the right ventricular apex. It was insulated with polyethylene, which deteriorated years after implantation as the result of being rubbed against the tricuspid valve. Silicone rubber was then introduced as an insulation material and continues in use today. Polyurethane insulation of a variety of different chemical characteristics has been most widely used since 1979 by several manufacturers.

Bipolar leads have had different configurations. Initially two parallel coils were encased in silicone rubber with insulation between the coils. This lead was large and difficult to insert into the venous system. Two such leads for a dual-chamber pacemaker might occupy and obstruct an entire subclavian vein. Monofilar and later multifilar coils increased durability and fracture resistance. Later evolution produced a coaxial (concentric) bipolar lead in which the two coils were insulated from each other. At present a still newer design remains in engineering evaluation in which a multifilar design has one of the coils insulated continuously with a thin coating from the other. As the multifilar leads are not concentric (coaxial) and the insulation is thinner than either silicone rubber or polyurethane, this design, if successful, will provide the thinnest bipolar lead design.

Whether an electrode system is unipolar or bipolar makes no difference in the current threshold of stimulation, which is a function of the surface area of the cathodal electrode. The voltage threshold is somewhat higher for the bipolar compared to the unipolar lead because of the lead wire required for the second, i.e., intracardiac (anode) electrode and the relatively smaller (therefore higher impedance) anode on the lead compared to the very large anode on the pulse generator. During unipolar pacing the cathode contacts cardiac tissues; during bipolar pacing both cathode and anode are in contact. In practice the unipolar anode is usually on the pacemaker case and is adjacent to the pectoral musculature. Other possibilities exist in which the anode is not against stimulatable tissue but along a lead, lying, perhaps, in the superior vena cava. This is simply another example of unipolar pacing, though in this instance both anode and cathode are intravascular. In a recent study of stimulation threshold and electrogram amplitude the mean atrial electrogram was found to be 4.38 mV in its

Table I
Electrogram (EGM) Amplitude (mVolts)

	Atrial			Ventricular	
Unipolar	Bipolar	P	Unipolar	Bipolar	P
4.38	4.56	NS	11.13	11.09	NS
n = 25					

unipolar version referenced to the subcutaneous tissue of the chest wall and 4.56 mV in the bipolar version. The ventricular electrogram was 11.13 mV in the unipolar and 11.09 mV in the bipolar, both were insignificant differences. The amplitude of the atrial and ventricular electrograms are therefore similar in unipolar and bipolar format (Table I). The amplitude of the far-field ventricular electrogram on the atrial channel is far larger in the unipolar than in a bipolar atrial electrogram. The remote atrial signal is small in both unipolar and bipolar ventricular electrograms. The unipolar and bipolar atrial and ventricular strength-duration curves are also similar, though the voltage stimulation threshold curve is higher in the bipolar than in the unipolar, reflecting the increased impedance of the bipolar lead (Figure 9).

The difference between the voltage threshold of unipolar and bipolar and the difference in lead impedance between unipolar and bipolar reaches statistical

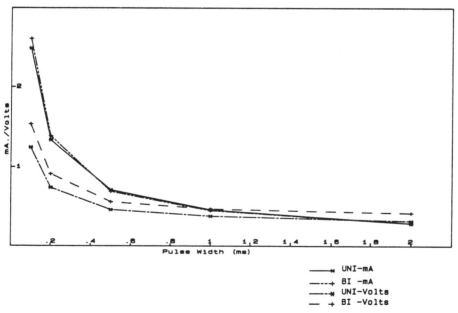

Figure 9. *Strength-duration curves for unipolar and bipolar ventricular stimulation show that current stimulation thresholds are equivalent unipolar and bipolar. The bipolar voltage threshold is slightly higher by a statistically significant margin.*

Table II
Stimulation Threshold Atrium

Pulse Duration (ms)	Volts			mA		
	Unipolar	Bipolar	P	Unipolar	Bipolar	P
0.1	1.47	1.90	<.0001	3.7	3.8	NS
0.5	0.54	0.72	<.0001	1.01	1.03	NS
1.0	0.43	0.57	<.0005	0.62	0.62	NS
n = 25						

	Pulse Duration	Unipolar	Bipolar
	0.1	397	500
Impedance	0.5	534	699
	1.0	693	919

Table III
Stimulation Threshold Ventricle

Pulse Duration (ms)	Volts			mA		
	Unipolar	Bipolar	P	Unipolar	Bipolar	P
0.1	1.14	1.38	<.00001	2.33	2.30	NS
0.5	0.42	0.51	<.00001	0.66	0.65	NS
1.0	0.34	0.42	<.00001	0.42	0.42	NS
n = 25						

	Pulse Duration	Unipolar	Bipolar
	0.1	489	600
Impedance	0.5	636	784
	1.0	809	1000

significance for the voltage threshold. The difference is statistically insignificant for current stimulation thresholds. The impedances, as expected, reflect the voltage threshold difference. The unipolar impedance at each pulse duration is significantly lower than the bipolar, reflecting the higher bipolar voltage threshold. Consequently, presently available unipolar and bipolar electrodes are, for all practical purposes, interchangeable in stimulation threshold and sensing electrogram. The bipolar far-field electrograms, both for interference signals and for the ventricular electrogram on the atrial lead, are significantly attenuated. Therefore aside from the slightly higher voltage threshold and impedance of the bipolar atrial lead no difference exists in stimulation capability. From this perspective alone unipolar and bipolar atrial and ventricular leads can be used interchangeably (Tables II, III).

D. Electrode Surface Area and Shape

The surface area of a stimulating electrode is directly and linearly related to the current threshold of stimulation. Though the shape of the stimulating surface plays a role, its clinical significance is not clear. Smaller surface area

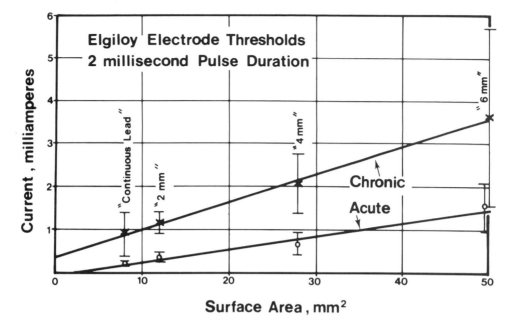

Figure 10. *A direct and linear relationship exists between current threshold and electrode size. The greater the electrode surface area the higher the current threshold.*

electrodes have lower current and charge thresholds than do larger electrodes and the current density threshold (mA/mm) remains relatively constant over a wide range of surface areas. Voltage threshold also decreases with surface area, though not as greatly as do current and charge thresholds. These phenomena exist both at implant (acutely) and chronically (Figure 10).

The chronic-to-acute threshold ratio depends on the size, shape, and material of the electrode and the thickness of the nonexcitable fibrous tissue that separates the electrode from excitable myocardium. In general, spherical solid tip electrodes have the highest chronic threshold evolution, cylindrical electrodes have lesser increases, and porous surface metal and carbon electrodes have even lower chronic threshold levels.

CHARACTERISTICS REQUIRED FOR A PACEMAKER ELECTRODE

1. electrochemical inertness;
2. low overvoltage during stimulation;
3. resistance to electrolytic destruction;
4. low electrical resistance;
5. low biological reactivity.

E. Electrode Material

The electrode should not go into solution during passage of an electric current, at least at conventional output levels for cardiac pacing. The metal itself should be nontoxic and salt formation should not occur. If a metal meets these criteria as a cathode, but not as an anode, then it may be used only for unipolar pacing. Materials usable for implanted pacing are the following:

1. Platinum with 10% iridium;
2. Elgiloy, an alloy of cobalt, iron, chromium, molybdenum, nickel, and manganese;
3. A silver and stainless steel combination;
4. Activated vitreous carbon.

Threshold is a function of the reactivity of the material and the overvoltage developed during passage of a current for cardiac stimulation. The more noble a metal, i.e., the less reactive, the lower this overvoltage and the lower the voltage and current pacing threshold. Platinum-iridium has consistently lower thresholds than the more reactive metal, Elgiloy; carbon lower than either. Nevertheless, both metals have been quite successful for long-term pacing and the difference in threshold is unimportant as a practical matter. The prolonged durability of metal electrodes is proven. Carbon, used for briefer periods, seems to behave equally well.

Steroid electrodes contain a very small amount of dexamethasone (about 1 mg). The steroid is slowly eluted into adjacent tissue, reduces the local tissue reaction, and maintains a low threshold acutely and chronically and moderates the early threshold rise compared to similar, nonsteroidal electrodes.

F. Lead Insulation

Insulation material for implantable leads has long been of concern. The material must be a good insulator, must be non- or minimally reactive, and noncarcinogenic. It must be durable and resist wear and the flailing of the tricuspid value. It must not undergo time-dependent spontaneous deterioration and must not be metabolized. It must not cause thrombosis.

The earliest lead material used was polyethylene. It served well and for prolonged periods, but there have been increasing reports that after a decade or more, insulation wear can be seen adjacent to the tricuspid valve from continual lead and valve contact. The second material introduced was silicone rubber. It is well tolerated in the soft tissue, i.e., as a myocardial lead and in the venous system. Wear seems to have been a very small problem and numerous leads have been in place for years without significant deterioration. A small and unknown number of chronically placed silicone rubber leads have provoked local venous calcification that may invade the lead itself (Figure 11). A significant problem is that silicone rubber leads were and are relatively large for the venous system and may be introduced into the cephalic vein with some difficulty. This is especially true for bipolar leads and even more if two leads are to be introduced for dual-chamber pacing. Smaller diameter silicone rubber leads have been introduced in the past few years and seem to be behaving well. If lubricated at manufacture, introduction of two silicone leads may be almost as friction free as the polyurethane leads.

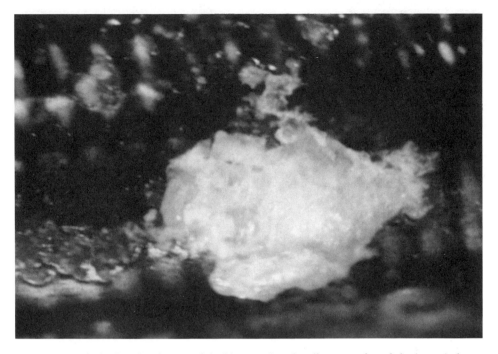

Figure 11. *The lead in the photograph had become densely adherent to the subclavian vein because of calcification that had invaded the silicone rubber insulation. The hard edge of the calcium deposit caused a fulcrum that contributed to a local lead fracture.*

Since 1979 a series of polyurethane insulated leads have been introduced by several manufacturers and now represent the largest group of leads implanted. The leads are smaller in diameter than older rubber leads. Two unipolar leads can easily be inserted into a moderate size cephalic or external jugular vein or via a plastic introducer. Of great importance is that polyurethane slides well against polyurethane while silicone rubber adheres to silicone rubber, though newer silicone leads are improved in this regard. These leads lend themselves especially well to dual-chamber implant. Since they are small, they are readily insinuated beneath a trabeculum and threshold has been low and stable.

Polyurethane is a category of synthetic polymer and different polyurethanes have different characteristics. Several models have been associated with a high early and late failure rate with insulation disruption, short circuit, and lead fracture (Figure 12). As this effect has been limited to several lead models from one manufacturer, ventricular models 6972, 4002, 4012 and atrial models 6990U and 6991U, either the material or the manufacturing process may have been at fault. Despite the polyurethane problems, the need for small diameter slippable leads will continue their popularity. Other polyurethane leads from a variety of manufacturers and simultaneous and successor leads from the same manufacturer have demonstrated longevity similar to silicone rubber leads over five to ten years (Figure 13). The original defective leads have caused severe clinical problems, but correction of the manufacturing problems has resulted in leads

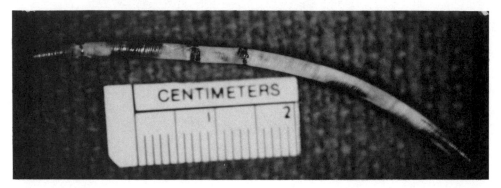

Figure 12. *A polyurethane lead is shown that has undergone deterioration by surface cracking, whitish opacification, and discoloration. Three areas of complete loss of insulation appear—two partially caused by a ligature holding the lead to the tissue. The third (left) was apparently spontaneous.*

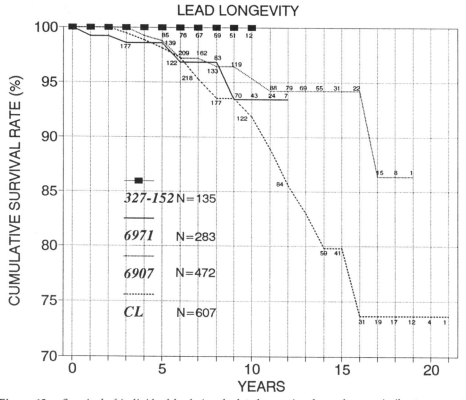

Figure 13. *Survival of individual leads is calculated on a time base of years similar to or greater than that of the longer lasting lithium anode powered pacemakers. Patterns of wear are readily apparent. Two older silicone rubber leads (CL and 6907) have had cumulative survivals at 14 years of over 74% and 86%, respectively. While some urethane leads have had very high failure rates, most have not. All urethane leads have had a far shorter exposure, but model 6971 had a survival of 94% at 12 years and 327–152 had almost 100% survival 9 years after implant by which time the older leads had already shown a substantial failure incidence.*

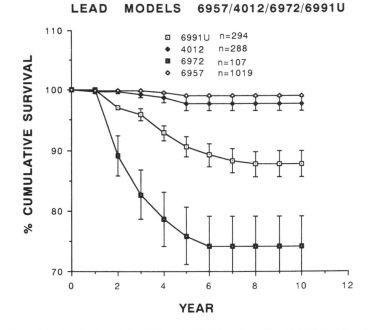

LEAD MODELS 6957/4012/6972/6991U

Figure 14. *Two defective lead models 6972 and 6991U and another (4012) that has behaved less well than a fourth model (6957). 6957 has a cumulative survival of 99.1 ± 0.43%; model 4012, 97.8 ± 1.2%; model 6972, 74.2 ± 4.9%; and model 6991U, 87.7 ± 2.2% 10 years after implant. Five years following implant and thereafter the additional failures were few (but late failures persisted) and the cumulative survival reached a relative plateau.*

with acceptable stability. Still, the experience over the past decade has been that lead failure in the vulnerable leads has been early and that at about five years the leads remaining in place have a more stable longevity projection (Figure 14).

G. Solid and Porous Electrodes

Earlier electrodes had been solid metal, whether in a tight coil, a corkscrew-like spiral, or at the end of a transvenous lead of platinum-iridium, Elgiloy, or silver alloy. In the past few years new configurations have become available. These are platinum-iridium or Elgiloy porous electrodes and those of sintered carbon. The porous electrode may be a coil of fine platinum-iridium wire with interstices into which tissue grows; or a porous surface bonded into a solid base.

The porous surface electrode has Elgiloy spherical powder particles bonded to each other and to a solid Elgiloy substrate. The surface is 30% porous and about 100μm thick. The totally porous electrode consists of a sintered platinum-iridium fiber of micrometers arranged randomly at a density of 10% and hemispherical in shape.

The activated vitreous carbon electrode produces a biocompatible porous surface electrode with pores about 10 angstroms in size and a depth of 10 microns. The fibrous capsule is thinner than that surrounding a metal electrode.

BENEFITS OF POROUS ELECTRODES

a. Ingrowth of fibrous tissue into the electrode interstices increases electrode anchoring;
b. A thinner fibrous capsule forms about the electrode to yield a smaller surface area "virtual electrode";
c. Increase of the effective surface area for sensing while maintaining a small area for pacing.

The overvoltage is about 10% of that of solid tip platinum electrodes. The sensing impedance of a porous activated vitreous carbon electrode is about of that of a solid tip platinum electrode. The porous Elgiloy, platinum-iridium, and carbon electrodes provide the following:

1. lower polarization caused by overvoltage;
2. fibrous ingrowth with enhanced attachment of electrode to tissue;
3. smaller fibrous capsule;
4. lower impedance for sensing;
5. lower current and voltage for stimulation acutely and chronically.

H. Steroid Leads

Maintenance of stable and low acute and chronic stimulation thresholds is highly desirable. Because of the effect of a fibrous tissue layer producing a "virtual" electrode, which increases stimulation threshold and reduces electrogram amplitude (ventricular and importantly atrial), a glucocorticoid steroid has been incorporated into a porous electrode to reduce the fibrous reaction and its consequences. Parenteral glucocorticoid administration has been shown to reduce threshold acutely and chronically in patients with a high threshold. An electrode (models 4003 and 4503 and many others) consists of a porous platinum surface with a silicone rubber plug containing approximately 1 mg of dexamethasone sodium phosphate. In contact with tissue fluids, steroid slowly elutes from the electrode and affects the inflammatory process of the cells immediately adjacent. There is no systemic effect of the steroid and the concentration is maximum at the electrode/tissue interface. Elution occurs over several years and 20% of the steroid remains in the electrode 4 years after implant. It seems that threshold will remain stable thereafter, and the ultimately late effects (i.e., 8–10 years postimplant) indicate a stable low threshold. In conventional solid and non-steroid porous electrodes, stimulation and sensing threshold is permanently stable after early threshold evolution. In patients in whom steroid electrodes have been implanted, the rise in stimulation threshold, usually seen in both atrium and ventricle, during the first month postimplant, is ameliorated and frequently completely eliminated. If any stimulation threshold increase has occurred, it has been smaller and returns to a lower level sooner than in the nonsteroid electrode. At approximately 16 weeks after implantation, threshold levels are statistically significantly lower for steroid electrodes than for identical nonsteroid electrodes. This difference persists chronically. The reduction of the size of the inflammatory shell surrounding the electrode seems to improve sen-

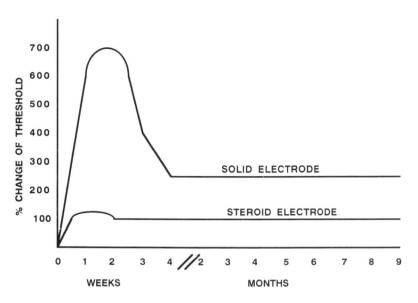

THRESHOLD-EARLY EVOLUTION

Figure 15. *Steroid-eluting electrodes have produced a distinct reduction in stimulation threshold acutely and chronically. Sensing characteristics have also improved. In this diagram similar solid tips, without steroid and steroid eluting electrodes, have been compared. The increase in stimulation threshold for the steroid lead early after implant is much reduced and the long-term stable threshold for both is characteristic.*

sing characteristics, especially in the atrium where the initially small electrogram makes improved sensing characteristics particularly important (Figure 15).

Following the successful introduction of the steroid-eluting electrode, further designs have been attempted. These include a smaller surface area electrode with a small surface area, i.e., 1.5 mm^2, and a high impedance, a surface button for epicardial use and a platinized endocardial screw-in steroid-eluting electrode. A steroid-eluting collar proximal to the electrode is also being investigated.

The benefit of the steroid electrode lies in the prolonged low level of stimulation threshold and high level of sensing. The occasional patient with recurrent high stimulation threshold in the early postimplant period or who progressively increases threshold until late after implant electrode revision is required seems to benefit from a steroid-eluting electrode. Chronic thresholds are sufficiently low so that long-term pacing at a 2.5 V output has been reliable, thus decreasing current drain from the battery and allowing prolonged longevity with the small and power-hungry pacemakers now in use. There seems to be no difficulty with the steroid-eluting electrode; there is no late increase in displacement, which might have been associated with poor fibrous tissue formation.

I. Lead Fixation

Myocardial. Epicardial and myocardial leads have, from first usage, been actively attached to tissue. Epicardial leads have been backed by a polyester mesh sutured to the epicardium. Leads introduced into the myocardium (5815, 6913) have been backed by a silicone rubber plate that allows suture to the epicardium. Myocardial sutureless electrodes (6917 and 6917A) are screwed into the myocardium and have a polyester mesh "skirt" that provokes fibrous ingrowth to fix the electrode. This electrode has been associated with high threshold evolution and has fallen into disuse. Another sutureless design has two horizontal metal projections holding the electrode which has no active attachment to the myocardium. The most recently introduced, 4951, is harpoonlike and rests in the myocardium. It too has a suture plate designed to fix the electrode to the epicardium. In this regard all of these electrodes can be considered as "active" fixation.

Endocardial.   Over 95% of all implantations and therefore leads, are endocardial, both for atrial and ventricular use. Attachment to the endocardium is by remote control because, unlike the "epimyocardial" lead in which the operator approaches the myocardium with the lead-electrode system, the operator never approaches the endocardial surface. The problem of displacement of the endocardial lead has existed since its earliest usage, despite its ease of application and relatively stress-free implantation.

The earliest (1958–1960) endocardial stimulating leads were relatively stiff and were held in place by that rigidity. Such a lead could be placed in the right ventricular apex or in the outflow tract and did not require intracardiac support. The problems of so rigid a catheter included ventricular perforation, loss of pacing, and hemopericardium. A lead must be sufficiently rigid, aside from the stylet used to guide it, if it is to be inserted in the right ventricular apex. Leads that are excessively limp have a higher displacement rate than those that are somewhat more rigid. If excessively rigid, perforation may result. The usual solution is to have a stiff guide wire within a more flexible lead. The guide wire is withdrawn after maneuver of the softer lead into position. Early leads were cylindrical and isodiametric. As the surface was smooth, fibrous ingrowth into the lead material never occurred and the tightly fitting fibrous layer could not grip the lead itself. Two early leads, the 5816 and the 588S had a larger diameter stimulating tip than the body of the lead. Fibrous tissue growth "glove fit" about the lead and provided a barrier to late displacement of the large tip through the fibrous neck. This provided the first, possibly inadvertent, passive fixation leads. A variety of flanges, fine tines, conical protrusions, and fins (some perforated for greater attachment) about the tip of the lead have provided more modern passive fixation devices. In each instance the basis for passive fixation was the delay in actual fixation until fibrous growth from the endocardium occurred.

The bulbous tip leads suffered from two defects: high threshold after implant and a high early displacement rate. although they were generally stable chronically. Parallel developments occurred that produced thinner leads, smaller electrodes, and greater capacity for early fixation. The first "passive" techniques were conical "shoulders" proximal to the stimulating electrode. Once in position a fibrous layer was laid down around the lead, trapping it in position because the fibrous "neck" is smaller than the "shoulder." Later developments included:

1. tines, or short 2–3 mm long protuberances proximal to the electrode;

2. fins in which a conical shoulder (which is a complete conical segment) is replaced by 3 or 4 rubber or plastic slivers arranged radially around the electrode;
3. ribbing of the lead insulation proximal to the electrode;
4. a small layer of polyester velour into which fibrous tissue will grow (not a commercial product).

In all of these designs the early fixation effect was less but the late effect more significant. The effect on early and late displacement was substantial. Probably the major residual problem is the difficulty or impossibility of late removal of the passively attached lead once the fibrous attachment has matured. Because of the infrequent but potentially lethal occurrence of endocarditis involving tissue and a retained lead, the problem of late irremovability may be the most serious clinical pacing problem.

Active fixation leads attempt to provide immediate fixation during implant.

ACTIVE FIXATION LEADS

1. A grasping jaw mechanism;
2. A complex helical coil that can wind itself about a trabeculum;
3. An exposed metal screw that is the electrode at the end of the lead;
4. A retractable metal screw that is the electrode and is manually expelled into the endocardium;
5. A retractable screw that holds the lead but is not the electrode. The electrode is conventional at the lead tip, the screw is a fixation device only;
6. Nylon whiskers that protrude from a perforated solid electrode to penetrate and grasp the endocardium. This design provided high local reactivity andunacceptably high threshold. This lead is obsolete;
7. A balloon proximal to the electrode. The electrode was slid (hopefully) beneath a trabeculum and was inflated. Once inflated with saline or contrast material the balloon held the lead in place much as a catheter in the urinary bladder. This lead had a high late dislocation rate and high threshold. When the balloon deflates, as it must when it ruptures because of ingress of body fluid via the balloon membrane, the lead remains in a cavity from which it can be displaced. This lead is obsolete.

Active fixation leads are useful in the ventricle and in the atrium where, in general, the early displacement rate is higher than in the ventricle. At best they provide immediate stable fixation with (a) low displacement rate and (b) potentially easy removal of a chronically implanted lead by reversal of the fixation mechanism, i.e., unscrewing it.

The leads, especially with the retractable screw mechanism, seem easy to use, relatively atraumatic, and live up to their promise. Active fixation leads are likely to be progressively used more widely.

J. Anodal or Cathodal Stimulation

The terms unipolar and bipolar refer to the presence of the anode and cathode in the heart (bipolar) or the cathode only in the cardiac position (unipolar) and the anode at a remote site. The cathode (negative terminal) must be stimulating in all instances and threshold is a function of cathodal characteristics.

Pacemaker-Induced Tachycardia

A pacemaker-induced tachycardia requires a stimulus from the pacemaker to be started. Once begun it continues spontaneously without the need for further pacemaker stimulation, such as supraventricular tachycardia, atrial fibrillation or flutter, or ventricular tachycardia or fibrillation (Figures 16 and 17). Stimulation threshold is ascertained during diastole when ventricular sensitivity has returned to a stable level before a new depolarization. During late diastole the myocardium is more sensitive to a cathodal than anodal stimulus and equally sensitive to cathodal and bipolar stimuli. Myocardial sensitivity to stimulation changes significantly immediately after the QRS complex during the relative refractory period. The phenomenon of pacemaker-induced ventricular fibrillation in which the stimulus falls into the vulnerable period of the cardiac cycle has been observed during bipolar stimulation except in a few published instances and is related to the anode of a bipolar electrode (Figure 18). (See Figure 17.)

The possibility of ventricular fibrillation increases during myocardial ischemia, infarction, metabolic imbalance, and drug intoxication. Completely satisfactory pacemaker sensing of all conducted, idioventricular, and aberrant cardiac foci, especially during myocardial deterioration and infarction, does not

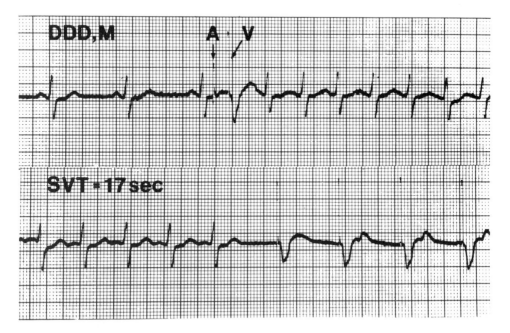

Figure 16. *Pacemaker programming placed an atrial channel stimulus in the vulnerable period of the atrium. Supraventricular tachycardia with a duration of 17 seconds was induced and ended spontaneously. This is an example of a pacemaker-induced atrial tachycardia.*

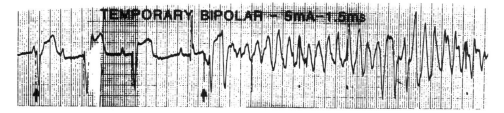

Figure 17. *A single-chamber temporary pacemaker was capable of stimulating the heart at a normal output, but sensed intermittently. A stimulus that fell at the end of the T wave of a spontaneous beat caused sustained ventricular tachycardia. In this instance both anode and cathode were stimulating the heart, i.e., in the bipolar mode.*

exist. The problem of pacemaker competition with spontaneous cardiac activity has not been eliminated. Competition between premature ventricular contractions and a bipolar stimulus is especially problematic during bipolar temporary pacing following acute myocardial infarction. Most temporary pacing is bipolar. Most of implanted pacing is unipolar cathodal, although bipolar pacing is becoming more common. In experimental canine cardiac stimulation during is-

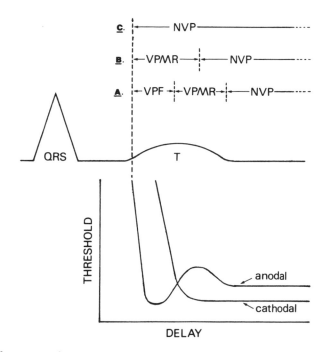

Figure 18. *Three types of myocardial response to suprathreshold stimuli after the refractory period are observed:* **A.** *The vulnerable period for fibrillation (VPF) followed by one for multiple responses (VPMR), followed by the nonvulnerable period (NVP).* **B.** *Stimulation early in the excitable period produces multiple responses followed by a nonvulnerable period.* **C.** *Some animals are nonvulnerable to arrhythmias and a single stimulus produces a single response. The cathodal and anodal excitation thresholds at different delays during the cardiac cycle (strength-interval curves) are also shown.*

chemia, at outputs which approximate those of conventional cardiac pacers, three distinct patterns follow the ventricular absolute refractory period:

A. Some animals are nonvulnerable to arrhythmia (NVP), and a single stimulus (anodal or cathodal) produces a single response (NVP = nonvulnerable period);
B. In others, the initial sensitivity produces multiple ventricular responses (VPMR) to a single stimulus, followed by a nonvulnerable period (VPMR = vulnerable period for multiple responses);
C. In still others the earliest response will be that of ventricular fibrillation followed by the vulnerable period for multiple responses and then the nonvulnerableperiod) (VF = ventricular fibrillation).

Sensitivity to anodal stimulation occurs earlier than cathodal after the absolute refractory period and because of the phenomenon of the "anodal dip," sensitivity is greater for a brief time during the vulnerable periods for multiple responses or ventricular fibrillation than it ever is to cathodal stimulation. In order to stimulate early with the cathode, a much higher stimulus level is required, effective only well after the beginning of anodal sensitivity (Figure 19).

The anodal refractory period is of shorter duration than the cathodal. If a bipolar electrode is in place and anodal and cathodal electrode surface areas are equal and lie on equally sensitive tissue, the refractory period for bipolar and anodal stimulation will be the same and shorter in duration than the cathodal

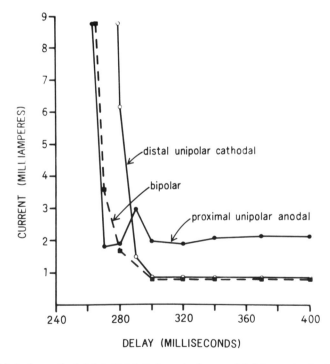

Figure 19. *Unipolar cathodal (at distal tip), unipolar anodal (at proximal ring), and bipolar strength-interval curves determined in a patient with a Cordis temporary 4F electrode. Note that the anodal and bipolar absolute refractory periods are equal and shorter than the cathodal refractory period.*

refractory period. Ventricular vulnerability will be equal for anodal and bipolar stimulation. A bipolar or anodal stimulus can therefore initiate an arrhythmia over a greater portion of the cardiac cycle and a a lower threshold than can a cathodal stimulus. The bipolar threshold equals the lower of the anodal or cathodal threshold so that early excitation is possible. Some temporary pacing leads are available in which the anodal surface is much larger than the cathodal and at least one in which the anodal (ring) surface is moved to a distance of 25 cm from the cathode (tip) so that it is removed from the heart to lie in the superior vena cava.

The importance of this data lies in the relative avoidance of bipolar pacing should significant irritability be present. The possibility exists of reducing irritability and therefore myocardial vulnerability by changing from bipolar to unipolar pacing where possible. When pacing is required during acute myocardial infarction, it is desirable to maintain either a large anode or one remote from the heart. Ventricular fibrillation is an uncommon occurrence during cardiac pacing, but it does occur.

FACTORS THAT REDUCE VENTRICULAR FIBRILLATION

1. Careful avoidance of excessive cardiac medication;
2. Electrolyte balance;
3. Administration of some antiarrhythmic drugs;
4. Good oxygenation and ventilation;
5. Unipolar cathodal or remote or large anodal stimulation;
6. Noncompetitive stimulation.

All newly introduced bipolar leads for implant have an anode ten times or more larger than the cathode to reduce the possibility of anodal stimulation and therefore the possibility of ventricular fibrillation.

K. Pulse Duration, i.e., The Strength-Duration Curve

Threshold varies as a function of impulse duration and the direction of this variation is dependent on the parameter measured. The strength-duration curve is the major basis for understanding cardiac stimulation threshold. Current, voltage, charge (the product of current and time), and energy (the product of current, voltage, and time ($E = IVT$) all vary as a function of pulse duration. A common method of variation of output of a programmable pulse generator is by change of pulse duration. Only through comprehension of the strength-duration curve, and awareness that it is not a linear function, can the basic factors of increase of output in the presence of high threshold and decrease of output to conserve energy be appreciated (Figure 20).

The lowest point on a stimulation curve at an infinitely long pulse duration is called **rheobase** and the pulse duration at which threshold is twice the rheobase value is the **chronaxie** time. The knowledge of rheobase is useful in pacemaker design as a pulse duration near or beyond rheobase is a relatively or totally useless expenditure of electrical capacity (Figure 21).

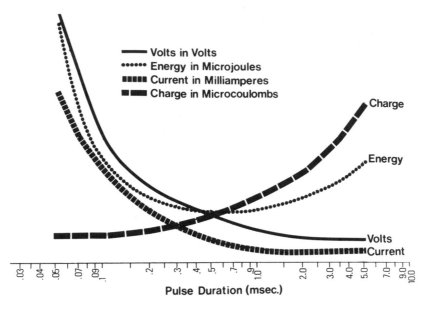

Figure 20. *Strength-duration curves of cardiac stimulation are shown. While current and voltage requirements increase to produce cardiac response as pulse duration shortens, charge is the most significant factor in stimulation efficiency, decreasing with pulse duration. Energy at threshold is lowest at 0.5 to 1.0 ms pulse duration, increasing at shorter and longer durations.*

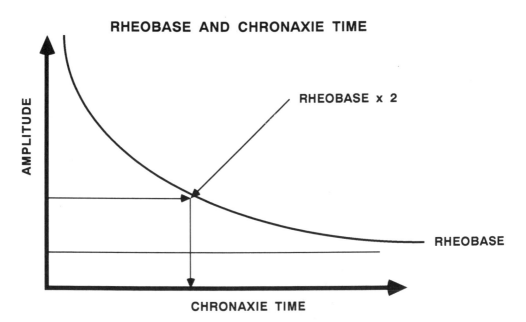

Figure 21. *Rheobase and chronaxie time are basic analyses of the strength-duration curve. **Rheobase** is the voltage or current stimulation threshold of an infinitely long pulse duration. The **chronaxie time** is the pulse duration of a stimulus double the value of **rheobase**. The chronaxie time approximates the most efficient stimulation pulse duration.*

Current.   The current flow at threshold is parallel (rheobase) to the abscissa from about 2.0 ms and onward. Threshold values rise as pulse duration shortens.

Volts.   Rheobase is reached between 1 to 2 ms; at shorter durations threshold rises.

Two derived functions, charge and energy, show a different pattern. Charge is perhaps the most useful single function, as it describes threshold in the same terms in which chemical battery capacity is measured (milliampere hours or ampere hours), and its consumption is inversely related to battery longevity. Charge expended at threshold decreases with shortened pulse duration, as the decline in time is far more rapid than increase in current flow per unit of time.

Quantification of Threshold.   The threshold of cardiac stimulation is the least cathodal electrical stimulus that, when delivered in diastole after the absolute, relative refractory, and the hypersensitive periods, is able to maintain consistent capture of the heart.

At a given pulse duration the mean current per pulse in milliamperes (mA) is the electrical impulse parameter that has been used, and should continue to be used, to quantify the threshold stimulus. The mean current is independent of the lead-heart circuit impedance. It is equally appropriate to quantify threshold by using the quantity of electricity or charge per pulse in microcoulombs (μC). Charge is found by multiplying the mean current by the pulse duration (mean current [I] $\times$ time [T]).

Voltage is an indirect measurement of threshold. The actual voltage drop across responsive myocardium and other interelectrode tissue cannot be separated from the voltage drop across lead resistance and the nonlinear polarization drop across the electrode-tissue interface. For practical purposes, only voltage threshold may be obtainable because most manufacturers produce pulse generators with capacitor-coupled constant voltage output. If pulse duration is kept constant, then the variation of output voltage can be an effective means of finding threshold.

The energy threshold in microjoules (μJ) has been the most common measure of threshold and is approximated by multiplying mean current by mean voltage by pulse duration (mean current [I] $\times$ mean voltage [V] $\times$ time [T]). This is an unfortunate measure of stimulation threshold because the voltage that actually contributes to the excitation process is unknown.

Strength-duration Curves.   The strength-duration curve of stimulation is the quantity of charge, current, voltage, or energy required to stimulate the heart at a series of pulse durations. These values vary significantly as a function of pulse duration and, of these, only charge is approximately linear (Figure 22). In order to set a voltage or pulse duration for parameter output programming, the position that a specific voltage or pulse duration occupies on the curve must be known. At a 2.7-volt output approximately 0.5 ms, pulse duration may be required to capture. The threshold of stimulation at a fixed voltage (2.7 or 5.0 V) is the point of intersection of the threshold and output curves. Similarly, if output voltage is varied at a constant pulse duration, the voltage threshold can

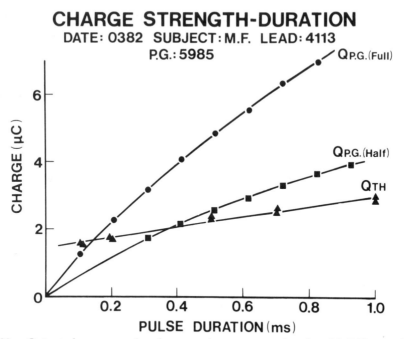

Figure 22. *Output charge per pulse of a pacemaker programmed to 5 and 2.7 V, superimposed on the charge strength-duration curve. The points of intersection of the threshold with output curves determines minimum pulse duration at which capture occurs for the programmed output voltage.*

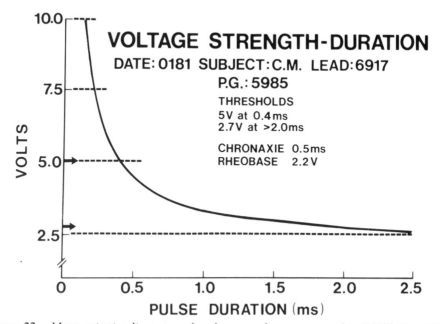

Figure 23. *Mean output voltage per pulse of a pacemaker programmed to 5 V (full) and 2.7 V (half) superimposed on the voltage strength-duration curve. Capture was consistent for programmed pulse durations equal to or greater than 0.4 ms at 5 V or 2.0 ms at 2.7 V. Rheobase is at 2.2 V which means that below that output voltage no pulse of any duration would produce capture, even though output charge and energy may be very large at long pulse durations.*

be determined (Figure 23). In the instance cited, the rheobase is 2.2 V. If the pacemaker had an output below 2.2 V then no stimulus, of any duration, would capture despite increasing output charge and/or energy.

A similar situation exists for current threshold. The analysis of output-to-threshold variation can be made as described above (Figure 24). During constant voltage pacing the current output decreases as the pulse duration increases. The decrease occurs because of increasing polarization and, therefore, impedance at longer pulse durations is greater than at shorter durations (Figure 25).

The relationship between threshold charge and output chargeper pulse as a function of pulse duration may be easier to visualize than either the voltage or the current output-to- threshold relationships because the charge curves are nearly linear over the range of relevant pulse durations.

Safety Factor. Safety factor refers to the amount by which the pulse generator's output exceeds the threshold at a given pulse duration.

Safety Factor:

$$= \frac{\text{Pulse Generator Output} - \text{Threshold Value}}{\text{Threshold Value}}$$

$$= \frac{\text{Pulse Generator Output}}{\text{Threshold Value}} - 1$$

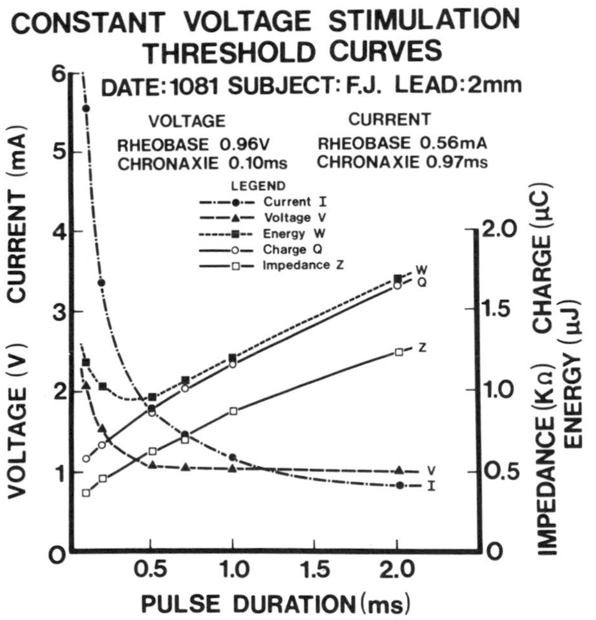

Figure 24. *A typical set of chronic strength-duration curves for constant voltage stimulation are shown. As pulse duration increases, charge increases, mean current and voltage threshold fall, and energy threshold is at a minimum at approximately 0.5 to 0.8 ms. The shortest pulse duration requires the least charge at threshold.*

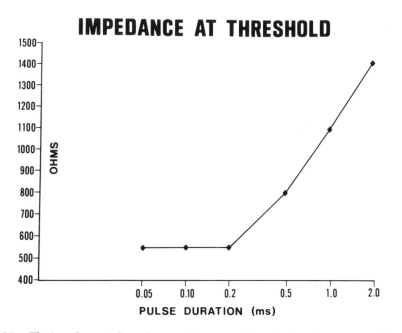

Figure 25. *The impedance to flow of current increases with pulse duration increase. Shorter pulse durations produce much lower impedances and are therefore more efficient for stimulation. The impedance can double over the pulse duration programmable range of conventional pulse generators.*

As the aim of pacing is to capture the heart each time a stimulus is produced, the safety factor is used to set the output at a sufficiently high level to accommodate the variation in threshold that may occur during daily activities such as sleeping, eating, and exercise, and that which may also be due to medications.

The question remains of how great the safety factor should be under various circumstances, including the period early after implantation when threshold evolution occurs. Since the threshold peak may be five times the charge at implant, the initial output setting should be at least five times the threshold charge. The second period for which a safety factor must be considered is that of the chronic, stable threshold. As the normal physiological variation in charge threshold is no more than 30%–50%, doubling the charge threshold should be adequate. The third circumstance is that of the high and, even unstable threshold. In this situation the actual threshold may be unknown (except during programming) and unpredictable. Pacemaker output should be set at a very high level to provide for maximum safety, and the patient should be seen at sufficient time intervals to ascertain if and when stability occurs.

The use of a safety margin of 100% of threshold charge will provide adequate patient safety if the long-term threshold is stable. As the long-term threshold is almost always stable when chronic (6 months or more after implant) and can be expected to vary within a narrow range, 100% charge margin will be satisfactory. Even if threshold is high, but stable, a safe margin can be found depending on the output capability of the pulse generator used. If threshold is actually unstable, then only very great outputs will suffice, many beyond the capability of any implantable pulse generator. In that case it is clearly desirable to revise electrode status so that a new, hopefully low and stable threshold will result.

The reasons for setting an output at some reasonable level above threshold are the reduction of output and the consequent prolongation of pulse generator longevity and the reduction of the likelihood of local muscle stimulation if a unipolar pacer is in use. Output programmable single-chamber pacemakers can increase or decrease the anticipated longevity by as much as 5–8 times depending on programmability capability and output setting. For dual-chamber pacemakers the longevity range is far greater.

All output programming is based on understanding of the strength-duration curve and the various portions of the curve: the portion for voltage and current at short pulse durations, i.e., less than 0.3 ms in which relatively small changes in pulse duration make large differences in threshold; the knee in which relatively proportional changes are made between pulse duration and voltage or current threshold; and the flat portion of the curve at longer pulse durations in which large changes in pulse duration make very small changes in threshold. The charge threshold, i.e., the product of time (pulse duration) and current is low at short pulse durations and high at long pulse durations. Since it is charge that produces a cardiac event, the charge threshold should be determined and charge output kept at a minimum to reduce battery drain. All battery capacity is calculated in charge, i.e., 1 ampere hour, etc.

Atrial and ventricular thresholds are similar in principal and no difference exists in determining threshold or setting output between atrium and ventricle. For implant of dual-chamber pacemakers similar procedures should be undertaken for atrium and ventricle if output is independently programmable. If output is not independently programmable it is likely that threshold will be lower in one chamber than the other. The output for both must be set to meet the needs of the chamber with the higher threshold, thus using battery capacity that might otherwise be conserved. If different output settings can be established, it is desirable to set each chamber individually.

DETERMINATION OF THRESHOLD AND SETTING OF OUTPUT

There are several different means of controlling output in an output programmable pacemaker. While a few implantable constant current pulse generators remain in service, no new ones are being manufactured and those implanted are undergoing attrition by battery depletion and patient death. All newly manufactured pulse generators are of constant voltage output and four different output voltage combinations are possible. Two different combinations are possible for constant current generators and need not be described further.

1. Single Voltage—Multiple Pulse Durations

This had been the most commonly available mode for single-chamber pacemakers until about eight years ago. Many remain implanted. Output voltage is

5.0 V and pulse duration commonly from 0.05—2.0 ms. With pulse duration as the only variable, threshold is determined by a progressive decrease in pulse duration until the shortest pulse duration that will consistently capture the heart is found. If 0.3 ms or less, tripling the pulse duration will provide a 100% threshold margin. A threshold pulse duration of 0.1–0.2 ms allows an output of 0.5 ms with safety. (Remember that as the pulse duration is increased threshold increases as does output.) If the threshold is 0.4 ms (the approximate voltage chronaxie) or greater, then the pulse duration should be set at 4 times threshold. So great an increase may not be available and even when it is, a full 100% safety margin may not be possible.

2. Dual Voltage—Multiple Pulse Durations

Many pulse generators provide this capability. The two voltages are the traditional 5.0 V and 2.5 V, which is also the battery voltage before it is doubled to produce 5.0 V. Two alternative approaches are possible. Formerly the 5.0 V setting alone was used, as in the single voltage unit (see above), and the volt setting was disregarded except when special low output or great longevity was required. Because of the recent introduction of low threshold (i.e., carbon, porous, and steroid) electrodes, many models are delivered at 2.5 V output and the 5.0 V setting is used only as a "high output" setting.

A useful approach is to set the output at 2.5 V and determine the minimum threshold pulse duration. Programming the output voltage to 5.0 V at that pulse duration will provide an adequate safety margin. If 2.5 V never captures no matter what the pulse duration, i.e., rheobase is above 2.5 V, threshold must be determined at 5.0 V, but it will certainly be high and a full 100% safety margin may not be attainable. If threshold is at 0.05–0.3 ms pulse duration at 2.5 V, then tripling the pulse duration at 2.5 V will be safe, effective, and will allow efficient battery consumption.

3. Triple Voltage—Multiple Pulse Durations

The pulse durations usually available are similar to those of single voltage, multiple pulse duration generators. For some generators only four pulse durations are available corresponding to the parts of the standard deviation curve in which change in pulse duration has a significant effect on threshold, i.e., 0.25 to 1.0 ms. The actual voltages available are 2.5, 5.0, 7.5–8.2 or 10.0 V. These represent battery voltage, the conventional doubling of battery voltage, and its tripling or quadrupling. The 7.5 to 10.0 V output should be used as a short-term expedient only. Battery capacity is consumed so rapidly at these outputs that pulse generator longevity will necessarily be very short.

The voltage setting should be at 2.5 V. Pulse duration threshold is found and the final voltage may be left at or 2.5 or 5.0 V as above. If capture is not 2.5 V, threshold is determined at 5.0 V and the final setting is at prolonged pulse duration and 5.0 V or at the threshold pulse duration at 10.0 V. If capture is possible at a relatively short pulse duration at 5.0 V, it may be better to use

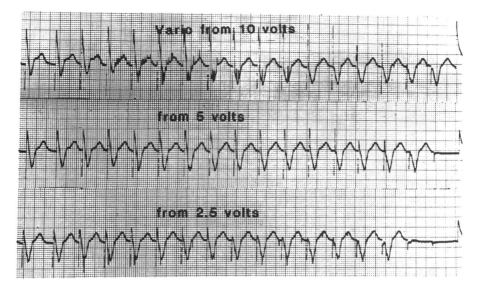

Figure 26. *Threshold can often be very accurately determined noninvasively if multiple pulse durations and output voltage settings are available. Use of the "Vario" system at three output voltages 10 V, 5 V, and 2.5 V at a pulse duration of 0.5 ms allows accurate determination of the voltage threshold. ABOVE: Each step is 0.64 V and capture is consistent through the fifteenth step. Threshold is below 0.64 V. MIDDLE: Each step is 0.32 V. One stimulus does not capture so that threshold must lie between 0.64 and 0.32 V. BELOW: Each step is 0.15 V. As two steps are missed, threshold is at 0.45V. A strength-duration curve can be constructed easily if desired.*

a longer pulse duration at 5.0 V knowing that a 100% margin is not possible but also recognizing the high battery drain of 7.5–10.0 V.

Several pulse generators have a special autothreshold procedure. One such is named "Vario." In this test process a pulse duration and voltage are set. Application of a magnet to the generator begins a progressive reduction of output voltage by $\frac{1}{16}$ output steps. Removal of the magnet immediately restores the output to its full voltage setting. Threshold voltage is readily determined at a specific pulse duration. If this technique is available, select the shortest pulse duration and the 5.0 V setting. If the voltage threshold determined during the Vario process is less than half that voltage setting, leave output at 5.0 V. If not, increase the pulse duration until the voltage threshold is half or less than the 5.0 V setting. If such a setting cannot be found, a judgment will have to be made, but if possible, maintain output voltage at 5.0 V (Figure 26).

4. Multiple Voltage—Multiple Pulse Durations

The present generation of CMOS circuits allows very small steps in output voltage, i.e., 0.1 V, and smaller steps in pulse duration, 0.01 ms. Multiple voltage outputs are progressively more common in modern pulse generators. These steps are too fine to have any practical benefit in setting output. Determining threshold, using all of this capability, can become excessively burdensome. It's probably wisest to treat such an excess of pulse duration and voltage steps as if they represented three voltage steps, i.e., 2.5, 5.0, and 7.5–10.0, and no more than 20 pulse duration steps.

Output voltage of less than 2.5 V will not represent significant benefit in reduction of battery drain and so should be used for special purposes only, such as the elimination of stimulation of extracardiac tissue or local pectoral muscles. Probably situations will be found in which such low voltages will be useful.

ENERGY SOURCES

Many different energy sources have been used to power cardiac pacemakers. The energy to stimulate the heart under optimal and even usual circumstances is small, approximately 3 μJ, though several times that amount is required for consistent, long-term stimulation.

```
EVALUATED ENERGY SOURCES

1. Biogalvanic;                      7. Rechargeable   nickel-cadmium
2. Piezo-electric energy;               cells;
3. Photoelectric cells with transcu-  8. Mercury-zinc cells;
   taneous light;                     9. Carbon-zinc cells;
4. Energy of glucose oxidation;      10. Nuclear converters;
5. Skeletal muscle contraction;      11. Cells with a lithium anode and a
6. Fuel cells;                           variety of different cathodes.
```

Nuclear pacemakers powered by plutonium and promethium have been implanted. All promethium pacemakers have been removed, and none are now being implanted. The longevity of promethium pacemakers was no more than that of middle longevity lithium pulse generators because the half-life of promethium is 2.7 years. Very few (if any) plutonium pacemakers continue to be implanted, none have been recently manufactured, and all are the technology of the 1970s. The longevity expectation of these units was 20–40 years, and longevity experience is 82% cumulative survival 16 years after implantation. None of the developments of the past decade in cardiac pacing is available in nuclear units. Associated malignancy has not been reported. About 3000 units have been implanted worldwide and many remain functioning.

Lithium cells power all new, nonnuclear pacemakers now implanted. Five different lithium chemistries had reached commercial availability and four already are obsolete, although some pacemakers with obsolete cells (in practice only the LiCuS) still remain in service. A variety of battery sizes and capacities and therefore potential longevities exist for the remaining lithium power source (LiI) chemistry. The user should carefully evaluate patient needs and the selection of the appropriate power source and battery capacity (Table IV). Knowledge of the depletion characteristics of each of the cell types is important in under-

Table IV

Chemistry	Nominal Capacity Ah	Voltage	Estimated Longevity (Years)	Problems
LiI	0.8–3.5	2.8	4–15	1. Variable capacity
LiAgCr (Obsolete)	0.6	3.4	3–4	1. Small capacity 2. Short longevity at high drain
LiCuS (Obsolete)	0.9–1.8	2.1	4–12	1. Nonhermetic
LiPb (Obsolete)	0.9	1.9 (5.7 as manufactured)	2–3	1. Small capacity
LiSOCl (Obsolete)	0.75–1.5	3.6	3–6	1. Rapid depletion @ EOL
NiCd (Obsolete)	0.19	1.3	10(?)–20(?) Recharge monthly	1. Small capacity 2. Monthly recharge 3. Voltage & rate instability 4. Rapid self-discharge
HgZnO (Obsolete)	1.0	1.35	3–5	1. Large volume/ weight 2. High self-discharge 3. Wide scatter of failures—Early/Late

standing the management of the pulse generators they power. For example, the mercury-zinc cell maintained its output voltage until virtually complete depletion occurred. Then the battery voltage fell rapidly, within several days to 1 week, from the stable normal 1.35 V to zero. Monitoring such pacemakers required weekly observations. They are, of course, obsolete. The lithium cupric sulfide cell, no longer used in new pacemakers, but with units still in service behaves similarly, holding the output voltage until it is largely depleted when there is rapid voltage decline and pulse generator end-of-life.

The lithium iodine cell now powers all newly introduced pulse generators. It's depletion characteristic is by slow increase in internal cell impedance as the chemical reaction occurs which produces electricity. The output voltage of a fresh cell (BOL or beginning-of-life) is 2.8 V and the internal resistance is 10,000 ohms. At end-of-life (EOL), the output voltage is 1.8 V and the internal resistance is some 40,000 ohms. At this time the cell may not have either sufficient output voltage or current delivery capacity to operate the pulse generator electronics properly or to deliver its rated output to the lead. Those pacemakers that can telemeter battery voltage and cell resistance indicate the state of the cell and can give an estimate of the remaining longevity of the device. The elective replacement interval (ERI) occurs when the cell is substantially depleted, its voltage is 2.0–2.2 V, and the impedance is 20,000 to 30,000 ohms. The pulse generator cell which has reached the elective replacement interval should be replaced (Figure 27).

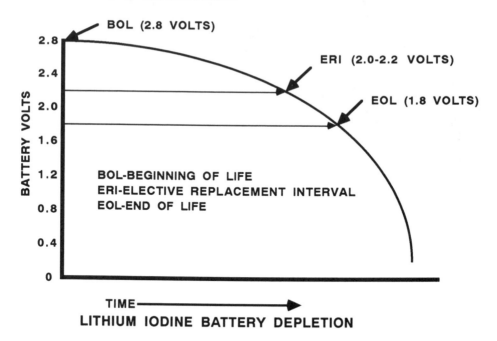

Figure 27. The output voltage of a fresh lithium iodine cell is 2.8 V. As electricity is generated the internal impedance progressively increases and when it reaches about 40,000 ohms the end of its useful life has occurred. The elective replacement interval (ERI) is reached when the output voltage is 2.2 V. The end of life (EOL) is reached at 1.8 V. The unit powered by such a battery should be replaced at that time.

PULSE GENERATOR LONGEVITY

Pacemaker longevity after implantation depends on many factors. Certainly it depends on the battery drain required to operate the electronic circuit; the drain required for the programmed output and the continuous drain from the battery, the component which establishes the entity known as "shelf-life". All three factors have been improved. "Shelf-life" improvement and efficient circuit operation have been progressively accomplished and have been discussed earlier. Pulse generator output needed to achieve cardiac capture has also been reduced over the three decades since implanted stimulation was first used (Figure 28).

The electrodes used in 1960 required a pulse generator output of 675 µJ and longevity was about 6 months. Output required in 1992 for consistent stimulation is 3–6 µJ and the longevity of the implantable pulse generators has increased correspondingly. Even during the mercury battery era it was known that a small surface area, high impedance electrode, would reduce the current required for stimulation and increase the effective longevity of a pulse generator. At least one manufacturer of pulse generators and leads achieved the de facto programmable reduction in output during pulse generator replacement following battery depletion by inserting a resistor in series between the lead and a

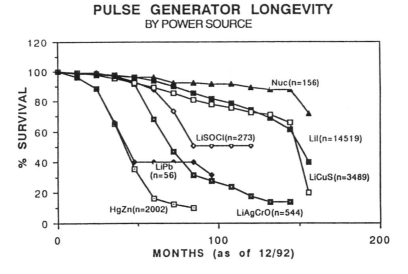

Figure 28. *The overall longevity of pulse generators with various power sources used for implantable cardiac pacemakers is given for mercury batteries, nuclear converters, and the five different lithium batteries that have been used in devices implanted in humans. Each power source has a characteristic longevity even if used in different pulse generator designs. The longest duration source was the nuclear with a cumulative survival of 72% 217 months after implantation. The briefest was mercury-zinc, no longer in use, with a 0% cumulative survival 100 months after implant and 50% survival after 36 months.*

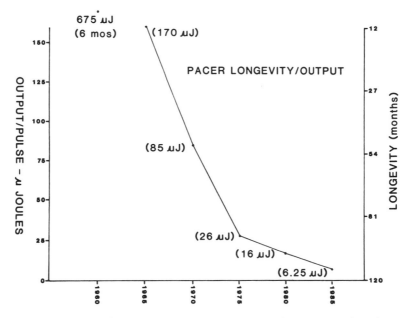

Figure 29. *The longevity of implantable pacemakers is inversely proportional to the continuous battery drain. In this diagram the continuous battery drain is listed on the left vertical axis, the longevity is on the right vertical axis. The actual battery drain from a "typical" pulse generator of year of its manufacture (horizontal axis) is a function of decrease in output. A modern, programmable output pulse generator, drained at a 1960 level would last as long.*

constant voltage pulse generator. The higher resistance reduced pulse generator current output (Ohm's law). As current output determines battery drain, increased longevity occurred.

As stimulation threshold is directly related to electrode size, the progressive reduction in cathodal size and increase in stimulation efficiency through the introduction of porous and steroid electrodes have been as important in increasing pulse generator longevity as improvements in battery and electronic technology. In the case of steroid and porous electrodes the reduction in current threshold has been achieved simultaneously with a reduction of electrode impedance. Consequently, the same current can stimulate tissue but at a lower voltage. (High impedance steroid electrodes are now in clinical evaluation.) This has allowed lower voltage pacemakers, operating at the battery voltage (2.5–2.8 V) rather than at a higher voltage requiring a transformer. As voltage transformation is less than 100% efficient, some decrease in pulse generator longevity occurred (Figure 29).

CALCULATION OF PULSE GENERATOR LONGEVITY

The functional longevity of an implantable pulse generator depends on a number of factors, which are discussed in the following paragraphs.

1. Capacity of the Battery in the Implanted Generator

Until almost the end of the mercury-zinc era only one battery capacity was available, i.e., each mercury cell had a capacity of 1 ampere hour. As the cells (six, five, and later four) were in series, the output voltage was additive but the overall charge capacity was not. A 3-ampere hour mercury zinc cell was used in one generator and had a prolonged longevity, but the manufacturer nevertheless stopped its manufacture. During the lithium era batteries of different chemistry have different capacities, and batteries of the same chemistry are constructed in different sizes. For example, lithium iodine batteries used in commercial pulse generators are of 0.8- to 3.0-ampere hour capacity.

The useful battery longevity as used is always less than the nominal capacity. As its capacity is consumed the battery voltage falls, and at some point the output voltage and current delivering capacity is insufficient to deliver the rated pacemaker output or to operate the pacemaker circuit. The useful battery capacity as opposed to its total capacity then becomes the capacity available to operate the pacemaker at settings consistent with normal function.

2. Battery Self-discharge

The mercury cell had a very high self-discharge, approximating 10% of useful capacity per year, so that efficient operation of the pacemaker circuit and reduction of output could produce only a limited benefit in prolongation of pulse generator longevity. Lithium batteries have a self-discharge of less than 1% per year so that efficiency of pulse generator design and operation can be translated into increased longevity.

3. Output Impedance

For a constant voltage pulse generator the impedance of the lead-electrode system influences pacemaker output. Within the limits of conventional lead impedance, lower impedance increases output and battery drain while a higher impedance lead decreases drain. In limiting instances, a lead fracture with cessation of output preserves pulse generator longevity; lead insulation defect or conductor short circuit accelerates battery depletion. An impedance of 510 ohms is used as the standard during calculation of output impedance and battery drain.

4. Circuit Efficiency

Discrete component circuits were inefficient in operation, and a great deal of battery drain was consumed in operation of the sensing and pulse forming circuits. Complementary metal oxide semiconductor (CMOS) circuits are far more efficient and even far more complex circuits than those previously available and operate at far lower battery drain. Single channel sensing pacemakers drain far less than dual channel and triple channel, which will soon be available.

5. Percent Operation

The drain to operate the pulse generator sensing circuit is small as such circuits are efficient. The output circuit consumes much larger energies in stimulating the heart, especially at higher outputs. A pacing system that senses almost continuously will have a far greater longevity than one that paces continuously. In general, calculations of projected longevity consider stimulation 50% of the time. Wide variations in longevity can be anticipated based on the actual proportion of pacing.

6. Output Programming

The most important longevity consideration during normal pulse generator operation is the output programmed for the pulse generator. Many modern single-chamber pulse generators may be programmed from 5–200 μJ. The longevity of the generator will be directly related to the output selected. Dual-chamber pulse generators and those in which the stimulation rate changes with atrial rate or with sensor input drain the power source more than single-chamber, single rate devices. An increase in stimulation rate increases the rate at which a higher output is delivered. Increase in output voltage has a major effect on charge output. Doubling output voltage doubles the charge and the drain from the power source.

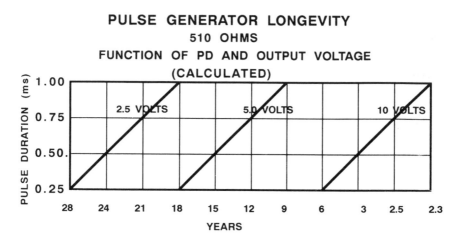

Figure 30. *The effect of programming on pulse generator longevity is shown in this calculation of estimated longevity of model 155 as a function of output voltage and pulse duration programming. At 2.5 V and 0.25 ms pulse duration the estimated longevity with a 510-ohm load is 28 years. At 10 V and 1.0 ms output the calculated longevity is 2.3 years.*

The effect of programming output is quite significant. A single model with four pulse durations (0.25, 0.50, 0.75, and 1.0 ms) and three output voltage settings (2.5, 5.0, and 10.0 V) can, at a stimulation rate of 70 bpm, have an estimated longevity through a standard 510-ohm load of 23 years at the least output (0.25 ms at 2.5 V) to 2.3 years at the greatest output (1.0 ms at 10 V). Increasing or decreasing the stimulation rate will also affect the current drain (Figure 30).

7. Continuous Battery Drain

Considering all of the enumerated factors a continuous battery drain is calculated and used in a formula to calculate pulse generator longevity. Obviously it is subject to significant variation from the calculation.

The formula for the longevity of a pulse generator is therefore:

$$\text{Longevity}_{PG} = \frac{\text{Useful battery capacity}}{\text{Continuous battery drain}}$$

Continuous battery drain = Self-discharge + continuous drain for sensing + continuous drain for circuit operation + drain for stimulation (converted to a continuous output number) + miscellaneous additional drain

$$\text{Longevity}_{PG} \ (\text{Years}) = \frac{\text{Useful battery capacity (Ah)}}{(\text{Continuous drain}) \ (24^*) \ (365^{**})}$$

* hours per day
** days per year

While accurate calculation of the longevity of a specific pacemaker unit depends on the factors listed and possibly others, most implanted units are set at nominal rates and outputs, and with nominal impedance leads so that, from a practical point of view, longevities fall within a relatively narrow range and projections can be given that will be broadly accurate.

ATRIOVENTRICULAR AND VENTRICULOATRIAL CONDUCTION

Pacemakers are implanted because of failure of atrioventricular conduction, impulse formation, or both. The interval from the sensed or paced atrial event to the ventricular event is an important consideration in dual-chamber pacing. The appearance of the intrinsic deflections of the atrium and ventricle is different for each different atrial or ventricular focus, and the timing of the various events depends on the site at which they are sensed in the atrium and ventricle and the site of origin of the atrial or ventricular depolarization. For example, the setting of an AV interval of 150 ms from pacing the right atrial appendage to pacing or sensing the right ventricular apex will produce timing consequences quite different from pacing the left atrial appendage and sensing or pacing the right ventricular apex. The description of AV conduction and VA conduction timing cycles are all based on the conventional implant sites of right atrial appendage and right ventricular apex. Were the implant sites different, the timing measurements would be different. None of the timing cycles will mimic closely the normal PR interval which is not measured from intracardiac events but from the surface. The PR interval is, of course, the time from the earliest appearance of the P wave to the earliest appearance of the QRS complex in any ECG lead.

The PR Interval

The AV interval is the time that allows ventricular filling following atrial contraction. In the dual-chamber pacemaker the AV interval starts with a stimulus to the atrium from the pacemaker atrial channel or from sensing of the atrial intrinsic deflection. The intrinsic deflection begins at the SA node so that its earliest appearance is there. Atrial sensing usually occurs via a lead in the right atrial appendage which means that by the time the atrial depolarization is sensed the atrial contraction will have begun. If sensing is from the left atrium the atrial contraction (at least of the right atrium) will be even further advanced when the intrinsic deflection is sensed.

There are four possible AV intervals depending on different circumstances of atrial and ventricular sensing and pacing (Figure 31).

Should AV conduction exist, programming the implanted dual-chamber pacemaker will allow selection of any one of these possibilities. Each change will have a different physiology to some degree. The physiological effect of changing the PR interval is not yet entirely understood though it is being investigated intensively. Nevertheless, the duration of the PR interval is under physician control by programming the AV interval and the physician should

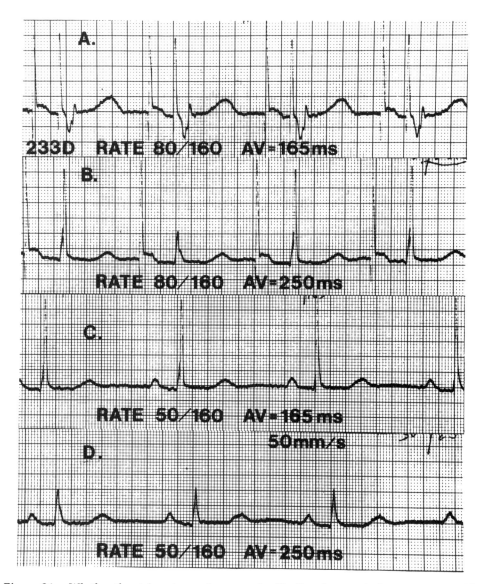

Figure 31. *Whether the atrium is paced or sensed will affect the ventricular response.* **A.** *The atrium is continually paced and at an AV interval of 165 ms the ventricle is paced as well. Not enough time has elapsed for the ventricle to depolarize via AV conduction.* **B.** *The atrium is continually paced but at an AV interval of 250 ms the QRS complexes are conducted. Still, the intrinsic deflection of the QRS complex is sufficiently late so that fusion beats occur.* **C.** *By slowing the pacing rate the intrinsic deflection of the atrial depolarization is sensed and at 165 ms AV interval spontaneous AV conduction occurs, pseudo fusion ventricular beats occur.* **D.** *At 250 ms AV interval, begun by atrial sensing, both atrial and ventricular stimuli are inhibited as the ventricular intrinsic deflection falls within the AV interval.*

comprehend the changes that can be made and the possible physiological consequences of AV interval programming. (See Sensing and Timing The Cardiac Electrogram, Chapter 3.)

AV INTERVALS

1. The sensed atrium to the sensed ventricle; in this instance the best AVI calculation will be from the intrinsic deflection of the atrium to the intrinsic deflection of the ventricle;

2. The sensed atrium to the paced ventricle; i.e., from the intrinsic deflection of the spontaneous P wave to the ventricular channel stimulus;

3. From the paced atrium to the sensed ventricle. In this instance timing starts with the atrial stimulus and the P wave occurs entirely within the AV interval and to obtain a conducted QRS a prolonged AV interval may be required;

4. From the paced atrium to the paced ventricle; the timing cycle starts with the atrial stimulus and ends with the ventricular stimulus. The atrial contraction is wholly within the AV interval and the effective filling time will be short.

Antegrade Conduction

Those implanted for sinus node dysfunction often have normal or moderately impaired AV conduction. About half of patients implanted for sinus node dysfunction have prolonged AV conduction defined as an interval of greater than 450 ms from the ID_A to the ID_V or the presence of Wenckebach conduction or AV block with atrial pacing below 120 bpm. The prolonged interval, i.e., 450 ms was selected because of the normally greater duration of ID_A ID_V from the right atrial appendage to the right ventricular apex than the PR interval. It is, of course, only the $ID_A \rightarrow ID_V$ that is sensed by the pacemaker. The interval from the two spontaneous depolarizations is 40–60 ms shorter than the interval from a stimulus to the right atrial appendage to the conducted ventricular ID at similar rates. The depolarization latency is added to the AV interval during any conduction process following atrial stimulation. Because of this variation of AV interval caused by sensing or pacing the atrium some pulse generators allow different AV intervals when pacing or sensing the atrium, longer when pacing, shorter when sensing (Figure 32).

Because of the time difference between the paced atrium and the sensed atrium, the AV interval will be of different duration depending on whether the atrium has been paced or sensed. As the AV interval begins with the atrial stimulus or sensing the atrial intrinsic deflection, the difference in duration of the AV interval can be as much as 40–60 ms. Consequently, the programmed AV interval will be shorter or longer depending on whether the timing cycles are started by atrial pacing or sensing. Thus a physiological hysteresis of the PR interval will exist unless the pacemaker responds with a longer interval when the cycle is started by a stimulus and a shorter interval when it is started by a

AV DELAY AND PR INTERVAL

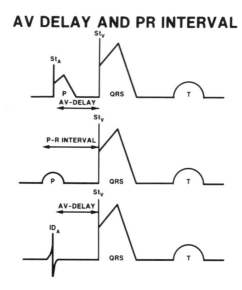

Figure 32. *The AV interval starts at the atrial stimulus or sensing of the atrial intrinsic deflection.* **Above.** *The AV interval contains the entire P wave and a briefer interval from the end of the P wave to the ventricular stimulus.* **Below.** *The P wave has begun spontaneously and the sensed intrinsic deflection begins the AV interval providing a longer time from the beginning of atrial contraction to the ventricular stimulus.* **Middle.** *Represents a spontaneous P wave.*

sensed event. Thus, either there will be hysteresis of the electronic AV interval or there will be a hysteresis of the physiological PR interval. Many modern dual-chamber pulse generators now allow a programmable option of different AV intervals depending on whether the atrium is sensed (shorter interval) or paced (longer interval). This capability eliminates the hysteresis described earlier. In addition, some dual-chamber generators also decrease the AV interval at more rapid paced (sensor driven) or sensed rates in order to mimic the natural condition.

Retrograde (VA) Conduction

While the existence of retrograde conduction has been recognized since 1913, its effect on the implanted dual-chamber pacemaker was unexpected at the time of introduction of the first pacemakers able to sense in the atrium and the ventricle. Measurement of antegrade and retrograde conduction during pacemaker implant has demonstrated that 45% of patients who require pacemaker implantation, for any indication—ventricular or supraventricular tachycardia, sinus node dysfunction, or AV block—have retrograde conduction at some paced rate if paced from the ventricle. If paced in the AV sequential mode by testing with extrastimuli, the incidence is even higher. Sixty-seven percent of patients paced for sinus node dysfunction have retrograde conduction, and 14% of those with fixed complete antegrade heart block have retrograde conduction. Even patients who have had AV block for many years may retain retrograde conduction. The mean retrograde conduction time from the ventricular

Table V

Primary Diagnosis	Total No. Pts.	1:1 VA Conduction Pts.	1:1 VA Conduction %	VA Conduction Time at Lowest Rate
Sick sinus syndrome	6	4	67	222
Sinus brady/arrest	16	11	69	214
Incomplete AV block	14	5	36	293
Complete AV block	16	4	25	210
Ventricular tachycardia	1	1	100	NA
TOTAL	53	25	47	235 ms

stimulus to the atrial intrinsic deflection (ID_A is 235 ± 50 ms and the range is 110 ms to 450 ms (Table V).

The presence of retrograde (VA) conduction and the status of antegrade (AV) conduction is determined during pacemaker implantation. With the definitive pacemaker leads in place, the interval of the passive $ID_A \rightarrow ID_V$ is measured. If AV conduction exists, a clearly defined number will be found, if AV block exists, this will be apparent. The atrium is paced and the interval from the atrial pacemaker stimulus (St_A) to the ventricular (ID_V) response is evaluated at a number of paced rates, i.e., 80, 100, 120, 140, and 160 bpm. The rate for the onset of AV block is ascertained (Figures 33 and 34).

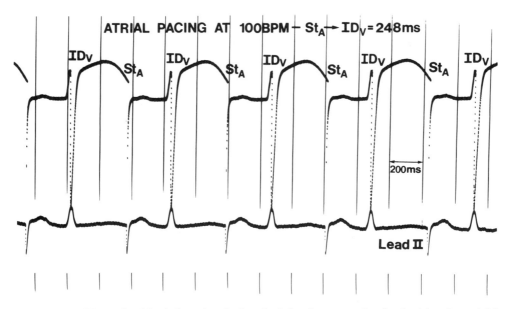

Figure 33. *Electrophysiological testing during dual-chamber pacemaker implant involves atrial pacing to determine the stability of AV conduction. The atrial lead is used for stimulation while the ventricular response is recorded. The interval from atrial stimulus to ventricular response can be measured readily at each paced rate. Here at a coupling interval of 600 ms (100 bpm) the conduction interval is 248 ms.*

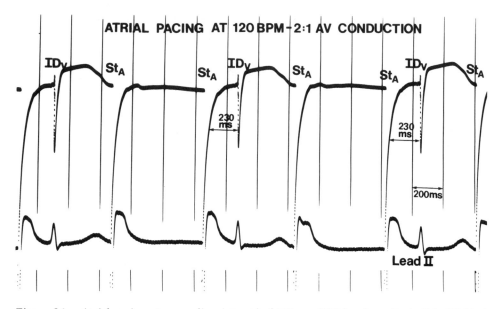

Figure 34. *Atrial pacing at a coupling interval of 500 ms (120 bpm) results in 2:1 AV block. The consistent atrial capture and 2:1 response are clearly apparent.*

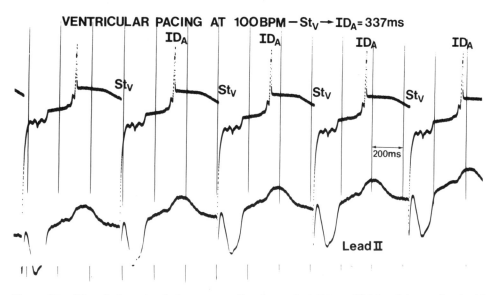

Figure 35. *Ventricular stimulation at a coupling interval of 600 ms (120 bpm) is associated with consistent retrograde conduction at an interval of 337 ms. The measurement is from the ventricular stimulus to the intrinsic deflection of the retrograde P wave.*

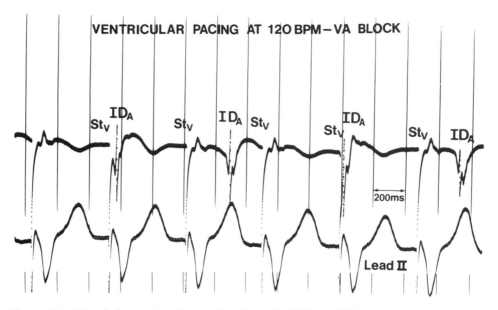

Figure 36. *Ventricular pacing at a coupling interval of 500 ms (120 bpm) results in complete retrograde block. Here the atrial intrinsic deflections are completely dissociated from the paced QRS complexes.*

The ventricle is then paced (St$_V$) at the same rates (above), the retrograde P wave recorded from the atrial channel, and retrograde conduction intervals determined (Figures 35 and 36). Measurement of antegrade and retrograde conduction intervals allows evaluation of the state of AV and VA conduction as supporting evidence for pacemaker implantation and to allow the setting of the atrial refractory interval after the ventricular event to avoid retrograde conduction and the onset of the endless loop tachycardia.

Pacemaker-Mediated Tachycardia

Pacemaker-mediated tachycardias (PMT) require the presence of a dual-chamber pacemaker in order to exist. If the dual-chamber pacemaker did not exist or if atrial sensing were suddenly lost, the tachycardia would cease. PMTs result from ventricular stimulation as a result of triggering via the atrial channel. Sensor-mediated pacemaker tachycardias have also been recognized and are described in Chapter 11 (Rate Modulated Pacing). There are several pacemaker-mediated tachycardias, caused by different events and not requiring similar management. The sensing of atrial fibrillation or flutter will increase the rate of ventricular stimulation and result in a PMT (Figure 37). Sensing of electromagnetic or electromyographic interference can trigger the ventricular channel and produce PMT. Possibly the most common cause of pacemaker-mediated tachycardia is the sensing of retrograde P waves. This event is properly termed an endless loop tachycardia (ELT).

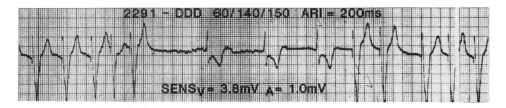

Figure 37. *An example of both pacemaker-mediated tachycardia and electromyographic interference (EMI). A patient with a dual-chamber unipolar pacemaker developed atrial fibrillation, which caused irregular ventricular stimulation, occasionally at the upper rate limit coupling interval, i.e., 150 bpm. With arm movement, EMI also occurred (center) that briefly inhibited ventricular output. With cessation of arm movement the pacemaker-mediated tachycardia resumed. (Pulse generator model = 2291, mode DDD, lower rate limit = 60 bpm, AVI = 140 ms, upper rate limit = 150 bpm, atrial refractory interval = 200 ms, ventricular channel sensitivity = 3.8 mV and atrial channel sensitivity = 1.0 mV.*

Endless Loop Tachycardia

The existence of retrograde conduction via the natural pathway and antegrade conduction via the implanted dual-chamber pacemaker provides a reentry circuit which mimics the natural situation in which an accessory pathway allows a circuit movement tachycardia. This reentry tachycardia has been variously called **"pacemaker reentry tachycardia," "pacemaker circus movement tachycardia," "pacemaker-mediated tachycardia,"** and **endless loop tachycardia."** The basis of the tachycardia is the ability of the atrial channel to sense a P wave displaced from its natural position before the QRS complex. The P wave can be displaced by a ventricular premature contraction with retrograde conduction, an atrial premature contraction, a ventricular pacemaker channel escape following an ineffective atrial stimulus, a ventricular escape in an atrial synchronous pacemaker, or atrial channel triggering by electromagnetic or electromyographic interference.

Once displacement of the P wave has occurred, the atrial refractory interval (ARI) after the ventricular event must be sufficiently short so that the retrograde P wave falls after the ARI ends. Endless loop tachycardia cannot exist in any pacemaker without atrial sensing. Endless loop tachycardia was described on a theoretic basis for the original atrial synchronous (VAT) pacemaker, and cases apparently occurred but may not have been recorded in the medical literature. As most of the VAT pacemakers were limited in upper rate to 100, 105, or 120 bpm with an AV interval of 165 ms, the atrial refractory interval after the ventricular event was 435, 406, or 335 ms, ample in the vast majority of patients with the only rhythm then paced, complete heart block, to avoid the reentry mechanism. With the need to increase the allowed upper rate, the atrial refractory interval was correspondingly abbreviated and the possibility increased that a retrograde P wave would occur beyond the refractory interval.

Should the P wave be displaced but fall within the atrial refractory interval, it will be unsensed and no further event will occur. (Some models allow it to be sensed but not used to start a timing cycle.) If the P wave falls into the sensitive portion of the pacemaker cycle it will be sensed and begin an AV interval. As

AV conduction will be via the pacemaker the, ventricular stimulus may occur when natural VA conduction does not exist. There will then be no retrograde P wave to continue the cycle and endless loop tachycardia will die out. If retrograde conduction persists another P wave will occur and the reentry loop will be sustained. The existence of a short AV interval tends to continue VA refractoriness and a long interval to allow VA conduction recovery. Thus if a psuedo-Wenckebach mechanism is programmed with a low upper rate limit the consequent prolongation of the AV interval allows recovery of VA conduction and maintenance of the endless loop tachycardia. The circus movement or loop occurs by ventricular escape with retrograde conduction which produces a P wave sensed by the pacemaker atrial channel which, in turn, causes a ventricular channel stimulus followed by a retrograde P wave and so forth (Figure 38). The

---

MECHANISMS FOR TERMINATION OF AN ENDLESS LOOP TACHYCARDIA

1. Programming the ARI beyond the measured retrograde conduction time;
2. Automatic extension of the ARI after a VPC (the most common cause of a displaced P wave). This does not deal with any of the other onset mechanisms of ELT;
3. Atrial insensitivity for a single event if the pacemaker operates at its upper rate limit for a specific number of paced ventricular events, 16 in one algorithm (Figure 39);
4. Atrial insensitivity for more than one atrial event such as the DVI mode followed by a full atrial refractory interval before the restoration of normal atrial sensing. This brief operation in the DVI mode may allow competition with an unsensed P wave, followed by a ventricular stimulus, a retrograde P wave and the resumption of the tachycardia;
5. Atrial insensitivity for many events, that is the resumption of the ventricular inhibited (VVI) mode which then returns to a preselected rate (fallback) with resumption then of atrial sensing (Figure 40).
6. It has been gradually recognized that antegrade and retrograde P waves have different electrical characteristics in morphology, amplitude and slew rate. Given sufficiently sophisticated analysis of all three parameters, about 95% of antegrade and retrograde P waves can be distinguished. Considering amplitude distinction only, almost 90% of antegrade P waves can be distinguished from the retrograde mate. Several pacemaker models have many atrial sensitivity levels, one has more than 20 settings, another has ten levels at each of two different frequency settings. Almost all antegrade P waves are larger than the retrograde mate. It is, therefore, possible to select a sensitivity level in which an antegrade P wave will drive the ventricle while the retrograde P wave will be too small to be sensed and cause endless loop tachycardia. Selective atrial sensing is possible and, when accomplished, very useful.

ALL MECHANISMS OF MANAGING ENDLESS LOOP TACHYCARDIA ARE BASED ON ONE OF THESE MECHANISMS, ALL OF WHICH INVOLVE LOSS OF ATRIAL SENSITIVITY IN ONE OF A VARIETY OF FORMATS (Figure 41.)

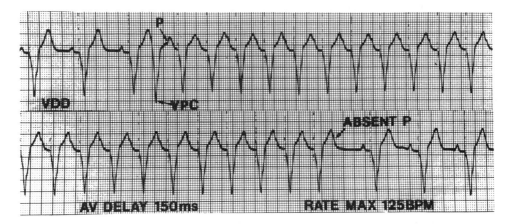

Figure 38. *Endless loop tachycardia is started by a VPC that displaces a P wave and is then sustained by sensing the retrograde P at a prolonged AV interval. After progressive prolongation of the VA interval, indicative of fatigue of the retrograde conduction pathway, a P wave is not conducted and the tachycardia is terminated.*

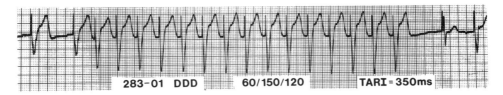

Figure 39. *This algorithm for termination of an endless loop tachycardia causes a loss of atrial sensing for a single event after 16 ventricular channel stimuli at the upper rate limit.*

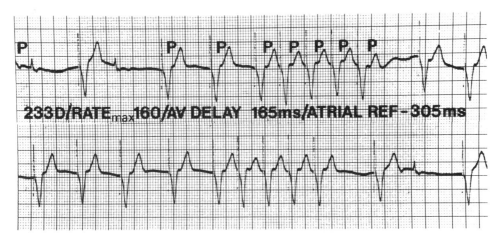

Figure 40. *The fallback response to endless loop tachycardia involves return to VVI pacing at a lower rate when the upper rate limit is reached. In this ECG the lower rate is 80 bpm, sufficiently rapid to entrain the atrium so that when atrial sensing is automatically restored the endless loop tachycardia is immediately resumed.*

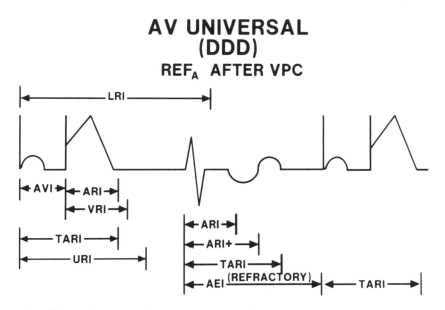

Figure 41. *The various pacemaker responses to terminate endless loop tachycardia all involve atrial insensitivity following a VPC. Several are diagramed. ARI involves the setting of atrial refractoriness adequate to have a retrograde P wave fall within. ARI+ is the production of a prolonged ARI for a single beat started by a VPC (defined as a sensed ventricular event not preceded by a sensed or paced atrial event). TARI is the establishment of a still more prolonged atrial refractory interval, now including the duration of the programmed AV interval after a VPC. AEI is the start of an atrial escape interval followed by an atrial insensitive stimulus and a total atrial refractory interval. All means of preventing or terminating an endless loop tachycardia involve atrial refractoriness at the time of a retrograde or dissociated P wave.*

cycle continues until:

1. retrograde conduction is lost;
2. the atrial refractory interval (ARI) is extended beyond the retrograde conduction time;
3. the atrial channel becomes refractory for a single atrial event;
4. the atrial channel becomes refractory for more than a single atrial event.

ANTEGRADE AND RETROGRADE ENDLESS LOOP TACHYCARDIAS

As an endless loop tachycardia is commonly begun by a premature ventricular beat with a retrograde P wave, one method evaluated for its prevention is the emission of an atrial channel stimulus synchronously with the sensed ventricular beat. This stimulus is intended to depolarize the atrium and cause its contraction during the atrial refractory period begun by the sensed ventricular event. The atrium will then be refractory to activation via the retrograde conduction mechanism. Several dual-chamber pulse generators have this mode as a programmable option. However, if a patient has **sustained antegrade con-**

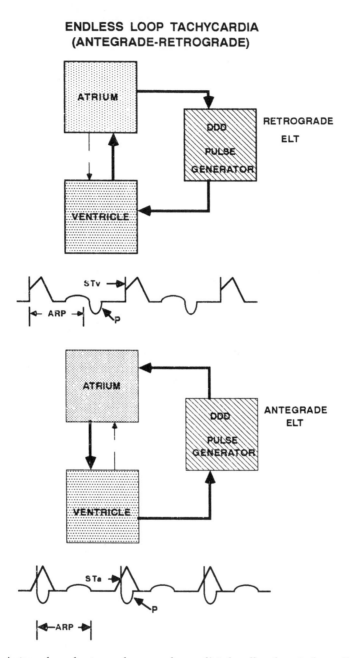

Figure 42. *Antegrade and retrograde pacemaker-mediated endless loop tachycardias are shown. The conventional tachycardia is above and dependent on retrograde conduction with the P wave falling after the end of atrial refractoriness. The unusual antegrade tachycardia depends on the existence of antegrade conduction and absent retrograde conduction with the atrium being activated by the atrial stimulating mechanism of the pacemaker response to an ectopic ventricular beat. The tachycardia is sustained as the paced atrial event is conducted to the ventricle, but the resultant ventricular beat is considered ectopic as it is not preceded by a normally timed or sensed atrial event.*

duction (for example, in the presence of sinus bradycardia) but **absent retrograde conduction**, then atrial stimulation depends not on a normal retrograde pathway but on pacemaker-mediated stimulation of the atrium. The next ventricular stimulus will be in response to the atrial paced event, and each ventricular event will be categorized by the pacemaker as ectopic so that an atrial stimulus will follow (as the endless loop avoidance mechanism) and maintain the tachycardia loop. In contradistinction to the usual endless loop tachycardia, which can be called a **retrograde tachycardia** as it is based on retrograde conduction, this endless loop tachycardia is an **antegrade tachycardia** (von Knorre and colleagues) (Figure 42).

AV DESYNCHRONIZATION ARRHYTHMIA

Another dual-chamber arrhythmia recently described has been called the AV desynchronization arrhythmia (AVDA) by Barold. It is, in some ways, an analog of the endless loop tachycardia as it depends also on the presence of retrograde, i.e., ventriculoatrial conduction for its mechanism. The arrhythmia occurs when a ventricular stimulus produces a ventricular contraction and a consequent retrograde P wave. If this P wave falls into an interval of atrial refractoriness it will be unsensed. Should the dual-chamber pacemaker be atrially refractory because of magnet placement or because of the DVI mode, the event will be continuous. In either mode the absence of atrial sensing will cause the emission of an atrial stimulus preceding the effective ventricular stimulus. If the VA conduction time is prolonged, then the atrial stimulus will fall early and ineffectively after the retrograde atrial depolarization during refractoriness of the atrial myocardium. Should this combination of events occur, the P wave cannot be replaced into its physiological position. When atrial refractoriness ends, e.g., when the magnet is removed, the retrograde P wave persists and an endless loop tachycardia may start, usually at a more rapid rate. Such an endless loop will not end with magnet application as the AVDA will recur with magnet application as will the endless loop when the magnet is removed. Termination of the endless loop will be by programming of the mode to single-chamber operation. The AVDA is encouraged by the presence of prolonged retrograde conduction; a relatively short lower rate limit interval (rapid lower rate) and prolonged AV interval so that the atrial escape (i.e., ventricular stimulus to atrial stimulus) interval is also brief. The AVDA can be induced by any technique that loses atrial capture in the presence of sustained retrograde conduction, including a stimulus below capture threshold.

BIBLIOGRAPHY

Albert H, Glass B, Pittman B, et al: Cardiac stimulation threshold: Chronic study. Ann NY Acad Sci 1964; 3:889–892.
Amundson DC, McArthur W, Mosharrafa M: The porous endocardial electrode. PACE 1979; 2:40–50.

Anderson N, Mathivarnar R, Skasky M, et al: Activee: fixation leads—long term threshold reduction using a drug-infused ceramic collar. PACE 1991; 14:639 (abstract).

Ausubel K, Klementowicz P, Furman S: Interatrial conduction during cardiac pacing. PACE 1986; 9:1026–1031.

Barold SS, Ong LS, Heinle RA: Stimulation and sensing thresholds for cardiac pacing: Electrophysiologic and technical aspects. Progr Cardiovasc Dis 1981; 24:1–24.

Barold SS, Roehrich DR, Falkoff MD, et al: Sources of error in the determination of output voltage of pulse generators by pacemaker system analyzers. PACE 1980; 3:585–596.

Barold SS, Winner JA: Techniques and significance of threshold measurement for cardiac pacing. Relationship to output circuit of cardiac pacemakers. Chest 1976; 70:760–766.

Basu D, Chatterjee K: Unusually high pacemaker threshold in severe myxedema, decrease with thyroid hormone therapy. Chest 1976; 70:677–679.

Bink-Boelkens M, Ross B, Gillette P, et al: The incidence of retrograde conduction in children. PACE 1984; 7:618–621.

Bisping HJ, Kreuser J, Birkenheier H: Three year clinical experience with a new endocardial screw-in lead with introduction protection for use in the atrium and ventricle. PACE 1980; 3:424–435.

Bluhm G, Larsen FF, Nordlander R, et al: Long-term comparison of the electrical characteristics of polyurethane and polyethylene insulated ventricular leads. PACE 1990; 13:583–587.

Brandt J, Attewell R, Fahraeus T, et al: Atrial and ventricular stimulation threshold development: A comparative study in patients with a DDD pacemaker and two identical cargon-tip leads. PACE 1990; 13:859–866.

Breivik K, Ohm OJ, Engedal H: Acute and chronic pulse-width thresholds in solid versus porous tip electrodes. PACE 1982; 5:650–657.

Breivik K, Ohm OJ, Engedal H: Long term comparison of unipolar and bipolar pacing and sensing, using a new multiprogrammable pacemaker system. PACE 1983; 6:592–600.

Brewer G, Mathivanar R, Skalsky M, et al: Composite electrode tips containing externally placed drug releasing collars. PACE 1988; 11:1760–1769.

Burgess MJ, Grossman M, Abildskov JA: Fibrillation threshold of a patient with myocardial infarction treated with a fixed-rate pacemaker: Case report. Am Heart J 1970; 80:112–115.

Castellanos A, Lemberg L: Pacemaker arrhythmias and electrocardiographic recognition of pacemakers. Circulation 1973; 42:1381–1391.

Conti J, Curtis A: Atrial fixation leads a visual aid confirming actual fixation. PACE 1992; 15:126–127.

Curzio G, Multicenter Study Group: A multicenter evaluation of a single-pass lead VDD pacing system. PACE 1991; 14:434–442.

Davies JG, Sowton E: Electrical threshold of the human heart. Br Heart J 1966; 28:231.

Dekker E, Buller J, Van Erven FA: Unipolar and bipolar stimulation thresholds of the human myocardium with chronically implanted pacemaker electrodes. Am Heart J 1966; 71:671–677.

Dekker E: Direct current make and break thresholds for pacemaker electrodes on the canine ventricle. Circ Res 1970; 27:811.

Ector H, Witters E, Tanghe L, Aubert A, DeGeest H: Measurement of pacing threshold. PACE 1985; 8:66–72.

Erlanger J: The physiology of heart block in mammals with especial reference to the causation of Stokes-Adams disease. J Exper Med 1905; 7:676.

Erlanger J, Hirschfelder AD: Further studies on the physiology of heart block in mammals. Am J Physiol 1905; 15:153–206.

Flammang D, Renirie L, Begemann M, et al: Amplitude and direction of atrial depolarization using a multipolar floating catheter: Principles for single lead VDD pacing. PACE 1991; 14:1040–1049.

Furman S, Benedek ZM, The Implantable Lead Registry: Survival of implantable pace-maker leads. PACE 1990; 13:1910–1914.

Furman S, Cooper JA: Atrial fibrillation during AV sequential pacing. PACE 1982; 5:133–135.

Furman S, Fisher JD: Endless loop tachycardia in an AV universal (DDD) pacemaker. PACE 1982; 5:486–489.

Furman S, Garvey J, Hurzeler P: Pulse duration variation and electrode size as factors in pacemaker longevity. J Thorac Cardiovasc Surg 1975; 69:382–389.

Furman S, Hurzeler P, Mehra R: Cardiac pacing and pacemakers IV. Threshold of cardiac stimulation. Am Heart J 1977; 94:115–124.

Furman S, Hurzeler P, Parker B: Clinical thresholds of endocardial cardiac stimulation: A long term study. J Surg Res 1975; 19:149–155.

Furman S, Mehra R: Anodal influence on ventricular fibrillation. (abstract) Am J Cardiol 1974; 33:137.

Furman S, Parker B, Escher DJW: Decreasing electrode size and increasing efficiency of cardiac stimulation. J Surg Res 1971; 11:105–110.

Furman S, Parker B, Escher DJW, et al: Endocardial threshold of cardiac response as a function of electrode surface area. J Surg Res 1968; 8:161–166.

Gettes LS, Shabetai R, Downs TA, et al: Effect of changes in potassium and calcium concentrations on diastolic threshold and strength-interval relationships of the human heart. Ann NY Acad Sci 1969; 167:693–705.

Haffajee C, Murphy J, Love JC, et al: Is routine testing for retrograde ventriculo-atrial conduction helpful prior to DDD pacemaker implantation. (abstract) PACE 1983; 6:311.

Hamilton R, Bahoric B, Griffiths J, et al: Steroid eluting epicardial leads in pediatrics: Improved epicardial thresholds in the first year. PACE 1991; 14:633.

Hayes D, Graham K, Irwin M, et al: A multicenter experience with a bipolar tined poly-urethane ventricular lead. PACE 1992; 15:1033–1039.

Hellestrand K, Nathan A, Bexton R, et al: The effect of the antiarrhythmic agent flecainide on acute and chronic pacing thresholds. (abstract) PACE 1983; 6:318.

Henglein D, Gillette PC, Shannon C, et al: Long-term follow-up of pulse width threshold of transvenous and myo-epicardial leads. PACE 1984; 7:203–214.

Hiller K, Rothschild JM, Fudge W, et al: A randomized comparison of a bipolar steroid-euluting lead and a bipolar porous platinum coated titanium lead. PACE 1991; 14:695 (abstract).

Hirshorn HS, Holly LK, Hales JRS, et al: Screening of solid and porous materials for pacemaker electrodes. PACE 1981; 4:380–390.

Horowitz LN, Spear JF, Josephson ME, et al: The effects of coronary artery disease on the ventricular fibrillation threshold in man. Circulation 1979; 60:792–797.

Hughes HC Jr, Tyers GFO, Torman HA: Effects of acid-base imbalance on myocardial pacing thresholds. J Thorac Cardiovasc Surg 1975; 69:743–746.

Hynes JK, Holmes DR Jr, Meredith J, et al: An evaluation of long-term stimulation thresh-olds by measurement of chronic strength duration curves. PACE 1981; 4:376–379.

Irnich W: Elektrotherapie des Herzens—physiologische und biotechnische Aspekte. Berlin, Fachverlag Schiele & Schon, 1976.

Irnich W: The chronaxie time and its practical importance. PACE 1980; 3:292–301.

Jacobs LJ, Kerzner JS, Diamond MA, et al: Pacemaker inhibition by myopotentials de-tected by Holter monitoring. PACE 1982; 5:30–33.

Johns J, Fish F, Burger J, et al: Steroid-eluting epicardial pacing leads in pediatric patients: Encouraging early results. PACE 1991; 14:633–633.

Jones M, Geddes LA: Strength-duration curves for cardiac pacemaking and ventricular fibrillation. Cardiovasc Res Cent Bull 1977; 15:101–112.

Kastor JA, Sanders CA, Leinbach RC, et al: Factors influencing retrograde conduction: Study of 30 patients during cardiac catheterization. Br Heart J 1969; 31:580.

Kelen GJ, Bloomfield D, Hardage M: Holter monitoring the patient with an artificial pacemaker—A new approach. Amb Electrocardiol 1978; 1:1–4.

Kelen GJ, Bloomfield DA, Hardage M, et al: A clinical evaluation of an improved Holter monitoring technique for artificial pacemaker function. PACE 1980; 3:192–197.

Kistin AD, Landowne M: Retrograde conduction from premature ventricular contractions: A common occurence in the human heart. Circulation 1951; 3:738.

Klementowicz P, Ausubel K, Furman S: The dynamic nature of ventriculoatrial conduction. PACE 1986; 9:1050–1054.

Kruse IBM: Long-term performance of endocardial leads with steroid-eluting electrodes. PACE 1986; 9:1217–1219.

Kruse IM, Terpstra B: Acute and long-term atrial and ventricular stimulation thresholds with a steroid-eluting electrode. PACE 1985; 8:45–49.

Kugler JD, Fetter J, Fleming W, et al: A new steroid-eluting epicardial lead: Experience with atrial and ventricular implantation in the immature swine. PACE 1990; 13:976–981.

Lagergren H, Edhag O, Wahlberg I: A low-threshold, non-dislocating endocardial electrode. J Thorac Cardiovasc Surg 1976; 72:259–264.

Lapicque L: La chronaxie et ses applications physiologiques. Paris, Hermann & Cie, 1938.

Levy S, Corbelli JL, Labruni P, et al: Retrograde (ventriculoatrial) conduction. PACE 1983; 6:364–371.

Lindemans FW, Zimmerman ANE: Acute voltage, charge and energy thresholds as functions of electrode size for electrical stimulation of the canine heart. Cardiovasc Res 1979; 13:383–391.

Llewellyn M, Bennett D, Heaps C, et al: Limitation of early pacing threshold rising using a silicone insulated, platinized, steroid-eluting lead. PACE 1988; 11:496 (abstract).

Longo E, Catrini V: Experience and implantation techniques with a new single-pass lead VDD pacing system. PACE 1990; 13:927–936.

Luceri RM, Furman S, Hurzeler P, et al: Threshold behavior of electrodes in long-term ventricular pacing. Am J Cardiol 1977; 40:184–188.

Mahmud R, Denker S, Lehmann MH, et al: Effect of atrioventricular sequential pacing in patients with no ventriculoatrial conduction. J Am Coll Cardiol 1984; 4:273–277.

Mahmud R, Lehmann M, Estrada A, et al: Facilitation of retrograde conduction with atrioventricular sequential pacing. (abstract) J Am Coll Cardiol 1983; 1:674.

Mehra R, Furman S: Comparison of cathodal, anodal, and bipolar strength-interval curves with temporary and permanent electrodes. Br Heart J 1979; 41:468–476.

Mehra R, Furman S, Crump JF: Vulnerability of the mildly ischemic ventricle to cathodal, anodal, and bipolar stimulation. Circ Res 1977; 41:159–166.

Mehra R, McMullen M, Furman S: Time dependence of unipolar cathodal and anodal strength-interval curves. PACE 1980; 3:526–530.

Michelson EL, Spear JF, Moore EN: Effects of procainamide on strength-interval relations in normal and chronically infarcted canine myocardium. Am J Cardiol 1981; 47:1223–1232.

Michelson EL, Spear JF, Moore EN: Strength-interval relations in a chronic canine model of myocardial infarction. Circulation 1981; 63:1158–1165.

Mines GR: On dynamic equilibrium in the heart. J Physiol 1913; 46:349–383.

Mitamura H, Ohm OJ, Michelson EL, et al: Importance of the pacing mode in the initiation of ventricular tachyarrhythmia in a canine model of chronic myocardial infarction. J Am Coll Cardiol 1985; 6:99–103.

Mond H, Stokes K, Helland J, et al: The porous titanium steroid eluting electrode: A double blind study assessing the stimulation threshold effects of steroid. PACE 1988; 11:214–219.

Mond H, Stokes K: The electrode-tissue interface: The revolutionary role of steroid eluting. PACE 1992; 15:95–107.

Mund K, Richter G, Weidlich E, et al: Electrochemical properties of platinum, glassy carbon, and pyrographite as stimulating electrodes. PACE 1986; 9:1225–1229.

Nernst W: Zur Theorie des elektrischen Reizes. Pflugers Arch 1908; 122:275–314.

Overdijk AD, Dekker E: Comparison of thresholds in epicardial and endocardial stimulation of the human heart by chronically implanted pacemaker electrodes. Am Heart J 1969; 77:172.

Parsonnet V, Hesselson AB, Harari DC: Long-term functional integrity of atrial leads. PACE 1991; 14:517–521.

Preston TA: Anodal stimulation as a cause of pacemaker-induced ventricular fibrillation. Am Heart J 1973; 86:366–372.

Preston TA, Barold SS: Problems in measuring threshold for cardiac pacing. Am J Cardiol 1977; 40:658–660.

Preston TA, Fletcher RD, Lucchesi BR, et al: Changes in myocardial threshold. Physiological and pharmacologic factors in patients with implanted pacemakers. Am Heart J 1967; 74:235–242.

Preston TA, Judge RD: Alteration of pacemaker threshold by drug and physiological factors. Ann NY Acad Sci 1969; 167:686–692.

Preston TA, Judge RD, Bowers DL, et al: Measurement of pacemaker performance. Am Heart J 1966; 71:92–99.

Preston TA, Judge RD, Lucchesi BR, et al: Myocardial threshold in patients with artificial pacemakers. Am J Cardiol 1966; 18:83–89.

Radovsky AS, Van Vleet JF, Stokes KB, et al: Paired comparisons of steroid-eluting and nonsteroid endocardial pacemaker leads in dogs: Electrical performance and morphologic alterations. PACE 1988; 11:1085–1094.

Ripart A, Mugica J: Electrode-heart interface: Definition of the ideal electrode. PACE 1983; 6:410–421.

Schallhorn R, Oleson K: Multi-center clinical experience with an improved steroid-eluting pacemaker lead. PACE 1988; 11:496 (abstract).

Schamroth L, Friedberg HD: Significance of retrograde conduction in AV dissociation. Br Heart J 1965; 27:896.

Scherf D: Retrograde conduction in the complete heart block. Dis Chest 1959; 35:320.

Schuchert A, Hopf M, Kuck KH, et al: Chronic ventricular electrograms: Do steroid-eluting leads differ from conventional leads? PACE 1990; 13:1879–1882.

Smyth NPD, Tarjan PP, Chernoff E, et al: The significance of electrode surface area and stimulating thresholds in permanent cardiac pacing. J Thorac Cardiovasc Surg 1976; 71:559–565.

Somerndik JM, Ostermiller WE: Sleeping threshold change causing failure of artificial cardiac pacing. J Am Med Assoc 1971; 215:980.

Sowton E, Barr I: Physiological changes in threshold. Ann NY Acad Sci 1969; 167:679–685.

Spear JF, Moore EN, Horowitz LN: Effects of current pulses delivered during the ventricular vulnerable period upon the ventricular fibrillation threshold. Am J Cardiol 1973; 32:814–822.

Stamato N, O'Toole M, Fetter J: The safety and efficancy of chronic ventricular pacing at 1.6 volts using a steroid eluting lead. PACE 1992; 15:248–251.

Starke ID: Long-term follow-up of cardiac pacing threshold using a noninvasive method of measurement. Br Heart J 1978; 40:530–533.

Starr DS, Lawrie GM, Morris GC Jr: Acute and chronic stimulation thresholds of intramyocardial screw-in pacemaker electrodes. Ann Thorac Surg 1981; 31:334–338.

Stokes K, Bird T: A new efficient nanoTip lead. PACE 1990; 13:1901–1905.

Stokes KB: Preliminary studies on a new steroid eluting epicardial electrode. PACE 1988; 11:1797–1803.

Surawicz B, Chlebus H, Reeves JT, et al: Increase of ventricular excitability threshold by hyperpotassemia. J Am Med Assoc 1965; 191:1049.

Svenson RH, Clark M, Hall D, et al: Analysis of manifest and latent retrograde conduction in patients with AV sequential pacemakers. Implications for pacer induced tachycardias. (abstract) J Am Coll Cardiol 1983; 1:674.

Takeshita A, Tanaka S, Nakamura M: Study of retrograde conduction in complete heart block using His bundle recordings. Br Heart J 1974; 36:462–467.

Thiele G, Lachmann W, Eschemann B, et al: Modification of stimulus threshold increase following heart pacemaker implantation. Zeitschrift Fur Die Gesamte Innere Medizin 1980; 35:863–866.

Timmis GC, Gordon S, Westveer D, et al: A new steroid eluting low threshold lead. (abstract) PACE 1983; 6:316.

Timmis GC, Helland J, Westveer D, et al: The evolution of low threshold leads. CPPE 1983; 1:313–334.

Timmis GC, Westveer DC, Helland J, et al: Pacemaker stimulation thresholds and the Wedensky effect. PACE 1983; 6:320 (abstract).

Varriale P, Pilla AG, Tekriwal M: Single-lead VDD pacing system. PACE 1990; 13:757–766.

Von Knorre GH, Ismer B, Voss W, et al: Orthodromic and antidromic pacemaker circus movement tachycardia. PACE 1991; 14:1233–1238.

Wahlberg I, Edhag O, Lagergren HR: Low threshold endocardial electrodes for permanent cardiac pacing. Comparison between one large and two small surface electrodes. Acta Med Scand 1977; 201:337–343.

Wainwright R, Davies W, Tooley M: Ideal atrial lead positioning to detect retrograde atrial depolarization by digitization and slope analysis of the atrial electrogram. PACE 1984; 7:1152–1158.

Walker WJ, Elkins JT, Wood LW: Effect of potassium in restoring myocardial response to a sub-threshold cardiac pacemaker. N Engl J Med 1964; 271:597.

Walls JT, Maloney JD, Pluth JR: Clinical evaluation of a sutureless cardiac pacing lead: Chronic threshold charges and lead durability. Ann Thorac Surg 1983; 36:328–331.

Weiss G: Sur la possibilite de rendre comparable entre eux les appareils cervant a l'excitation electrique. Arch Ital Biol 1901; 35:413.

Wiggers CJ, Wegria R, Pinera B: The effects of myocardial ischemia on the fibrillation threshold: The mechanism of spontaneous ventricular fibrillation following coronary occlusion. Am J Physiol 1940; 131:309.

Winkle RA, Stinson EB, Bach SM Jr, et al: Measurement of cardioversion/defibrillation thresholds in man by a truncated exponential waveform and an apical patch-superior vena caval spring electrode configuration. Circulation 1984; 69:766.

Wish M, Swartz J, Cohen A, et al: Steroid-tipped leads versus porous platinum permanent pacemaker leads: A controlled study. PACE 1990; 13:1887–1890.

Yee R, Jones DL, Jarvis E, et al: Changes in pacing threshold and R wave amplitude after transvenous catheter countershock. J Am Coll Cardiol 1984; 4:543–549.

Chapter 3

SENSING AND TIMING THE CARDIAC ELECTROGRAM

Seymour Furman

INTRODUCTION

Aside from the basic function of cardiac stimulation, all pacemaker complexity and flexibility is based on the cardiac chambers sensed and the variety of pacemaker response. Pacemaker utility and flexibility have increased over the years in direct proportion to the number of cardiac, noncardiac, and even nonphysiological structures sensed and the increase of the variety of response to sensed events. The earliest pacemakers, asynchronous ventricular pacemakers, stimulated the heart but did not respond to cardiac activity. The simple timing cycles those pacemakers produced were single unmodified intervals between stimuli. If the pacemaker rate were set to be 60 bpm, a stimulus was emitted once each second. No variation existed. While stimulation is basic to pacemaker function, the ability to sense cardiac function, and the mode of response to a sensed event defines the pacemaker mode of operation.

All decisions concerning pacemaker design are based on the comprehension of the various intervals and timing cycles desired and on the sensing of one or both chambers. All analyses of the ECGs of pacemaker and cardiac interaction are based on the understanding of stimulation intervals (i.e., rates), refractory and blanking intervals, and timing cycles of both the heart and the pacemaker. The basic principles of all pacemaker operations are identical, as are the principles of ECG interpretation. Examples concerning specific devices or ECG patterns will be used for illustrative purposes only, not to emphasize the quality of one device compared to another. The actual operation of each of the devices can be obtained from the manufacturer's literature and readily compared to the principles enunciated and analyses proposed. Without adequate sensing, all of the benefits will be unavailable.

Single-chamber pacemaker timing cycles and intervals are relatively simple, no matter how complex the device may seem, even compared to earlier pacemakers. Dual-chamber devices add far greater complexity because intervals are set for both atrium and ventricle individually; both chambers must be sensed and an interval is set between the function of the two chambers and then additional intervals, such as upper and lower rate limits, are set, as are intervals when the generator is insensitive (refractory or blanked) to one chamber or the other or both. The most recent pacemakers both single- and dual-chamber, have one or two rate modulating sensors and therefore add an additional sensing channel(s). In such single chamber pacemakers two (or three) sensing channels now exist where only one existed previously, and in dual-chamber pacemakers three (or four [i.e., atrium, ventricle, sensor #1, and sensor #2) sensing channels exist where only two existed before. Some dual-chamber pacemakers (e.g., DVI) have a single timing cycle derived from sensing one chamber only (though both chambers are stimulated) and are therefore simpler than the designation "dual-chamber" would imply. In some units a few intervals are programmable, but others are fixed (e.g., the committed DVI) during manufacture. The operation of some pacemakers can be extensively modified following implantation, while in others, such modification is limited. More recent dual-chamber pacemakers have tended to have broadly programmable timing as well as output functions and should be used in preference to less programmable devices. Sensing atrial and ventricular electrograms successfully is required because each timing cycle begins and ends with a sensed intrinsic deflection or emission of a stimulus, and programming for consistent and reliable sensing is mandatory for appropriate pacemaker cycling. An electrogram that is unsensed will not inhibit or trigger pacemaker output, and a competitive stimulus will result.

ARTIFICIAL TEST SIGNALS

Test signals for pulse generator design have been developed by the Association for the Advancement of Medical Instrumentation (AAMI) to assist when an actual electrogram cannot be used. Such an approach provides a consistent and electronically reproducible signal to emulate the electrogram. Sensing circuits can then be designed to a standard. The standard, however, does not resemble the physiological event closely, and it may be that some undersensing occurs because of design to an artificial rather than a natural signal (Figure 1).

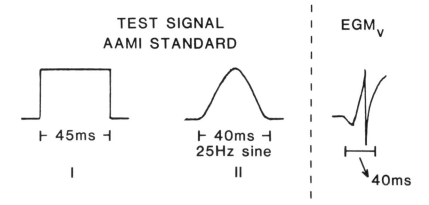

Figure 1. *AAMI recommended two standard test signals that reflect diversity in the engineering community. Standard (I) is rectangular, and standard (II) is a half sine wave of approximately the same duration. The ventricular electrogram, drawn to the same scale, shows the difference between the various test signals and the electrogram.*

SENSING THE CARDIAC ELECTROGRAM

The endocardial or epicardial electrogram (EGM) is the electrical signal emitted by the depolarization-repolarization process of the heart and detected from within or upon its surface. This signal should be measured during each pacemaker implantation and pulse generator replacement. Such measurement is best done by direct recording on a physiological recorder with a band width of 0.1–2000 Hz. At the very least, a pacing systems analyzer (PSA) should be used to determine the amplitude of the electrogram. Some analyzers are now sufficiently sophisticated to approach the value of a physiological recorder. As there is no uniformly accepted standardization of the sensitivity of any pacemaker circuit, it is best to measure the electrogram with an analyzer made by the manufacturer of the pacemaker to be implanted. It should also have the same electrode configuration (unipolar or bipolar) as the pacemaker lead that is to be used. Even then a significant difference may exist as sensing standards may have changed and a previous generation PSA may be used. If the electrogram is recorded on a physiological recorder, it should be analyzed for:

1. Configuration (morphology) of the depolarization waves (QRS or P).
2. Amplitude, duration, and timing relative to the peripheral QRS or P waves of that component of the electrogram that is called the "intrinsic deflection" (ID).
3. Slew rate (dV/dt or rate of development) of the intrinsic deflection.
4. The presence of injury current and repolarization (S-T segments and T) waves.

If possible, the electrogram should be referenced to an ECG lead in order to relate intracardiac to surface events (Figure 2).

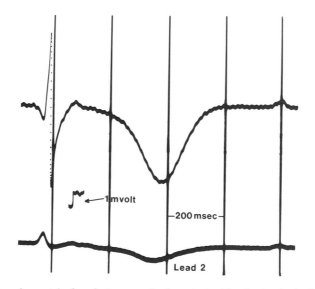

Figure 2. *A chronic ventricular electrogram is characterized by the intrinsic deflection, i.e., the rapidly moving portion of the depolarization wave as it passes the electrode in contact with tissue. An isoelectric ST segment and a deeply inverted T wave are recorded. The intrinsic deflection may appear early or late compared to the simultaneously recorded ECG.*

The "intrinsic deflection" (ID) is the rapid biphasic portion of the electrogram that occurs as the cardiac muscle adjacent to the electrode becomes electronegative with the passing depolarization wave. The intrinsic deflection exhibits the highest slew rate (dV/dt) seen in the electrogram and is the only component of the electrogram with a sufficiently rapid voltage change to trigger a pacemaker. It bears only a variable relationship to the peripheral ECG as it indicates the electrical activity of only a very small area of the heart. A majority (58%) of acute unipolar ventricular electrograms have a biphasic intrinsic deflection with roughly equal R and S waves, while 30% are predominantly monophasic positive, and 12% are monophasic negative. In 88% of chronic implants the intrinsic deflection is biphasic, and in the remainder of electrograms it is monophasic negative.

"Far-field" potentials arise from electrical activity distant from the electrode and include contralateral ventricular activation, skeletal muscle potentials, and external electromagnetic interference (EMI). In the atrial electrogram, the intrinsic deflection indicates atrial activation while the ventricular potentials constitute far-field signals and vice versa (Figure 3).

The "current of injury" appears as an elevation in electrical potential that follows the ID immediately in acute electrograms and represents a small area of damaged endocardium caused by electrode irritation. The current of injury appears as an elevated S-T segment during the acute period of implantation and later disappears, leaving an isoelectric chronic S-T segment (Figure 4).

A statistically significant decrease in the slew rate of about 40% occurs as an electrode enters the chronic phase; the decrease in amplitude is not signif-

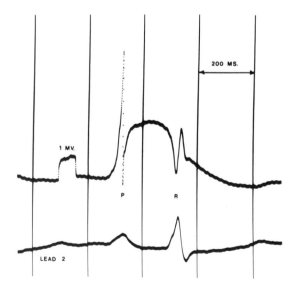

Figure 3. *An atrial electrogram is quite similar to a ventricular electrogram, but its overall amplitude is smaller. In this instance, the coronary sinus electrogram is recorded approximately halfway into the lead 2 P wave. The QRS complex is seen approximately 250 ms after the discrete atrial electrogram as a far-field signal.*

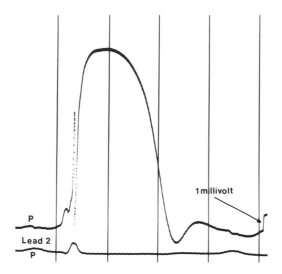

Figure 4. *An acute ventricular electrogram is characterized by the intrinsic deflection recorded simultaneously with the surface QRS complex and a current of injury, which is the dome-shaped elevation of the ST segment. The T wave is lost in the ST segment elevation. In transition from acute to chronic, the ST segment elevation will disappear.*

icant. The maturing electrode may, therefore, have a subthreshold signal (electrogram), i.e., lacking an adequate amplitude or slew rate, or both, to trigger a pulse generator properly (Figure 5). The atrial intrinsic deflection is morphologically similar to the ventricular intrinsic deflection, differing only in overall

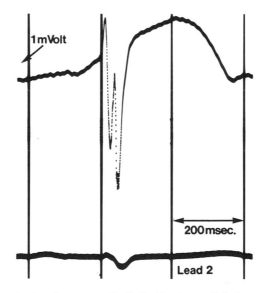

Figure 5. *A poor ventricular electrogram in distinction to a satisfactory one (see Figure 2) with a QRS complex in which the intrinsic deflection is of low amplitude, is split, and reverses itself, resetting the timing mechanism of the pulse generator.*

amplitude. Its timing relative to the peripheral P wave depends on the electrode's proximity to the S-A node. Far-field ventricular potentials may be comparable in amplitude but not in slew rate to the atrial intrinsic deflection. Such far-field ventricular potentials may be of sufficient amplitude when sensed by a unipolar atrial electrode to be sensed via the atrial channel and may then inhibit and recycle the stimulation rate during atrial pacing. Injury currents appear in 14% of acute atrial electrograms (Figure 6).

If lead and electrode placement is satisfactory, the best electrogram and stimulation threshold will usually coincide at one anatomical position. The amplitude of the ventricular sensing signal should be at 4 mV at a slew rate of at least 1.5 mV per millisecond (mV/ms) to accommodate the expected 40% acute-to-chronic decrease in the slew rate. A dome shaped S-T segment (injury potential) of at least 2 mV, measured at the time of electrode placement, is a further favorable indication of adequate placement. In the absence of a suitable recorder, a pacing systems analyzer or an external pacemaker with adjustable sensitivity may be used to estimate the electrogram to be sensed.

It has been recommended, and may be common practice, to evaluate sensitivity settings for an implanted pulse generator from electrogram telemetry. The two amplifiers, for telemetry and for sensing the cardiac electrogram, may have different characteristics, and in some models do have different character-

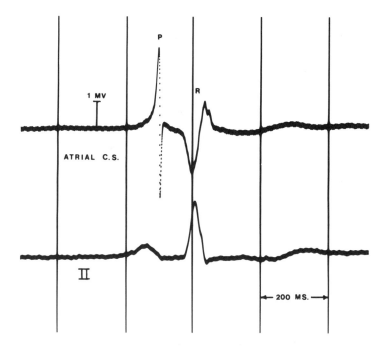

Figure 6.   *A unipolar atrial electrogram recorded from the coronary sinus also records a large far-field ventricular electrogram. In this instance, the ventricular electrogram is sufficiently large so that it may be sensed from the coronary sinus lead. Note also that the atrial electrogram appears virtually at the end of the surface P wave. This would be an example of late sensing of the atrial electrogram, far later than the beginning of the P wave in lead 2.*

istics, so that assessing what the pulse generator will, or will not sense, by measurement of the telemetered electrogram is fraught with the possibility of error.

ANTEGRADE AND RETROGRADE ATRIAL ELECTROGRAMS

Antegrade and retrograde atrial electrograms are recognizably different. It is visually possible to discriminate a recording of the two electrograms. In instances of amplitude difference, the pacemaker atrial sensing channel will be able to discriminate between the two and reduce the likelihood of endless loop tachycardia (see Chapter 4). In an evaluation of 34 patients undergoing dual-chamber pacemaker implantation, 31 had unipolar systems, 3 had bipolar. All antegrade and retrograde pairs were measurably different. All 34 had measurable antegrade/retrograde amplitude differences, and 30 of the unipolar pairs (96.8%) and all bipolar cases displayed antegrade/retrograde amplitude differences of at least 0.25 mV. Thirty of the unipolar cases (96.8%) and two of the bipolar cases had measurable slew rate differences. Overall configuration differed in 14/31 (45.2%) of unipolar and all 3 bipolar cases. Using criteria of both 0.25-mV sensitivity discrimination and 0.5-V/s slew rate discrimination, all 34 antegrade atrial electrograms could be discriminated from their retrograde mates. Therefore, electronic means alone would allow the differentiation of antegrade from retrograde atrial electrograms. This approach is potentially very

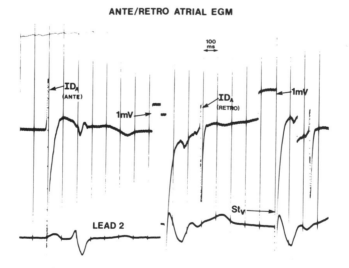

ANTE/RETRO ATRIAL EGM

Figure 7. *An example of an antegrade atrial electrogram (left) and two retrograde atrial electrograms (right) from the same patient. The antegrade EGM (ID_A) is approximately twice the amplitude of the retrograde. The slew rate, directly related to the distance between the dots forming the intrinsic deflection, is also about twice as great. These two electrograms can be readily discriminated by presently available pulse generators.*

important as discrimination of tachycardias becomes progressively more important and antegrade and retrograde, and ectopic atrial and conducted and ectopic ventricular activity must be accurately discriminated (Figure 7).

LATE SENSING

The electrocardiographic phenomenon of "late sensing" of a QRS complex is readily explained as sensing of the intrinsic deflection (ID) only. The intrinsic deflection is usually not coincident with the leading edge of a QRS complex or P wave in any peripheral lead. Indeed, it is likely that the position of the intrinsic deflection will be different in each lead, so that "late sensing" may appear in one lead and not in another, simultaneously recorded. In each different focus, conducted and idioventricular, the intrinsic deflection will appear at a different point in the QRS or P complex and give the impression of different pacemaker

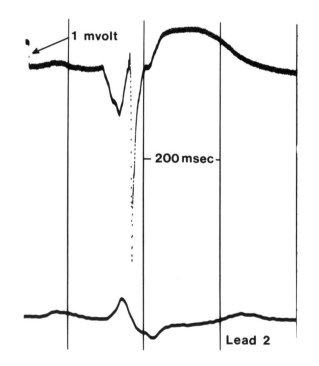

Figure 8.   *The ventricular electrogram is recorded close to the end of the surface ECG. If one assumes that sensing of the surface ECG will occur at its beginning, then this electrogram will produce late sensing. Late sensing does not exist, it is simply a misinterpretation that what the pacemaker senses is the beginning of the surface QRS complex.*

escape intervals if it assumed that the generator senses the leading edge of the peripheral signal. Once comprehended, "late sensing" becomes a nonevent and does not represent malfunction (Figure 8).

THE BIPOLAR ELECTROGRAM

The bipolar electrogram is the result of the potential difference between the two intracardiac poles (electrodes), each exhibiting a unipolar pattern. If the bipolar axis is at a right angle to the depolarization pathway, simultaneous identical signals at each pole can cancel each other, yielding a small or zero bipolar result. If the bipolar axis is oriented parallel to the depolarization pathway, there will be a signal delay at one pole relative to the other, and this can result in an augmented bipolar signal greater than either unipolar component. When the proximal pole of a catheter electrode is separated from the endocardial wall, the intrinsic deflection is small, so that the tip intrinsic deflection alone dominates the bipolar waveform. Simultaneous comparison of the group of ventricular bipolar and tip unipolar signals from a single lead shows that bipolar sensing offers the following:

1. Either enhanced or attenuated intrinsic deflection without a difference between mean unipolar and bipolar values;
2. Intrinsic deflection durations shortened by 28%;
3. Injury currents attenuated by 37%;
4. T waves attenuated by 34%.

The only disadvantage of the bipolar sensing configuration is the possibility of intrinsic deflection attenuation or cancellation if the two electrodes become oriented 90° to the direction in which the depolarization waves are propagated. In one clinical series, the bipolar intrinsic deflection was smaller than the simultaneous tip unipolar signal in 51% of cases, with 2% of the bipolar signals being too small to be sensed, while the simultaneous unipolar signal was of adequate amplitude. In 43% of cases in this series, the bipolar intrinsic deflection was larger than the tip unipolar signal, and in 6% the unipolar and bipolar signals were equal. Bipolar injury current (S-T elevation) and far-field potentials were smaller than the unipolar signal in 96% of cases. Atrial endocardial bipolar electrodes attenuate adjacent ventricular potentials by 80%, relative to simultaneous corresponding unipolar signals. When an atrial electrode is implanted for the automatic termination of supraventricular tachycardia, only a bipolar electrode should be used. Dual-chamber pacing systems now available use unipolar leads for both atrial and ventricle, some use bipolar leads, and others allow programming between unipolar and bipolar (Figures 9 and 10).

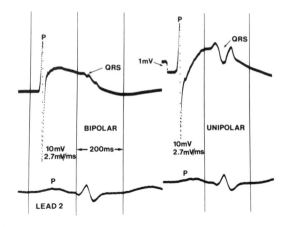

Figure 9.   *The major difference between atrial unipolar and bipolar electrograms is the presence of a large QRS complex in the unipolar recording and a smaller (invisible) complex in the bipolar recording. In this recording from the right atrial appendage, the unipolar electrogram has a much larger QRS complex as a far-field signal than the bipolar electrogram. The amplitude and frequency content of the two electrograms (other than far-field signals) are approximately equal.*

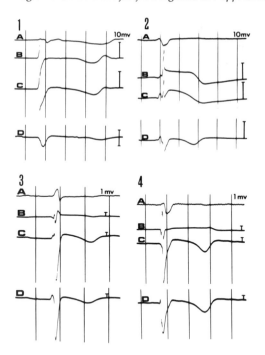

Figure 10.   *Four bipolar ventricular electrograms: Tracing (A) shows a simultaneously recorded lead 2 of the surface ECG; Tracing (B) the bipolar electrogram; (C) the electrogram from the tip electrode; (D) the electrogram from the ring or proximal electrode. In the first electrogram, the ring signal (D) is small and the bipolar (B) and tip (C) signals are almost identical. In the second, the bipolar signal (B) is larger than either the tip (C) or the ring (D) signal. Summation has occurred. In the third, the bipolar signal (B) is the subtraction of the tip (C) and the ring (D) signals and is somewhat smaller than either. The bipolar signal (B) in the fourth tracing is midway between the tip (C) and ring (D) signals. This is the usual situation.*

BIPOLAR SENSING

To demonstrate the superior rejection of electromyographic interference, twenty pacemakers that could be programmed into unipolar or bipolar sensing and pacing were evaluated in unipolar and bipolar modes of operation. All implants were conventional and were free of technical or physiological complications. Four upper extremity provocative maneuvers were performed on the side of the implant. They were:

1. pushing the implant side fist into the opposite hand;
2. pulling hands (placed at mid-chest) apart with the patient's maximum effort;
3. adduction of the arm on the pacemaker side, against resistance;
4. vigorous scratching of the implant side arm across the abdomen.

There were three categories of positive response:

a. inhibition—pacemaker output inhibited (Figure 11);
b. triggering—ventricular stimulation resulted from myopotentials sensed in the atrial channel (Figure 12);
c. reversion asynchronous (noise mode)—operation in either atrial or ventricular channel or both caused by sensed myopotentials (Figure 13).

The results of this evaluation were that no evidence of myopotential inter-

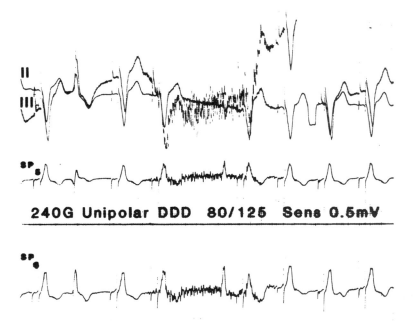

Figure 11.   *Inhibition of ventricular output occurs at atrial channel sensitivity of 2.5 mV and ventricular channel sensitivity of 0.5 mV, both in the unipolar lead configuration. Onset of myopotential interference inhibits atrial and ventricular output. Following 1300 ms of asystole, the first ventricular capture is an escape beat followed by a pacemaker escape (25 mm/s). All leads 2, 3, SP5, and SP6 are simultaneous.*

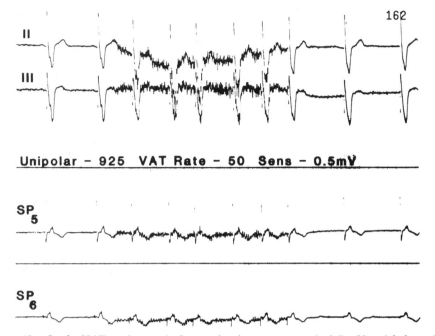

Figure 12.   *In the VAT mode ventricular sensing is not present. At 0.5-mV atrial channel sensitivity, myopotential interference triggers the ventricular response above the automatic ventricular rate (25 mm/s).*

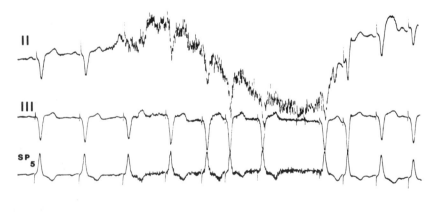

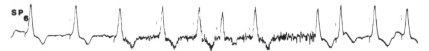

Figure 13.   *In the VAT mode ventricular sensing does not exist. Atrial channel sensitivity was set at 1.3 mV in the unipolar lead configuration. With the onset of myopotential interference, the ventricular response is increased in rate by triggering from the sensed atrial events. In the interference mode, a single ventricular stimulus is emitted at the noise escape interval and atrial triggering then resumes for a single beat (25 mm/s).*

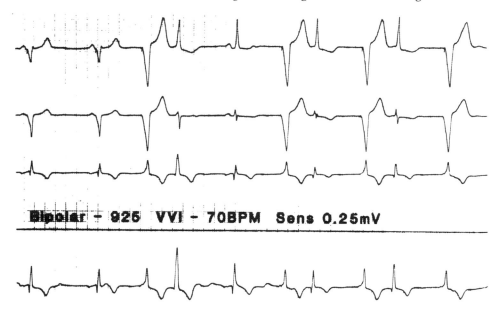

Figure 14. *Oversensing of the T wave can occur in either the unipolar or bipolar lead configuration. In the VVI mode and bipolar configuration at the maximum sensitivity (0.25 mV), the interval between beats 4 and 5 and is prolonged because of recycle from the T wave (25 mm/s). All leads 2, 3, SP5, and SP6 are simultaneous.*

ference existed at any sensitivity setting in the bipolar configuration of either tested pacemaker in atrium or ventricle. In the unipolar configuration, all patients (20/20) had myopotential interference at the highest atrial or ventricular sensitivity setting. T wave sensing occurred at the maximum sensitivity in four patients, two only in the bipolar configuration, one in unipolar only, and one in both unipolar and bipolar (Figure 14). Twenty-five percent of patients had myopotential interference at the unipolar atrial sensing threshold, which did not allow a setting that would reject myopotential interference while providing satisfactory atrial sensing. Twenty percent (2/10) of one model had ventricular inhibition at the least sensitivity setting (2.5 mV) of the ventricular channel, so that myopotential interference could not be avoided in the unipolar mode no matter how large the electrogram. It can be concluded from these evaluations and from the known behavior of the cardiac bipolar electrogram compared to its unipolar mate that discrete sensing and the absence of myopotential inhibition and electromagnetic interference is a characteristic of bipolar pacing, and such interference occurs substantially, even at moderate sensitivity levels during unipolar pacing.

UNIPOLAR AND BIPOLAR PACING AND SENSING

Unipolar and bipolar pacing have been available since the beginning of pacemaker technology. Unipolar and bipolar sensing, via the stimulating electrode, has been used since the introduction of sensing during cardiac pacing. The relative merits of the two approaches have been argued ever since. The benefits of bipolar pacing and sensing compared to unipolar are:

1. Pacing is only of the heart and stimulation of extracardiac tissue is rare. Pectoral muscle stimulation does not occur;
2. Stimulation thresholds of unipolar and bipolar electrodes are essentially identical (though the bipolar voltage stimulation threshold may be marginally higher);
3. A benefit of unipolar pacing is the smaller size of the lead system so that two intravascular unipolar leads are smaller than two intravascular bipolar leads. Though bipolar lead systems being developed are so small that this may eventually no longer be true;
4. A benefit of unipolar stimulation is that the stimulus artifact on the ECG is larger and therefore allows easier interpretation of pacemaker function.

The benefits of bipolar sensing over unipolar, described in the following list, are important:

1. There is minimal sensing of noncardiac signals. Neither electromyographic nor electromagnetic interference is as important an issue as it is with unipolar sensing;
2. The sensed electrogram is clean, i.e., free from far-field signals. The frequent sensing of pectoral muscle signals during unipolar pacing occurs because the anode of the system is located on the pulse generator, which is usually adjacent to the pectoral musculature. In a bipolar system the anode is within the heart.
3. As described above, the bipolar electrogram may be smaller than the unipolar or larger than the unipolar. The presence of a bipolar lead provides greater potential options for sensing configuration. Many pulse generators allow programming polarity to unipolar or bipolar, and if unipolar, whether the sensing electrode is the tip or the ring both referenced to the pulse generator case.

Presently available pulse generators have a variety of configuration options including:

1. Fixed unipolar—The electrode within the heart is a unipolar cathode, the anode is universally on the pulse generator;
2. Fixed bipolar—The electrode tip is the cathode and the proximal ring is the anode. In a modern implantable bipolar electrode the anodal ring is much larger than the cathodal tip so that anodal induced ventricular tachycardia/fibrillation is unlikely. It is possible to program a sensing configuration in which the ring is the cathode and the tip the anode. This configuration is not safe for stimulation.
3. Bipolar sensing and unipolar pacing—A nonprogrammable option used in some pacemakers takes advantage of the discrete sensing of the bipolar mode. Stimulation is unipolar with the pulse generator as the anode and the electrode tip as the cathode. Pectoral muscle electromyographic interference is not possible, but stimulation of the pectoral muscle is possible;
4. Programmable unipolar/bipolar—In this instance a conventional bipolar lead is used but the pulse generator has a programmable option, either conventional bipolar with the tip cathodal or unipolar with the tip cathodal and the pulse generator case anodal;
5. Multiprogrammable unipolar/bipolar—In this option the bipolar may be tip cathodal, ring anodal, or it may be reversed, i.e., ring cathodal-tip anodal. If the unipolar mode is selected then either the tip or the ring may be used for sensing while the pulse generator is the anodal ground.

ELECTROMYOGRAPHIC INTERFERENCE AND BIPOLAR SENSING

The bipolar electrode rejects electromagnetic interference because the electrogram or electromagnetic signal that results from sensing on the two electrodes is too small to reach the level of programmed sensitivity. Nevertheless, it is possible for a bipolar far-field electrogram to be sufficiently large (though nonetheless small) to be sensed at a high pacemaker sensitivity setting. One such event was recorded (Figure 15) during programming of a bipolar atrial antitachycardia pacemaker to its highest sensitivity when used to manage recurrent supraventricular tachycardia. The lead was in the atrial appendage, quite close to the chest wall and the patient was thin. Pectoral movement was detected and

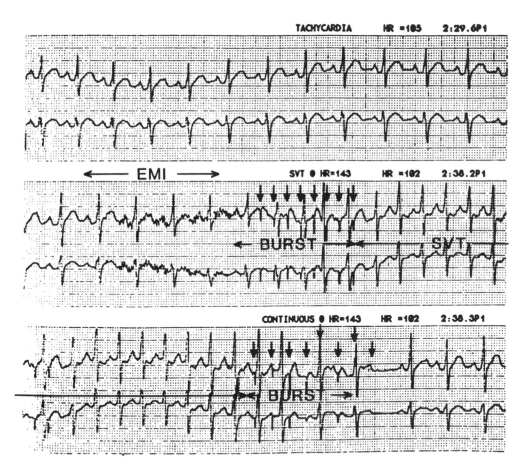

Figure 15. *The tracing is a bedside monitor recording of a patient with an implanted 262–12 bipolar atrial antitachycardia pacemaker. Because of a small electrogram associated with the supraventricular tachycardia, a sensitivity of 0.4 mV was programmed. During pectoral muscle movement and normal sinus rhythm (marked EMI) a stimulus burst (arrows) was emitted that caused a recurrence of the supraventricular tachycardia. The device detected the episode and emitted a second burst (arrows) that terminated the supraventricular tachycardia. No pacemaker or lead defect was found.*

interpreted as atrial activity. The antitachycardia mode was activated and caused supraventricular tachycardia. When that supraventricular tachycardia was subsequently detected, it was terminated by the same stimulus burst that had initiated it.

Other recorded electromyographic interference in the presence of a bipolar lead has been caused by some variety of malfunction, i.e., perforation of the electrode through the right ventricular wall to detect diaphragmatic movement or lead insulation defect.

NONCONTACT ATRIAL SENSING

Noncontact atrial sensing leads are a special case of atrial bipolar lead systems and have proven to be especially useful. In conventional atrial bipolar leads, the tip and ring are circumferential, detect the electrogram in all directions, and are separated one from the other by an insulated length along the lead system. This separation has traditionally been 1 centimeter or 1 inch but, may, of course, be any distance. A noncontact lead may use two or three electrodes circumferentially about a lead. One version of the noncontact lead has the electrodes entirely circumferential, another uses split ring electrodes on opposite sides of the lead and separated by several millimeters or more along the lead (Figure 16).

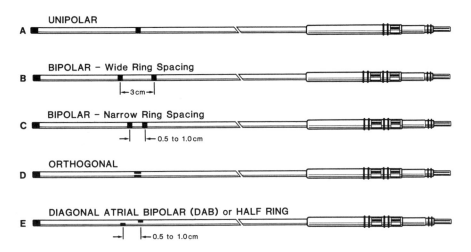

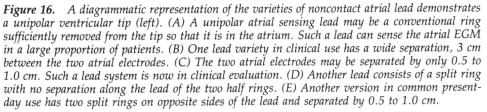

Figure 16. A diagrammatic representation of the varieties of noncontact atrial lead demonstrates a unipolar ventricular tip (left). (A) A unipolar atrial sensing lead may be a conventional ring sufficiently removed from the tip so that it is in the atrium. Such a lead can sense the atrial EGM in a large proportion of patients. (B) One lead variety in clinical use has a wide separation, 3 cm between the two atrial electrodes. (C) The two atrial electrodes may be separated by only 0.5 to 1.0 cm. Such a lead system is now in clinical evaluation. (D) Another lead consists of a split ring with no separation along the lead of the two half rings. (E) Another version in common present-day use has two split rings on opposite sides of the lead and separated by 0.5 to 1.0 cm.

Noncontact atrial sensing has been a goal for over a decade. In 1979, sensing of the atrial electrogram by a 60-mm^2 unipolar intraatrial electrode, part of the ventricular lead, was introduced. That and subsequent systems have provided an atrial electrogram 2- to 3-mV amplitude, adequate to assure consistent atrial synchrony. During the 1980s the orthogonal lead was introduced that was also able to sense the atrium while floating within the intraatrial blood pool. The initially described lead was in several versions, each with a group of circular (dot) electrodes, 0.8 mm^2, spaced 90° around a 2-mm diameter lead. In Type I atrial sensors, three and four such electrodes were designed. In Type II, three electrodes were placed circumferentially with an additional electrode 2 mm proximal to one of the three. P wave amplitudes of 2.47 ± 1.6 mV were found. In an evaluational version (which never reached commercial release), these electrodes were modified into two split semi-circular, partially circumferential rings with insulation between. The two rings were each 6 mm^2 in surface area, located at the same level (13 cm from the tip) of the lead on which they were located.

A system now commercially available consists of a triaxial lead with the distal tip, the unipolar ventricular electrode, and two conductors connected to two atrial partially circumferential flat patch electrodes 6 mm^2 surface area located 180° apart on the lead and insulated one from the other, separated by 5 mm from each other. This system has been named the diagonal atrial bipolar (DAB) configuration (Figures 17 and 18). Another system now in clinical evaluation has a bipolar ventricular electrode and two atrial ring electrodes, each 25 mm^2 in surface area, separated by 5 mm along the lead. The atrial electrodes are (in three different versions) 11, 13, and 15 cm from the ventricular electrode. Initial reported results are similar to those already described. The atrial electrogram is sensed as two unipolar electrograms when referenced to the pulse generator case. The two unipolar electrograms are then constructed into a bipolar by the differential amplifier within the pulse generator. In such a configuration, it is possible to sense two independent electrograms. In that instance the first electrogram that reaches the sensitivity level of the pacemaker device will be sensed and will determine timing (Figures 19 and 20). These electrodes are highly directional and reject far-field signals very effectively. Consequently, because interference is so much less likely to occur, pulse generator sensitivity can be set at a much higher level. Atrial sensitivities of 0.1, 0.2, 0.3 to 1.0 mV are programmable. Nevertheless lead movement within the atrium may result in extreme fluctuation in the amplitude of the electrogram finally detected. Small far-field electrograms require high sensitivity settings to detect the smallest of the signals (Figure 21).

Another system clinically available has two circumferential atrial ring electrodes on the ventricular lead. Each is 3.5 mm in diameter with a surface area of 16 mm^2 with the two electrodes separated by 3 cm. The more distal of the pair is 13 cm from the ventricular electrode which is sited in the right ventricular apex, although other separations are available. Each electrode detects the unipolar atrial electrogram referenced to the pulse generator, and the bipolar atrial electrogram is generated as the potential difference between the two atrial electrograms and constructed through the pulse generator's differential amplifier.

Twenty-six (now 43 patients) who had been implanted with a single lead

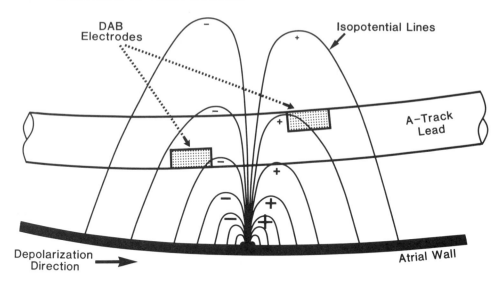

Figure 17.   *Dipole field associated with depolarization. This diagram of a floating, i.e., noncontact atrial sensing electrode shows the depolarization wave front crossing both portions of the DAB electrode so that they are sensed simultaneously.*

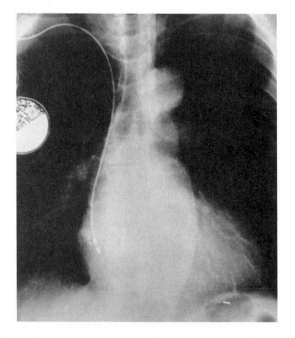

Figure 18.   *A radiographic demonstration of a floating atrial lead demonstrates it in the mid-right atrium relatively near the atrial wall. The electrode tip is in the right ventricular apex. This is a common position for such a lead.*

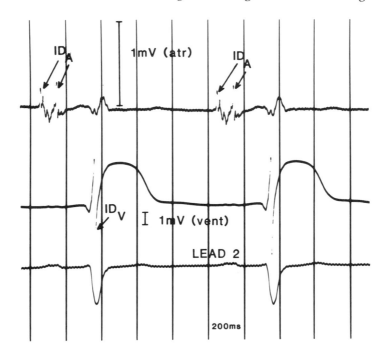

Figure 19. *A dual atrial bipolar lead electrogram (above) recorded simultaneously with a unipolar ventricular electrogram (middle) and lead 2 (below). The lead had the atrial sensing electrodes separated along its length. Two atrial electrograms were recorded, separated by about 75 ms. Because of the small size of the far-field ventricular electrogram, high sensitivity can be set to sense the diminutive atrial electrogram while rejecting the ventricular depolarization.*

(DAB) VDD pacemaker had had normal atrial function, defined as an atrial rate with activity of at least 100 bpm and a minimum rate of at least 50 bpm. None had a history of atrial fibrillation, flutter, or other supraventricular tachycardia. None developed an atrial arrhythmia following pacemaker implant. The mean atrial electrogram at implant was 3.54 mV, the minimum 0.8 mV, and the maximum 11.1 mV. The mean atrial electrogram slew rate was 1.6 mV/ms with ten

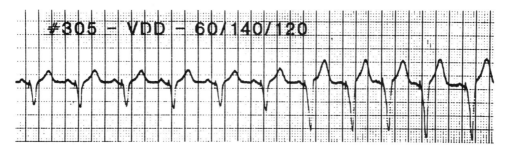

Figure 20. *An ECG of atrial synchrony with a split atrial EGM demonstrates apparent variation in the duration of the AV interval, depending on fluctuation of the amplitude of the first of the two EGMs. When the first EGM is unsensed (left) the AV interval appears to be longer. When it is sensed the AV interval appears to be briefer.*

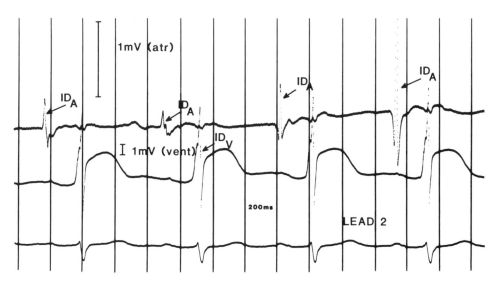

Figure 21.   *This is a three-channel recording of a noncontact atrial bipolar lead with the unipolar tip referenced to the subcutaneous tissue of the chest wall and the right ventricular apex. The atrial electrode is a dual atrial bipolar, i.e., partially bipolar electrode, in the mid-right atrium. The lead position is quite stable as indicated by the constancy of the unipolar ventricular electrogram. Because of movement of the atrial electrode relative to the atrial wall, the amplitude of the atrial electrogram is highly variable. Atrial electrograms recorded vary between approximately 0.25 mV and 3 mV. On the atrial channel the ventricular depolarization is small relative to the ventricular electrogram so that atrial sensitivity can be made extremely high to produce satisfactory sensing of the atrial electrogram.*

measured atrial electrogram slew rates less than 1.0 mV/ms and the mean of that group was 0.41 mV/ms. The mean ventricular stimulation threshold was 0.68 mA and 0.46 V at 0.5 ms. Consistent atrial sensing was characteristic of the postoperative course, providing satisfactory VDD function.

ATRIAL AND VENTRICULAR ELECTROGRAM TIMING

The electrogram (EGM) and the electrocardiogram (ECG) indicate intracardiac events and body surface events, respectively. They have different characteristics and the qualities of one cannot be inferred from the other. In the absence of pacemaker telemetry, the only occasion at which the electrogram will be available is at the time of implant or pulse generator replacement. The electrograms and surface leads should be recorded simultaneously to determine the relationship between the two. The progressively increasing availability of electrogram telemetry allows post-implant determination of the quality and timing characteristics of the electrogram and improves acumen for different diagnostic problems. Electrocardiogram interpretation channels now available in several pacemaker models trigger on the intrinsic deflection and can give an accurate indication of the exact instant of sensing. As electrocardiogram interpretation channels and a stimulus are accurate to 1 ms, pacemaker timing cycles can then be accurately determined (Figure 22). Some generators provide markers that indicate the end of a particular (atrial or ventricular) refractory interval as well as the EGM and additional assistance in ECG interpretation (Figure 23). Some dual-chamber generators allow the triggered mode in the atrium or the ventricle or both, allowing the marking of either P wave or QRS complex with an indication of the exact instant of sensing. When considering any timing cycles or analyzing any ECG for pacemaker function, it is necessary to analyze function as a series of intervals between sensed or paced events rather than as a continuous rate. Rate is a relatively simple designation during continuous pacing or continuous inhibition but is worthless and confusing if pacing and sensing alternate. Each event must be analyzed discretely. It must be recognized that rate is a continuum of a series of discontinuous events.

Atrial and ventricular electrograms are readily determined via the implanted lead system. Each different site in the heart, either in the atrium or ventricle, will have a different electrogram. The electrocardiogram is the sum of multiple electrograms recorded from the body surface. The electrogram of importance during cardiac pacing is that sensed by the lead system in the atrium and/or ventricle. Exact measurements of AV and VA conduction times can only be determined by recording and comparing the atrial and ventricular electrograms from one intrinsic deflection to the other. It is therefore necessary to record the atrial and ventricular electrograms during paced and unpaced cardiac activity.

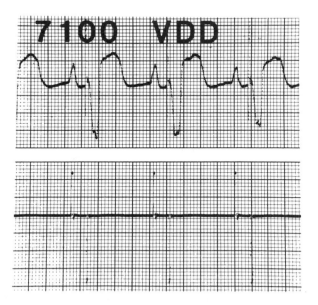

Figure 22. *An ECG interpretation channel was recorded simultaneously with lead 2 for an atrial synchronous (VDD) pacemaker. In the ECG interpretation channel the sensed P wave produces an upward going stimulus at the instant of atrial sensing. The ventricular stimulus also produces a downward mark. The interval between atrial sensing and ventricular stimulus emission can be accurately determined as can the instant of atrial sensing.*

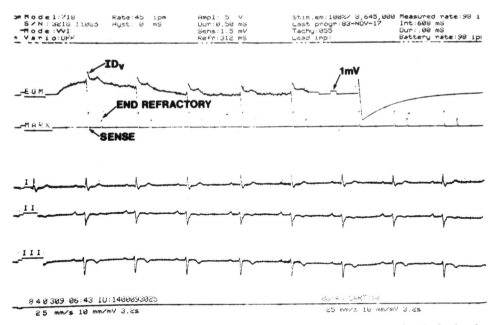

Figure 23. *A multichannel recording of pacer testing shows an electrogram of a single-chamber ventricular pacemaker simultaneously with a mark for ventricular sensing and a mark for the end of the refractory period after ventricular sensing. This information is recorded simultaneously with telemetry from the pacemaker memory (above) and 3 ECG surface leads.*

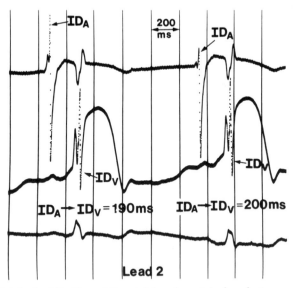

Figure 24. *The intrinsic deflection of the atrial and ventricular electrograms are the elements sensed to recycle a pacemaker. In the dual lead system the atrial and ventricular electrograms are recorded simultaneously with the ECG (lead 2). As each focus, atrial and ventricular, produce a unique electrogram, the timing of the interval from the atrial to the ventricular intrinsic deflection varies with different cardiac foci. In this three-channel recording the two intervals of ID_A to ID_V are different as each electrogram originates at a different focus.*

Each of the intervals determined is important to the proper setting of an implantable dual-chamber pacemaker.

With leads in place, the following measurements can be made on a multichannel recorder with oscilloscope and hard copy recording:

1. interval from intrinsic deflection of the atrial depolarization ID_A to intrinsic deflection of ventricular depolarization ID_V ($ID_A{\rightarrow}ID_V$) (Figure 24);
2. interval from the atrial pacemaker stimulus St_A to the intrinsic deflection of ventricular depolarization ID_V ($St_A{\rightarrow}ID_V$). Optimally patients should be paced at rates of 60, 80, 100, 120, and 140 bpm and atrioventricular conduction time assessed (Figure 25) and the rate for onset of AV block ascertained (Figure 26);3. interval from the ventricular pacing stimulus St_V to the intrinsic deflection of atrial depolarization ID_A ($St_V{\rightarrow}ID_A$). Optimally, patients should be paced at rates of 60, 80, 100, 120, and 140 bpm and ventriculoatrial conduction intervals assessed and (Figure 27) the rate for onset of VA block ascertained. Retrograde (VA) conduction can only be evaluated adequately when the ventricular rate (paced or unpaced) is more rapid than the atrial rate (Figure 28);
4. routine measurement of atrial and/or ventricular stimulation thresholds;
5. recording and measurement of the atrial and ventricular electrograms independently.

In examining the recordings when the ventricle was paced, the absence of orderly atrial depolarizations, i.e., atrial depolarization that occurred independently of any ventricular activity, documents the absence of retrograde conduction (Figure 29).

The mean antegrade conduction interval at rest ($ID_A{\rightarrow}ID_V$) is 212 ± 33 ms

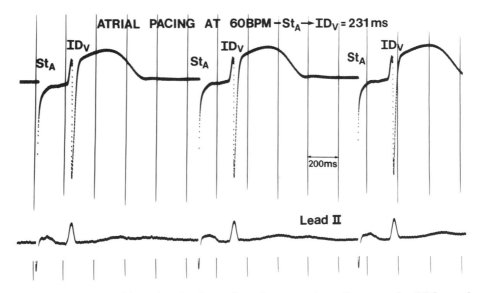

Figure 25. *The interval from the stimulus to the atrium to produce a P wave and a QRS complex that is produced in response is the interval for antegrade conduction. Here, the ventricular electrogram and ECG lead 2 are recorded simultaneously. Antegrade conduction is between the stimulus (St_A) to the ventricular response (ID_V). This varies as a function of the atrial stimulated rate. In this instance, at a cycle length of 1,000 ms (60 bpm), the interval $St_A{\rightarrow}ID_V$ is 231 ms.*

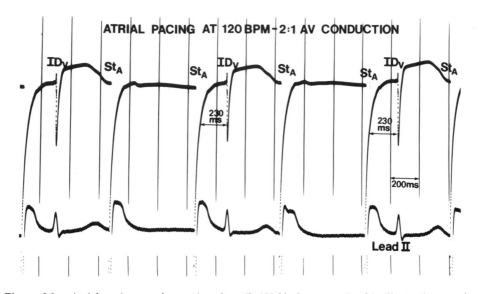

Figure 26. *Atrial pacing can be continued until AV block occurs. In this illustration, surface lead 2 is recorded simultaneously with the ventricular electrogram. The coupling interval of atrial stimulation is 500 ms (120 bpm); the atrial response to stimulation is clearly recorded, but conduction from the P wave to the QRS is at 2:1 AV block.*

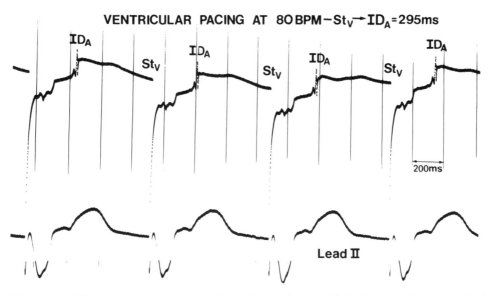

Figure 27. *The measurement of retrograde conduction is accomplished by recording surface lead 2 and the atrial electrogram. The ventricle is paced at a coupling interval of 750 ms (80 bpm), and the interval between the ventricular stimulus and the retrograde recorded P wave can be measured readily. In this instance $St_V \rightarrow ID_A$ is 295 ms.*

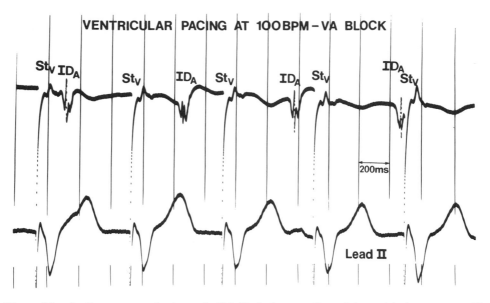

Figure 28. *In the presence of retrograde VA block the recording of the atrial electrogram will demonstrate P waves moving independently of the QRS complex. Just as with antegrade conduction this will demonstrate the absence of a relationship between ventricular depolarization and atrial depolarization.*

prolonged to a mean interval ($St_A \rightarrow ID_V$) of 312 ± 62 ms at the highest atrial pacing rate before AV block occurred. Twenty-five percent of patients with AV conduction at rest developed AV block at the lowest rate of atrial capture, 70 and 80 bpm; 25% developed AV block at 100 bpm; 20% of patients at 120 bpm; 20% of patients at 40 bpm; 4% at 160 bpm; 4% never do develop AV block. About 50 ms of the increase in the interval during pacing can be attributed to the $St_A \rightarrow ID_A$ latency during pacing from the right atrial appendage.

A variety of retrograde conduction responses exist. In 47% of patients, 1:1 retrograde conduction is present at some ventricular paced rate; 6% of patients had retrograde Wenckebach block, and 47% of the patients had retrograde block (Figure 30). Of those patients with complete antegrade block during atrial pacing, 14% had 1:1 VA conduction at a mean VA conduction time of 235 ± 50 ms (range 110–380 ms). Of additional patients who demonstrated 2:1 AV conduction with atrial pacing, i.e., no 1:1 antegrade conduction, 25% had intact 1:1 retrograde conduction. Therefore, 17% of patients had 1:1 retrograde VA conduction when no 1:1 antegrade conduction could be demonstrated (Figure 31).

Considering all indications for pacing, 47% of patients had some level of intact 1:1 retrograde conduction. The proportion of patients with intact VA conduction varied considerably when patients were analyzed by rhythm disturbance. In those patients with sinus node dysfunction, 67% had intact VA conduction and 69% of patients with sinus bradycardia or sinus arrest had intact VA conduction. Thirty-six percent of patients with incomplete atrioventricular block and 17% of patients with complete atrioventricular block (spontaneously and during atrial pacing) had intact VA conduction.

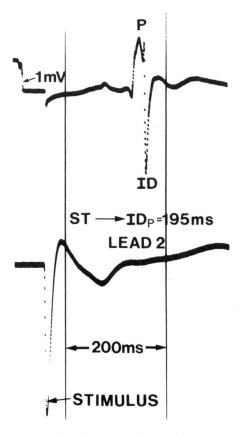

Figure 29. Accurate measurement for the retrograde conduction time can be accomplished by measurement between the ventricular stimulus and the intrinsic deflection of the retrograde atrial depolarization. In this illustration, taken from a sequence of similarly timed retrograde atrial depolarizations, the conduction time is 195 ms.

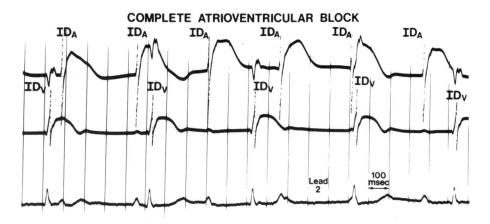

Figure 30. An electrogram of complete AV block was recorded simultaneously from atrium and ventricle. Lead 2 is below and indicates the absence of association between P waves and ventricular response. Above, the intrinsic deflection of the ventricle occurs at an approximate coupling interval of 1000 ms and the intrinsic deflection of the atrium at coupling intervals of 800 ms. While the two rates are relatively close, the dissociation between atrial and ventricular activity is clearly indicated.

114

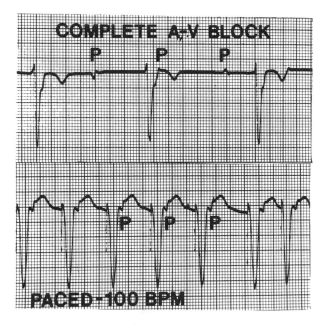

Figure 31. *Complete antegrade AV block may coexist with retrograde 1:1 conduction. In this example, the upper strip is unpaced showing complete AV block; the lower is the same patient paced at 100 bpm with consistent 1:1 retrograde conduction.*

The interaction between the two chambers during implantation of a dual-chamber pacemaker is all important. This interaction is based on the appropriate pacing and sensing of the two chambers and of the setting of the intervals between the atrial and ventricular channels. A variety of refractory and sensitive intervals determines the means of dealing with atrial and ventricular premature contractions and minimum and maximum atrial tracking rates. The complexity is substantial. Three intervals are of critical importance to successful management of an implanted pulse generator that senses in two chambers.

Once the pacing and sensing characteristics of the two chambers individually have been established, attention should be directed to the intervals that determine the interaction of the two chambers. The four measurements made allow determination of the spontaneous AV conduction time (if it exists) and allow the optimal setting for automatic pacemaker rate and AV delay that will permit sensing spontaneous atrial activity and AV conduction to drive the ventricle as frequently as is feasible. If spontaneous AV conduction varies from a desirable AV interval (probably between 140–200 ms) for the interval between the atrial and ventricular intrinsic deflection ($ID_A \rightarrow ID_V$) the pulse generator can be set at that interval deemed to be appropriate. Measurement of the atrially paced interval to the intrinsic deflection of the ventricle $St_A \rightarrow ID_V$ is determined by two distinct timing events. These are the atrial pacemaker stimulus (St_A) and the ventricular intrinsic deflection (ID_V). Two intervals are also defined. These are the latent interval between the atrial pacer stimulus (St_A) and the intrinsic deflection of the atrium (ID_A) and the interval between that stimulus (St_A) and the ventricular intrinsic deflection (ID$_V$), which is significantly rate-dependent. The atrial latent interval does not seem to vary with the pacing rate.

The significance of recognition of the difference between ID$_A$→ID$_V$ and St$_A$→ID$_V$ is in maintenance of a constant PR interval. As there is a latent period of atrial stimulation and as all pacemaker timing cycles begin with a sensed event (always an intrinsic deflection) or a stimulus, always followed by a latent period, it is obvious that the interval from intrinsic deflection of the atrium (ID$_A$) to the intrinsic deflection of the ventricle (ID$_V$) is shorter than from atrial pacing stimulus (St$_A$) to the ventricular intrinsic deflection (ID$_V$) (Figure 32). In order to maintain a constant PR interval, the dual-chamber pacemaker timing cycles must be different when sensing the P wave than when pacing the atrium. If only one AV interval is available, starting with a sense or pace event, paced and sensed PR intervals will be of different duration (Figure 33).

The last measurement should be of the interval for retrograde (VA) conduction following a ventricular stimulus once the two leads are in place. Intact retrograde conduction allows a pacemaker-mediated endless loop tachycardia and determination of its possibility, presence, and duration is required (Figure 34). Only a few conclusions can be drawn from the unpaced surface ECG concerning the existence and nature of retrograde conduction. Although the sequence of retrograde atrial activation may result in an inverted P wave in leads II, III, and AVF, the presence and morphology of a P wave is almost impossible to discern when inscription of the QRS occurs simultaneously, and even in the

AV DELAY AND PR INTERVAL

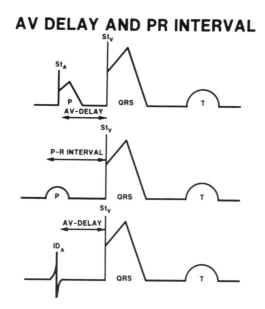

Figure 32. *Each timing cycle for an implanted pacemaker starts and ends with a sensed intrinsic deflection or the emission of a stimulus. Because the atrial electrogram recorded from the right atrial appendage is sensed well into the P wave, the AV interval between an atrial stimulus and a ventricular stimulus or a sensed atrial intrinsic deflection and a ventricular stimulus will be of different durations.*

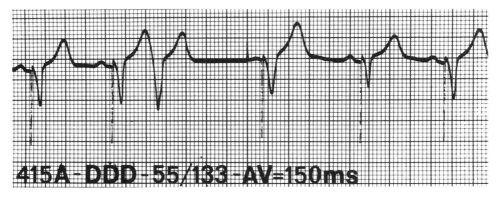

Figure 33. *In this dual-chamber pacemaker, a ventricular premature contraction after the second ventricular paced beat resets the timing cycle and the next stimulus produces a P wave and then a succeeding QRS complex. As the timing of the AV interval starts with the atrial stimulus, the P wave occurs much closer to the ventricular stimulus than it does when it is spontaneous, as it is for all other P waves seen in this ECG. Then, the P wave precedes the ventricular stimulus by a longer interval because the P wave is sensed near its peak on the ECG.*

ST and T segments, the presence and polarity of a P wave may be difficult to determine. Retrograde AV nodal conduction cannot be predicted from knowledge of the state of antegrade conduction. Nevertheless, during temporary or single-chamber pacing, an assessment of the state of VA conduction can sometimes be made and may be useful (Figure 35).

The characteristic arrhythmia of the pacemaker that senses the atrium and ventricle is the artificial reentry tachycardia, a pacemaker-mediated tachycardia of the "endless loop" variety. One of the most important intervals of the VDD or DDD pacemaker is the time during which the atrial channel will be refractory after a paced or sensed ventricular event. As 47% of all patients who require

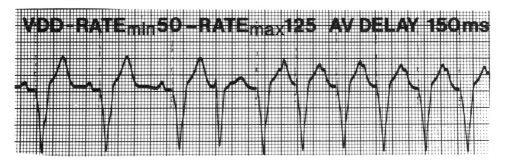

Figure 34. *Endless loop tachycardia exists because of retrograde conduction of the P wave following ventricular stimulation. Almost invariably, the endless loop tachycardia occurs at the upper rate limit and the AV interval is prolonged. The first prolongation of the AV interval occurs immediately following the VPC, the fourth ventricular complex from the left. The retrograde P wave, seen approximately 160 ms after the beginning of the VPC, causes the next ventricular stimulus that is delayed until the entire upper rate interval of the pacemaker (480 ms) has passed. Because of this requirement of delay of the ventricular stimulus, the AV interval is prolonged well above the programmed setting.*

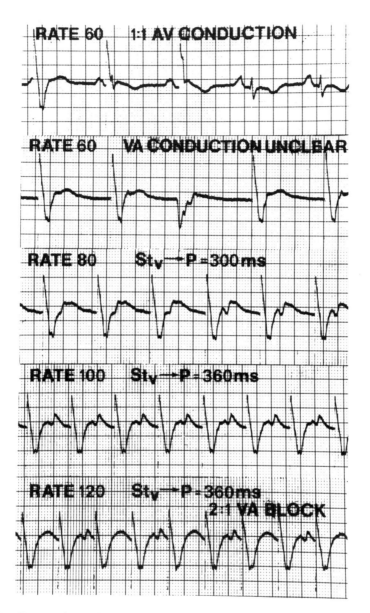

Figure 35. *Retrograde conduction is readily seen on the surface ECG when a single-chamber ventricular pacemaker is in place. Ventricular pacing must be at least 10 bpm faster than the spontaneous atrial rate. In this recording, retrograde conduction and even 2:1 retrograde block is visible. At a ventricular paced rate similar to that of the spontaneous cardiac rate, ventricular capture is seen once and 1:1 AV conduction predominates. Even with ventricular pacing (ECG #2), the ventricular paced rate is too slow to indicate whether VA conduction is present or not. As the ventricular paced rate increases to 80 bpm, the retrograde P waves are clearly seen with the peak of the P at approximately 300 ms after the ventricular stimulus. At a ventricular paced rate of 100 bpm, the retrograde conduction time increases to approximately 300 ms, and at a ventricular paced rate of 120 bpm, 2:1 VA block occurs. The state of retrograde conduction can be evaluated preoperatively in some instances.*

pacemaker implantation and 21% of those whose indication is high-degree AV block have retrograde conduction, the problem is not small. The duration of the VA conduction time demonstrates that a short atrial refractory interval after a ventricular event allows sensing of the retrograde P wave (see below).

THE AV TIMING BASIS OF PACEMAKER SYNDROME (PROLONGATION OF THE AV INTERVAL)

Pacemaker syndrome is the complex of disabilities caused by single-chamber ventricular pacing or displacement of the atrial contraction to a time early after the preceding ventricular contraction during dual-chamber pacing. Three causes have been recognized:

1. The loss of atrioventricular synchrony;
2. Sustained retrograde conduction;
3. A single ventricular rate when rate modulation is required for exercise.

Rate modulation is discussed in Chapter 11 and the loss of atrial synchrony with random synchronization in Chapter 4. Sustained retrograde conduction or its equivalent, the presence of a P wave early after a QRS complex with a prolonged delay to the next QRS, occurs in a variety of ways, including during VDD and DDI modes and the DDD mode with pseudo-Wenckebach operation, which produces an AV interval beyond any normal duration. Pacemaker syndrome is, in this instance, associated with prolongation of the AV interval well above any normal duration.

Retrograde or ventriculoatrial conduction positions the atrial contraction after the ventricular contraction, effectively reversing the normal pathway of cardiac depolarization. In the normal, cardiac depolarization begins at the sinoatrial (SA) node, followed by the depolarization of the atrium, the AV node, bundle of His, and ventricle. During ventricular pacing only, this pathway is reversed. The right ventricular apex is first depolarized and (assuming the absence of any block of the conduction pathway) the SA node is depolarized last.

The hemodynamic effect of retrograde conduction occurs because of the prolonged AV interval between the atrial contraction and the next ventricular contraction. For example, VVI pacing at 70 bpm (interval of 857 ms) associated with consistent retrograde conduction at an interval of 300 ms will produce an effective AV interval of 557 ms. Such an AV interval is associated with substantial reduction of cardiac output and in many (but not all) patients, the symptomatic concomitants of pacemaker syndrome. It is a common observation that retrograde atrial entrainment occurs with less symptomatic compromise at more rapid rate modulated ventricular rates. In a patient as above, pacing at 100 bpm (interval of 600 ms) is likely to be associated with a longer retrograde interval, i.e., 350 ms. As the stimulation interval is 600 ms, the AV delay produced will be only 250 ms, within a more normal and therefore less symptomatic timing relationship. For example, pacing at 100 bpm (cycle length ms) with retrograde conduction at 160 ms produces an effective AV delay of 440 ms. Correction may be achieved by converting to dual-chamber pacemaker operation (Figure 36).

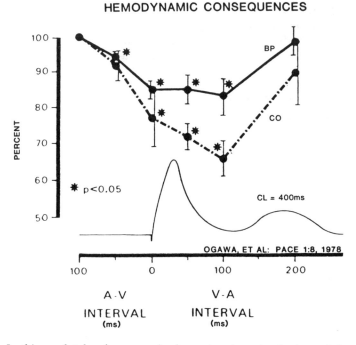

Figure 36. *In this graph taken from an animal experiment, pacing is at a cycle length of 400 ms (150 bpm). Cardiac output and blood pressure fall at AV intervals of less than 50 ms in duration and are most pronounced at VA intervals of 100 ms, decreasing as the VA interval is prolonged. Different intervals would exist in humans, although the overall effect would be similar. (Courtesy of Dr. Leonard Dreifus.)*

A prolonged AV delay may be produced in several other ways. During atrial (AAI) pacing alone, the AV delay may be prolonged, even at lower rates (i.e., 60 bpm) and especially at higher rates. If AV conduction is sufficiently prolonged, an AV interval of 300–500 ms may be produced with the P wave early after the conducted QRS, yielding the same effect as in retrograde conduction described above (Figure 37). Actual retrograde conduction is not required. Correction is accomplished by conversion to dual-chamber pacing in which ventricular stimulation allows programming the AV delay.

An alternative mechanism is the presence of a retrograde conduction with a programmed low upper rate limit. (See Chapter 4, Figure 32.) With an upper rate interval of 400 ms (150 bpm), the AV delay following a retrograde atrial beat is about 150 ms. When the upper rate interval is increased to 480 ms (125 bpm), the AV delay becomes 200 ms, and when the upper rate interval is 600 ms (100 bpm), with the retrograde conduction interval remaining constant, the effective AV delay is forced to prolong, in this instance to about 380 ms, as a programmed upper rate interval of 600 ms (100 bpm) prohibits a ventricular channel stimulus from occurring sooner than 600 ms after a previous ventricular channel stimulus. In this instance the AV interval can be markedly prolonged in the presence of DDD pacing. This effect is most visible during pseudo-Wenckebach operation with a large disparity between the programmed upper rate limit

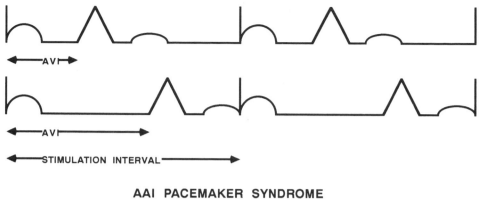

AAI PACEMAKER SYNDROME
(PROLONGATION OF AV INTERVAL)

Figure 37.   *This diagram demonstrates atrial pacing with prolonged PR interval caused by first-degree AV block. (Top) The AV interval is of relatively normal duration and is followed by a ventricular depolarization. (Bottom) AV conduction is prolonged. As the atrial stimulation rate is fixed, (and even if it is rate modulated) the P wave precedes the QRS such that it acts as if it were a retrograde P wave.*

interval and the upper rate limit based on atrial refractoriness. That time disparity, termed the pseudo-Wenckebach interval is moved, during upper rate limit operation, into the AV interval, prolonging it beyond its programmed value. Correction is accomplished by programming an upper rate limit sufficiently high so that the programmed AV delay can be maintained.

Still another mechanism for the prolongation of the AV delay exists during operation of a DDI pacemaker. Despite differences in blanking and refractory intervals, the DDI mode can be considered to be a DDD mode in which the upper and lower rate limits are identical. This then becomes the limiting case of low upper rate limit pacing of a DDD pacemaker. Consider, for example, that the DDI pacing rate is 70 bpm (857 ms), retrograde conduction occurs 350 ms after the ventricular stimulus, and the atrial refractory interval after the ventricular event is 325 ms in duration. The retrograde P wave will be sensed and inhibit an atrial channel stimulus, but the ventricular channel stimulus must be delayed until the lower rate limit has elapsed (857 ms) producing an effective AV delay of 507 ms (Figure 38). Correction may be difficult in this instance as the reason for selecting the DDI mode was, presumably, the desire to maintain AV synchrony at a low upper rate limit. Still, if a moderately higher upper rate limit can be tolerated, then every millisecond (ms) subtracted from the upper rate limit interval (increasing the upper rate limit) can also be subtracted from the total duration of the AV delay.

In any of these mechanisms the normal operation of the single- or dual-chamber pacemaker produces a sufficiently prolonged AV delay so that hemodynamics are disturbed. Retrograde conduction is required for some of the mechanisms, such as in ventricular pacing or low upper rate DDD or DDI pacing. During AAI pacing with prolonged first-degree AV block, retrograde conduction is not necessary. In effect, the typical arrhythmia of DDD pacing associated with

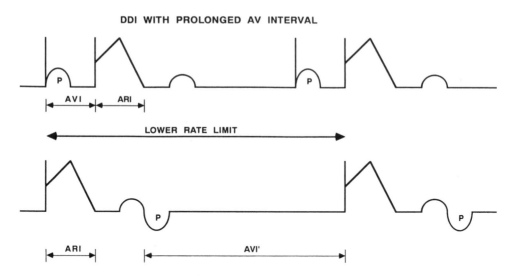

DDI WITH PROLONGED AV INTERVAL

Figure 38. During DDI pacing the atrium is sensed and the atrial channel output may be inhibited, but an AV interval is not begun. If the atrial rate is less than the lower limit of the pacemaker (above) then an atrial channel stimulus will be followed by the ventricular channel stimulus at the programmed AV interval (above). If a ventricular contraction is followed by a retrograde P wave that falls after the end of the atrial refractory period, it will inhibit atrial channel output, but the ventricular stimulus will fall at the end of the lower rate limit (escape interval) yielding a very prolonged AV interval (below).

retrograde conduction is the endless loop tachycardia, while the typical arrhythmia of DDI pacing with retrograde conduction is the marked prolongation of the AV delay with pacemaker syndrome.

INTERATRIAL CONDUCTION DURING CARDIAC PACING

DDD pacemakers sense and pace right-sided chambers of the heart. The activity and timing of the left atrium and left ventricle are only inferred from the sensing of right-sided events. The relationship of left-sided atrial and ventricular systole is most important for systemic hemodynamics, and effective atrioventricular synchrony is partially determined by the interatrial conduction time (IACT). At the time of DDD pacemaker implantation, interatrial conduction can be measured with an intraesophageal pill electrode to determine left atrial depolarization and to detect right atrial depolarization from the right atrial appendage. During stimulation of the right atrial appendage, the interatrial conduction time can thus be measured from the right atrial stimulus to the left atrial response. Mean interatrial conduction time for all patients is 95 ± 18 ms during sinus rhythm and 122 ± 30 ms during right atrial pacing (P>0.001). This confirms the finding described above of the difference in AV interval between paced and sensed AV interval. In patients with P wave duration less than 110 ms, interatrial conduction prolonged from 85 ± 10 ms during sinus rhythm to 111 ± 9 ms during right atrial pacing (P<0.01) compared to 114 ± 20 ms prolonging to 141 ± 17 ms (P<0.01) in those patients with a P wave duration greater than 110 ms. In each

Table I
Relative Constancy of Interatrial Conduction Time (IACT) with Increasing Rate of Atrial Stimulation

	Sinus Rhythm		Atrial Pacing			
Rate (bpm)	65	80	100	120	140	160
IACT (ms)	95	115	118	120	122	122

Values in this table were obtained from results of 20 patients who were studied at all of the listed pacing rates.

patient, atrioventricular conduction prolonged with incremental right atrial pacing, but interatrial conduction times did not vary.

Interatrial conduction prolongs from the sinus rhythm baseline during atrial pacing, probably because of a latent interval between the stimulus and the local atrial depolarization, and remains constant at all paced rates from 60–160 bpm (Table I). In addition to longer interatrial conduction times during sinus rhythm, patients with electrocardiographic P wave prolongation have longer interatrial conduction times during right atrial pacing than do normals (P<0.001). Based on interatrial conduction times alone, the AV interval during DDD cardiac pacing with right atrial stimulation should be approximately 25 ms longer than when the atrium is tracked (Figures 39–41).

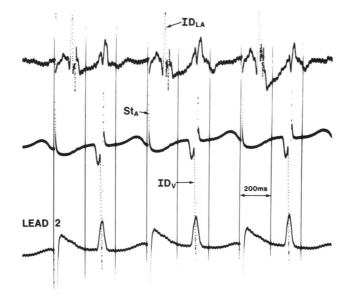

Figure 39. *Intracardiac and surface recordings during pacing from the right atrial appendage. The upper tracing was recorded from the esophageal pill electrode; middle tracing from right ventricular electrode; and lower tracing from surface ECG lead 2. Interatrial conduction time was measured during atrial pacing from the atrial pacing stimulus (St$_A$) to the ID$_{LA}$.*

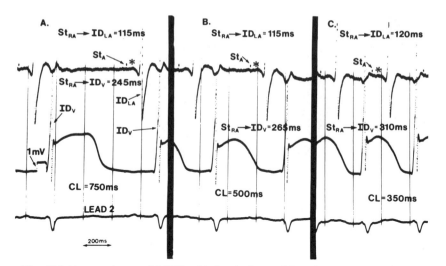

Figure 40. *Relative constancy of IACT with increasing atrial pacing rates. In all three panels, upper tracing was recorded from intraesophageal pill electrode, middle tracing from right ventricular electrode, and bottom tracing from surface ECG lead 2. Interatrial conduction time measured from $St_{RA} \rightarrow ID_{LA}$ and noted with an asterisk (*) in the tracings was approximately the same (115–120 ms) despite increasing the atrial pacing rate from 80 bpm (panel A: cycle length [CL] = 750 ms) to 120 bpm (panel B: CL = 500 ms) to 170 bpm (panel C: CL = 350 ms). Atrioventricular conduction (measured from $St_{RA} \rightarrow ID_V$) Prolonged with decreasing cycle lengths.*

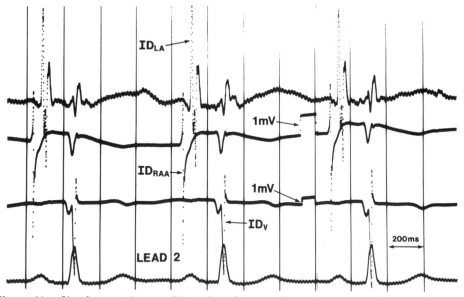

Figure 41. *Simultaneous intracardiac and surface recordings during sinus rhythm. The upper tracing was recorded from an intraesophageal pill electrode demonstrating the intrinsic deflection (ID) of the left atrial (LA) signal. The second tracing is from an electrode in the right atrial appendage (RAA) and records right atrial activity. The third tracing, recorded from an electrode in the right ventricular apex, shows the ventricular intrinsic deflection (ID_V) coinciding with the QRS complex recording on the surface ECG lead 2 on the bottom tracing. The ID_{LA} comes at a fixed interval after the ID_{RAA} during sinus rhythm and both are coincident with the P wave on the surface ECG. Interatrial conduction time was measured during sinus rhythm from onset of the P wave in surface ECG lead 2 to ID_{LA}.*

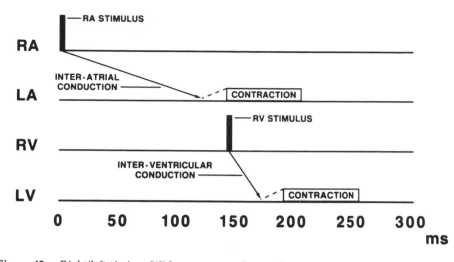

Figure 42.   *Right/left timing. With a programmed AVI of 150 ms from right atrial (RA) to right ventricular (RV) pacing stimulus, the relationship of left atrial (LA) to left ventricular (LV) contraction is dependent on interatrial conduction and to a lesser degree on interventricular conduction (represented as arrows). The electromechanical delay is depicted by the dotted lines.*

Several factors should be considered when determining the optimum programmable AV interval during DDD pacing. Among them is the interatrial conduction time (IACT). The IACT influences the relationship between left atrial filling and contraction on the one hand, and left ventricular systole on the other (Figure 42). Interatrial conduction time prolongs during atrial pacing from values obtained during sinus rhythm and remains constant in the face of increasing atrial pacing rates. This prolongation presumably represents (right-sided) intra-atrial propagation of the pacing stimulus that prolongs only minimally at increasing pacing rates. This data correlates well with earlier studies in which patients with normal P waves have had interatrial conduction times measured at 77 ± 8 ms via coronary sinus catheters compared to the present value of 95 ± 18 ms. Patients with prolonged P waves on the surface electrocardiogram had prolonged interatrial conduction times also comparable to previously reported values (112 ± 14 ms vs 122 ± 30 ms). Of most importance is the recognition that interatrial conduction times have been constant in all studies and that a differential of approximately 25 ms between the allowed interatrial conduction time when the patient's atrial depolarization is sensed and when atrial depolarization is stimulated will produce approximately equal hemodynamic intervals.

PACEMAKER VARIATION OF AV INTERVAL

The AV interval during dual-chambered pacing can vary in four separate ways:

1. A paced atrial event to a sensed ventricular event;
2. An atrial stimulus followed by an AV interval and a ventricular stimulus;

AV PACING SEQUENCES

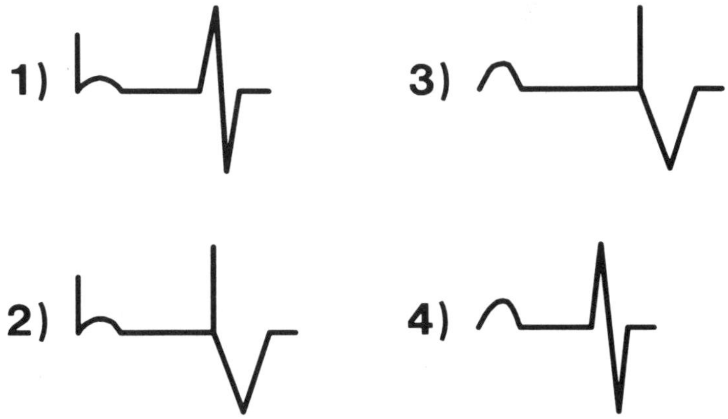

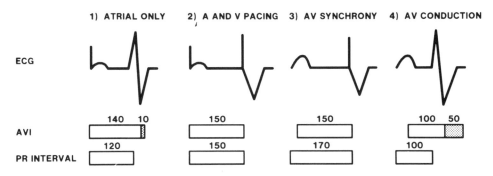

Figure 43. *Four possible timing cycles exist during dual-chamber pacing. These are: (1) atrial stimulation with AV conduction; (2) atrial and ventricular stimulation; (3) atrial sensing and ventricular stimulation; (4) atrial sensing and ventricular sensing. The hemodynamic AV interval of the four circumstances differs. In order to have equivalent AV intervals for hemodynamics, the intervals for each of the paced to sensed events must vary.*

Figure 44. *AV/PR intervals. The diagrammatic representation of variation in AV timing based on an unvarying programmed AV interval of 150 ms shows significant variation in the PR or physiological interval. (1) In the presence of AV conduction at a shorter interval than allowed (i.e., 150 ms), the PR interval will be briefer than programmed; (2) during pacing of both atrium and ventricle, the interval between both stimuli will be as programmed; (3) if the timing cycle begins with a sensed atrial event and ends with a paced ventricular event, the effective PR interval will be prolonged; while (4) in the presence of both atrial and ventricular sensing, the effective PR interval may be the shortest of all.*

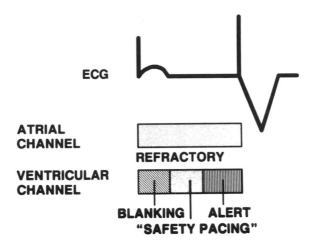

Figure 45. *AV interval. During pacing the AV interval is broken down into several subintervals. Commonly, these are a brief blanking interval in which the atrial stimulus cannot inhibit ventricular output, followed in some pacemakers by a "safety pacing" interval in which a sensed event, whether an atrial stimulus, a VPC, or noise produces a "committed" stimulus at some time thereafter, allowing some sensing but avoiding ventricular stimulation, and then a fully alert interval in which a sensed event normally recycles the pacemaker.*

3. A sensed atrial event to a paced ventricular event;
4. A sensed atrial event to a sensed ventricular event (Figures 43–45).

The hemodynamic consequences of these four circumstances are distinctly different. As indicated in the text (concerning interatrial conduction time), the conduction between the right atrium and left atrium is prolonged if a timing cycle starts at an atrial stimulus rather than starting at a sensed atrial event. Several available DDD pacemakers have pairs of programmable AV intervals: one for timing cycles that start with an atrial stimulus, the other with a sensed atrial event. Because of latency following atrial stimulation and latency following ventricular stimulation, a difference of approximately 50 ms will produce the most appropriate timing cycle. Dual AV intervals of this variety are appropriate, especially at more rapid atrial rates where stimulation does not occur and sensing is continuous. Determination of hemodynamics as a function of AV interval should always be performed with the knowledge of whether the AV interval has been started by a paced or a sensed event and ends with a paced or sensed event.

ABBREVIATION OF THE AV INTERVAL

Atrioventricular intervals (AVI) may prolong via the mechanism of pseudo-Wenckebach upper rate limitation and may vary because of atrial and ventricular sensing or pacing. AV intervals may also be abbreviated via several mechanisms during normal pacemaker operation. This is an attempt to mimic the normal abbreviation of the AV interval with increasing rate. These should not be misinterpreted as pacemaker malfunction.

1. Rate Modulated AV Interval In the past few years ratemodulation of the A9 interval has become available on rate modulated dual-chamber (DDDR) and more conventional dual-chamber (DDD) pacemakers. During such operation there may be two or more possible AV intervals. Usually the longer interval occurs between the lower rate limit and some intermediate rate, such as 100 bpm at which a briefer AV interval may be associated with atrial sensing or pacing. At still higher atrial rates still briefer AV intervals may exist. The customary rate modulation of the AV interval is a step function as above, though there is no reason that continuous variation may not eventually exist (Figure 41, Chapter 11).

2. Premature Ventricular Beat in the AV Interval A P wave may start the normal timing cycle in a DDD/VDD pacemaker. An early premature ventricular beat, entirely independent of the atrial event, may fall into the pacemaker AV interval to inhibit ventricular output and recycle. The apparent AV interval will be correspondingly abbreviated (Figure 46).

3. VDD Operation During normal operation of one variety of VDD mode, the lower rate limit (i.e., the ventricular escape interval) has precedence over the AV interval. Should the sensed P wave occur sufficiently late that establishment of the programmed AV interval will prolong the ventricular escape interval, that escape will occur at the lower rate limit and the AV interval will be abbreviated (Figure 47). The alternate mode of VDD operation gives the AV interval precedence over the lower rate limit, and the emission of a ventricular stimulus will begin an AVI and prolong the ventricular escape interval, producing a lower rate. In such an instance the lower rate interval might be, for example 1000 ms, i.e., 60 bpm and the AV interval, 200 ms. In the first instance the longest interval between ventricular stimuli must be 1000 ms, i.e., 60 bpm. In the latter the lower rate interval may be prolonged to 1200 ms, a rate of 50 bpm.

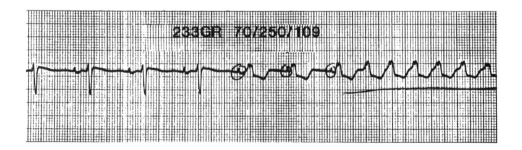

Figure 46. *Abbreviation of the AV interval can also occur with the beginning of a ventricular tachycardia in which three ventricular premature contractions fall during the AV interval and inhibit and recycle the pacemaker. Thereafter the tachycardia accelerates and inhibits pacemaker output and clarifies the nature of the "abbreviated" AV interval.*

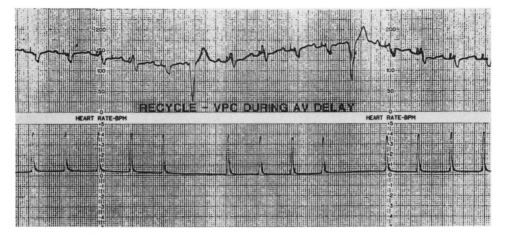

Figure 47. *This Holter recording with a single ECG channel above and the pacemaker stimuli shown below demonstrates intermittent ventricular capture. In addition, two ventricular premature contractions (center and right-center) occur during the AV interval following a P wave, causing pacemaker recycle and a shortened AV interval.*

4. Crosstalk Crosstalk is the sensing of the output of one channel by the other. In practice, the output of the atrial channel is that which may be sensed by the ventricular channel, misinterpreted for a spontaneous ventricular event, and produce ventricular asystole. This can occur in two ways. The atrial or ventricular lead may be displaced either because of deficient fixation at the point of introduction or for any of the other reasons for displacement of either lead. If the two leads are in proximity it becomes more likely that atrial output will be sensed by the ventricular channel. This variety of event is more likely during temporary compared to implanted pacing. During implanted pacing unipolar leads project the stimulus over a larger field so that crosstalk is more likely when compared to bipolar stimulation that projects across a more restricted field. As high an incidence of crosstalk as 21% has been observed in some unipolar DDD pacemakers. Nevertheless, crosstalk with bipolar implanted pacing does occur. In model 284–02, a model using bipolar sensing and unipolar pacing, an incidence of 17% of crosstalk has been observed. Crosstalk has been observed in other dual-chamber pacemaker systems. In the instance of some unipolar and bipolar devices, crosstalk exists within the circuit so that proximity of the electrodes and high output are not necessary to allow crosstalk to occur (Figure 48).

As ventricular asystole is potentially lethal, it must be absolutely avoided (Figure 49). Two approaches have been designed into the pulse generator. One is the duration of ventricular channel insensitivity beginning with the emission of the atrial stimulus. This is the blanking period. A blanking period is one of insensitivity to avoid sensing of a hardware event; a refractory period is one designed to avoid sensing a physiological event, e.g., a retrograde P wave. In some devices the ventricular blanking period beginning with the atrial stimulus is fixed in duration, in others it is programmable.

The second approach is that of **safety pacing** or **nonphysiological AV delay** in which the sensing of an early event in the early portion of the AV interval following the atrial stimulus and the end of the blanking period produces an early ventricular channel stimulus (Figure 50). In one formulation, the blanking

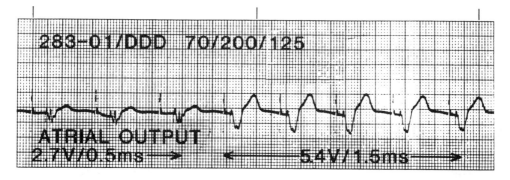

Figure 48. *Crosstalk is shown with the nonphysiological AV interval compared to the programmed duration. To the left the output was 2.7 V and 0.5 ms, a moderate output which is not sensed in the ventricular channel and does not cause AV interval shortening. To the right a higher output of 5.4 V and ms pulse duration was programmed. This output was sensed in the ventricular channel and the AV interval consequently reduced in duration.*

period is brief, 12–16 ms. This is followed by a safety pacing interval during which a sensed event in the ventricular channel (the atrial channel is refractory during the entire AVI) produces a ventricular channel stimulus 110 ms later. This mechanism may abbreviate the programmed AV, increase the actual stimulation rate of the pacemaker by reducing the interval between stimuli, and even produce pacemaker syndrome if the duration of the abbreviated AV interval is too short (the latter is not common). the rate of stimulation in ventricular based timing results from the duration of the AV interval and the ventricular escape interval, the effective abbreviation of the AVI because of crosstalk may produce an occult increase in pacemaker rate. Should safety pacing or nonphysiological AV delay not be operational, crosstalk may, nevertheless abbreviate the AVI and a conducted ventricular event may begin the VA escape interval producing an overall abbreviated cycle length and, therefore, an increase in rate. A similar mechanism in other dual-chamber devices is named the nonphysiol-

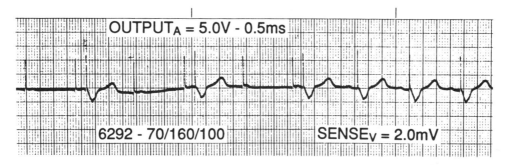

Figure 49. *In the absence of a safety response such as "safety pacing" or "nonphysiological AV delay" inhibition of ventricular channel output is possible with serious consequences. Atrial output of 5 V and 0.5 ms is moderately high but not beyond that of common programming. The sensitivity of 2 mV is a common setting. Atrial pacing causes a P wave and inhibition of ventricular output.*

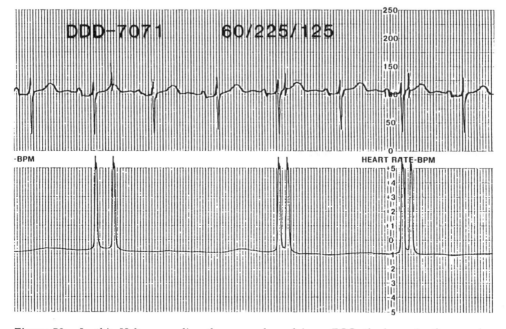

Figure 50. *In this Holter recording the upper channel is an ECG, the lower is of pacemaker stimuli. Because of atrial undersensing some atrial stimuli fall directly on the QRS complex (first stimulated pair) and because the QRS intrinsic deflection falls during ventricular blanking, the programmed AV interval (225 ms) is allowed to occur. In other situations the QRS intrinsic deflections falls milliseconds thereafter in the safety pacing interval. This causes the abbreviated AV interval (second and third paced pairs).*

ogical AV delay. The interval between sensing the event defined as crosstalk and the response may be programmed in duration, so that anticipated crosstalk may not produce an abbreviated AVI.

The means of ending crosstalk are the following:

1. **Programmable blanking**—The repolarization of an atrial stimulus may be sensed following the end of the blanking period. A programmable blanking period may be prolonged.
2. **Safety pacing**—Safety pacing may be programmed **on** or **off** in some models. In others it is always present as a nonprogrammable feature.
3. **Nonphysiological AV delay**—As with safety pacing.
4. **Reduce atrial channel output**—A reduced atrial channel amplitude is less likely to be sensed in the ventricular channel. Crosstalk may occur following increase in atrial channel output required by high threshold. If so, this mechanism may not be available.
5. **Reposition a lead**—If the atrial and ventricular leads are too close, then repositioning the atrial higher into the atrial appendage or the ventricular further into the right ventricular apex may resolve the problem. If the leads are already properly positioned, this may not be possible.
6. **Reduce ventricular sensitivity**—As crosstalk is based on ventricular sensing of atrial activity, reducing the sensitivity of the ventricular channel may be sufficient to eliminate sensing of the atrial stimulus while retaining sensitivity

to conducted or ectopic ventricular activity. In rare and carefully considered instances an asynchronous ventricular channel may be considered.

7. **Committed AV interval**—A committed AV interval is one in which the ventricular channel is refractory during the entire interval between the atrial stimulus and the ventricular stimulus, i.e., if an atrial stimulus is emitted a ventricular channel stimulus is "committed." This approaches the ultimate blanking interval and clearly can be competitive with a premature ventricular beat or a conducted ventricular beat at an interval briefer than the programmed AV interval. This mode is a programmable option in some DDD pacemakers and the only mode of operation in others. It was in clinical use in earlier "committed" DVI pacemakers.

8. **Reduction in frequency of atrial stimulation**—If the rate of atrial stimulation has been set relatively rapidly, i.e., 70–80 bpm, stimulation may occur frequently, especially with the patient at rest. If the lower rate of atrial stimulation is reduced to 40–50 bpm it is less likely that atrial channel stimulation will occur. As the occurrence of crosstalk requires atrial channel stimulation it will not occur in the absence of such stimulation.

9. **Pulse generator replacement**—If crosstalk cannot be eliminated by any of the listed mechanisms, programming to single-chamber pacing, atrial only if possible, or ventricular only may be attempted. Finally, a different pulse generator may be more resistant.

BIBLIOGRAPHY

Antonioli GE, Grassi G, Baggioni GF, et al: A simple P-sensing ventricle stimulating lead driving a VAT generator. In C Meere (ed.): Cardiac Pacing. Pace Symp Montreal Canada 1979, chaps 34–39.

Aubert AE, Ector H, Denis BG, et al: Sensing characteristics of unipolar and bipolar orthogonal floating atrial electrodes: Morphology and spectral analysis. PACE 1986; 9:343–359.

Ausubel K, Klementowicz P, Furman S: The AV interval in DDD cardiac pacing. CPEP 1986; 4:60–66.

Bagwell P, Pannizzo F, Furman S: Unipolar and bipolar right atrial appendage electrodes: Comparison of sensing characteristics. Med Instrum 1985; 19:132–135.

Barold SS, Gaidula JJ: Failure of demand pacemaker from low-voltage bipolar ventricular electrograms. JAMA 1971; 215:923.

Breivik K, Engedal H, Ohm OJ: Electrophysiological properties of a new permanent endocardial lead for uni- and bipolar pacing. PACE 1982; 5:268–274.

Breivik K, Ohm OJ: Myopotential inhibition of unipolar QRS-inhibited (VV) pacemakers assessed by ambulatory Holter monitoring of the electrocardiogram. PACE 1980; 3: 470–478.

Brownlee RR: Toward optimizing the detection of atrial depolarization with floating bipolar electrodes. PACE 1989: 12:431–442.

Castillo C, Castellanos A: Retrograde activation of the His bundle in the human heart. Am J Cardiol 1971; 27:264–271.

Castillo C, Samet P: Retrograde conduction in complete heart block. Br Heart J 1967; 29: 553–558.

Curzio G and the Multicenter Study Group: A multicenter evaluation of a single pass lead VDD pacing system. PACE 1991; 14:434–442.

DeCaprio V, Hurzeler P, Furman S: Comparison of unipolar and bipolar electrograms for cardiac pacemaker. Circulation 1977; 56:750–755.

Furman S, Gross J, Andrews C: Single-lead VDD pacing. In G Antonioli (ed.): Pacemaker Leads-1991 Ferrara, Italy. Amsterdam, Elsevier Science Publishers, 1991, pp. 183–197.

Furman S, Hurzeler P, DeCaprio V: Cardiac pacing and pacemakers. III. Sensing the cardiac electrogram. Am Heart J 1977; 93:794–801.

Furman S, Hurzeler P, DeCaprio V: The ventricular endocardial electrogram and pacemaker sensing. J Thorac Cardiovasc Surg 1977; 73:258–266.

Gabry MD, Behrens M, Andrews C, et al: Comparison of myopotential interference in unipolar-bipolar programmable DDD pacemakers. PACE 1987; 10:1322–1330.

Goldreyer BN, Olive AL, Leslie J, et al: A new orthogonbal lead for P synchronous pacing. PACE 1981; 4:638–644.

Griffin JC: Sensing characteristics of the right atrial appendage electrode. PACE 1983; 6: 22–25.

Griffin JC, Finke WL Jr: Analysis of the endocardial electrogram morphology of isolated ventricular beats. PACE 1983; 6:315 (abstract).

Kleinfeld M, Barold SS, Rozanski JJ: Pacemaker alternans: A review. PACE 1987; 10:924–933.

Klementowicz PT, Furman S: Selective atrial sensing in dual chamber pacemakers eliminates endless loop tachycardia. JACC 1986; 7:590–594.

Klementowicz PT, Furman S: Stability of atrial sensing and pacing after dual-chamber pulse generator implantation. JACC 1985; 6:1338–1341.

Longo E, Catrini V: Experience and implantation techniques with a new single-pass lead VDD pacing system. PACE 1990; 13:927–936.

McAlister HF, Klementowicz PT, Calderon EM, et al: Atrial electrogram analysis: Antegrade versus retrograde. PACE 1988; 11:1703–1707.

Mymin D, Cuddy TE, Sinha SN, et al: Inhibition of demand pacemakers by skeletal muscle potentials. JAMA 1973; 223:527.

Nielsen AP, Cashion R, Spencer WH, et al: Long-term assessment of unipolar and bipolar stimulation and sensing thresholds using a lead configuration programmable pacemaker. JACC 1985; 5:1198–1204.

Ohm OJ, Bruland H, Pedersen OM, et al: Interference effect of myopotentials on function of unipolar demand pacemakers. Br Heart J 1974; 36:77–84.

Pannizzo F, Amikam S, Bagwell P, et al: Discrimination of antegrade and retrograde atrial depolarization by electrogram analysis. Am Heart J 1986; 112:780–786.

Pannizzo F, Furman S: Automatic discrimination of retrograde p waves for dual chamber pacemakers. JACC 1985; 5:393.

Pannizzo F, Mercando AD, Fisher JD, et al: Automatic methods for detection of tachyarrhythmias by antitachycardia devices. JACC 1988; 11:308–316.

Secemsky SI, Hauser RG, Denes P, et al: Unipolar sensing abnormalities: Incidence and clinical significance of skeletal muscle interference and undersensing in 228 patients. PACE 1982; 5:10–19.

Tomaselli GF, Nielsen AP, Finke WL, et al: Morphologic differences of the endocardial electrogram in beats of sinus and ventricular origin. PACE 1988; 11:254–262.

Varriale P, Pilla AG, Tekriwal M: Single-lead VDD pacing system. PACE 1990; 13:757–766.

Wirtzfeld A, Lampadius M, Schmuck L: Unterdruckung von Demand-Schrittmachern durch Muskelpotentiale. Dtsch Med Wschr 1972; 97:61.

Wish M, Fletcher RD, Gottdiener JS: Importance of left atrial timing in the programming of dual-chamber pacemakers. Am J Cardiol 1987; 60:566–571.

Wish M, Gottdiener JS, Cohen AI, et al: M-mode echocardiograms for determination of optimal left atrial timing in patients with dual chamber pacemakers. JACC 1988; 11: 317–322.

Chapter 4

COMPREHENSION OF PACEMAKER TIMING CYCLES

Seymour Furman

All comprehension of pacemaker electrocardiography depends on the interpretation of pacemaker timing cycles. What should a pacemaker channel sense and when should an event be sensed? When is either the atrial or ventricular channel refractory to an incoming electrogram? When is it sensitive? If an event is sensed, what are the primary cycles, i.e., the lower and upper rate limits? What are the atrial and ventricular refractory intervals? When will an event remain unsensed and what will be the consequences? Timing cycles must be individually interpreted. Only collectively do they make up a pacing rate. When considering any timing cycles or analyzing any ECG for pacemaker function it is necessary to analyze function as a series of intervals between sensed or paced events rather than as a continuous rate. Rate is a relatively simple designation during continuous pacing or continuous inhibition but is of little worth and confusing if pacing and sensing alternate. Each event must be analyzed discretely. It must be recognized that rate is a continuum of a series of discontinuous events. Interpretation of the paced ECG has become considerably more difficult in the past few years with the advent of sensor drive, as well as dual-chamber pacing with atrial drive and pacemakers with both atrial and sensor drive simultaneously. Atrial based timing has also added a new dimension as ECG interpretation will be erroneous or impossible if the operation of the device is unknown or if incorrect assumptions are made. For example, during ECG interpretation, especially upper rate determination, it must be known whether the sensor drive is operative; whether atrioventricular interval (AVI) or atrial refractory interval (ARI) modulation with rate or both are operative; and whether the timing system used is atrial based, ventricular based, or modified atrial based, i.e., in which a conducted ventricular event is timed differently than a premature ventricular beat. The effect of all of these operational circumstances may not be apparent on ECG interpretation. For all of these circumstances the ECG interpretation channel has become far more important than ever before (see Chapter 16).

Both atrial and ventricular electrograms (EGMs) are readily sensed via the implanted lead system. Each different site in the heart, either atrium or ventricle, will have a different electrogram. The ECG is the sum of multiple electrograms recorded from the body surface. The ECG and EGM have different characteristics and those of one cannot be inferred from the other. The EGM of importance during cardiac pacing is that sensed by the lead system in the atrium and/or ventricle. Exact measurements of atrioventricular (AV) and ventriculoatrial (VA) conduction times can only be determined by recording and comparing the atrial and ventricular EGMs from one intrinsic deflection to the other. This can best be done during the procedure of pacemaker implantation.

TIMING CYCLES

All pacemaker timing cycles begin and/or end with a sensed intrinsic deflection or a pacemaker stimulus. If a chamber is not sensed, its electrical output (ID_A or ID_V) will not start a timing cycle and all timing in relation to the unsensed chamber will be initiated by the chamber sensed. In a DVI pacemaker, atrial activity (ID_A) is never sensed and never initiates a timing cycle. All timing thus originates from the sensing of the ventricle, i.e., ID_V. If the interval between a pacer stimulus or sensed intrinsic deflection and the next ventricular ID is less than the escape interval of the ventricular pacemaker channel, then the ventricular channel will be inhibited and a new timing cycle begun. In the single-chamber pacemaker, all timing cycles start and end by sensing the same chamber (Figure 1). In a ventricular sensing single-chamber pacemaker (VVI or VVT) that chamber determines all timing events. The generator is set at an escape interval between one event and another. The escape interval between any two events, sensed or paced, may be equal or two separate intervals may be set; one if the timing cycle is begun by a sensed event, the other if the timing cycle is begun by a pacer stimulus. Such variation is called hysteresis (Figure 2). The interval after the paced or sensed event which has begun a timing cycle is further divided into a refractory period, an insensitive portion of the interval, designed to avoid sensing the QRS complex (including the T wave) produced by a stimulus. It is usually 250–300 ms in duration for ventricular pacing, longer for atrial pacing and sensing (in order to avoid sensing the far-field ventricular complex). This is usually followed by an additional interval in which a sensed event is defined as noise and causes the emission of the pacemaker stimulus at the end of the

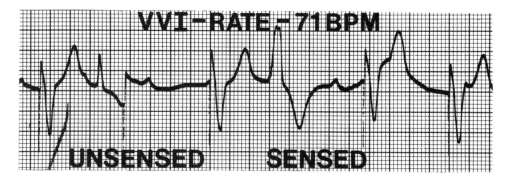

Figure 1. *The recycle of a ventricular inhibited pacemaker is always from the intrinsic deflection of the ventricular event. In this ECG the amplitude and/or the frequency content of the second QRS complex (the conducted beat) is inadequate to recycle the pacemaker and a ventricular stimulus falls harmlessly onto the T wave. The fourth QRS complex is a ventricular premature contraction which is sensed with pacemaker recycle at the escape interval: approximately 850 ms later. Pacemaker function is normal, the electrical quality of the conducted beat is inferior to that of the VPC and below the level of sensing.*

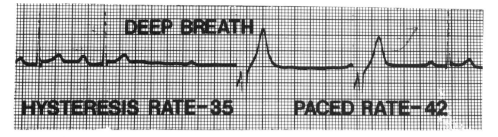

Figure 2. *The ECG of a patient with AV block is shown during a deep breath. the pacing rate was said to be at an interval of 1440 ms (42 bpm), while the onset was set at an interval of 1680 ms (25.7 bpm). Hysteresis available in implanted pacemakers allows a longer interval from the last sensed event to the first paced event than between successive paced events.*

escape interval, by extending the insensitive portion of the cycle through the normally sensitive period. Some designs make each of the three lesser intervals (refractory, noise sampling, and alert) a fixed proportion of the programmed interval between two events (i.e., the programmed pacemaker rate). In others only the sensitive interval is increased or decreased in duration by programming the rate; the refractory and noise sampling intervals are of fixed duration (Figure 3).

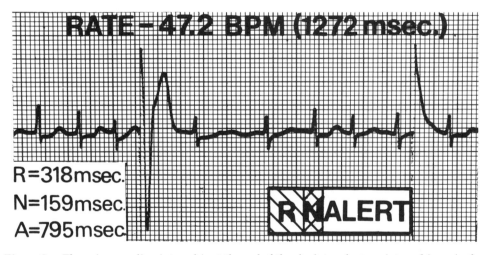

Figure 3. *The noise sampling interval is at the end of the absolute refractory interval in a single-chamber pacemaker, whether atrial or ventricular. Should a sensed event occur during the noise sampling interval, the emission of a stimulus at the escape interval will occur rather than being inhibited by succeeding sensed events during the pacemaker alert interval. In this ECG, both ventricular stimuli have been committed by previous QRS complexes, one of which fell during the noise sampling interval. Following the ventricular stimulus (left), the next QRS, approximately 600 ms later, inhibited and recycled the pacemaker. The second QRS once again inhibited and recycled the pacemaker. The third QRS fell during the noise sampling interval and forced pacemaker insensitivity during the alert interval. At its conclusion, the second ventricular stimulus was emitted competitively with a QRS. As the refractory interval and the noise sampling intervals are functions of the stimulus-to-stimulus interval, in some pulse generators the response seen above may be modified by changing the pacemaker interval (i.e., programming rate).*

If rate hysteresis is present and allows a longer interval after a sensed than a paced beat, the overall cardiac rate that inhibits such a generator will be lower (i.e., longer intervals between spontaneous cardiac events) than the pacing rate. Another version of pacemaker "hysteresis" provides a shorter interval after a sensed event thus attempting to preempt a tachycardia. In each instance, the difference between timing cycles may be a fixed amount or variable but is comprehensible only in terms of the interval between events.

DUAL-CHAMBER PACING

The single-chamber pacemaker has relatively simple timing cycles as described above. The dual-chamber pacemaker can be far more complex because, at maximum, the atrium and ventricle will both be sensed and will start timing cycles that will be both independent of each other but substantially interrelated. Each of the timing cycles begun by each chamber will have its own blanking, refractory, noise sampling, and alert periods. Both sets of timing cycles, atrial and ventricular, interact with the lower rate limit, which is similar to the interval that causes onset of pacing in a single-chamber unit. The lower rate limit is the longest duration without a sensed ventricular event that will be tolerated before a stimulus is emitted. In a VDD pacer, the escape will be by a ventricular stimulus. In a DVI or DDD pacemaker, escape will be by an atrial stimulus. As other intracardiac positions become timed during automatic management of tachyarrhythmias, timing cycles and their interrelationships will become evermore complex.

Both single- and dual-chamber rate modulated pacemakers have far more complex timing cycles than their single- and dual-chamber mates. Single-chamber (atrial or ventricular) rate modulated pacemakers have two sensing channels, one for the chamber and the second for the sensor. The system complexity is therefore greater than for a single rate single-chamber pacemaker. The rate modulated dual-chamber pacemakers have three sensing channels, atrium, ventricle, and sensor. Some have two sensors and atrial and ventricular sensing—four sensing channels in all. The timing cycle complexity for these units is far greater than in any earlier pacemakers. Such pacemaker function is described in Chapter 11, Rate Modulated Pacing.

The complexity of dual-chamber pacemaker timing is further enhanced by the programmability of the various portions of each timing cycle and of the mode of operation. Definitions of the various timing elements are necessary.

    a. Lower rate limit—the longest interval between sensed events without a pacemaker stimulus.

    b. Upper rate limit — the shortest interval between ventricular paced events or a sensed event followed by a paced event.

    c. AV interval — the interval between an atrial pace or sense event and the succeeding ventricular pace or sense event. It is the electronic analog of the PR interval. Some pacemakers have different AV intervals depending on whether the interval is begun by a sensed or paced atrial event, i.e., AV interval hysteresis. Others have an AV interval that abbreviates as either the sensor or atrial rate increases.

d. Atrial refractory interval — the interval after an atrial sense or pace event during which the atrial channel is insensitive to any incoming signal. The atrial refractory interval always consists of two consecutive portions, the AV interval and a time following a ventricular pace or sense event. The atrial refractory interval after a ventricular event may be fixed or programmable and may be equal whether preceded by an atrial event or not, i.e., it may be of longer duration when initiated by a ventricular premature contraction (Figure 4).

e. Ventricular refractory interval — the interval, after a ventricular pace or sense event during which the ventricular amplifier is insensitive to incoming signals (Figure 5). The ventricular refractory interval also sets the noise sampling period. During a rapid tachycardia, sensed QRS complexes may fall into the ventricular refractory interval, be unsensed and allow the pacemaker to function in the asynchronous and competitive or underdrive mode. While such an event normally occurs at very rapid tachycardia rates, approaching 200 bpm (if the ventricular refractory period is 300 ms), it is possible to lengthen the ventricular refractory interval so that slower rates will cause asynchronous stimulation especially if the duration of the refractory interval is linked to the pacing interval and changes with programmed rate. Producing competitive or "underdrive" pacing at the pacemaker "noise rate" during a tachycardia has been given the designation "dual demand" because pacing occurs if the spontaneous atrial or ventricular intervals are longer than the allowed lower rate limit, and if the tachycardia intervals are sufficiently short to fall into the prolonged refractory period. Several generators can have the programmed single-chamber (atrial or ventricular) refractory set to 437 ms after the ventricular event, effectively producing a "dual demand" upper rate or onset setting of 138 bpm. (See Automatic Mode Change, below).

The duration of the atrial refractory interval determines whether a specific atrial intrinsic deflection (P wave) will be sensed or not. It is obviously undesirable for a second atrial event to be sensed once the AV delay has begun. It is undesirable for an atrial event to be sensed early after the ventricular event

THE ATRIAL REFRACTORY PERIOD

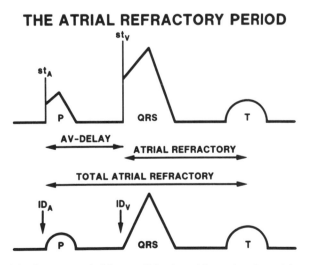

Figure 4. *The atrial refractory period (interval) begins with sensing the atrial event (here indicated at the beginning of the P wave) or the emission of the atrial stimulus. This instant also begins the AV interval, always refractory in the atrial channel. The ventricular event, paced or sensed, begins the atrial refractory interval after the ventricular event. Both of these independently programmable, but continuous events always comprise the total atrial refractory period (interval).*

THE VENTRICULAR REFRACTORY PERIOD

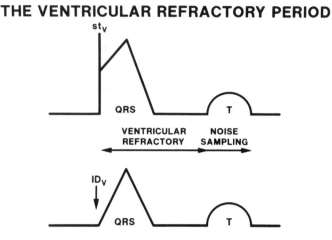

Figure 5.   *The ventricular refractory interval starts with the ventricular event. In some designs, the duration of the refractory interval may be shorter if the ventricular event is sensed than if a ventricular stimulus emitted. At the conclusion of the ventricular absolute refractory interval, a noise sampling interval occurs during which a sensed event causes the emission of the next scheduled stimulus.*

for two reasons. The first is that some limitation must exist on the brevity of the interval allowed between two sensed atrial events. If no lower limit of the interval existed, then the ventricle could be stimulated at an infinite rate. Thus, one use for the atrial refractory interval after a ventricular event is to limit the upper rate of pacemaker response (Figure 6). The second use is that it is possible to have a retrograde conducted P wave occur following ventricular

THE ATRIAL REFRACTORY PERIOD

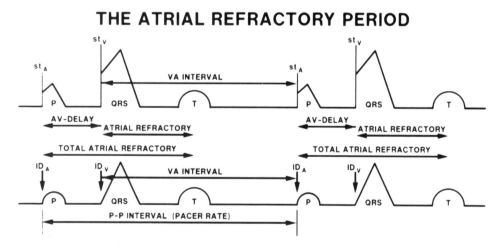

Figure 6.   *The diagrammatic representation is of two P-QRS sequences linked together, including the AV delay, atrial refractory interval. If the sensed P wave were to increase in rate, and therefore move progressively closer to the total atrial refractory interval, the upper rate of pacemaker response would be limited by the interval of total atrial refractoriness. Once the P wave entered a time of total atrial refractoriness it would be unsensed and would not begin a new cardiac cycle. The atrial refractory interval after the ventricular event is part of the total atrial refractory interval and establishes the upper rate limit.*

stimulation, even in the presence of fixed antegrade block. The atrial refractory interval after a ventricular event should be sufficiently long to eliminate sensing of such an atrial event. The elimination of sensing retrograde or aberrant atrial events and the setting of the level of the upper rate limit are the two critical functions of the atrial refractory period.

f. Blanking intervals — the need for accurate timing requires a clean signal from the chamber being sensed. It is particularly upsetting to satisfactory normal timing and recycle to sense an atrial stimulus via the ventricular channel or vice versa. The consequences can be disastrous if an atrial stimulus is sensed as a ventricular event via the ventricular channel. In that event, the ventricular channel may be inhibited producing ventricular asystole. A blanking interval is in place to avoid sensing pacemaker stimuli directed at one chamber in the opposite chamber. Blanking intervals can be considered as insensitive portions of the pacemaker cycle designed to avoid sensing hardware activity. Refractory intervals are insensitive to avoid sensing physiological activity.

UPPER RATE BEHAVIOR

During bradyarrhythmia management, a pacemaker rate is set below which the ventricular rate cannot fall. This lower rate limit (LRL), i.e., the longest interval a pacemaker will allow, is basic and obvious to pacemaker operation. Equally, a pacemaker that senses and tracks the atrium requires an upper rate limit (URL), i.e., the shortest interval (between ventricular stimuli or from a spontaneous QRS to the next ventricular stimulus) at which the pacemaker will stimulate the heart. This limit is mandatory to avoid sensing or responding to excessively rapid atrial events, such as atrial fibrillation or flutter or electromagnetic or myographic interference (EMI), to produce an excessively rapid ventricular response (Figure 7). Upper rate management incorporates efforts to limit the maximum rate while maintaining the benefits of atrial synchrony throughout a range that will provide physiological benefits for a wide range of patients. A young athlete who needs a pacemaker can tolerate and even require a ventricular rate of 175–200 bpm, i.e., ventricular coupling intervals of 300–343 ms, while the usual patient is better managed at a maximum ventricular rate of 100–150 bpm, a coupling interval of 400–600 ms. In both, the benefits of rate increase and of AV sequence are required.

A further complexity is that the implanted dual-chamber pacemaker functions as an AV conduction system, but it may not be the only functioning AV conduction system. The natural AV conduction system may function as an antegrade system or a retrograde system or both, continually or intermittently, while implantation of a dual-chamber pacemaker, which senses the atrium, is the equivalent of the implantation of an antegrade-only atrioventricular (AV) bypass tract. In managing the lower rate behavior (longest allowable interval), it is implicit that (at least) antegrade conduction by the natural AV system is interrupted or inactive. Retrograde conduction ability may be, paradoxically, intact. Pacemaker design criteria, therefore, include management under all of these circumstances. It has been recognized with the advent of dual-chamber pacemakers that the AV interval, the electronic analog of the PR interval, should be kept at physiological durations and AV interval modulation is now widely

EGM$_A$– ATRIAL FLUTTER

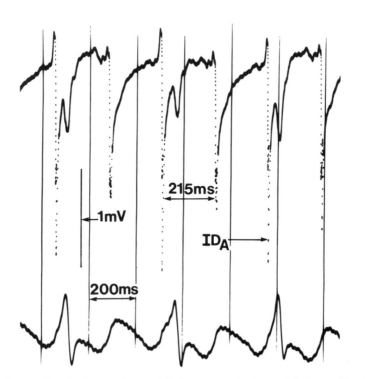

Figure 7. *A recording is shown of an atrial electrogram during atrial flutter. The intrinsic deflections are a cycle length of 215 ms (279 bpm) with each ID of adequate amplitude to be sensed by the atrial channel. The ventricular response is limited by the atrial refractory interval and the upper rate limit established independently of the atrial refractory interval in some pacemaker pulse generators.*

available. The upper rate design of each of these pacemakers must therefore accommodate all of the enumerated circumstances, i.e.,

1. Maximum rate, i.e., minimum interval appropriate for the patient;
2. Maintenance of AV synchrony;
3. Maintenance of the rate response of atrial tracking;
4. Avoidance of sensing retrograde P waves;
5. Gentle termination of a tachycardia produced by atrial arrhythmia, normal sinus activity or by sensing retrograde P waves.

The upper rate limit design is basic to all of these requirements. It must accommodate a single P wave or QRS, which may be sensed, and a continuous atrial or ventricular rate, which may be stable, accelerating, or decelerating. Avoidance of sensing of retrograde atrial P waves is, at present, only accomplished by making the atrial channel insensitive when the anticipated P wave is to occur. Selective sensing of the atrial EGM may be attempted. A variety of mechanisms have been developed, all based on this approach. Each of these mechanisms involves loss of AV synchrony either for a single or several P waves. Review of all timing cycles for all pacemaker systems is useful.

ATRIAL SENSING

Stability of Atrial Sensing

Atrial leads are somewhat less reliable than ventricular leads. Displacement from the atrial appendage occurs more commonly than from the right ventricular apex and atrial EGMs are far smaller than ventricular, so that slight decrease in atrial EGM amplitudes or slew rate may cross the line dividing adequate from insufficient sensing.

In evaluating the stability of atrial sensing and stimulation, patients were evaluated over the long-term, and it was found that stimulation threshold increased by about 40% from 3 days to 1 week after implant and remained elevated for 1 to 3 months, declining thereafter and remaining stable over a year of observation. Atrial sensitivity also remained stable though considerable patient variation existed. For 54% of patients atrial sensing either improved, i.e., a lesser sensitivity was necessary, or remained stable as measured during atrial sensitivity programming. Twenty-six percent of patients required higher sensitivity programming, while for 20% the sensitivity threshold fluctuated both up and down within the programmable sensitivity range. Thus atrial charge threshold tends to follow a predictable pattern while sensing is more erratic. Atrial electrograms have been found to decrease in amplitude during activity, further necessitating as large an atrial electrogram as possible to avoid loss of atrial sensing and atrial synchrony during exercise.

Selective Atrial Sensing

Whenever antegrade and retrograde atrial activation exist the amplitude of the antegrade atrial EGM is consistently larger than the retrograde event. While the reason for this difference is unclear, pacemaker sensitivity can be set to respond to antegrade atrial EGMs while rejecting retrograde EGMs. This circumstance allows the selective rejection of retrograde P waves and provides an additional means of avoiding a pacemaker-mediated tachycardia based on sensing of retrograde P waves and without the undue extension of atrial refractoriness.

TIMING INTERVALS OF DIFFERENT MODES OF PACEMAKER OPERATION

Asynchronous (VOO/AOO)

Only one timing interval exists, that between successive stimuli. While the duration of this interval may be varied, once set it is not modified by any sensed

VENTRICULAR ASYNCHRONOUS
(VOO)

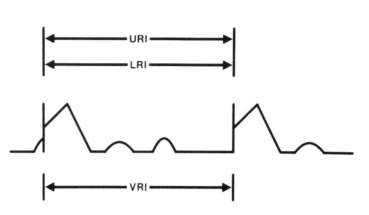

Figure 8. *During ventricular asynchronous (VOO) pacing there is no sensitivity to any cardiac activity. The upper and lower rates and ventricular refractory intervals are identical. Only the ventricle is stimulated. URI = upper rate interval; LRI = lower rate interval; VRI = ventricular refractory interval).*

event. As no sensing occurs, the upper and lower rate intervals are the same as the pacemaker escape interval (Figure 8).

AV Sequential Asynchronous (DOO)

Atrial and ventricular pacing is performed at fixed intervals between the atrial and ventricular stimuli and between the ventricular stimulus and the succeeding atrial stimulus. No sensing exists and no reset of timing occurs. Upper and lower rate and escape intervals are all equal (Figure 9).

Inhibited (VVI, AAI)

Stimulus emission is at the set escape rate in the absence of spontaneous activity. If spontaneous activity is sensed after the end of the pacemaker refractory interval, pacer output is inhibited and a new timing cycle begun. The new timing cycle may be of different duration depending on whether it was begun by a paced or sensed event. This differential timing is referred to as hysteresis. The lower and upper rate intervals may be equal unless hysteresis exists (Figures 10 and 11).

Triggered (VVT, AAT)

The same operation exists as in a single-chamber inhibited pacemaker. The difference is that a spontaneous cardiac event produces a pacemaker stimulus

AV ASYNCHRONOUS
(DOO)

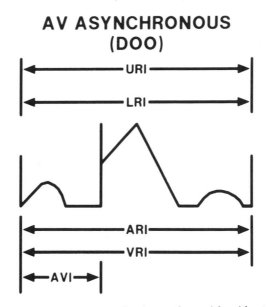

Figure 9. *AV sequential (DOO) pacing is of atrium and ventricle without sensing either chamber. The atrial and ventricular refractory intervals extend throughout the cardiac cycle. The upper rate interval (URI) and lower rate intervals (LRI) are equal, and both equal the atrial and ventricular refractory intervals. The atrial ventricular interval (AVI) is between the atrial refractory interval (ARI) and the upper rate interval (URI).*

VENTRICULAR INHIBITED
(VVI)

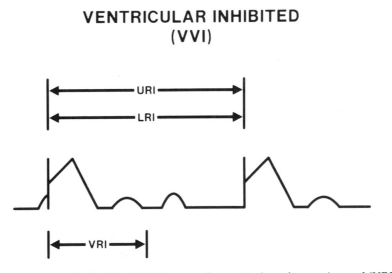

Figure 10. *In ventricular inhibited (VVI) pacing the ventricular refractory interval (VRI) extends for part of a cycle beginning with the ventricular event. During the ventricular alert interval, ventricular activity is sensed and can recycle the pulse generator. Upper rate and lower rate intervals are identical unless hysteresis is designed into the system.*

ATRIAL INHIBITED
(AAI)

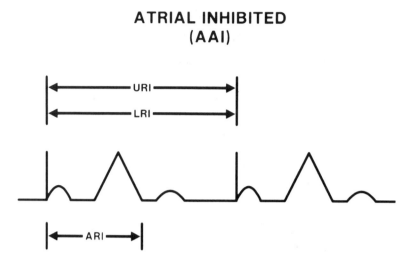

Figure 11.   *During atrial inhibited pacing, all timing cycles begin and end with the sensed atrial event. The upper and lower rate intervals are equal as pacemaker output is inhibited by the sensed atrial event. The atrial refractory interval starts with an atrial sensed or stimulated event and ends before the lower rate interval ends. This allows for an alert interval between the end of the atrial refractory interval and the end of the lower rate interval, when the next atrial stimulus must be emitted.*

onto the P or QRS, simultaneously with the intrinsic deflection. The unit is not inhibited. There is a lower rate interval (i.e., the pacemaker escape interval) and an upper rate interval beyond which the pacemaker will not respond to a sensed event.

AV Sequential Ventricular Inhibited (DVI)

The atrium is paced and then the ventricle is paced after a set AV interval (AVI). The atrium is never sensed and all cycles are begun by a ventricular pace or sense event. There are two different versions of this mode of operation; one allows ventricular sensing after the atrial stimulus (during the AVI), the other must stimulate the ventricle if the atrium is stimulated and is therefore referred to as "committed."

In the "noncommitted" version the timing cycle begins with the establishment of the AV interval upon emission of an atrial stimulus. As the atrium is never sensed, no timing cycle ever begins with atrial sensing. Sensing continues in the ventricular channel throughout the AV interval. A sensed ventricular event during the AV interval inhibits ventricular output and begins the fixed duration ventriculoatrial (VA) interval. The VA interval consists of the ventricular refractory interval during which no ventricular (and of course no atrial) activity will be sensed, and the ventricular alert interval during which ventricular activity will inhibit and recycle both atrial and ventricular channels. Once the ventricular event is sensed, the VA interval is begun. Competition between atrial stimuli and atrial contraction is possible if a P wave falls during the ventricular

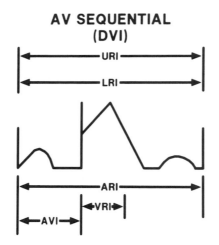

Figure 12. *The AV sequential (DVI) pacemaker has no atrial sensing, i.e., the atrial refractory interval (ARI) extends throughout the pacemaker timing cycle. As the ARI sets the upper rate interval (URI), the ARI and URI are equivalent and the pacemaker does not increase its rate in response to atrial activity. Only one rate exists for pacing, i.e., URI = LRI. The ventricular refractory interval (VRI) occurs after the ventricular event. Thereafter, the ventricular channel is alert, i.e., during the AVI, the interval between the atrial paced event and the ventricular paced or sensed event.*

refractory or alert intervals of the ventricular interval. Thus, there are two major intervals, the AV interval and the VA interval (Figure 12).

In the "committed" version of the AV sequential (DVI) pacemaker, a single timing cycle begins with the atrial stimulus. The ventricular channel is refractory during the AV interval and for the ventricular refractory interval thereafter. As the atrium is never sensed and the AV interval is refractory for both atrium and ventricle, this pacemaker has only one timing cycle that is begun by the ventricular pace or sense event. The single timing cycle may be of different duration depending on whether it starts from a pace or sense event (Figure 13). Both "committed" and "noncommitted" units can be competitive with atrial activity as the atrium is never sensed, but as an atrial stimulus forces a ventricular stimulus after the AV interval, a committed device is readily competitive with spontaneous ventricular activity (Figure 14).

All pacemakers that do not sense the atrium or if they do, then stimulate the ventricle (without tracking the atrium) have an upper rate limit interval that equals the stimulation interval. Except in the instance of pacemaker lower rate hysteresis (in which a longer interval without a sensed event is allowed than between two paced events), the lower rate interval equals the upper rate interval, which in turn equals the pacing interval and the pacemaker escape interval.

AV Sequential, Atrial, and Ventricular Inhibited (DDI)

An additional mode of pacer operation is analogous to the DVI mode in which the atrium is unsensed and all sensing and recycling derives from the

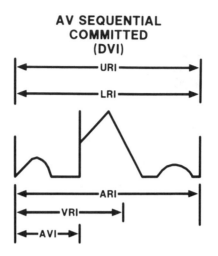

Figure 13. *The committed AV sequential (DVI) pacemaker has no atrial sensing, i.e., the atrial refractory interval (ARI) extends throughout the pacemaker timing cycle. It differs from the noncommitted DVI unit by extension of the ventricular refractory interval (VRI) throughout the AV interval (AVI). Consequently, once the atrial stimulus has been emitted, neither atrial nor ventricular sensing occurs during the AV interval. Absence of sensing of ventricular activity during the AV interval is the timing cycle difference between committed and noncommitted DVI modes.*

ventricular channel. The major benefit of the DVI mode is that the ventricular rate cannot increase above the programmed pacemaker rate because the atrium is unsensed and ventricular activity can inhibit both ventricular and atrial output. The major defect is that the atrium is not sensed and that therefore, pacemaker atrial channel activity can be competitive with spontaneous atrial activity. This is so because the emission of a ventricular stimulus in either the committed or

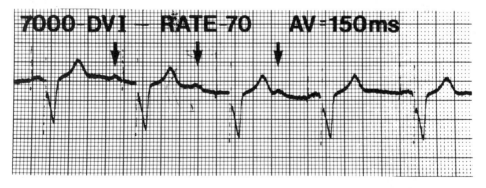

Figure 14. *Because of the lack of atrial sensing in the DVI mode, competition with spontaneous atrial activity can readily occur. If a ventricular stimulus is emitted, unless an event is sensed during the alert portion of the ventricular cycle, the next atrial stimulus must be emitted. In this instance, competition between spontaneous atrial activity and pacemaker stimuli in the atrial channel exists.*

noncommitted DVI modes forces the next atrial stimulus unless there is an intervening ventricular event that inhibits and recycles the generator.

In dual-chamber pacemakers that sense the atrium, a dual function traditionally has been present, atrial sensing with inhibition of atrial channel output and the start of the AV interval. This allows an increase in the ventricular stimulation rate in response to a sensed atrial event. In the DDI mode, sensing of the atrium only inhibits atrial channel output, it does not start an AV interval. Thus, a spontaneous P wave falling during the alert interval of the atrial cycle inhibits atrial output but does not start an AV interval and does not increase the ventricular rate in response to the atrial rate (Figure 15).

During DVI pacing, continuous stimulation in the ventricular channel will produce continuous stimulation in the atrial channel and, if the spontaneous atrial rate is more rapid than the pacemaker rate, competition with atrial activity will result. In the DDI mode, atrial activity will inhibit atrial channel output. In both DVI and DDI there is no ventricular rate response. If the atrial rate is slower than the pacemaker rate, AV synchrony is restored, and if the atrial rate is more rapid than the ventricular rate, competition occurs in DVI and does not occur in DDI pacing. The more rapid the atrial rate the less AV synchrony exists with either mode (Figure 16). Pacing rate change can occur in rate modulated dual-chamber pacemakers operation in the DDI (i.e., DDIR mode) so that while the atrium is not tracked it may be driven to an increase in rate by sensor drive. A very early P wave after a preceding QRS complex may inhibit the atrial channel without producing an AV interval. The P wave may then act, hemodynamically, as a retrograde atrial event producing an effective pacemaker syndrome (Figure 17).

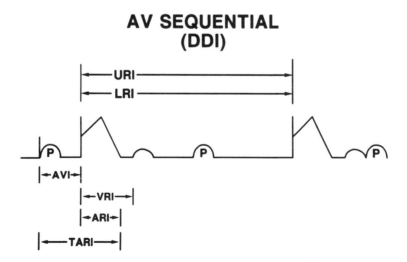

**AV SEQUENTIAL
(DDI)**

Figure 15.   *The AV sequential (DDI) mode differs from the DVI mode as the atrium is sensed. It differs from the DDD mode in that sensing a spontaneous atrial event does not begin a timing cycle, which must end with a sensed or paced ventricular event. Atrial competition is thus avoided, but the rate response of the DDD pacemaker is also avoided. An atrial event after the atrial refractory interval causes inhibition of atrial output but does not trigger a ventricular response.*

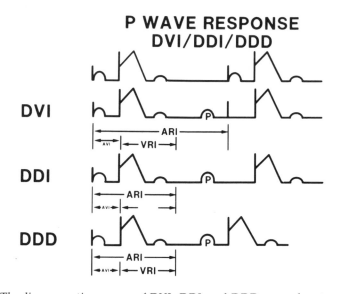

Figure 16. *The diagrammatic response of DVI, DDI, and DDD pacemakers to a spontaneous P wave shows that in DVI, a spontaneous P wave is unsensed and an atrial stimulus may occur at the atrial escape interval. In the DDI mode, the P wave is sensed and the atrial channel is inhibited and recycled, and an AV interval is not begun. In the DDD mode, the atrial channel output is inhibited, an AV interval is begun, and the ventricular rate is increased.*

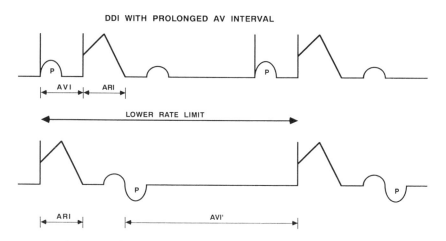

Figure 17. *Prolongation of the AV interval during DDI pacing can occur when an early P wave, spontaneous or following retrograde conduction, falls after the end of atrial refractoriness but well before the next ventricular escape. Atrial channel stimulation is inhibited, but the resultant interval between the sensed P wave and the ventricular channel stimulus may be so long that the effect is that of producing a sustained and entrained retrograde P.*

Atrial Synchronized (VAT)

This dual-chamber pacemaker senses the atrium and stimulates the ventricle. The ventricle is never sensed. There are two timing cycles. One cycle begins with the sensed atrial event. After the set AV interval the ventricular stimulus is emitted. If no P wave is sensed, stimulation returns to a second interval established between ventricular stimuli, the lower rate, or ventricular escape interval. The atrial refractory interval (ARI) (the upper rate limit interval) begins at atrial sensing and continues beyond the ventricular event. The upper rate limit may be set by the atrial refractory interval only or it may be set independently of the ARI, with the upper rate limit as one interval and the atrial refractory period as another yielding a pseudo-Wenckebach response at the upper rate limit. This was the first unit to sense only a single chamber in which both a lower rate limit interval between ventricular stimuli and an upper rate limit interval between ventricular events was required (Figure 18).

Management of the upper rate response is a problem in any pacemaker that senses the atrium. The problem existed in the atrial synchronous (VAT) pacemaker, which did not sense the ventricle, but as the unit is now obsolete, it need not be considered further. In modern devices, upper rate management is a problem for the atrial synchronous (VDD) and AV universal (DDD) pacemakers. These will be discussed and analyzed further.

AV SYNCHRONOUS
(VAT)

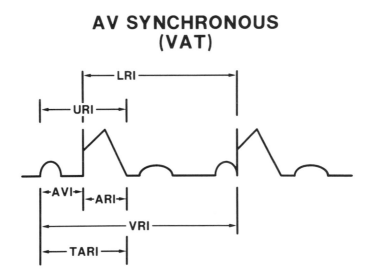

Figure 18. *Atrial synchronous pacing without ventricular sensing establishes an upper rate interval, which is equivalent to the duration of the total atrial refractory interval and a lower rate interval between ventricular events. The ventricular refractory interval (VRI) extends throughout the entire timing cycle so that ventricular sensing does not occur at any time.*

Atrial Synchronized, Ventricular Inhibited (VDD)

This dual-chamber pacemaker senses the atrium and paces and senses the ventricle. It is inhibited and recycled by a ventricular contraction. There are four major timing cycles:

1. The AV interval (AVI) starting at an atrial event;
2. The VA interval (VAI) starting at a ventricular pace or sense event;
3. The lower rate interval (LRI) between ventricular events;
4. The upper rate interval (URI) between ventricular events.

The AV, lower, and upper rate intervals begin with the sensed atrial event. During the AV interval the atrial channel is refractory, as it is for a time after the ventricular event. The ventricular pace or sense event begins the VA interval, of which the ventricular refractory interval and the atrial refractory interval are part. The atrial and ventricular refractory intervals are coincident in part, but one may be longer than the other. In the absence of atrial activity, the AV interval is not begun and ventricular stimuli are emitted at the ventricular lower rate interval—if no ventricular activity is sensed during the ventricular alert interval. The upper rate, at which atrial activity will be tracked, is limited by the sum of the atrial refractory interval before the ventricular event (the AV interval) and that after the ventricular event, which together add up to the total atrial refractory interval (Figure 19).

Formula 1

Atrial Refractory + AV Interval = Total Atrial Refractory
Interval   Interval
ARI   +   AVI   =   (TARI)

If, for example, the AV interval is fixed at 150 ms and the atrial refractory interval after a ventricular event is 250 ms, the total atrial refractory interval will be 400 ms and the maximum tracking rate 150 impulses per minute. Calculation of the upper rate interval, if the TARI is known, is by formula 2.

Formula 2

60,000/TARI = Upper Rate Limit (BPM)

Two different approaches exist for the upper rate limit. One is that of setting the upper rate limit independently of the TARI, the other is to set the TARI and allow the upper rate limit to result from the TARI. A consequence of the independent upper rate limit is the pseudo-Wenckebach mode in which the AV delay cannot be fixed but consumes the time differential between the TARI and the upper rate limit interval. While the AV interval cannot be abbreviated below its programmed setting (unless a nonconducted, aberrant, or early conducted contraction occurs), it can lengthen. In the AV block approach no prolongation of the AV delay occurs and a P wave that falls into any part of the TARI is unsensed, and sudden AV block results without previous lengthening of the AV interval (Figure 20). The pseudo-Wenckebach approach produces a plateau at the upper rate limit before AV block occurs. In both, a P wave that falls into

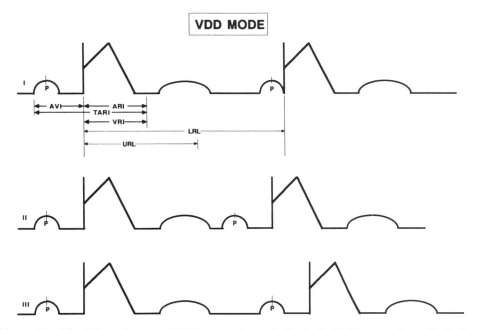

Figure 19. *The AV synchronous (VDD) pacemaker is similar to the VAT pacemaker with similar upper and lower rate intervals but with, in addition, ventricular sensing. Cardiac sensing thus exists in the atrial and ventricular channels. The total atrial refractory interval (TARI) consists of the AV interval (AVI) and the atrial refractory interval (ARI). The upper rate interval (URI) is here coincident with TARI and the lower rate interval (LRI) is via a ventricular stimulus escape, i.e., from one ventricular stimulus to the next. The major timing difference between VAT and VDD is that the ventricular channel is refractory throughout the entire pacemaker timing cycle in the VAT mode. A second variety of operation of the VDD mode is in use. (I) As the second P wave occurs so late that establishment of the programmed AV interval would produce a ventricular rate less than the programmed lower rate limit, the ventricular stimulus abbreviates the AV delay. The AV interval is sacrificed and the lower rate limit is maintained. (II) In this instance the two P waves occur sufficiently early so that the programmed AV interval can exist without a ventricular stimulation rate below the lower rate limit. (III) In an alternate mode of VDD operation the AV interval is hierarchically superior to the lower rate limit. The P wave occurs sufficiently late and the programmed AV interval places the ventricular stimulus at a longer V-V interval than the lower rate limit. The AV interval is retained, the lower rate limit is not.*

the TARI will be unsensed and will be blocked. In the pseudo-Wenckebach approach, one more interval exists, the Wenckebach interval between the TARI and the independently programmed URI of greater duration than TARI. The maximum ARI after a ventricular event is kept short to allow high upper rates, generally in the range of 175–180 bpm (coupling interval of 333–343 ms). The TARI will be as long as in the AV block mode because of the lengthening of the AV interval (which is part of the TARI). When the AV interval prolongs in the pseudo-Wenckebach mode of Upper rate behavior, the TARI is being prolonged. When the ARI after the ventricular event and the minimum AV interval are set to limit the upper rate, AV block will result. If the total of the minimum AV interval and the ARI after a ventricular event allow a higher rate than the independently set upper rate limit, then the pseudo-Wenckebach response, i.e., prolongation of the AV interval, will result. The degree of prolongation will be

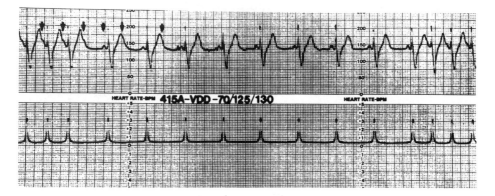

Figure 20. *A VDD pacemaker operating in the AV block mode has been recorded during Holter monitoring. As the P waves move closer to the preceding ventricular stimulus, they eventually fall into the atrial refractory interval after the ventricular event. The second P wave (arrow) is unsensed as are the marked fourth and sixth P waves. The patient remains in 2:1 AV block until the atrial rate slows and atrial synchronization returns. Paradoxically, the ventricular rate increases as the atrial rate decreases. The AV interval between a sensed P wave and a ventricular stimulus it causes is constant.*

the difference between the upper rate interval and the minimum TARI (Figure 21).

Formula 3

Upper Rate Limit Interval (URI) − TARI = Prolongation of AV Interval

= Wenckebach Interval (WI)

The upper rate limit can be set by one of two intervals. The first is the total

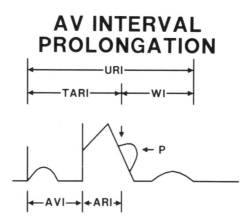

Figure 21. *The Wenckebach upper rate limit response is the result of an upper rate interval that is longer (therefore setting a lower rate) than the total atrial refractory interval. The difference between the two intervals (TARI-URI) is the Wenckebach interval. It is the equivalent of the duration of the rate plateau from the onset of the upper rate interval to the onset of AV block, and it is the duration of the potential prolongation of the AV interval during upper rate operation. TARI = atrial refractory interval; URI = upper rate interval; AVI = AV interval; ARI = atrial refractory interval; WI = Wenckebach interval.*

atrial refractory interval (TARI). As no P wave falling during any part of the TARI can be sensed, total atrial refractory interval = upper rate limit interval (TARI = URI). The other possibility is that the desired upper rate limit will be lower (URI will be longer) than that imposed by the TARI. In that event, the upper rate interval (URI) will be set independently of the TARI. The difference between the two intervals can be called the Wenckebach interval (WI). A P wave that falls into the TARI will be unsensed; one that falls after the upper rate limit interval will start a timing cycle that incorporates an AV interval of programmed duration. A P wave that falls into the Wenckebach interval (the difference between TARI and URI) will be sensed and will start a timing cycle, the ventricular stimulus of which cannot be emitted until the URI has passed. Depending on duration and when the P wave is sensed in the Wenckebach interval, the AVI may actually be prolonged or nevertheless, be of normal duration (Figure 22).

If the TARI sets the upper rate (i.e., TARI = URI), sudden AV block will result. If the URI sets the upper rate below that set by the TARI, then pseudo-Wenckebach results. For example, if the independently set URI is at a cycle length interval of 343 ms (175 bpm) and that interval is of shorter duration than the TARI, e.g., 400 ms (150 bpm), a P wave will fall into the TARI before it can fall into the upper rate interval. AV block results and Wenckebach block is impossible. Formula 3 can be further interpreted so that if a positive number results, pseudo-Wenckebach behavior can occur; if a negative number results (negative time is impossible), AV block occurs (Figure 23).

Pseudo-Wenckebach AV behavior depends on a short ARI after a ventricular event. If the ARI is programmable, then the longer it is made, the less will be the extension of the AVI, and the more likely it will be that the AV block mode will occur. The unique mode of behavior of pseudo-Wenckebach operation is that of a rate plateau between the upper rate limit and the rate at which AV block occurs. Once again, this is a matter of the timing cycles involved. For example, if the TARI is 385 ms (156 bpm), and the upper rate interval is 480 ms (125 bpm), then the interval between 480 ms and 385 ms (a rate of 125–156 bpm) will be one of a rate plateau with prolongation of the AV interval. When the P

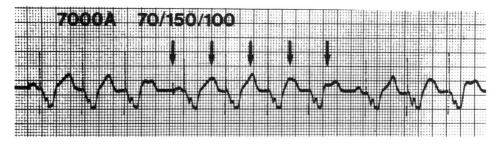

Figure 22.   *Wenckebach upper rate behavior occurs when the atrial rate is more rapid than the controlled ventricular pacemaker response. The minimum response is 70 bpm, the maximum is 100 bpm, and the AV interval is 150 ms. As the atrial rate is more rapid than the allowed ventricular response, the P waves (marked by a vertical arrow) move progressively closer to the preceding ventricular stimulus, prolonging the AV interval until the fifth P wave falls into the atrial refractory interval after the ventricular event and is blocked, i.e., produces no response. The next, spontaneous P wave, begins the cycle again.*

WENCKEBACH

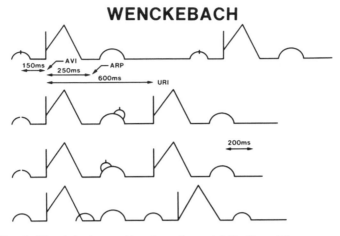

Figure 23. *Pseudo-Wenckebach operation depends on stabilization of the upper ventricular rate below the actual atrial rate, i.e., with the upper rate limit interval longer than the total atrial refractory interval. In this diagram, the P wave is sensed at the mark. ABOVE: TARI (AVI + ARP) is 400 ms giving a maximum follow rate of 150 bpm. As the upper rate limit interval is 600 ms, the maximum allowed ventricular response will be 100 bpm. There is a 200 ms Wenckebach interval (URI-TARI). The P wave is sensed after TARI and URI and provokes a normal ventricular response. NEXT: The P wave falls within the URI, at a time when a response at the normal AV interval will not violate the URI. No prolongation of the AV interval occurs. NEXT: The P wave occurs earlier but beyond the TARI. A normal AV interval would cause a stimulus that would violate the URI; the stimulus is, therefore, delayed. BELOW: The P wave falls into the atrial refractory interval, it is unsensed and the next P wave produces the ventricular response.*

wave falls into TARI, i.e., at an interval less than 385 ms, it will be blocked (Figure 24).

In the pseudo-Wenckebach approach, the atrial refractory interval after a ventricular event is fixed (though it may be programmable). The AV interval is flexible and may be extended but not shortened. In the hierarchical design of such a unit, the set upper rate limit is at a higher priority than the constancy of the AV interval. If the shortest interval between ventricular stimuli is set at 600 ms (URI), but that allowed by the TARI is 300 ms, any sensed atrial event that occurs after the end of the atrial refractory interval but which, after the set AV interval would cause a ventricular stimulus before the end of the upper rate interval, will be delayed so that a stimulus does not occur before 600 ms (from one ventricular event to the next) have elapsed. This delay is added to the programmed AV interval so that in this instance, the time to the AV interval (possibly programmed to 150 ms) from the sensed atrial event would have been prolonged from the programmed 150 to 450 ms. Time is moved from after the ventricular event to before the ventricular event (the AVI), but the TARI still determines the upper rate limit (Figure 25). Two additional events occur: The sudden production of AV block after a stable AVI, characteristic of the AV block upper rate limit, is replaced by a prolonged Wenckebach period between the programmed upper rate limit and the upper rate limit imposed by the actual refractory intervals. The ventricular rate is stabilized by prolongation of the AV interval while the AVI is prolonged.

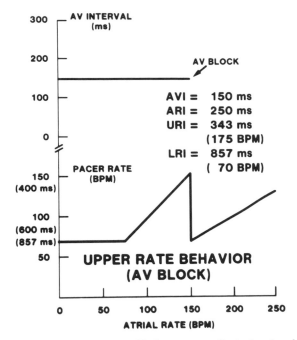

Figure 24. *A graphic illustration of the AV block upper rate limitation in which the total atrial refractory interval is the upper rate interval. Two simultaneous events, the ventricular rate and AV interval, are dependent upon the actual numerical settings. In this instance, taken from a commercially available pacemaker, the AV interval is set at 150 ms and the atrial refractory interval at 250 ms. The total atrial refractory interval is 400 ms and the maximum follow rate is 150 bpm. The URI has been independently set at 343 ms (175 bpm), a number which is, in this setting, irrelevant, as the pacemaker cannot track at an atrial coupling interval of 343 ms. At an atrial rate of less than 70 bpm (857 ms) the atrium is driven. Between 70 and 150 bpm (857–400 ms) there is a 1:1 response at a constant AV interval (above). When a P wave falls into the atrial refractory interval it is unsensed and the ventricular response is to the next P wave, i.e., AV block.*

The AV interval may also be shorter than programmed if the atrial event occurs at a time when emission of a ventricular stimulus, following the programmed AV interval, would occur after the passage of the entire lower rate interval. In this circumstance, the lower rate interval (which is between ventricular events) takes hierarchical precedence over the evolution of the entire AV interval. The AV interval will appear to be short but only because the pacemaker has not allowed a full AV delay to occur, i.e., has disregarded the P wave as a time-setting event (Figure 26). In some designs the AV interval takes hierarchical precedence over the lower rate limit. A sensed P wave will start the AV interval and can extend the lower rate interval beyond its set duration. In most designs, an atrial event that occurs so late that a cycle which it starts would occur after the end of the lower rate limit will be sensed but disregarded in the timing of the ventricular stimuli.

Because lower rate limit escape is by a ventricular (not an atrial) stimulus, it is readily possible for the atrium to be entrained retrograde. If the spontaneous atrial coupling interval is longer than the pacemaker ventricular escape, the

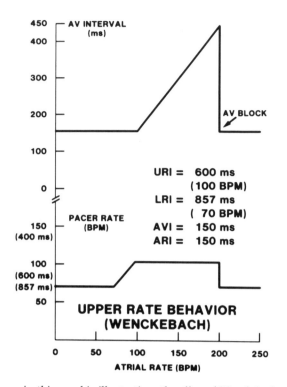

Figure 25. *As shown in this graphic illustration, the effect of Wenckebach upper rate limitation involves two simultaneous events and is dependent upon the actual settings and numerical relationships of the various intervals. In this interval, the upper rate limit is at an interval of 600 ms, the lower rate interval is 857 ms, the AV interval and the atrial refractory interval each equal 150 ms and total 300 ms. If not for the independent rate limitation at 100 bpm, this pacemaker could respond at 200 bpm. BELOW: Until the atrial rate exceeds 70 bpm (857 ms) the atrium is paced. Between an interval of 857 ms and 600 ms (rate of 70–100 atrial bpm) there is a 1:1 ventricular response and the AV interval remains as programmed, in this instance, 150 ms. As the ventricular rate is stabilized at an interval of 600 ms, this will be maintained as the P-R interval decreases. Simultaneously, the AV interval prolongs (above) with the addition of each millisecond of Wenckebach interval, which is consumed by a P wave moving toward the ventricular event and added to the AV interval. Because of the numbers chosen in this example (taken from the capability of a formerly commercially available pulse generator) the maximum duration of the AV interval can be 450 ms. When a P wave falls into the ARI, it is unsensed, the rate plateau ends, and the AV interval returns to normal. If the atrial rate maintains its relationship to the URI, the cycle resumes.*

ventricle will be stimulated, and in the presence of retained retrograde conduction the atrium may be entrained (Figure 27).

AV Universal (DDD)

The AV universal pacemaker senses and paces both atrium and ventricle. There are at least four different timing cycles:

1. The AV interval (AVI), starting at a sensed or paced atrial event;
2. The VA interval (VAI), starting at a sensed or paced ventricular event;

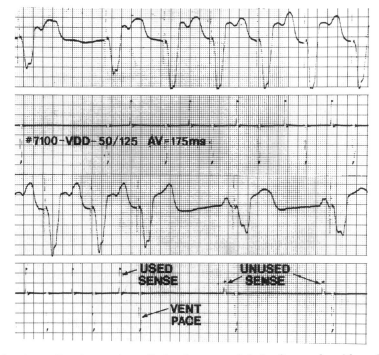

Figure 26. *An endless loop tachycardia has been recorded simultaneously with an ECG interpretation channel in a VDD pacemaker. The lower rate limit is 60 bpm (1000 ms), the paper speed is 50 mm/sec. The onset of the tachycardia is by a ventricular escape and a retrograde P wave (upper left). The marks below the line are ventricular channel stimulation indicators. The upward marks are atrial channel sensing indicators. The taller marks indicate an atrial event sensed by the pacemaker, in this instance the retrograde P, which is sensed 260 ms after the ventricular stimulus. The AV interval is also clearly indicated as 220 ms, prolonged beyond the programmed 175 ms. At the lower right retrograde conduction fatigues, the tachycardia ends with a ventricular escape. The P waves occur too late to start the timing cycle as an AV delay after a sensed P would have required a longer interval than 1000 ms between ventricular stimuli. Though the P waves are sensed, they are not used to start a timing cycle and the marks are, therefore, lower to indicate a sensed but unused event.*

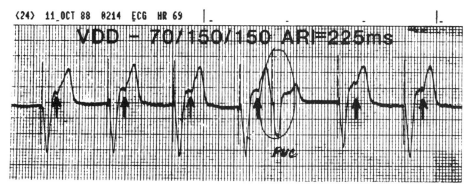

Figure 27. *A VDD pacemaker in which the spontaneous atrial escape is longer than the programmed ventricular escape will stimulate the ventricle. The atrium may be entrained retrograde as occurs in this illustration. One retrograde P wave (fourth from the left) fell beyond atrial refractoriness and, at the programmed AV interval, caused a ventricular stimulus. Ventricular escape with retrograde conduction then returned. (The handwritten "PVC" is likely in error.)*

3. The lower rate interval (LRI) between atrial events;
4. The upper rate interval (URI) between ventricular events.

In addition to these basic timing cycles, each channel has refractory and blanking periods that determine the response to atrial and ventricular events at a particular time in the cardiac or pacemaker cycle. In effect, the pacemaker is a combination of the AV sequential (DVI) and AV synchronous (VDD) pacemakers. The combination of sensing and pacing two chambers leads to far greater complexity of function than pacing and sensing in one channel, i.e., single-chamber pacing or pacing in two channels and sensing in one (AV sequential-DVI) or even sensing in two channels and pacing in one (VDD).

DDD pacing shares with DVI and VDD the restoration of AV synchrony, but the lower rate interval is started either from the atrial event (paced or sensed) or from a ventricular event rather than from the ventricular event only as it is in VDD pacing. Like the VDD mode it has an additional capability, that of the production of a tachycardia that is mediated by the pacemaker when the two parallel conduction systems allow antegrade conduction in the pacemaker and retrograde conduction via the natural AV conduction system (the endless loop tachycardia).

In the VDD mode, atrial pacing does not exist so that pacemaker escape is only in the ventricular channel. Should retrograde conduction exist, a retrograde conducted P wave may occur, be sensed, and cause a consequent ventricular stimulus. If the P wave is closely coupled to the ventricular event but beyond the ARI, it will be sensed, and if the URI is set to produce a low upper rate, (prolonged URI), the AVI will be prolonged via the pseudo-Wenckebach mode so that the mechanism for recovery of VA conduction and endless loop tachycardia exists. This mechanism is likely for the VDD mode but less likely for the DDD mode because the pacemaker escape is not via the ventricular channel, but via the atrial channel. The atrial stimulus produces a P wave before the ventricular stimulus produces a QRS complex. The result is a greater likelihood of avoiding the tachycardia because displacement of the P wave is limited. Nevertheless, if the ventricular event is idioventricular, i.e., not produced by the pacemaker or conducted from a preceding P wave, then a retrograde P wave is possible and will initiate the tachycardia. If retrograde conduction exists and the P wave is closely coupled to the ventricular event and within the ARI, consistent retrograde conduction can occur.

Modern DDD pacemakers now include all of the single- and dual-chamber modes described. Any one can be selected as is appropriate to the occasion. Many modern DDD pacemakers also have a rate modulated capability (along with all of the modes described above) so that rate modulation as well as AV synchrony can be achieved. While rate modulation in the VDD and DDD pacing systems is integral to their capability to track the P wave, modes previously unassociated with rate modulation capability, single chamber VVI and VOO and dual chamber DVI and DDI can now provide both AV synchrony and rate modulation (Figure 28).

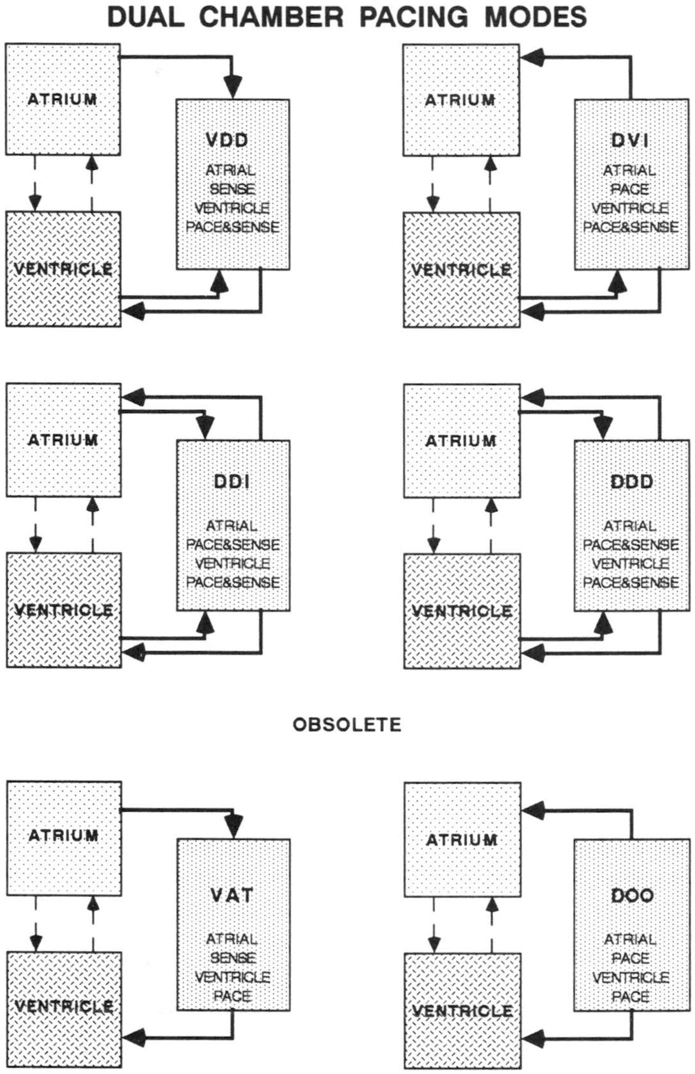

Figure 28. *Modern DDD pulse generators can be programmed to a variety of single-chamber modes such as VVI, VVT, AAI, AAT, and many dual-chamber modes. If the pulse generator has rate modulation capability, still more modes are possible. The dual-chamber modes are shown with the ability to pace and or sense the ventricle and, or, the atrium. Any mode should be sensitive to the activity of the chamber paced, but especially if it is the ventricle. Consequently the two modes, which remain possible, but do not have ventricular sensing are now obsolete, except in the most unusual and carefully determined circumstances.*

ATRIAL AND VENTRICULAR BASED TIMING

The diagrammatic representations earlier in this text were based on ventricular based timing. An alternative approach, in more common use since the advent of sensor-driven dual-chamber pacemakers, is that of atrial based timing. During ventricular based timing, atrial escape intervals (AEI) and ventricular escape intervals are of constant duration. This approach can introduce variation in the ventricular pacing rate depending on whether atrium and ventricle are both being paced, whether the atrium alone is paced and the ventricle is being driven by atrioventricular conduction, and whether the AV interval is being modulated with the sensor (or atrial) driven rate, which is now common. At the maximum tracking or sensor-driven rate limit, the difference in rate between atrial and ventricular based timing may be 10 bpm or more. ECG interpretation may be confusing if it is unclear which timing mechanism is operative (Figure 29).

Atrial based timing attempts to stabilize the atrial and ventricular rates by maintaining the interval between atrial paced events constant. During atrial based timing the overall atrial rate is primary, within the limits of the upper

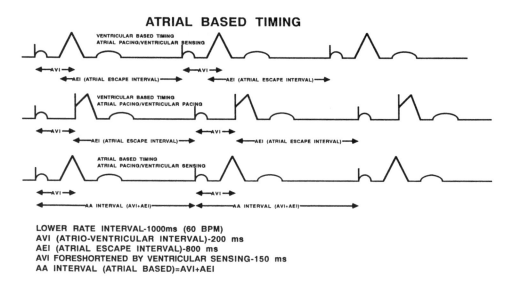

ATRIAL BASED TIMING

LOWER RATE INTERVAL-1000ms (60 BPM)
AVI (ATRIO-VENTRICULAR INTERVAL)-200 ms
AEI (ATRIAL ESCAPE INTERVAL)-800 ms
AVI FORESHORTENED BY VENTRICULAR SENSING-150 ms
AA INTERVAL (ATRIAL BASED)=AVI+AEI

Figure 29.   Atrial and ventricular based timing are compared during atrial pacing with AV conduction producing the ventricular depolarization during atrial and ventricular based timing and with ventricular based timing and pacing of atrium and ventricle. In this diagram it is assumed that sensing of the ventricular event is at its beginning (infrequently true, in reality) and that the AV interval (AVI) is constant in duration. The intervals are set to produce a lower interval of 1000 ms (60 bpm). The top line is of ventricular based timing, with foreshortening of the AV interval by ventricular sensing to 150 ms. During ventricular based timing the interval between atrial stimuli thus becomes 950 ms (AVI$_{foreshortened}$ [150 ms] = AEI [800 ms]), the equivalent of a sustained rate of 63 bpm. If atrium and ventricle are both paced (middle line), then the interval between atrial stimuli is 1000 ms (AVI [200 ms] + AEI [800 ms]), the equivalents of a sustained rate of 60 bpm. During atrial based timing, with AV conduction, the interval is maintained at the lower rate interval of 1000 ms, the AA interval (AVI [200 ms] + AEI [800 ms]) the equivalent of a sustained rate of 60 bpm.

and lower rate limits. Within this range the ventricular rate will follow the atrial. During **ventricular based** timing a paced atrial event followed by a nonpaced ventricular event (conducted or idioventricular) during the programmed or modified (e.g., by AV interval modulation) AV interval will start an atrial escape interval at the end of which (assuming no other spontaneous atrial or ventricular activity) an atrial channel stimulus will be emitted. The effect will be to accelerate the ventricular rate by subtracting the difference between the duration of the programmed AV interval and the interval between the atrial channel stimulus and the sensed ventricular event. If, for example, the lower rate was set at 1200 ms (50 bpm) with an AV interval of 200 ms, the atrial escape interval would be 1000 ms. Were a conducted ventricular event to be sensed 150 ms following the atrial stimulus, the atrial escape interval would begin. As it is 1000 ms, the next atrial channel stimulus would occur 1150 ms later or (if it were sustained) at a rate of 52 bpm. During **atrial based** timing the next atrial stimulus would fall, despite the sensed ventricular event, 1200 ms after its predecessor, maintaining overall (atrial and ventricular) rate constant. In this instance, were atrium and ventricle both paced, the ECGs of both atrial and ventricular based timing would be indistinguishable. In an atrial based system, the atrial stimulation interval is constant while the atrial escape interval will vary as necessary. In a ventricular based system, the atrial escape interval is constant and the interval between atrial channel stimuli may vary (Figure 30).

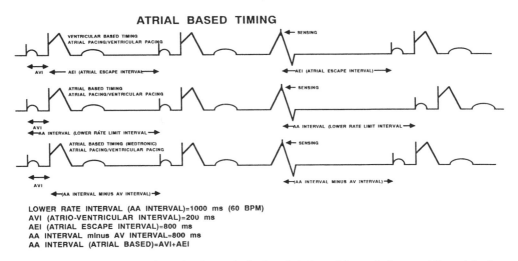

ATRIAL BASED TIMING

LOWER RATE INTERVAL (AA INTERVAL)=1000 ms (60 BPM)
AVI (ATRIO-VENTRICULAR INTERVAL)=200 ms
AEI (ATRIAL ESCAPE INTERVAL)=800 ms
AA INTERVAL minus AV INTERVAL=800 ms
AA INTERVAL (ATRIAL BASED)=AVI+AEI

Figure 30. *Comparison of atrial and ventricular based timing with recycle from an idioventricular event demonstrates the difference in interval produced by the two timing mechanisms. A conducted ventricular event is defined as a ventricular event preceded by an atrial event, an idioventricular event one not preceded by a sensed or paced atrial event. In this diagram sensing of the PVC is at the peak. ABOVE: During ventricular based timing the atrial escape interval (AEI) begins with the sensed PVC. MIDDLE: During atrial based timing, a lower rate interval begins with the sensing of the PVC resulting in a longer interval than during ventricular based timing. BELOW: To maintain the benefits of atrial based timing but to avoid the prolongation of the interval between PVC and the escape beat, the modified atrial based approach differentiates between a conducted ventricular event and an idioventricular event in which instance the AVI is subtracted from the AA (lower rate limit) interval.*

A modification by one manufacturer of atrial based timing is different management of a ventricular sensed event depending on whether that event had been preceded by an atrial paced or sensed event in which case the ventricular event is defined as a conducted beat. If not preceded by an atrial event, the ventricular event is defined as a premature beat. During ventricular based timing, a sensed premature beat (see definition above) is followed by an atrial escape interval, during atrial based timing by a lower rate interval (i.e., including an AV interval and an atrial escape interval), and in modified atrial based timing

ATRIAL BASED TIMING

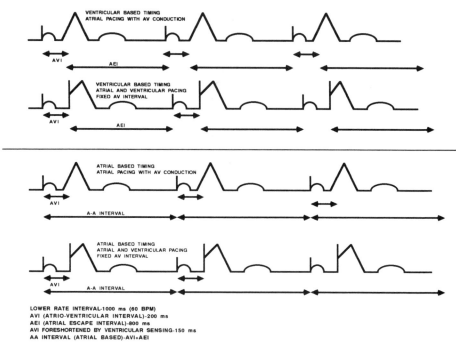

LOWER RATE INTERVAL-1000 ms (60 BPM)
AVI (ATRIO-VENTRICULAR INTERVAL)-200 ms
AEI (ATRIAL ESCAPE INTERVAL)-800 ms
AVI FORESHORTENED BY VENTRICULAR SENSING-150 ms
AA INTERVAL (ATRIAL BASED)-AVI+AEI

Figure 31. *Ventricular based and atrial based timing are illustrated both in atrial paced events with intact AV conduction and during atrial and ventricular pacing. In all instances, the AV interval (AVI) is 150 ms without modulation for rate changes and can only be abbreviated by a ventricular sensed event. ABOVE: The atrial escape interval after a sensed or paced ventricular event is 250 ms. If both atrium and ventricle are paced (at those intervals) the stimulation rate is at a coupling interval of 400 ms or 150 bpm (as would occur elsewhere in this chapter). With atrial pacing and conduction to the ventricle, the AV interval is abbreviated, perhaps by 25 ms (TOP)). As the atrial escape interval (AEI) is constant at 250 ms, the interval betwee one atrial stimulus and the next will be 375 ms (AVI + AEI [125 ms + 250 ms]) or a rate of 160 bpm.*

Below: In a similar situation with atrial based timing and the same programmed intervals, both without modulation by change in atrial stimulation rate as a result of sensor drive. The overall rate is not based on the sum of the AVI and that of the ARI, rather on the established interval between atrial stimuli, i.e., AA timing, which may be modified by sensor drive. In both tracings, an analogous circumstance exists as with the ventricular based tracings. The upper one is of atrial pacing with AV conduction, the lower of both atrial and ventricular pacing. Both rates are the same as the AA interval is constant, not the sum of AVI and ARI.

by a lower rate interval from which the AV interval has been subtracted. The atrial based timing approach will prolong the overall interval between paced events, while the ventricular based and modified atrial based intervals will be similar (Figure 31).

The importance of the difference between atrial and ventricular based timing results from the variations in rate which can occur in both systems and result from:

1. The time of sensing the atrial event;
2. The time of sensing the ventricular event (it is unusual for the ventricular event to be sensed, and start a timing cycle at the beginning of the electrocardiographic QRS complex);
3. The duration of the AV interval, which in modern pulse generators has both a programmed duration and one modified by the atrial rate and the sensor-driven rate;
4. The lower rate limit interval which is programmed and also modified by sensor function.

It may be difficult or impossible to ascertain the exact timing to be anticipated because of different influences of the various timing cycles. Telemetry of an ECG interpretation channel with timing cycles is very helpful.

ENDLESS LOOP TACHYCARDIA

The endless loop tachycardia (ELT) is the pacemaker analog of a natural reentry tachycardia. As the reentry tachycardia depends on the presence of two pathways, antegrade and retrograde, a pacemaker-mediated reentry arrhythmia (the endless loop tachycardia) usually requires the pacemaker as the antegrade pathway and the natural pathway as the retrograde conduction pathway. Retrograde conduction via the pacemaker is extremely unusual (Figure 32). (See retrograde endless loop tachycardia). Several dual-chamber pacemakers do have a mode intended to prevent endless loop tachycardia in which a ventricular premature beat (the most common initiator of an endless loop tachycardia), defined as a ventricular event not preceded by an atrial channel pacemaker stimulus or a sensed P wave, is followed without delay by an atrial channel stimulus. This is intended to allow that paced P wave to fall into a period of atrial refractoriness so that it does not begin an AV delay and to make the atrium refractory for a retrograde conducted P wave. In the presence of retained antegrade conduction and blocked retrograde conduction, this mode allows the pacemaker to act as a retrograde pathway.

Endless loop tachycardia is only one of a series of pacemaker-mediated tachycardias. Other such tachycardias include pacemaker electronic tachycardias, autonomic pacemaker tachycardia in which the pulse generator timing circuit senses P and QRS at a time when a pacemaker tachycardia is produced and the circuit is caught or "latched" in that mode. Echo beats, atrial premature contractions, and atrial fibrillation and flutter in the presence of heart block are other possible pacemaker-mediated tachycardias.

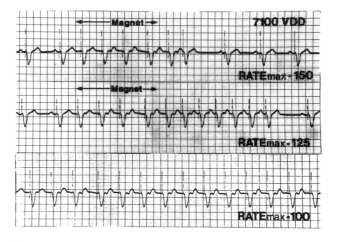

Figure 32. *In this atrial synchronous ventricular inhibited (VDD) pacemaker (model 7100), the atrial refractory period after a ventricular sensed or paced event is 120 ms, guaranteeing that any retrograde P wave will be sensed. The patient had antegrade 2:1 block. The duration of the endless loop tachycardia depends on the number of factors, including the ability to sustain retrograde conduction. In each of the three ECGs, the endless loop tachycardia is started by the application of the magnet, which converts the pacemaker to the asynchronous (VOO) mode of operation. Because the magnet rate of 85 bpm is faster than the spontaneous atrial rate, the P waves are forced into the retrograde position. The AV delay is set at 125 ms. The tachycardia, in each instance, is started by application of a magnet with entrainment of the P waves retrograde. The irregularity of ventricular stimuli with the magnet in place is caused by a timing cycle variation as part of magnet operation in this pulse generator. In the upper strip, in which the maximum allowed pacemaker rate is 150 per minute (400 ms), the tachycardia is sustained for only one beat because the P wave meets a refractory VA conduction pathway. The maximum pacemaker rate (minimum interval) is set by the total of the AV delay and the atrial refractory period. Because the atrial refractory period is fixed, the AV delay is prolonged by the pacemaker to meet the maximum programmed rate. As the allowed AV delay is shortest at the most rapid maximum rate, it is very likely that the conduction pathway will be refractory. The middle ECG has a maximum pacemaker rate of 125 bpm (480 ms). The AV delay is prolonged compared to that of the upper strip, because no two ventricular stimuli may be separated by less than 480 ms no matter where the retrograde P wave occurs. The AV delay is prolonged compared with that of the upper strip, and the retrograde pathway is less likely to be refractory. The endless loop tachycardia thus is briefly sustained, in this instance for six beats, before the retrograde pathway becomes refractory. The lowest ECG has a maximum pacemaker rate of 100 bpm (600 ms). The VA delay is prolonged as the retrograde conduction time remains the same as above but the delay between the sensed P and the next allowed ventricular stimulus is greater. Because recovery of the retrograde conduction system is possible, endless loop tachycardia is sustained. Initially it may be assumed that, in the presence of possible endless loop tachycardia, the minimum rate should be set to protect the patient. In this instance, as in others in which retrograde conduction exists but is unreliable, setting a higher rate may fatigue retrograde conduction fast enough to eliminate endless loop tachycardia (courtesy of Dr. S. Amikam).*

Endless loop tachycardia is most commonly initiated by a spontaneous ventricular premature contraction, electromagnetic interference or electromyographic interference, a programmed ventricular stimulus, an asynchronous ventricular stimulus (magnet), or a ventricular stimulus after a noncapture atrial stimulus. This latter may result in retrograde atrial activation during an alert period of the pacemaker cycle. The common denominator is that the P wave is displaced from its normal relation to the QRS complex. The endless loop tachycardia may also begin with an end diastolic, normally timed, atrial premature complex and a P wave that occurs retrograde after a normal antegrade P wave. In some instances, endless loop tachycardia may begin spontaneously, i.e., following a normally timed paced atrial beat or normally timed spontaneous P wave, in some cases followed by a paced QRS complex. Retrograde atrial activation may nevertheless be present in such instances. In other instances, in the absence of a pacemaker, a retrograde P wave may occur immediately after an antegrade P wave and a conducted QRS complex (Figure 33).

The events described above depend on the existence of retrograde conduction whether or not complete antegrade block exists. As an endless loop tachycardia has been described that depends on antegrade conduction and atrial channel stimulation simultaneous with a sensed ventricular premature beat, the usual endless loop tachycardia may be named **retrograde**. In a pacemaker with simultaneous atrial stimulation following a ventricular beat, once such an event is sensed, an atrial channel stimulus is emitted and, if antegrade conduction is absent and retrograde is present, then an endless loop tachycardia is effectively prevented by stimulation of the atrium and block of the retrograde pathway. If, however, the retrograde pathway is naturally blocked, but antegrade conduction exists, the atrial channel stimulus produces a P wave that may be conducted antegrade to the ventricle. As the pacer produced P wave will have fallen during atrial refractoriness it will be unsensed and the conducted ventricular

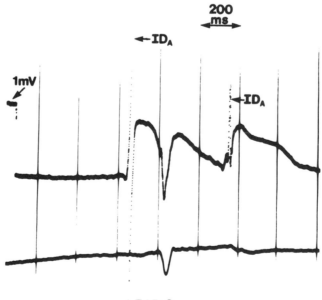

LEAD 2

Figure 33. *It is entirely possible for a retrograde P wave to occur after a normal spontaneous antegrade P wave. This electrogram is of an antegrade P wave of approximately 4 mV amplitude preceding a QRS by about 200 ms, to be followed by a retrograde P wave of approximately 1 mV amplitude about 350 ms later.*

beat will be pacemaker defined as a premature beat. It will once again provoke the simultaneous atrial channel stimulus, perpetuating this **antegrade** endless loop tachycardia (see Chapter 2, Figure 42).

Endless Loop Tachycardia Caused by an Atrial Premature Complex

During sinus rhythm with the right atrial appendage stimulating/sensing electrode, the atrial depolarization waveform reaches the AV node. Potential retrograde conduction finds the AV junctional tissue normally refractory. If an atrial premature complex arises from an atrial ectopic focus near the AV junction, the AV node depolarization may occur before the depolarization wave front reaches the atrial sensing electrode and the pacemaker interval will then be initiated. Should this occur, a significantly longer interval from AV node de-polarization to the arrival of the returning retrograde, i.e., ventriculoatrial im-pulse occurs and retrograde (VA) conduction is allowed. This retrograde P wave may be sensed and endless loop tachycardia will then follow. The same mech-anism is applicable to left as well as right atrial ectopic atrial activity (Figures 34, 35).

Differentiation of Endless Loop Tachycardia from Primary Supraventricular Tachycardia (SVT)

An endless loop tachycardia (or pacemaker-mediated endless loop tachy-cardia) differs from a supraventricular tachycardia, with conduction via the pace-maker, in a variety of ways:

1. The endless loop tachycardia is almost always **exactly** at the upper rate limit of the pacemaker, the coupling interval is **exactly** that of the upper rate limit interval. This exactness is caused by the highly accurate timing mechanism of the pacemaker and not by the exactness of the supraventricular tachycardia. Infrequently (see below) the endless loop tachycardia rate may be below the upper rate limit, never above.

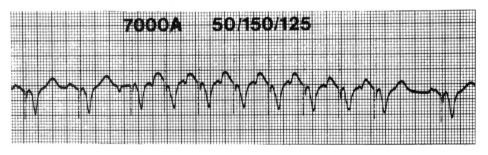

Figure 34.   Lead II. The third P wave is aberrant and starts an endless loop tachycardia that ends when the retrograde pathway is fatigued and a P wave is not conducted.

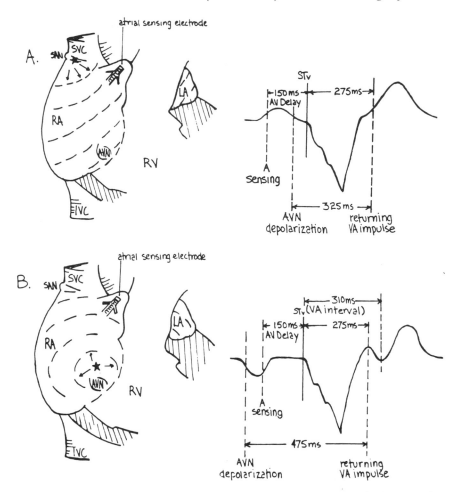

Figure 35. *Mechanisms of induction of tachycardia. A. During sinus rhythm, atrial sensing precedes AV node (AVN) depolarization. A relatively short interval (325 ms) elapses between AV node depolarization and the arrival of the retrograde (VA) impulse. B. If an atrial premature complex arises from the area of the AV node, AV node depolarization may precede atrial sensing. A longer interval elapses (475 ms) from AV node depolarization to the arrival of the retrograde (VA) impulse. The AV node has recovered and retrograde conduction is allowed. ASE = atrial sensing electrode; IVC = inferior vena cava; LA = left atrium; RA = right atrium; RV = right ventricle; SAN = sinoatrial node; STv = ventricular pacing stimulus; SVC = superior vena cava. (Courtesy of Dr. H. Frumin.)*

2. If the supraventricular tachycardia is slower than the upper rate limit, the pacemaker rate will be slower and the tachycardia can be sustained. The possibility of sustaining an endless loop tachycardia at a rate below the upper rate limit exists and the name given has been of a balanced endless loop tachycardia (BELT). Such a tachycardia is particularly important because the algorithms that exist in several pacemakers to terminate an endless loop tachycardia are based on the diagnostic criterion of stability at the upper rate limit interval.

3. If a supraventricular tachycardia is more rapid than the upper pacemaker rate,

a Wenckebach or AV block mechanism of upper rate limitation, depending on the variety of pacemaker implanted and its technique of upper rate management, is invoked. If the atrial rate substantially exceeds the upper rate limit, the Wenckebach mechanism may be obvious. If it exceeds the upper rate only marginally, the Wenckebach cycle may be so prolonged as to be almost invisible. In either event, whether at a rapid evolution, i.e., 3:1, 4:1, 5:1, etc., or at a very slow evolution, 15–20:1, it is a Wenckebach mechanism of upper rate limitation (Figure 36). Programming the upper rate limit down may produce Wenckebach operation and clarify the tachycardia.

An atrial rate below the upper rate limit does not prolong the AV interval; only when the upper rate limit has been reached does AV interval prolongation begin. At exactly the upper rate limit the AV interval is as programmed. A longer AV interval in the endless loop tachycardia is required to sustain the tachycardia because the endless loop tachycardia is based on retrograde conduction with a need to allow the AV conduction pathway to recover after the retrograde P wave so that it will conduct retrograde once again. No such prolongation of AV interval is necessary for supraventricular tachycardia in which the atrial rate is sustained on a basis other than the pacemaker-mediated reentry.

All of these characteristics, tachycardia rate exactly the same as the pacemaker upper rate limit, AV interval prolongation, absence of the Wenckebach mechanism, and prompt termination of a tachycardia when it is forced to be sustained at a lower rate, strongly suggest endless loop tachycardia instead of primary supraventricular tachycardia.

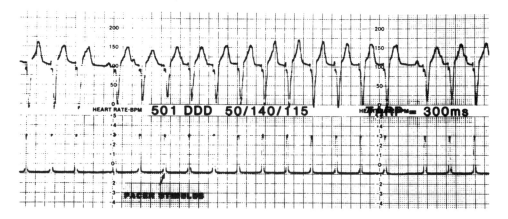

Figure 36.   *This Holter monitor recording of a relatively slow pseudo-Wenckebach cycle may not be recognized for what it is. The first three beats to the left are the end of the preceding cycle. Because the P wave is blocked, the fourth complex starts with a P wave and succeeding P waves are seen to move progressively closer to the pacemaker stimulus. As the atrial rate and the upper rate limit of the pacemaker are relatively close to each other, this progression is by only a few milliseconds for each beat, and the movement of the last P wave into the atrial refractory period after the ventricular event, to the right, occurs over twelve QRS complexes. The pseudo-Wenckebach cycle ends with a blocked P wave and the next cycle resumes with an escape P wave.*

Spontaneous Endless Loop Tachycardia

Spontaneous endless loop tachycardia may be initiated following a normally timed atrial event either spontaneous or paced and synchronized with a ventricular paced beat. Patients need not have a known or demonstrated bypass tract or other evidence of spontaneous reentry tachycardia. The spontaneous endless loop tachycardia may begin after a spontaneous P wave that produces a ventricular stimulus and then a retrograde P wave after the end of the atrial refractory period following the ventricular event. Such a tachycardia then can be sustained until fatigue terminates retrograde conduction (Figure 37). An endless loop tachycardia may begin following retrograde conduction following an atrial stimulus with atrial capture and a ventricular stimulus with ventricular capture. This will occur if retrograde conduction occurs at an interval greater than the programmed atrial refractory period after the ventricular event (Figure 38).

Spontaneous episodes of endless loop tachycardia may begin following a spontaneous P wave that precedes the ventricular stimulus by a somewhat prolonged AV interval, i.e., 200 ms. With a lower upper rate limit, i.e., 500 ms (120 bpm), an AV interval may be prolonged to 200 ms allowing easy maintenance of retrograde conduction. Should a tachycardia-terminating algorithm be in effect, the tachycardia may end only to begin a few beats later via the same mechanism (Figure 39).

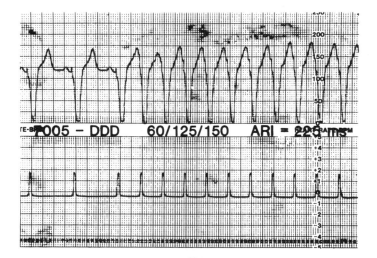

Figure 37. *Endless loop tachycardia begins after the third spontaneous P wave causes the third pacemaker-produced QRS complex. The retrograde P waves occur 200 ms after the ventricular stimulus, and as the upper rate limit interval is 400 ms, the resultant AV interval is also approximately 200 ms. (Model-Mode-lower rate/AV interval/upper limit-atrial refractory after ventricular event).*

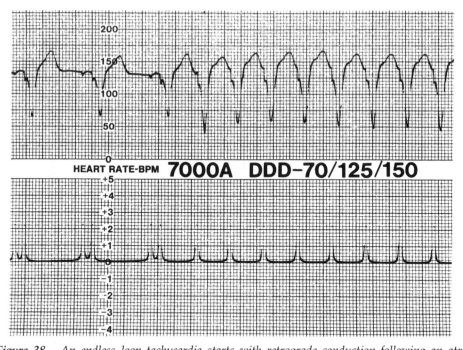

Figure 38. An endless loop tachycardia starts with retrograde conduction following an atrial stimulus with atrial capture and a ventricular stimulus with ventricular capture. Retrograde conduction occurred at an interval greater than 235 ms.

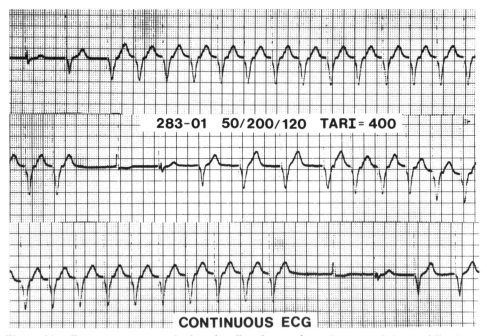

Figure 39. Two spontaneous episodes of endless loop tachycardia are each begun following a spontaneous P wave that precedes the ventricular stimulus by 200 ms. As the upper rate coupling interval is 500 ms, the AV interval is 300 ms. Each tachycardia is ended by the pacemaker after 15 intervals at the upper rate limit. The tachycardia terminating algorithm causes atrial channel insensitivity for one event after the sixteenth ventricular stimulus.

BALANCED ENDLESS LOOP TACHYCARDIA

As previously described, most endless loop tachycardias operate exactly at the upper rate limit. But this is not necessarily the case. The existence of endless loop tachycardia below the upper rate limit is important because it defeats those tachycardia terminating algorithms that depend on sustained ventricular stimulation exactly at the upper rate limit, and because of the recognition of the importance of exact timing in any decision-making process that uses a specific event (e.g., upper rate) as an absolute determinant of a tachycardia. The cycle length of a balanced endless loop tachycardia is determined by the sum of the ventriculoatrial conduction time and the atrioventricular interval (Figure 40). When an endless loop tachycardia occurs below the upper rate limit, ventriculoatrial conduction can be calculated by subtracting the atrioventricular interval from the tachycardia cycle length. The ventriculoatrial conduction time cannot be determined by this method when the tachycardia is at the upper rate limit because the AV interval may be extended to maintain the selected upper ventricular rate.

The necessary condition for occurrence of this tachycardia (Figure 41) is either preserved retrograde conduction at rapid pacing rates or a very long ventriculoatrial conduction time. Retrograde conduction can occur at higher pac-

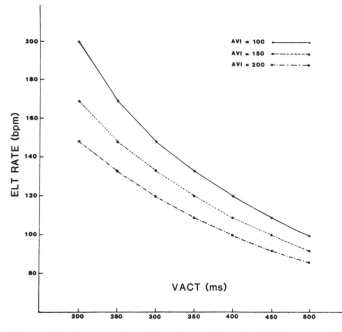

Figure 40. *Relationship between the endless loop tachycardia (ELT) rate and the programmed atrioventricular interval (AVI) and the ventriculoatrial conduction time (VACT). With longer ventriculoatrial conduction time for each atrioventricular interval, the tachycardia rate is slower. Similarly, at a given ventriculoatrial conduction time, as the atrioventricular interval increases, the tachycardia rate decreases.*

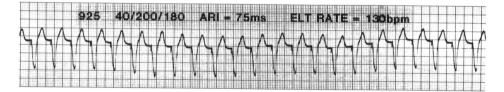

Figure 41. *Endless loop tachycardia (ELT) occurring at a rate slower than the pacemaker upper rate limit is shown. This tachycardia was induced in a patient with pacemaker model 925, programmed to a minimum rate of 40 bpm, an upper rate limit of 180 bpm, an atrioventricular interval of 200 ms and an atrial refractory interval (ARI) of 75 ms. The tachycardia is at an approximate rate of 130 bpm, well below the upper rate limit of 180 bpm.*

ing rates (140–160 bpm) in approximately 20% of patients tested at implant. Prolonged retrograde conduction times occur infrequently. Routine programming of long atrial refractory periods after a ventricular event will therefore avoid most but not all of these tachycardias. But, such prolongation will force a lower upper rate limit (Figure 42).

Consequently, during management of an endless loop tachycardia, its origin should be determined and may result from any one of the listed mechanisms. Further, a tachycardia may be spontaneous in that it may occur without any one of the mechanisms known to induce an endless loop tachycardia. It may be sustained over a prolonged period, especially if the upper rate limit is low, prolonged VA conduction exists, and prolonged AV conduction is encouraged. It may be at exactly the upper rate limit allowing the invocation of a tachycardia-terminating algorithm or it may be below the upper rate limit defeating efforts at its control and even making its diagnosis difficult if it is assumed that all such tachycardias operate exactly at the upper rate limit.

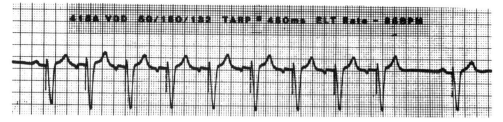

Figure 42. *A slow balanced endless loop tachycardia can be very much below the upper rate limit and can especially occur in the VDD mode, as atrial channel stimulation does not occur. In a pacemaker model in which the upper rate limit is determined by the total duration of atrial refractoriness, the fixed AV interval had been programmed to 150 ms and the atrial refractory interval to 300 ms, a total of 450 ms and an upper rate limit of 132 bpm. The retrograde conduction interval was about 550 ms, beyond the duration of atrial refractoriness. The retrograde P waves are inverted and the two antegrade P waves (at each end of the ECG) are upright. Each sensed retrograde P wave begins an AV interval of 150 ms duration which ends with a ventricular channel stimulus (until the retrograde channel is fatigued) with an overall cycle duration of 700 ms, a rate of 85 bpm. (0–180)*

In the endless loop tachycardia, depolarization of the ventricle may penetrate the His-Purkinje system and, if the pathway is not refractory, retrograde conduction can occur and another P wave will be produced. This P wave can, in turn, be sensed by the pacemaker atrial channel and stimulate the ventricle after the programmed AV interval. The reentry loop may thus be perpetuated as long as the retrograde pathway is not fatigued and as long as some algorithm designed to make the atrial channel refractory is not activated by the pacemaker circuit. In actual practice, the tachycardia may be incessant or prolonged as it is with natural reentry tachycardias or it may be self-limited after a brief episode.

The upper rate behavior of the pacemaker has a direct bearing on the existence of ELT. As in the natural tachycardia in which one pathway is used as the antegrade limb and the other as the retrograde, the natural pathway in the presence of a pacemaker acts as the retrograde limb. The retrograde pathway has a conduction refractoriness that is a function of a variety of factors, including the prematurity of the ventricular stimulus, the state of sympathetic and parasympathetic tone, the circulating catecholamine level, whether atrium and ventricle are being paced, and presumably others as well. Despite these factors, the retrograde (VA) conduction interval is well defined at any one time, though it may be no more constant than antegrade (AV) conduction. If retrograde conduction of a ventricular contraction produces a P wave after the ventricular event, it will be sensed or unsensed depending on whether the atrial channel is refractory at the time and the sensitivity setting of the atrial channel. If the atrial channel is refractory, it will be unsensed; if the atrial channel is not refractory and is adequately sensitive, the atrial contraction will be sensed.

The two conditions that encourage ELT are: (1) short atrial refractory interval (ARI) after a ventricular event; (2) prolongation of the AV interval (Figure 43).

The first allows sensing of a retrograde P wave; the second allows recovery

ENDLESS LOOP TACHYCARDIA

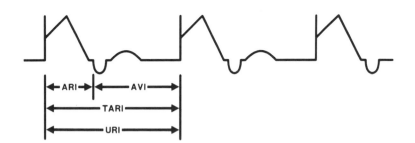

Figure 43. *A diagrammatic representation of the endless loop tachycardia involves a constant atrial refractory interval (ARI) and the establishment of an upper rate interval (URI) independently of the total atrial refractory interval (TARI). Because the retrograde P is sensed and produces the next ventricular stimulus, at the conclusion of the URI, the AV interval (AVI) is extended. As the AV interval is always part of the total atrial refractory interval, that interval is now prolonged to equal the upper rate interval. Once again, in this instance, the upper rate limit is set by the total atrial refractory interval, and in this instance, prolonged by the prolongation of the AV interval.*

of the tissue of the His-Purkinje system so that a ventricular contraction meets a nonrefractory retrograde pathway. Both factors are conditions of the pseudo-Wenckebach mode of upper rate limit management. Should ELT occur, management is by one of these means:

1. An algorithm that stops atrial sensing, restoring DVI or VVI pacing at the atrial rate with restoration of the AV synchrony later;
2. Recognition that a displaced P wave, i.e., one that does not precede a QRS complex is the most common cause of ELT, so that the ARI is prolonged after a ventricular event not preceded by an atrial event;
3. Programmed prolongation of the ARI for each ventricular event so that a retrograde P wave always falls into the ARI;
4. Programming atrial sensitivity so that antegrade atrial EGMs, almost always larger, are sensed, while retrograde EGMs, almost always smaller, are rejected;
5. Differentiation by pattern recognition by the pacemaker between an antegrade and retrograde P wave. This approach is only hypothetical at this time.
    If a retrograde or dissociated P wave is sensed, the AVI is begun. If the AVI is fixed, then a P wave will be followed by a ventricular stimulus after the programmed AV interval. If the AVI is at a "normal" interval then it is unlikely that a retrograde P wave can occur. If, however, the AVI is unfixed, i.e., the upper rate limit is the pseudo-Wenckebach mode, then the AVI will prolong, so that the next ventricular stimulus occurs after the entire upper rate interval. If this prolongation is sufficient, the retrograde AV pathway will not be refractory and continuation of the tachycardia will result. The only method that effectively stops ELT is by the first four means listed, effectively stopping sensing of P waves through one means or another.
6. One pulse generator defines an endless loop tachycardia by the stability of retrograde conduction. In this instance if the retrograde interval is less than 453 ms (but exceeds the atrial refractory interval after the sensed or paced ventricular event) and the event varies in duration by less than 31 ms for eight events, ELT is considered. The diagnosis is then tested by further stressing the conduction system and determining stability. If an ELT is confirmed by the pulse generator criteria, the atrial refractory period is prolonged to 453 ms for a single cycle. The pulse generator can also reprogram itself to a new and stable atrial refractory interval to avoid recurrent endless loop tachycardias.

All presently available choices designed to stop or prevent the endless loop pacemaker-mediated tachycardia involve loss of sensing of one or more retrograde atrial beats (Figure 44). The common feature of all endless loop tachycardia management techniques is the loss of atrial sensing. All of the approaches are attempts to combine a high upper rate capability with insensitivity to retrograde P waves and to ameliorate the sudden deceleration associated with reaching the upper rate limit. A technique referred to as "rate smoothing" is one such in which, at the upper rate limit and potential AV block onset, the ventricular rate is slowly decelerated by allowing a programmable percentage of rate change only. Rate smoothing is a technique that modifies the atrial escape interval by a programmable percentage of the previous atrial escape interval. Sudden halving of the rate with onset of AV block becomes a programmable feature and may be replaced, for example, by a 3% or 12.5% allowable decline. After all fallback and smoothing operations have been completed, endless loop tachycardia may resume unless a P wave falls into a refractory interval. In at least one reported instance, ELT occurred with intermittent third-degree AV block

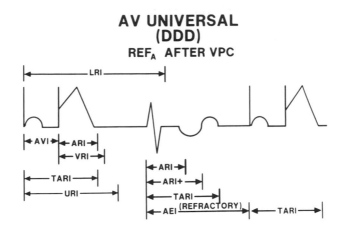

Figure 44. *Four different approaches are illustrated for the prevention of endless loop tachycardia (ELT) by making the atrial channel refractory. As most (but not all) ELT starts with a P wave displaced by a ventricular premature contraction, atrial channel refractoriness begins with a VPC. ARI is used in pacemakers with AV block upper rate limitation and provides that the atrial refractory interval is programmed to exceed the retrograde conduction interval after each ventricular event. ARI + is used in Wenckebach upper rate limitation with the atrial refractory interval kept relatively short but prolonged by a set duration after a VPC. After each VPC a total atrial refractory interval is begun. This approach is often used in devices in which no clear programming distinction is allowed between the ARI before the ventricular event (i.e., the AVI) and that after the ventricular event. An entire atrial escape (ventriculoatrial) interval is made refractory succeeded by the establishment of a new TARI, following which normal atrial sensitivity is resumed.*

and retained prolonged retrograde conduction. As management with retention of a satisfactory upper rate was difficult, ablation of the AV conduction system eliminated retrograde conduction.

PSEUDO-WENCKEBACH AND AV BLOCK

From the previous discussion it is now clear that whether an atrial-sensing pacemaker operates in the pseudo-Wenckebach or the AV block mode is a function of the timing cycles selected during upper rate behavior. Briefly stated, the upper rate limit of any pacemaker can be set by the TARI only; if this is so then the AV block mode will be present (Figure 45). If the TARI is sufficiently short so that the upper rate interval is set independently, then the difference between URI-TARI = Wenckebach Interval. In a pulse generator in which the ARI is fixed, i.e., not programmable, the only part of the TARI that will be programmable is the AVI. As long as the TARI is of shorter duration than the URI, a Wenckebach interval will exist. If a P wave falls during this interval, prolongation of the AVI can occur.

If, however, the ARI is programmable then the upper rate limit may be set by the TARI or by the URI depending on whether the ARI is programmed to be of shorter or longer duration. If the total of ARI and AVI, i.e., the TARI, is less than the URI, then the upper rate mode will be pseudo-Wenckebach as a

AV UNIVERSAL (DDD)

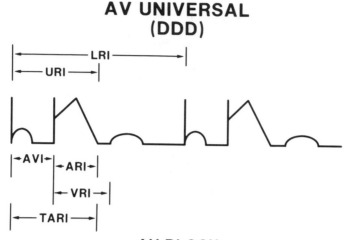

AV BLOCK

Figure 45. *The AV universal (DDD) pacemaker can consist of a variety of modes all of which have the common denominator of sensing and pacing atrium and ventricle. Diagram of the usual mode in which a spontaneous event in either chamber inhibits its output and in the atrium triggers a ventricular response. In the AV block mode of upper rate limitation, the AV begins with the sensed or paced atrial event. It ends with a sensed or paced ventricular event. The ARI begins with a sensed or paced ventricular event and together they add up to the TARI, which establishes the upper rate limit (URI). The VRI begins with a ventricular event, though they need not be of similar duration. The lower rate interval (LRI) is programmed independently and is the interval between the ventricular event and the next atrial event or between two atrial events. Unlike the VDD mode, escape is from the atrial not the ventricular channel. Note that the TARI establishes the upper rate limit (URI); it is not established independently of atrial refractoriness.*

P wave will enter the Wenckebach interval before entering the completely re-fractory interval (Figure 46).

If by programming the ARI the TARI becomes longer than the URI, a P wave will enter a zone of absolute refractoriness from one of complete sensitivity. AV block will result. Thus programmability of the ARI will allow a pacemaker to operate in the AV block or pseudo-Wenckebach modes.

As an example, if the AVI is set to be 150 ms and the ARI 155 ms, the TARI will be 305 ms as will the URI, and the upper rate limit will be 197 bpm. If the upper rate limit is independently programmed to 150 bpm, i.e., 400 ms, the Wenckebach interval is 95 ms, which is also the maximum prolongation of the AVI. If now the ARI is prolonged from 155–250 ms the TARI becomes 400 ms yielding an URL of 150 bpm. No Wenckebach interval can exist and no prolon-gation of the AVI is possible. If the ARI is prolonged beyond 250 ms the TARI becomes longer than the URI. A P wave will enter a zone of absolute refrac-toriness, the TARI, before it reaches the independently programmed URI. No Wenckebach function is possible.

With the introduction of ARI programming in all atrial sensing dual-cham-ber pacemakers, the physician is able to select between two upper rate behaviors, pseudo-Wenckebach or AV block. This option will add flexibility to patient man-agement. In the presence of retrograde conduction, pseudo-Wenckebach is less

AV UNIVERSAL
(DDD)

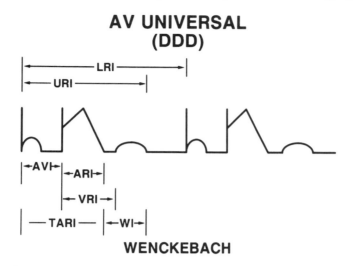

WENCKEBACH

Figure 46. *The AV universal (DDD) pacemaker in which the upper rate limit is via the pseudo-Wenckebach mechanism operates in a similar fashion to that of the AV block mode. Both AV block and the pseudo-Wenckebach approaches are interchangeable upon selection of the appropriate timing cycles. Unlike the AV block mode in which the URI is established by the TARI, in this mode the URI is programmed independently. As an independently programmed URI must be at a lower rate (longer interval) than TARI, the difference between the two intervals is the Wenckebach interval (WI). If a P wave falls in the Wenckebach interval, the subsequent ventricular stimulus is delayed until the end of the URI. AV block and pseudo-Wenckebach upper rate management are interchangeable depending on the duration of the URI and the TARI. As the TARI occupies a greater portion of the URI, the WI correspondingly decreases in duration. When TARI equals URI, no pseudo-Wenckebach effect exists.*

desirable than AV block and will be less likely because a prolonged AVI will be selected to encompass the retrograde conduction time. For those patients, usually without retrograde conduction, in whom a relatively low maximum ventricular rate is desired and in whom a moderate prolongation of AVI can be tolerated hemodynamically, the pseudo-Wenckebach mode can be programmed. As long as programmability of both AVI and ARI is possible, the physician can select one or the other.

AUTOMATIC MODE CHANGE

The operational mode of an implanted pacemaker may require change depending on alteration in rhythmic circumstances. Mode change in response to the rhythmic change and not induced by programming has been important since modes other than asynchronous were introduced. The earliest ventricular inhibited pacemakers were extremely sensitive to electromagnetic and electromyographic interference and could be inhibited with resultant asystole. In a primitive fashion, reversion of a pacemaker from normally sensitive, i.e., inhibited operation, to brief asynchronous operation was then designed into the pulse generator function. Such approaches were based on a "noise sampling" period as part of the pulse generator timing cycle so that several or even a single event falling during a brief portion of the cycle would produce an asynchronous stimulus at the normal pacemaker escape (or at some other predetermined) interval. An example of such an event is Figure 3 in this chapter. Sustained interference resulting from 60-Hz interference would then produce repetitive events during the "noise sampling" period and yield a sustained asynchronous rate. While this approach in various modifications remains in use, it is most suitable for single-chamber pacing. Absence of a sensed event during the "noise sampling" period permits return to inhibited function (Figure 47).

Another automatic mode change from inhibited to asynchronous was the dual demand approach intended for the underdrive of tachyarrhythmias in which pacing was set at a programmed rate, e.g., 70 bpm. The refractory period of the pacemaker could be set so that a tachycardia at a coupling interval briefer than a specific duration would fall into the pacemaker refractory interval. Operationally this occurs because of the existence of an absolute and nonprogrammable refractory interval of 125 ms duration and an additional and continuous relative refractory interval of programmable duration. During relative refractoriness a sensed event does not inhibit and recycle the pacemaker so that at the escape interval a stimulus is emitted. This mode is intended to stimulate and possibly terminate the tachycardia. Single-chamber pulse generators with programmable refractory periods are available and can readily be programmed into this capability. If, for example, the total refractory period is set to 450 ms, change from inhibited to asynchronous function will occur at a tachycardia rate of 133 bpm. If refractoriness is set to be 250 ms, then conversion will occur at 240 bpm, a tachycardia less likely to be manageable by underdrive pacing. An earlier mode named "fallback" involved a change from DDD operation to VVI operation at a rate other than the lower rate limit of the DDD pacemaker in the presence of a tachycardia which might be an ELT. The mode was unsuccessful in managing ELT as the intermediate rate might be able to entrain the atrium retrograde so that with the automatic restoration of DDD function a retrograde P wave would be sensed and the ELT would resume (see Chapter 2, Figure 40).

The usual management of a patient requiring atrial pacing in whom AV block is not anticipated (without sufficient conviction that only the AAI mode will be maintained) has been to set a DDD mode with a prolonged AV interval, hoping that AV conduction will continually maintain the ventricular channel inhibited. A pulse generator recently introduced manages this situation by mode change. It is programmed to the AAI mode, but ventricular sensing is maintained. If a spontaneous ventricular event is not sensed during a time interval window, the duration of which is the mean of the preceding eight intervals between the atrial paced or sensed event to the ventricular sensed event (measurable because ventricular channel sensing has persisted) plus 47 ms, with a maximum of 350 ms, the pacemaker reverts to the DDD mode and paces the ventricle. It remains in the DDD mode until a ventricular event is sensed, atrial pacing ceases and sensing atrial activity begins, or after 100 paced ventricular events. When one of these criteria have been met, the AV interval is prolonged to allow spontaneous ventricular events and if one occurs, the mode is returned to AAI as described above (Figure 48).

NOISE SAMPLING PERIOD

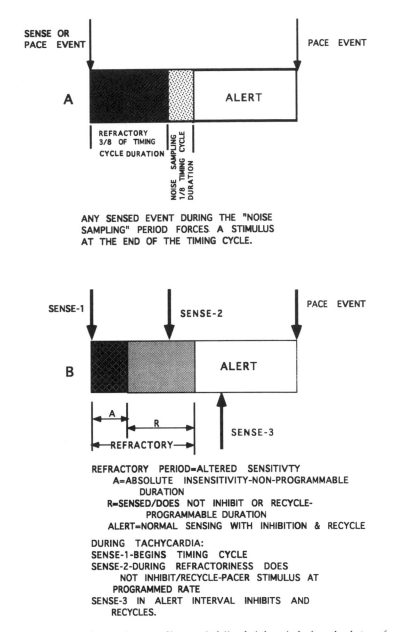

SENSE OR PACE EVENT

PACE EVENT

A

ALERT

REFRACTORY
3/8 OF TIMING
CYCLE DURATION

NOISE SAMPLING
1/8 TIMING CYCLE
DURATION

ANY SENSED EVENT DURING THE "NOISE
SAMPLING" PERIOD FORCES A STIMULUS
AT THE END OF THE TIMING CYCLE.

SENSE-1

SENSE-2

PACE EVENT

B

ALERT

A   R

REFRACTORY

SENSE-3

REFRACTORY PERIOD=ALTERED SENSITIVTY
 A=ABSOLUTE INSENSITIVITY-NON-PROGRAMMABLE
  DURATION
 R=SENSED/DOES NOT INHIBIT OR RECYCLE-
  PROGRAMMABLE DURATION
 ALERT=NORMAL SENSING WITH INHIBITION & RECYCLE

DURING TACHYCARDIA:
SENSE-1-BEGINS TIMING CYCLE
SENSE-2-DURING REFRACTORINESS DOES
  NOT INHIBIT/RECYCLE-PACER STIMULUS AT
  PROGRAMMED RATE
SENSE-3 IN ALERT INTERVAL INHIBITS AND
  RECYCLES.

Figure 47. *A. During the "noise sampling period," a brief period after absolute refractoriness, a sensed event causes loss of the next alert interval, changing the mode from VVI to VOO for a single cycle. If following the next pacer stimulus an event once again falls into the "noise sampling period," the mode change is continued. B. In this increasingly common modification of refractoriness, a substantial portion does sense. The sensed event is not used to start a timing cycle, but may be demonstrated on an ECG interpretation channel or may cause a change in operating mode as in "A" above.*

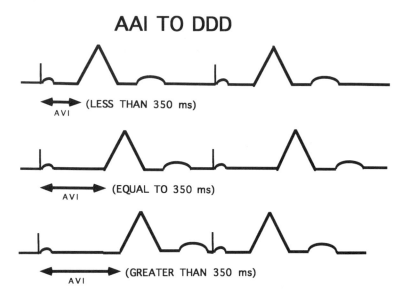

AAI TO DDD

(LESS THAN 350 ms)
AVI

(EQUAL TO 350 ms)
AVI

(GREATER THAN 350 ms)
AVI

Figure 48. *In the AAI mode with continued monitoring of the ventricular response, continued AV conduction maintains the ventricular channel inhibited. The maximum limit for AV conduction is 350 ms. If nothing is sensed after the elapse of 350 ms, ventricular channel stimulation begins at a preprogrammed AV interval.*

Dual-chamber pacing with atrial tracking requires the ability to control the upper rate response of ventricular stimulation via the mechanism of an independent programmed upper rate limit or by the establishment of an upper rate limit dependent on the duration of atrial refractoriness. (Both mechanisms have been described elsewhere in this text.) Instability of atrial rhythm presents another problem. Most atrial tachyarrhythmias (supraventricular tachycardia, atrial fibrillation, and atrial flutter) are sufficiently rapid so that conduction of rapid (physiological or pathological) atrial events to the ventricle must be limited to a desired maximum. Atrial rates deemed too rapid for a desired ventricular response were controlled by the independently programmed upper rate limit of the duration of atrial refractoriness, limiting the maximum ventricular response under all circumstances, by the mechanism of change of the pacing mode of 1:1 atrial tracking to 2:1 or higher degrees of AV block or by the pseudo-Wenckebach mechanism. In this circumstance, pacemaker response to atrial events was such that tracking occurred at the upper rate limit and then slowed by conversion to a mode of tracking other than 1:1.

Dual-chamber pacemakers have been used in progressively greater numbers of patients with episodic tachyarrhythmias during the past few years, resulting from an ability to manage them with medications and pacing or following ablation of the AV conduction system. In both instances the risk to dual-chamber function is that an atrial tachyarrhythmia will be transmitted to the ventricle. Several approaches have been attempted. One is the use of the DDI mode in which atrial sensing and pacing exist but without atrial tracking. Only a lower rate limit, usually, but not invariably with AV synchrony, is established. A difficulty with this approach is that despite the potential for physiological atrial rate variation there is no corresponding response in ventricular stimulation rate, and if the atrial rate is sufficiently more rapid than the automatic pacemaker rate, AV synchrony is lost. This limitation can be partially overcome in rate modulated dual-chamber pacemakers with a sensor-driven rate. Even AV synchrony may tend to be restored.

As the major difficulty is the development of atrial fibrillation or flutter in such patients, the preferred present means of controlling ventricular rate is automatic mode change in the presence of rapid, recurrent atrial events. These functions have been named by manufacturers as "Automatic Mode Switching" (AMS) and "Automatic Mode Conversion" (AMC). Other names are certain to appear. The pacemaker, in the sensor-driven mode determines an appropriate atrial rate and if atrial events are sensed during a mode change interval, the mode is changed from DDDR to VVIR. Atrial activity continues to be monitored, and if atrial events no longer fall into the mode change interval, the device returns to the DDDR mode of operation (Figure 49).

MODE CHANGE-RETRO P

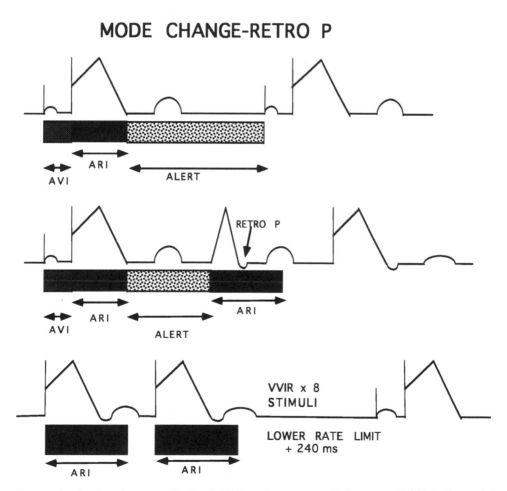

Figure 49. *In the minute ventilation DDDR mode, a retrograde P wave will fall during atrial refractoriness and change the pacing mode to VVIR. If the P wave remains entrained retrograde it will not emerge from atrial refractoriness. After 8 such sensed events, the pacing interval will be extended by 240 ms and return to DDDR function. Another retrograde P wave will restart the cycle.*

The value of such a mechanism depends on its precision and accuracy in determining when mode change is appropriate and when it may not be. Frequent episodes of change when unnecessary or lack of change when necessary vitiate much of its value. In order to operate automatic mode change, atrial activity must continue to be monitored during both DDDR and VVIR functions, as must the sensor determined rate (interval). In a presently constituted format, a single atrial event sensed during the relative atrial refractory period after a ventricular event is sufficient to induce change from DDDR to VVIR (Figure 50).

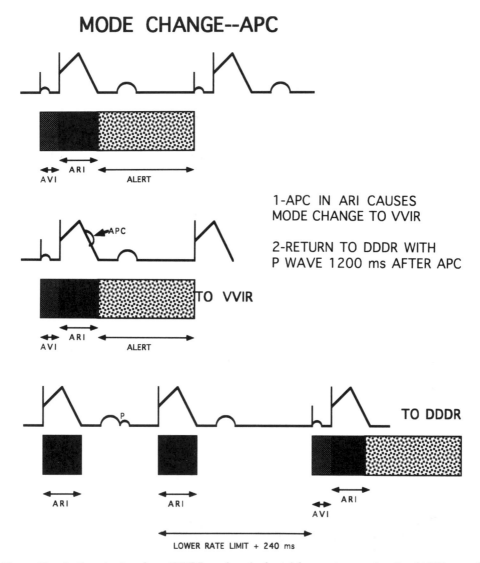

Figure 50.   *In the minute volume DDDR mode a single atrial premature contraction (APC) sensed during atrial refractoriness will change the pacing mode to VVIR, but not start a timing cycle. In the absence of consistent timing for the atrial event, the next P wave sensed 1200 ms after the P wave in atrial refractoriness will not start a timing cycle (sensed P waves do not start a timing cycle during VVIR function) but will change the pacing mode (to DDDR).*

Equally, during VVIR operation, should a single P wave fall beyond the duration of the sum of the adaptive AV interval and the adaptive ARI, then DDDR pacing will resume. As both conditions readily can occur with slight atrial arrhythmia, rapid acceleration or deceleration of atrial rate, or selection of a poorly responsive setting for determining the most appropriate rate with activity, there have been reports of inappropriate mode change.

ATRIOVENTRICULAR INTERVAL (AVI) MODULATION

Modification of Atrial Refractoriness

Atrial refractoriness can be modified automatically to achieve a change in the upper rate limit of a dual-chamber pacemaker, or a change in upper rate limit can occur as a consequence of a change in atrial refractoriness for another reason. The reasons for increasing atrial refractoriness after the ventricular event are to limit sensing retrograde atrial events and to establish an upper rate limit. The total atrial refractory interval (TARI) establishes the absolute upper rate limit, and it consists of the sum of the atrioventricular interval (AVI) and the atrial refractory interval following the ventricular sensed or paced event. If either component is abbreviated, the sum is decreased and the upper rate limit will be increased if total atrial refractoriness and not an independent upper rate limit establishes the upper rate limit.

The AV interval may be modified in several ways:

1. In ventricular based timing, a conducted or idioventricular event during the AV interval that inhibits and recycles ventricular timing will increase the lower rate limit.
2. A rate modulated AV interval usually is abbreviated at higher atrial sensed or sensor-driven atrial rates. As the AV interval is part of atrial refractoriness, total atrial refractoriness is reduced. The AV interval may be reduced progressively so that a still higher atrial or sensor rate will reduce atrial refractoriness even more.

The AV interval may be prolonged via the pseudo-Wenckebach mechanism for upper rate limitation. It is then added to the total atrial refractoriness and the upper rate is reduced. If the independently programmed upper rate limit is unchanged and is at a lower rate than atrial refractoriness will allow, the disparity will increase and the pseudo-Wenckebach effect will increase. If the independently programmed upper rate limit is higher than atrial refractoriness will allow, then the new abbreviated atrial refractory interval will allow the actual upper rate limit to move toward the independently set limit. The atrial refractory interval after the ventricular event has not been automatically reduced below that programmed. Prolongation of this interval is automatically performed in several pacemaker models after a ventricular premature event (defined as a spontaneous ventricular event not preceded by an atrial sense or pace event). Abbreviation has not been established as an automatic event, but there is no electronic reason why abbreviation of atrial refractoriness cannot be done at a specific atrial or ventricular rate. That change would also increase the upper rate limit. If the AV interval and atrial refractoriness after the ventricular event were both reduced simultaneously the upper rate limit would be increased. As the occurrence of retrograde conduction (when it exists at all) is reduced at upper rates, the reduction in duration of atrial refractoriness may have little effect.

The AVI may be modulated as part of the tachycardia detection mechanism to distinguish between a sinus tachycardia and an endless loop tachycardia which is based on retrograde, i.e., VA conduction. If the tachycardia persists at the upper rate limit, the AV interval is automatically modulated on alternate cycles by 47 ms. The interval between the paced ventricular event and the sensed atrial event is monitored. In the presence of an endless loop tachycardia the interval is constant (until fatigue occurs) and retrograde conduction is likely. If reduction in duration of the AV interval by the 47 ms modulations abbreviates the interval from one ventricular stimulus to the next by 47 ms, then sinus tachycardia is confirmed. Should endless loop tachycardia be determined, the device automatically extends the ARI to 453 ms for one cycle to block a retrograde P wave.

INCREASING THE UPPER RATE LIMIT

In recent dual-chamber units the absolute upper rate limitation imposed by TARI, i.e., total atrial refractoriness (the AV interval plus the atrial refractory interval after the ventricular event) has been partially circumvented by the mechanism of automatic reduction of TARI. As delineated earlier, retrograde conduction commonly (but not universally) disappears at more rapid ventricular paced rates. Consequently, the atrial refractory interval after the ventricular stimulus can be reduced in duration. As the PR interval is normally reduced in duration at more rapid rates, this can be mimicked by reduction of the AV interval during atrial tracking in DDD (or VDD) pacing or during rapid atrial pacing in rate modulated, i.e., DDDR pacing. The abbreviation of the AV interval is translated into an equivalent abbreviation of TARI and thus to a higher upper rate limit. For example, if the TARI is 450 ms consisting of 150 ms of AV interval and 300 ms of PVARP (postventricular atrial refractory period), the absolute upper rate limit will be 133 bpm. As that rate is approached, were the AV interval to be abbreviated to 125 ms, TARI would be 425 ms and upper rate 141 bpm. If AVI were reduced to 100 ms, TARI would be 350 ms and URL 150 bpm. Further extensions of the URL might be achieved by simultaneous reduction in the duration of PVARP to take advantage of the reduction in retrograde conduction at more rapid rates. However, this might cause some difficulty were retrograde conduction time to increase with increasing paced rate rather than resulting in VA block (Figure 51).

Lower Rate Behavior

In a single- or dual-chamber pacemaker the intervals begun by paced or sensed events can be equal or unequal. Formerly, most intervals were equal in

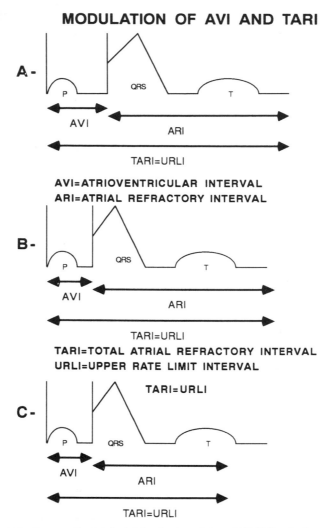

MODULATION OF AVI AND TARI

Figure 51. *In this diagram the total atrial refractory interval (TARI) sets the upper rate so that TARI = URLI (upper rate limit interval). A. The sum of the atrioventricular interval (AVI) and the atrial refractory interval after the ventricular stimulus (ARI) is equal to the total atrial refractory interval (TARI), which in turn equals the upper rate limit interval (URLI). B. The AVI has been modulated and is shorter in duration, the ARI has not been modulated, but the sum of two, i.e., TARI is now briefer in duration as is the URLI. The possible upper rate is now higher. C. In this diagram the AVI and ARI have both been abbreviated. The TARI and URLI are now both briefer and the upper rate limit has been increased.*

duration. With the advent of electronic circuits in which it is easy to provide either an unequal or equal interval, many single-chamber pacemakers provide a programming capability for hysteresis. All that is changed is the interval between successive events, depending on whether the cycle begins with a paced or sensed event. Hysteresis usually allows a longer interval between successively sensed events. An interval that ends with a paced event starts a shorter interval before emitting a stimulus and requires a still shorter interval for a spontaneous beat to begin a longer cycle. Hysteresis can be available in a DDD pacemaker as a longer escape interval in the atrial channel.

HYSTERESIS

During customary hysteresis operation, a lesser rate (i.e., longer coupling interval) inhibits the pacemaker. Should a single allowed interval be exceeded, pacing begins at a shorter coupling interval (i.e., a greater rate). During continuous pacing, a single ventricular interval shorter than the pacing interval is required to resume the lower rate. Because such a single event may be infrequent, prolonged, possibly unnecessary pacing may occur. A hysteresis variant named "search hysteresis" extends the pacing interval to the duration of the hysteresis interval every 256 continuous pacing cycles (Figure 52). With such prolongation a spontaneous event may occur and inhibit pacing. If a spontaneous event does not occur, pacing resumes at the usual interval. If an event

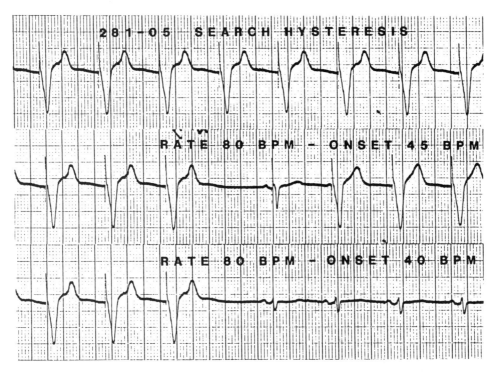

Figure 52. *Search hysteresis is intended to overcome a major limitation of ordinary hysteresis in which once pacing has started it may not end even if it may be unnecessary. UPPER ECG: Ventricular pacing at 80 bpm is continuous, with atrial entrainment retrograde. MIDDLE ECG: A single cycle of 1333 ms duration allows an atrial escape with a conducted ventricular beat. As this event is marginally too late, a ventricular stimulus fuses with the ventricular beat and starts stimulation again. LOWER ECG: With lowering of the hysteresis rate to an interval of 1500 ms the pacemaker pause is sufficiently long that the spontaneous ventricular event inhibits stimulation.*

does occur, the pacemaker is inhibited until the hysteresis interval is exceeded when pacing will resume, testing once again after each 256 consecutive paced events.

In the DDD mode, escape is by an atrial stimulus that occurs at the ventricular escape interval minus the AVI. This interval is the VA interval. For example, if the ventricular escape interval (which is the same as the lower rate interval) is 1000 ms and the AVI is 150 ms, the ventriculoatrial interval (VAI) (assuming no hysteresis) will be 850 ms from the preceding ventricular event. A P wave that occurs during the ventricular escape interval, i.e., during that 850 ms interval will start a new AVI, a new LRI, and a new URI. Rate hysteresis, possibly combined with search hysteresis, recently has been introduced in dual-chamber pacing so that one spontaneous rate maintains the pulse generator inhibited, while once pacing has begun, it will be at another rate. The dual-chamber hysteresis capability is being evaluated in the management of symptomatic vagal syndromes in which it may be especially effective.

In the DVI mode, the absence of atrial sensing means that during LRI and URI which, in the absence of deliberate or accidental hysteresis, are identical, all sensing is from the ventricular channel, but the atrial channel escape is at the VA interval, that is, the ventricular escape interval minus the AVI.

SENSOR- DRIVEN INTERVALS

The newly available sensor-driven, (rate modulated, adaptive rate, or rate responsive) pacemakers have an interval in addition to those that now are used to operate the device. The normal operation of a single-chamber, SSI device or a dual-chamber DDD device is as usual. In the single-chamber device, the lower rate or escape interval is as in an AAI or VVI pacemaker. In such a device there is no means of abbreviating the escape interval. In the rate modulated single-chamber device, a sensor allows abbreviation of the escape interval just as the sensed P wave causes abbreviation of the escape interval in a VDD pacemaker. Indeed, the most widely used rate modulated (activity sensing) device was a direct modification of an atrial synchronous, ventricular inhibited pulse generator. As the sensor is not sensitive to a stimulus visible on the ECG, there may be no clear indicator of why a specific response occurs. Nevertheless, the lower rate limit is the escape interval and the sensor-driven interval (SDI) and the upper rate interval (URI) are identical (Figure 53).

The dual-chamber sensor-driven pacemaker is similar to the DDD pacemaker. In this instance, the lower rate limit is an atrial escape stimulus. Two stimuli set the upper rate limit. Should the sensor-driven (SDI) upper rate interval be shorter than the atrial coupling interval (i.e., the atrial rate) the atrium will be paced and spontaneous atrial activity will be suppressed. If AV conduction occurs from the spontaneous or paced atrial event, the ventricular stimulus will be suppressed. If the atrial coupling interval is briefer than the SDI, it will take precedence and the sensor rate modulation and spontaneous atrial synchrony will occur (Figure 54).

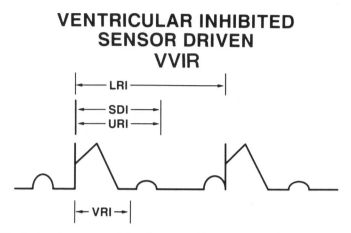

Figure 53. *Single-chamber rate modulated, sensor-driven pacing differs from single-chamber in-hibited pacing by the presence of an upper and lower rate. The lower rate is the analog of the set rate of the single rate pacemaker. In the rate modulated device, the set duration of the interval between stimuli can be modified by the sensor of physiology. The timing diagram is similar to that of the VVI device with the addition of a sensor-driven interval (SDI), which is the equivalent of the upper rate interval (URI).*

Other options exist. For example, the programmed AV interval may be a function of the atrial or sensor-driven rate or both. In that event, the AVI may be one value at the lower rate limit and another at the upper rate limit. This feature is likely to become more common as new devices are made available.

Another possibility is that atrial synchrony during dual-chamber pacing will be preserved at relatively lower rates and will then be sacrificed at higher rates.

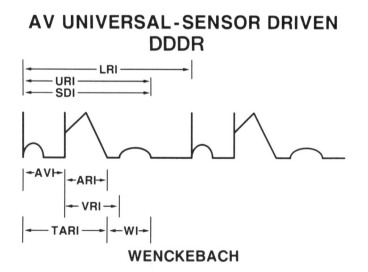

Figure 54. *The dual-chamber rate modulated device provides a sensor-driven interval (SDI), the equivalent of the upper rate interval. In the dual-chamber device diagramed, the timing cycles are those of the conventional dual-chamber pacemaker. In the DDD device, the atrium drives the ventricular stimulus to the upper rate interval (URI). In the rate modulated device, the upper rate interval is driven by the sensor and by the atrium, which is sensed or paced depending on whether sensor drive or atrium is at the briefer interval.*

In such an instance, for example, the mechanism described above of dual sensors, atrium, and another physiological sensor may be used up to a rate of perhaps 100 bpm, i.e., a coupling interval of 600 ms. Thereafter, if the sensor directs a shorter coupling interval, i.e., a higher rate, the atrial channel would be inactive and neither sensing nor stimulation would occur. The ventricular drive will then be from the sensor and no attempt at atrial synchrony would exist. Other timing events are likely as single-chamber and dual-chamber sensor-driven, i.e., rate modulated pacemakers are developed.

MULTIPLE SENSING CHANNELS

With the introduction of sensor-driven dual-chamber pacing, an additional channel of sensitivity has been added to pacemaker capability. It is possible to view evolution in pacing as relative to the increase in the amount of data received via the sensing channels rather than in any other way. It is readily possible to stimulate via one or many channels. However, sensing and correlating the responses of more than one channel becomes progressively more complex. Sensing a single channel, first the atrium and then the ventricle, was critical in pacemaker development. Until two channels could be sensed and logically handled, dual-chamber pacing and the practical restoration of atrial synchrony was not possible. The single-chamber rate modulated pacemaker was not more complex than dual-chamber pacing. Sensitivity to atrial activity was replaced by sensitivity to another event. The introduction of three channels of sensitivity, i.e., ventricle, atrium, and an additional sensor marks a new level of complexity and sophistication (Figure 55).

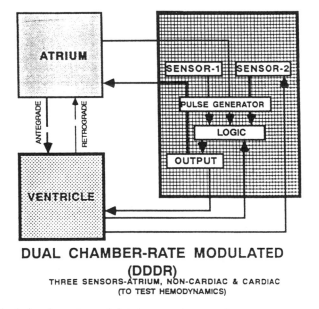

DUAL CHAMBER-RATE MODULATED (DDDR)
THREE SENSORS-ATRIUM, NON-CARDIAC & CARDIAC (TO TEST HEMODYNAMICS)

Figure 55. *A dual-chamber rate modulated pacemaker may have one sensor or two in addition to the atrium (three sensors in all). The interaction of the three may be complex. Such a unit now in clinical evaluation has a nonphysiological sensor, e.g., activity coupled with a physiological sensor, QT interval, designed for rapid and prolonged response.*

BIBLIOGRAPHY

Ausubel K, Gabry MD, Klementowicz PT, et al: Pacemaker-mediated endless loop tachycardia at rates below the upper rate limit. Am J Cardiol 1988; 61:465–467.

Barold SS, Carroll M: "Double reset" of demand pacemakers. Am Heart J 1972; 84:276–277.

Barold SS, Falkoff MD, Ong LS, et al: Interpretation of electrocardiograms produced by a new unipolar multiprogrammable "committed" AV sequential demand (DVI) pulse generator. PACE 1981; 4:692–708.

Barold SS, Gaidula JJ: Evaluation of normal and abnormal sensing functions of demand pacemakers. Am J Cardiol 1971; 28:201–210.

Barold SS, Levine PA: Autointerference of demand pulse generators. PACE 1981; 4:274–280.

Barold SS, Gaidula JJ, Banner RL, et al: Interpretation of complex demand pacemaker arrhythmias. Br Heart J 1972; 34:312.

Barold SS, Gaidula JJ, Castillo R, et al: Evaluation of demand pacemakers by chest wall stimulation. Chest 1973; 63:589–606.

Barold SS, Gaidula JJ, Lyon JL, et al: Irregular recycling of demand pacemakers from borderline electrographic signals. Am Heart J 1971; 82:477.

Barold S, Linhart J, Samet P: Reciprocal beating induced by ventricular pacing. Circulation 1968; 38:330–340.

Barold SS, Ong LS, Falkoff MD, et al: Inhibition of bipolar demand pacemaker by diaphragmatic myopotentials. Circulation 1977; 56:679–683.

Barold SS: Clinical significance of pacemaker refractory periods. (editorial) Am J Cardiol 1971; 28:237–239.

Batey RL, Calabria DA, Shewmaker S, et al: Crosstalk and blanking periods in a dual chamber (DDD) pacemaker: A case report. CPPE 1985; 3:314–318.

Bathen J, Gundersen T, Forfang K: Tachycardias related to atrial synchronous ventricular pacing. PACE 1982; 5:471–475.

Bertuso J, Kapoor AS, Schafer J: A case of ventricular undersensing in the DDI mode: Cause and correction. PACE 1986; 9:685–689.

Burchell HB: Analogy of electronic pacemaker and ventricular parasystole with observations on refractory period, supernormal phase, and synchronization. Circulation 1963; 27:878–889.

Castellanos A, Bloom MG, Sung RJ, et al: Mode of operation induced by rapid external chest wall stimulation in patients with normally functioning QRS-inhibited (WI) pacemakers. PACE 1979; 2:2–10.

Castellanos A, Lemberg L: Disorders of rhythm appearing after implantation of synchronized pacemakers. Br Heart J 1964; 26:747–754.

Castellanos A, Lemberg L: Pacemaker arrhythmias and electrocardiographic recognition of pacemakers. Circulation 1973; 42:1381–1391.

Castellanos A, Lemberg L, Arcebal AG, et al: Repetitive firing produced by pacemaker stimuli falling after the T wave. Am J Cardiol 1970; 25:247–251.

Castellanos A, Lemberg L, Jude JR, et al: Repetitive firing occurring during synchronized electrical stimulation of the heart. J Thorac Cardiovasc Surg 1966; 51:334–340.

Castellanos A, Lemberg L, Jude JR: Depression of artificial pacemakers by extraneous impulses. Am Heart J 1976; 73:24–31.

Castellanos A, Lemberg L, Rodriguez-Tocker L, et al: Atrial synchronized pacemaker arrhythmias: Revisited. Am Heart J 1968; 76:199–208.

Castellanos A, Maytin O, Lemberg L, et al: Part VIII. Rhythm disturbances and pacing. Pacemaker induced cardiac rhythm disturbances. Ann NY Acad Sci 1969; 167:903–910.

Castellanos A, Ortiz JM, Pastis N, et al: The electrocardiogram in patients with pacemakers. Prog Cardiovasc Dis 1970; 13:190–205.

Castellanos A, Spence M: Pacemaker arrhythmias in context. (editorial) Am J Cardiol 1970; 25:372.

Castellanos A, Waxman HL, Moleiro F, et al: Preliminary studies with an implantable multimodel AV pacemaker for reciprocating atrioventricular techycardias. PACE 1980; 3:257–265.

Castillo A, Berkovits BV, Castellanos A, et al: Bifocal demand pacing. Chest 1971; 59: 360–364.

Castillo C, Lemberg L, Castellanos A, et al: Bifocal (sequential atrioventricular) demand pacemaker for sinoatrial and atrioventricular conduction disturbances. (abstract) Am J Cardiol 1970; 25:87.

Center S, Samet P, Castillo C: Synchronous, standby, and asynchronous pervenous pacing of the heart. Ann Thorac Surg 1968; 5:498–507.

Den Dulk K, Lindemans FW, Bar FW, et al: Pacemaker related tachycardias. PACE 1982; 5:476–485.

Den Dulk K, Lindemans FW, Wellens HJJ: Noninvasive evaluation of pacemaker circus movement tachycardias. Am J Cardiol 1984; 53:537–543.

Echeverria HG, Luceri RM, Thurer RJ, et al: Myopotential inhibition of unipolar AV sequential (DVI) pacemaker. PACE 1982; 5:20–22.

Edwards LM, Hauser RG: Dual mode sensing by a variable cycle ventricular synchronous pulse generator. PACE 1981; 4:309–312.

Falkoff M, Ong LS, Heinle RA, et al: The noise sampling period: A new cause of apparent sensing malfunction of demand pacemakers. PACE 1978; 1:250–253.

Freedman RA, Rothman MT, Mason JW: Recurrent ventricular tachycardia induced by an atrial synchronous ventricular-inhibited pacemaker. PACE 1982; 5:490–494.

Frohlig G, Dyckmans J, Doenecke P, et al: Noise reversion of a dual chamber pacemaker without noise. PACE 1986; 9:690–696.

Frumin H, Furman S: Endless loop tachycardia started by an atrial premature complex in a patient with a dual chamber pacemaker. JACC 1985; 5:707–710.

Furman S: Dual chamber pacemakers: Upper rate behavior. PACE 1985; 8:197–214.

Furman S: Inhibition of a ventricular synchronous pacemaker. Am Heart J 1977; 93:581–584.

Furman S: Retreat from Wenckebach. (editorial). PACE 1984; 7:1–2.

Furman S, Fisher JD: Endless loop tachycardia in an AV universal (DDD) pacemaker. PACE 1982; 5:486–489.

Furman S, Fisher JD: Repetitive ventricular firing caused by AV universal pacing. (letter) Chest 1983; 83:586.

Furman S, Hayes DL: Implantation of atrioventricular synchronous and atrioventricular universal pacemaker. J Thorac Cardiovasc Surg 1983; 85:839–850.

Furman S, Huang W: Pacemaker recycle from repolarization artifact. PACE 1982; 5:927–928.

Furman S, Reicher-Reiss H, Escher DJW: Atrio-ventricular sequential pacing and pacemakers. Chest 1973; 63:783.

Harthorne JW, Eisenhauer AC, Steinhaus DM: Pacemaker-mediated tachycardias: An unresolved problem. PACE 1984; 7:1140–1147.

Johnson CD: AV universal (DDD) pacemaker-mediated reentrant endless loop tachycardia initiated by a reciprocal beat of atrial origin. PACE 1984; 7:29–33.

Kristensson BE, Kruse I, Ryden L: Clinical problems in atrial synchronous ventricular inhibited pacing: A long-term follow-up of 54 patients. PACE 1984; 7:693–701.

Kruse I, Ryden L, Duffin E: Clinical evaluation of atrial synchronous ventricular inhibited pacemakers. PACE 1980; 3:641–650.

Lamas GA, Antman EM: Pacemaker-mediated tachycardia initiated by coincident P-wave undersensing and ventricular blanking period. PACE 1985; 8:436–439.

Levine PA: Confirmation of atrial capture and determination of atrial capture thresholds in DDD pacing systems. CPPE 1984; 2:465–473.

Levine PA: Postventricular atrial refractory periods and pacemaker mediated tachycardias. CPPE 1983; 1:394–401.

Levine PA, Brodsky SJ, Seltzer JP: Assessment of atrial capture in committed atrioventricular sequential (DVI) pacing systems. PACE 1983; 6:616–623.

Levine PA, Lindenberg B, Mace R: Analysis of AV universal (DDD) pacemaker rhythms. CPPE 1984; 2:54–73.

Levine PA, Seltzer JP: AV universal (DDD) pacing and atrial fibrillation. CPPE 1983; 1: 275–282.

Levine PA, Seltzer JP: Fusion, pseudo-fusion, pseudo-pseudofusion and confusion: Normal rhythms associated with atrioventricular sequential "DVI" pacing. CPPE 1983; 1:70–80.

Levine PA, Seltzer JP: Runaway or normal pacing? Two cases of normal rate responsive (VDD) pacing. CPPE 1983; 1:177–183.

Luceri R, Castellanos A, Zaman L, Myerburg R: The arrhythmias of dual-chamber cardiac pacemakers and their management. Ann Intern Med 1983; 99:354–359.

Luceri R, Parker M, Thurer R, et al: Particularities of management and follow-up of patients with DDD pacemakers. CPPE 1984; 2:261–271.

Luceri RM, Ramirez AV, Castellanos A, et al: Ventricular tachycardia produced by a normally functioning AV sequential demand (DVI) pacemaker with "committed" ventricular stimulation. JACC 1983; 1:1177–1179.

Medina-Ravell V, Castellanos A, Portillo-Acosta B, et al: Management of tachyarrhythmias with dual chamber pacemakers. PACE 1983; 6:333–345.

Nathan D, Center S, Wu C, et al: Synchronization of the ventricle and atrium in complete heart block by self-contained implantable pacer. Circulation 1962; 26:767.

Oseran D, Ausubel K, Klementowicz PT, et al: Spontaneous endless loop tachycardia. PACE 1986; 9:379–386.

Rozanski JJ, Blankstein RL, Lister JW: Pacer arrhythmias: Myopotential triggering of pacemaker mediated tachycardia. PACE 1983; 6:795–797.

Seltzer JP, Levine PA, Watson WS: Patient-initiated autonomous pacemaker tachycardia. Pace 1984; 7:961–969.

Spurrell RAJ, Sowton E: An implanted atrial synchronous pacemaker with a short atrioventricular delay for the prevention of paroxysmal supraventricular tachycardias. J Electrocardiol 1976; 9:89–96.

Sung RJ, Castellanos A, Thurer RJ, et al: Partial pacemaker recycling of implanted QRS-inhibited pulse generators. PACE 1978; 1:189–195.

Tolentino AO, Javier RP, Byrd C, et al: Pacer-induced tachycardia associated with an atrial synchronous ventricular inhibited (ASVIP) pulse generator. PACE 1982; 5:251–259.

Van Cleve RB, Sung RJ, Maytin O, et al: Notes on ventricular techycardia occurring during magnet waving and on the function of the Omni-Ectocor pacemaker. Eur J Cardiol 1978; 8:543–551.

Whalen RE, Starmer CF, McIntosh HD: Electrical hazards associated with cardiac pacemaking. Ann NY Acad Sci 1964; 111:922–931.

Yokoyama M, Wada J, Barold SS: Transient early T wave sensing by implanted programmable demand pulse generator. PACE 1981; 4:68–74.

Chapter 5

HEMODYNAMICS OF CARDIAC PACING

David L. Hayes, David R. Holmes, Jr.

The most physiological "pacing" system is normal sinus rhythm with intrinsic sinoatrial and atrioventricular conduction. In the absence of disease, this system provides atrioventricular (AV) synchrony and rate responsiveness based on a complex physiological sensor. As consideration is given to the hemodynamic effects of cardiac pacing, the goal should always be to mimic the normal conduction system as much as possible.

Circulatory hemodynamics are complex because of the many interrelationships of variables and the effect of disease states on these variables. The increasingly large body of literature dealing with the hemodynamics of cardiac pacing is at times confounding. Some of the agreements and disagreements are the result of small but significant differences in protocols or methodology used for the individual studies, some are the result of different patient populations included, for example, patients with left ventricular dysfunction versus structurally normal hearts with primary electrical problems, and, finally, some are the result of small numbers of patients. The problems are complicated by the difficulty of isolating various components that affect cardiac output, i.e., atrioventricular interval (AVI), atrial contribution, and cardiac rate, and determining their individual importance.

These difficulties notwithstanding, the hemodynamics of cardiac pacing have attracted increasing interest. This interest has been stimulated by the limitations of ventricular pacing, the ability to restore AV synchrony and rate responsiveness, and the possible decreased morbidity and mortality afforded by AAI or DDD pacing (both of which restore AV synchrony) compared to ventricular pacing.

PHYSIOLOGICAL CONSIDERATIONS

Determinants of Cardiac Output

Changes in cardiac output are an important means by which the normal cardiovascular systems respond to changing demands, such as exercise. The cardiac output is the product of heart rate and stroke volume. (Stroke volume can be defined as the amount of blood ejected with each ventricular contraction, that is, end-diastolic volume minus end-systolic volume.) The relationship of each of these is variable for a given patient and depends upon the level of exercise, the presence or absence of underlying cardiovascular disease, and the specific characteristics of the disease, for example, the degree of left ventricular

195

dysfunction and ventricular compliance. Demands for an increase in cardiac output, such as those with exercise, usually are met primarily by an increase in heart rate and to a lesser extent by an increase in stroke volume (Figure 1). During exercise, some persons, such as highly trained athletes, can further increase stroke volume proportionately to increase cardiac output. These highly trained athletes are able to increase both stroke volume and heart rate during exercise, but peak heart rate may be less than that seen during exercise in sedentary persons. However, in patients with left ventricular dysfunction secondary to coronary artery disease or cardiomyopathy, conditions not uncommon in patients requiring permanent pacemakers, the ability to increase stroke volume may be limited or even absent. In these persons, the ability to increase heart rate in response to increased demands is of paramount importance.

Factors affecting stroke volume are more complex. Stroke volume is dependent on both end-diastolic volume and end-systolic volume; the latter depends upon two other major factors—myocardial contractility and afterload. Myocardial contractility is difficult to assess alone as it depends upon both afterload and end-diastolic volume. In patients with decreased contractility, other compensatory mechanisms must be recruited to maintain cardiac output, and even these may not be sufficient.

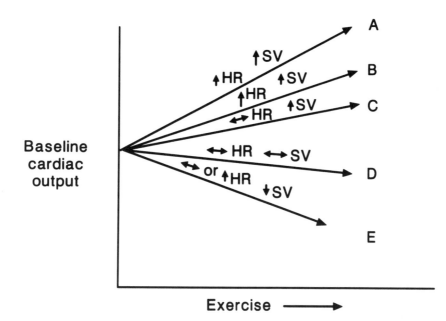

Figure 1.   Potential responses in heart rate (HR) and stroke volume (SV) to increasing exercise. A. Response in trained athletes during exercise. Large increase in cardiac output is the result of an increase in heart rate but a larger increase in stroke volume. B. Response in normal persons. There is a larger relative increase in heart rate but also some increase in stroke volume. C. Response in a patient with AV block or sinus node dysfunction but normal ventricular function who is chronotropically incompetent. D. Response in a patient with fixed heart rate and stroke volume who is unable to increase cardiac output with exercise or in whom cardiac output falls somewhat. E. Response of patient with markedly impaired ventricular function that worsens with exercise.

Afterload is a measure of the systolic ventricular wall stress required to eject blood. The resistance circuit into which the ventricle ejects blood is an important determinant of afterload. Although blood pressure is sometimes used to quantitate afterload, it is the peripheral vascular resistance that is more important. The relationship of cardiac output (CO), blood pressure (BP), and systemic vascular resistance (SVR) is shown in the following equation:

$$CO = BP/SVR$$

The concept of afterload is of particular importance in patients with hypertension or ventricular dysfunction. In the latter group, impaired contractility results in decreased cardiac output. This, in turn, results in compensatory physiological changes in an attempt to maintain perfusion by an increase in systemic vascular resistance. These changes, however, may further impair ventricular function by increasing the wall stress required to eject blood.

End-diastolic volume depends primarily on filling pressure, ventricular filling, and diastolic compliance. The well-known Frank-Starling curves (Figure 2) relate the degree of ventricular muscle stretch (preload) to a measure of performance, for example, cardiac output at a given level of myocardial contractility. Although the stretch of a muscle fiber (preload) can be easily measured experimentally, it cannot be quantitated clinically. Stretch can be correlated with diastolic volume. In turn, diastolic volume can be measured at angiography, by nuclear medicine techniques, or with echocardiography. More often, preload is assessed by measurement of the left ventricular end-diastolic pressure. The relationship between volume and pressure is a measure of the compliance of the ventricle. Patients with hypertrophied, stiff, noncompliant ventricles require a

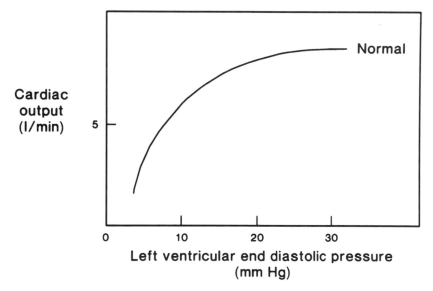

Figure 2. *Frank-Starling curve of cardiac output compared with left ventricular end-diastolic pressure.*

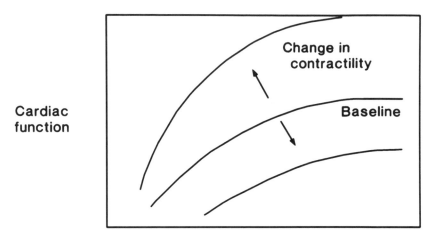

Myocardial fiber stretch

Figure 3.   *Schematic of ventricular function curves. Changes in contractility affect the relationship between myocardial fiber stretch (preload) and cardiac performance.*

higher pressure to achieve the same diastolic volume (stretch) as that required in a normal ventricle.

In addition to preload and afterload, ventricular function also affects cardiac output. Depending upon the underlying contractility, a change in the preload may significantly improve cardiac performance or change it very little (Figure 3). In a patient with significant left ventricular impairment and increased left ventricular end-diastolic pressure, increasing the preload further may not alter cardiac output.

The concept of ventriculoatrial (VA) conduction is essential to the understanding of the hemodynamics of cardiac pacing. Activation of mechanoreceptors (stretch receptors) within the walls of the atria and pulmonary veins results in peripheral vasodilatation and a decrease in systemic blood pressure. Either

Table I
Relationship among Stroke Volume (SV), Heart Rate (HR), and Cardiac Output (CO)

HR × SV = CO	
↑ HR × ↑ SV = ↑ CO	Usual response to exercise
↑ HR × ↑↑ SV = ↑ CO	Trained athlete
HR fixed × ↑ SV = ↑ CO	Response to exercise in patient with fixed-rate ventricular pacemaker and normal ventricle
HR fixed × SV fixed or ↓ = ↔ CO or ↓ CO	Response to exercise in patient with fixed-rate ventricular pacemaker and abnormal left ventricular function
↑ HR × SV ↑ or ↔ = ↑ CO	Response to exercise in patient with rate-responsive pacemaker

Table II
Maintenance of AV Synchrony

Resting State

Normal ventricular filling and normal or noncompliant ventricle
  a. maintains optimal preload
  b. contributes up to 20% of cardiac output compared to ventricular pacing
  c. prevents elevation of venous pressure seen with atrial systole against a closed AV valve or ventricular systole with an open AV valve
  d. prevents AV valve regurgitation seen with ventricular systole and an open AV valve
Left ventricular impairment and elevated filling pressure
  a. diminishing effect on cardiac output inversely proportional to the degree of left ventricular impairment
  b. prevents AV valve regurgitation seen with ventricular systole against an open AV valve

ventricular systole when the AV valves are open or atrial systole when the AV valves are closed can result in activation of these receptors.

In each patient, the relative roles of heart rate, stroke volume, and VA conduction vary. The relationship of these variables is confounded by the presence or absence of structural heart disease with impaired ventricular function, the fluid status of the patient, and the effect of cardioactive and vasoactive medications. In Table I some potential combinations of stroke volume and heart rate changes are shown. The importance of AV synchrony therefore depends upon the volume status, status of ventricular function, and the level of cardiac output required (Tables II and III).

The earliest indication for cardiac pacing was high-grade or complete heart block with recurrent Stokes-Adams attacks. In patients with this disorder, establishing a stable ventricular rhythm was lifesaving and prevented catastrophic asystole. This fact alone overshadowed the observation that although ventricular pacing improved cardiac output and/or patients' symptoms, normal function

Table III
Maintenance of AV Synchrony

Moderate-Maximal Exercise

Normal ventricular filling and normal or noncompliant ventricle
  a. maintains optimal timed preload
  b. contributes only small amount of increased cardiac output (<10%) compared to rate-matched asynchronous pacing
  c. prevents AV valve regurgitation seen with ventricular systole against an open AV valve
Left ventricular impairment and elevated filling pressure
  a. little effect on improving cardiac output
  b. prevents AV valve regurgitation seen with ventricular systole against an open AV valve

was not re-established with ventricular pacing. In addition, some patients with intermittent heart block actually experienced symptomatic hemodynamic deterioration with ventricular pacing (Figure 4). Adverse hemodynamics that are associated with a normally functioning pacing system resulting in overt symptoms or that limit the patients' ability to achieve optimal functional status is referred to as pacemaker syndrome. Pacemaker syndrome is the result of ventriculoatrial (VA) conduction and/or contraction of the atria against a closed AV valve that occurs when AV synchrony is lost. VA conduction may result in AV valve insufficiency and abnormal venous pulsations that may be symptomatic. VA conduction can result in activation of stretch mechanoreceptors in the walls of the atria and pulmonary veins. Vagal afferents transmit these impulses centrally, and the result is reflex peripheral vasodilatation, which may cause diz-

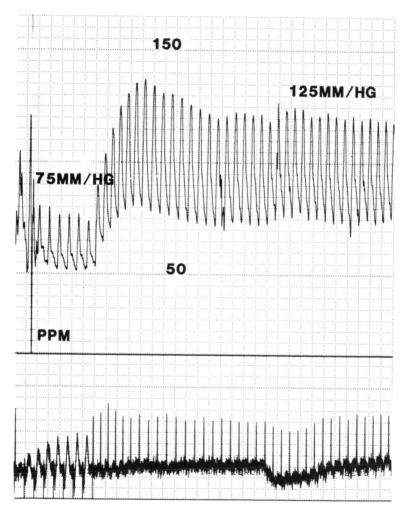

Figure 4. *Arterial pressure changes with and without ventricular pacing. Ventricular pacing of the first 7 beats results in a systolic arterial pressure of approximately 75 mm Hg. Subsequent intrinsic rhythm results in a systolic arterial pressure of approximately 125 mm Hg.*

Table IV
Potential Symptoms of Pacemaker Syndrome

Weakness	Chest pain
Near-syncope	Hypotension
Syncope	Congestive heart failure
Fatigue	Dyspnea
Lassitude	Jugular venous pulsations
Cough	Abdominal pulsations
Apprehension	

Table V
Potential Physical Findings in Pacemaker Syndrome

Cannon A waves
Blood pressure fall during ventricular pacing compared to normal sinus rhythm
Cyclic variation in cardiac output, arterial pressure, and peripheral vascular resistance
during hemodynamic monitoring.

---

ziness, near-syncope, or syncope. Pacemaker syndrome may therefore manifest with a variety of symptoms (Tables IV and V).

Pacemaker syndrome initially was identified as a complication of ventricular (VVI) pacing. However, pacemaker syndrome may occur anytime there is AV dissociation or where the AVI is so prolonged that atrial systole effectively occurs after ventricular systole. It has been described with AAI and DDI pacing modes as well as the rate adaptive counterparts of each of these modes, i.e., VVIR, AAIR, DDIR.

The incidence of pacemaker syndrome is difficult to determine and depends on how one defines pacemaker syndrome. If the definition is limited to patients with clinical limitations during any pacing mode that results in AV dissociation, the incidence is probably in the range of 7% to 10% of VVI paced patients as estimated in a review by Ausubel and Furman. In a study by Heldman et al., patients with DDD pacemakers were randomized to DDD versus the VVI pacing mode for 1 week and subsequently programmed to the alternate mode. The patients then completed questionnaires comparing 16 different symptoms during each pacing mode. With this approach some degree of pacemaker syndrome was felt to be present in 83% of those studied. The most common symptoms reported were shortness of breath, dizziness, fatigue, pulsations in the neck or abdomen, cough, and apprehension. It can be drawn from this study that if VVI paced patients have some basis for comparison, they may then be more aware of symptoms with VVI pacing.

IMPORTANCE OF AV SYNCHRONY IN PACED PATIENTS

In 1975 Karlof demonstrated a significant improvement in cardiac output in a group of 25 patients when paced in an atrial-triggered mode compared to fixed-rate VVI pacing. This study assessed the patients acutely and did not determine whether the hemodynamic improvement would be sustained chronically. We have shown similar results (Figure 5). Hartzler et al. confirmed these hemodynamic findings in an acute study in which cardiac output was measured in post-operative patients that were paced VVI versus AAI. In all patients the cardiac output improved when the atrium was paced maintaining AV synchrony (Figure 6). More recent studies have shown hemodynamic advantage of AAIR over DDDR pacing when the pacemaker was programmed so that DDDR pacing resulted in paced ventricular depolarization, demonstrating the hemodynamic importance of maintaining intrinsic ventricular depolarization, i.e., via AV conduction. However, it cannot be said that allowing the ventricle to depolarize via AV conduction is always superior. If the AVI were sufficiently prolonged some degree of hemodynamic compromise would result.

There has also been a suggestion of hemodynamic superiority of pacing the ventricle from a high septal position. Septal pacing may allow ventricular depolarization via the His-Purkinje system and avoid the altered depolarization pattern of right ventricular apical pacing.

Given the proven benefit of maintaining AV synchrony, who will benefit the most from restoration of AV synchrony? Is it the patient with normal left ventricular function or the patient with left ventricular dysfunction? The importance of atrial contribution to optimal left ventricular function, i.e., optimal

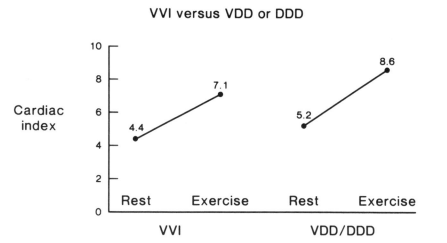

HEMODYNAMIC RESPONSE TO EXERCISE

Figure 5. *Hemodynamic response to exercise in 13 patients programmed to either VVI or VDD/DDD pacing. When programmed to VVI mode, with exercise the peak cardiac index was lower at 7.1 L/min/m², compared to 8.6 L/min/m² when the pulse generator was programmed to VDD/DDD mode.*

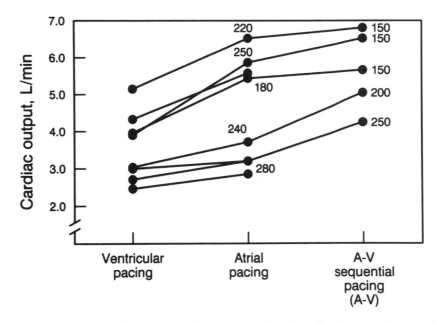

Figure 6. *Hemodynamic effect of ventricular versus atrial pacing. Cardiac output increased with atrial pacing when compared to ventricular pacing at identical heart rates in eight patients who were not pacemaker-dependent. The cardiac output was further improved by AV sequential pacing at shorter AV intervals compared with results of atrial pacing in five patients with intact AV conduction. Intrinsic PR intervals in ms are shown in the middle, and AV paced intervals in ms are shown on the right. From Hartzler GO, Maloney JD, Curtis JJ, et al: Hemodynamic benefits of atrioventricular sequential pacing after cardiac surgery. Am J Cardiol 40:234, 1977, with permission.*

cardiac output, in the presence of elevated left ventricular filling pressures has long been debated. Several investigators have reported that the contribution made by appropriately timed atrial systole is inversely proportional to the pulmonary capillary wedge pressure (Figure 7). Other investigators have reported improved hemodynamics with appropriately timed atrial systole regardless of left ventricular filling pressure.

If hemodynamic improvement is defined as an absolute improvement in measured cardiac output, then the patient with normal left ventricular function may realize the greatest improvement. Conversely, if hemodynamic improvement is defined as a relative improvement in measured cardiac output, then the patient with left ventricular dysfunction and a lower cardiac output may realize more relative benefit. In the patient with left ventricular dysfunction any improvement in cardiac output derived from appropriately timed atrial systole may be beneficial to the severely compromised patient. In addition to acute hemodynamic improvement, consideration also should be given to data from Alpert that has shown improved survival with dual-chamber pacing over single-chamber pacing in patients with congestive heart failure.

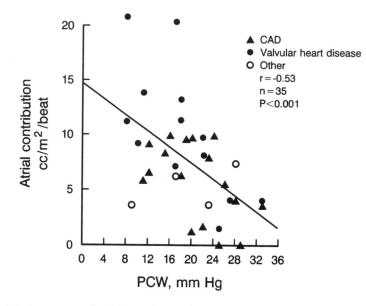

Figure 7. *The importance of atrial contribution depends on the filling pressure. There is an inverse relationship between absolute atrial contribution and the level of pulmonary capillary wedge pressure that reflects end-diastolic pressure. From Greenberg B, Chatterjee K, Parmley WW, et al: The influence of left ventricular filling pressure on atrial contribution to cardiac output. Am Heart J 98:742–751, 1979, with permission.*

A similar question can be posed for systolic versus diastolic left ventricular dysfunction. Which patient will derive the most benefit from restoration of AV synchrony? The patient with diastolic dysfunction and a stiff left ventricle or decreased compliance will gain more from AV synchrony. Maintaining AV synchrony will allow optimal left ventricular filling and maximal cardiac output. Even in the absence of underlying conduction system disease some investigators have found marked hemodynamic improvement by application of dual-chamber pacing to patients with hypertrophic cardiomyopathy. Presumably the benefit occurs because of the altered depolarization pattern with ventricular pacing in which the septum is not the first portion of the ventricle to be activated. Ventricular pacing alone would not result in the same benefit because loss of atrial systole in this clinical setting.

Following Karlof's initial study, a subsequent study by Kruse was able to demonstrate that the acute benefit shown by Karlof was maintained chronically. Kruse randomized a group of 16 patients to either ventricular pacing at 70 ppm or P-synchronous pacing for a 3-month period. Invasive hemodynamic studies were then performed with assessment at both rest and two levels of exercise. Chronically the patients with P-synchronous pacing demonstrated a significantly higher cardiac output, a lower systemic vascular resistance, lower serum lactate levels, and a smaller A-V O_2 difference at both levels of exercise (Figure 8).

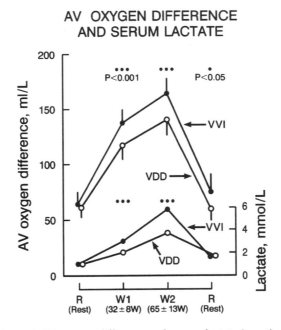

**AV OXYGEN DIFFERENCE
AND SERUM LACTATE**

Figure 8. *Comparison of AV oxygen difference and serum lactate in patients with VVI versus VDD pacing. The latter is associated with an improved hemodynamic response to the demands of exercise. From Kruse I, Arnman K, Conradson T-B, et al: A comparison of acute and long-term hemodynamic effects of ventricular inhibited and atrial synchronous ventricular inhibited and atrial synchronous ventricular pacing. Circulation 65:846,1982, with permission.*

The higher systemic vascular resistance with fixed rate ventricular pacing compared to P-synchronous pacing demonstrated by Kruse was interpreted as a response to greater sympathetic stimulation with fixed-rate ventricular pacing in a physiological attempt to boost cardiac output. Other studies have measured norepinephrine levels in fixed-rate ventricular pacing versus P-synchronous pacing and documented greater sympathetic stimulation in the absence of AV synchrony. In a study by Nordlander et al., VVI and VAT pacing modes were compared and myocardial oxygen uptake and coronary blood flow measured along with cardiac output. Although cardiac output was significantly higher with VAT pacing there was no significant difference between myocardial oxygen uptake and coronary blood flow between the two pacing modes. The investigators felt that the greater cardiac output with VAT pacing with similar myocardial oxygen uptake as VVI established VAT pacing as a more hemodynamically efficient pacing mode.

Numerous studies have also compared levels of atrial natriuretic peptide (ANP) when patients were paced VVI versus DDD and/or AAI (Figure 9). All studies have reflected a higher ANP level with VVI pacing. This has been explained by atrial distention, i.e., higher atrial pressures with the less physiological ventricular pacing mode. Many believe that the clinical sequelae of this atrial distention is facilitation of atrial fibrillation and an increased risk of throm-

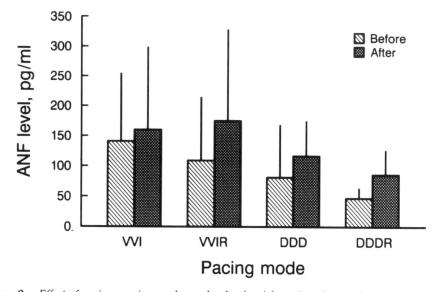

Figure 9.   *Effect of various pacing modes on levels of atrial natriuretic peptide (ANF) before and immediately after exercise. DDDR pacing resulted in the least elevation of ANF levels both at rest and following exercise.*

boembolic phenomena (see Importance for AV Synchrony on Morbidity and Mortality).

IMPORTANCE OF AV SYNCHRONY FOR MORBIDITY AND MORTALITY

The importance of AV synchrony in terms of morbidity and mortality must also be considered. Numerous investigators have retrospectively compared morbidity and/or mortality of patients after DDD or AAI pacing to patients receiving VVI pacing. Endpoints analyzed have included the incidence of atrial fibrillation, arterial thromboembolic events, incidence of congestive heart failure, and mortality. Table VI summarizes major studies to date. In patients with sinus node dysfunction, the incidence of atrial fibrillation and embolic events are significantly higher after VVI pacing than after DDD or AAI pacing. Rosenqvist et al. demonstrated a statistically significantly better survival in patients with sinus node dysfunction who received AAI pacing. Alpert et al. demonstrated improved 5-year survival rates for patients with congestive heart failure, both those paced for AV block and those with sinus node dysfunction, with dual-chamber pacing. Although the validity of any retrospective data can be questioned, it is impressive that similar findings have been reported by multiple investigators.

Table VI
Comparison of Morbidity and Mortality Between VVI Pacing and DDD or AAI Pacing

Investigators	No. of Pts.	Pacing Modality, No. of pts.			Atrial Fibrillation (%)				Mortality (%)				Thromboembolic Events (%)				Congestive Heart Failure (%)			
		AAI	DDD	VVI	AAI	DDD	VVI	P*	AAI	DDD	VVI	P*	AAI	DDD	VVI	P*	AAI	DDD	VVI	P*
Rosenqvist et al.	168	89		79	6.7		47	<0.0005	8		23	<0.05					15		37	<0.005
Santini et al.	339	135	79	125	4	13	47	<0.001	13	16	30	<0.001	2	2.5	8	NS				
Zanini et al.	110	53		57	3.8		17.5	<0.025	9.4		17.5	NS	0		7		1.9		5.3	
Stangl et al.	222	110		112	6		19		17		27	†								
Alpert et al. (1987)	128		49‡	79						22§	26	NS//								
Sasaki et al.	49	12	12	25	0	0	36	<0.01		25¶	43	<0.03//	0	0	20	<0.05				
Feuer et al.	220		110††	110		8	18	<0.05		7	15	‡‡					4.2#	27	28	NS**
Ebagosti et al.	90§§	45#		45	8.8///		24.4	<0.05**	15.4#		22.1	NS**	0	0	6.6				26	NS
Hayes et al.	1,092§§		649	443		5.5	9.2	=0.03¶¶	15	15	29	<0.003¶¶								
Alpert et al. (1986)	180##		48***	132						30§	27	NS//								
										31¶	53	<0.02//								

* For difference between VVI and AAI unless otherwise noted; † cumulative survival not statistically significant when overall groups compared. For subgroups without underlying heart disease, survival in AAI > VVI, P < 0.02. For subgroups with coronary disease, survival in AAI > VVI, P < 0.05; ‡ DDD, 11; DVI, 38; § without congestive heart failure; // For difference between VVI and DDD + DVI; ¶ With congestive heart failure; # value is for AAI and DDD together; ** for difference between VVI and AAI + DDD; †† DDD or DDI; ‡‡ not analyzed; §§ mixed conduction disturbances requiring pacing, not just sinus node dysfunction; /// classified as overall occurrence of atrial arrhythmias, not just atrial fibrillation; ¶¶ for difference between VVI and DDD; ## patients with atrioventricular block; *** DDD, 12; DVI, 36; NS = not significant.

IMPORTANCE OF OPTIMALLY TIMED ATRIOVENTRICULAR DELAY

Although there is some controversy in the pacing literature, there is a general consensus that optimal timing of the AVI will have a positive effect on hemodynamics (Figure 10). Daubert wrote "An optimal AV delay means that at each and every cycle, the AV interval produces exactly the delay required for the atrial systole to make its maximum contribution to stroke volume, should the patient be resting or exercising."

There are several aspects of the AVI to consider. First is the difference in the optimal AVI depending on whether it is initiated by a paced or sensed atrial event. This difference exists because of the electromechanical delay following a paced atrial event and the interatrial conduction time. The electromechanical delay is dependent upon multiple factors including atrial lead position and atrial size and function. Consider first the significance of the interatrial conduction time. It must be remembered that with a transvenous pacing system, it is the right atrial to right ventricular AVI that is being programmed. Cardiac output ultimately is affected by the left atrial to left ventricular AVI. The hemodynamic

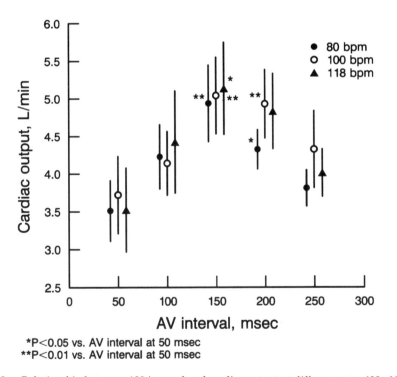

*P<0.05 vs. AV interval at 50 msec
**P<0.01 vs. AV interval at 50 msec

Figure 10.   *Relationship between AV interval and cardiac output at different rates (80, 100, 110 bpm). In this study, the maximal cardiac output was seen at an AV interval of 150 ms. From Haskell, RJ, French WJ: Optimum AV interval in dual chamber pacemakers. PACE 9:670–675, 1986, with permission.*

significance of the electromechanical delay lies in the fact that the programmed AVI begins simultaneously with the atrial pacing stimulus but it is the actual atrial depolarization that determines the onset of the effective delay between the atrium and ventricular depolarization, the AR or AV interval. That is, the effective interval is shorter than the programmed AVI. Conversely, during P-synchronous pacing, the programmed AVI begins with atrial sensing and the effective PV or PR interval begins with the native P wave. Therefore, the AVI should be programmed to reflect this difference. Multiple studies have shown the optimal AVI during DVI pacing to be longer than the optimal AVI during P-synchronous pacing. This difference at rest has been in the range of 30 to 50 ms. An increase in cardiac output when the AVI is optimized for P-synchronous pacing has also been demonstrated. A differential AVI is now available on many dual-chamber pacemakers as a programmable option.

In normal individuals the PR interval shortens as heart rate increases (Figure 11). (There is significant patient variability in PR shortening during exercise. An average shortening of the PR interval has been said to be 4 to 5 ms per 10 bpm increment in heart rate.) It follows then that for paced patients the optimal AVI at rest usually is not the optimal AVI during exercise. This introduces another hemodynamic variable for the AVI. In the paced patient, whether the atrium is being paced or sensed, the AVI has traditionally remained constant at the programmed AVI. In an effort to mimic the response of the normal conduction system a rate variable AVI is becoming a standard programmable option in dual-

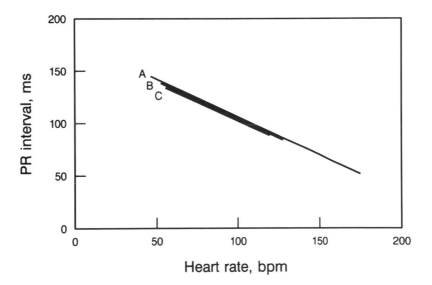

Figure 11. *Linear regression of PR interval (ms) and heart rate (beats/min) from electrocardiogram for young healthy subjects (group A), older healthy subjects (group B), and subjects following myocardial infarction (group C). From Rees M, Haennel RG, Black WR, et al: Effect of rate-adapting atrioventricular delay on stroke volume and cardiac output during atrial synchronous pacing. Can J Cardiol 6:447, 1990, with permission.*

chamber pacemakers. (There is significant variation in rate variable or rate adaptive AVI features among various pacemakers—See Chapter 17, Programmability.) Confirmation of hemodynamic benefit from a rate variable AVI has been repeatedly demonstrated. Hemodynamic benefit may occur not only because of the optimized AVI but also because a rate variable AVI may allow a higher ventricular rate depending on the timing circuit of the pacemaker. A higher paced ventricular rate may potentially maintain AV association to a greater workload and avoid untoward hemodynamic consequences of pseudo-Wenckebach or 2:1 block. It appears to be hemodynamically advantageous to implement the rate variable AVI when it is a programmable option.

Much has been learned about the hemodynamic importance of the AVI but the best way to program the AVI for the individual patient has yet to be determined. Some have advocated routine measurement of the interatrial conduction time in an effort to optimize the programmed AVI and others have advocated routinely doing repetitive cardiac output determinations at various AVI to determine the optimal value. This information could be meaningful, but collection of the data would be time consuming, expensive, and impractical for most physicians. To date there is not a quick, efficient, cost-effective way to establish the single most appropriate AVI for a given patient.

IMPORTANCE OF RATE RESPONSIVENESS

The importance of chronotropic competence was evident from the Karlof and Kruse studies already cited. These studies achieved rate responsiveness via VDD or VAT pacing.

When single-chamber rate adaptive pacing was introduced in the mid-1980s the importance of rate responsiveness was again questioned. The initial questions were aimed at comparing VVIR pacing (which provides rate responsiveness but not AV synchrony) to DDD or VDD pacing (which provides rate responsiveness and AV synchrony) and to VVI pacing (which provides neither rate responsiveness or AV synchrony). The hemodynamic studies that have been performed have demonstrated that rate responsiveness is the most important contributor to an increase in cardiac output and work capacity during exercise. Several studies warrant individual description. Prior to the clinical availability of VVIR pacemakers, Wirtzfeld and colleagues studied the relative importance of AV synchrony by determining cardiac outputs at rest and at multiple stages of exercise while pacing the patient in three different pacing modes. Patients were paced VVI at 70 ppm, VDD and VVI pacing at a rate matched to the rate achieved at each stage of exercise during the preceding VDD stress test. Cardiac outputs achieved were essentially identical during VDD and VVI rate-matched pacing (there was a slightly higher cardiac output with VDD during low-level exercise but no difference during higher level exercise). Both modes resulted in a significantly higher cardiac output than did VVI pacing (Figure 12). It was concluded that the increase in heart rate was the main contributor to improved cardiac output given the fact that the addition of AV synchrony (VDD) did not

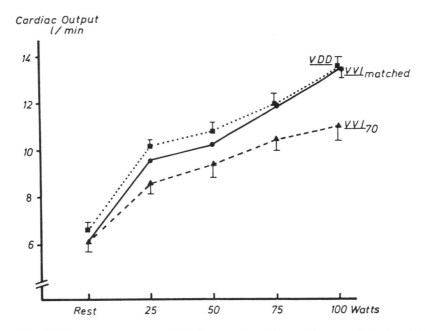

Figure 12. *Cardiac output at rest and during exercise in 11 patients paced in three different modes: VVI at 70 bpm (dashed line); VDD (dotted line); and VVI with the pacing rate at each stage of exercise programmed to match the ventricular rate achieved at the same stage of exercise during VDD pacing, i.e., VVIR equivalent (solid line). From Wirtzfeld A, Schmidt G, Himmler FC, et al: Physiological pacing: Present status and future developments. PACE 10:50; 1987, with permission.*

add significantly to the cardiac outputs obtained with rate responsiveness alone (VVI rate matched).

Fananapazir measured exercise capacity in a group of patients exercised in three different pacing modes: VOO (no rate responsiveness or AV synchrony), atrial synchronized ventricular pacing during chest wall stimulation (CWS) (for practical purposes this was equivalent to VVIR pacing in that it provided rate responsiveness but not AV synchrony), and VAT (rate responsiveness and AV synchrony). The VAT pacing mode resulted in a 44% increase in work capacity over VOO pacing and V-CWS-T pacing resulted in a 40% increase in work capacity proving that rate response is the most important factor in increasing work capacity (Figure 13).

Nordlander depicted the importance of chronotropic competence by summarizing 11 separate studies that had demonstrated the relative mean increase in work capacity by comparing fixed-rate ventricular pacing to some form of rate adaptive pacing (Figure 14). (This included VDD, VAT, rate-matched VVI, and VVIR both activity-sensing and QT rate adaptive pacing.) By linear regression analysis he demonstrated a highly significant positive linear correlation among the results of these 11 studies. This reinforces the fact that ventricular rate response is the single most important factor in increasing work capacity

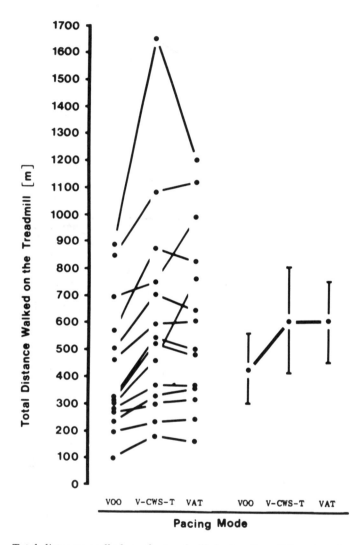

Figure 13.   *Total distances walked on the treadmill during three different pacing modes: VOO at 70 bpm; VAT; and V-CWS-T, a VVIR equivalent. From Fananapazir L, Bennet DH, Monks P: Atrial synchronized ventricular pacing: Contribution of the chronotropic response to improved exercise performance. PACE 6:604; 1983, with permission.*

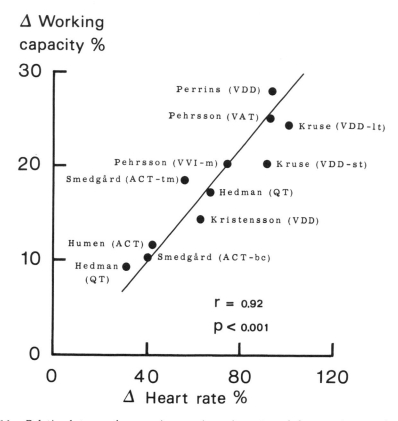

Figure 14.   *Relation between the mean increase in pacing rate and the mean increase in working capacity following the change from fixed rate to various types of rate responsive pacing. VDD and VAT = atrial triggered ventricular pacing; ACT = activity sensing rate responsive pacing; QT = QT interval sensing rate responsive pacing; lt = long-term; st = short-term; VVI-m = ventricular rate matched to atrial rate; tm = treadmill exercise; bc = bicycle ergometer exercise. From Nordlander R, Hedman A, Pehrsson SK: Rate responsive pacing and exercise capacity—a comment. PACE 12:750, 1989, with permission.*

and that the way in which rate responsiveness is achieved is relatively unimportant.

IMPORTANCE OF COMBINED AV SYNCHRONY AND RATE RESPONSIVENESS

The information cited regarding the importance of AV synchrony and the importance of rate responsiveness has unfortunately been used by some to advocate the importance of one over the other. Rate responsiveness and AV synchrony should not be considered mutually exclusive but as being complementary. AV synchrony is critical for avoidance of pacemaker syndrome and for optimizing cardiac output in patients with diastolic dysfunction as well as pro-

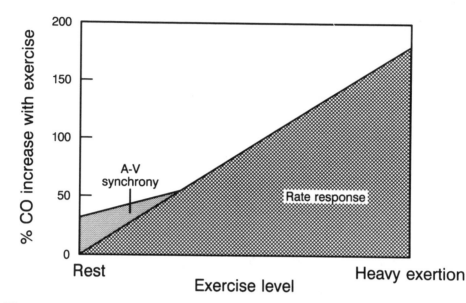

Figure 15. *Schematic representation of relative contribution of AV synchrony and rate response with increasing levels of exercise. At high levels of exercise rate response is largely responsible for the increase in cardiac output. AV synchrony is more important at rest and lower levels of activity. This should not be underestimated because the majority of the older paced population are at rest or low levels of exercise most of the time. Modified from D. Benditt MD, University of Minnesota, with permission.*

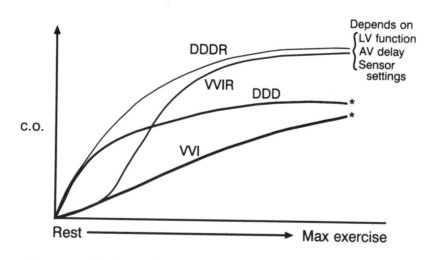

*Assuming significant chronotropic incompetence

Figure 16. *Schematic representation of potential differences in achieved cardiac output (C.O.) with various pacing modes. Cardiac output is represented on the X axis and level of exercise on the Y axis. DDDR should theoretically optimize cardiac output at both rest and peak exercise because AV synchrony is maintained at rest and low levels of exercise and rate response maintained throughout exercise. Although VVIR and DDDR may achieve similar cardiac outputs at peak exercise, cardiac output may be less in the VVIR mode at rest and during low levels of exercise due to the absence of AV synchrony.*

viding hemodynamic benefit for patients with systolic dysfunction. In patients with relatively normal ventricular function the contribution to cardiac output by AV synchrony is probably most important during sedentary and low-level activities at which most paced patients spend the majority of their time. As previously discussed, maintenance of AV synchrony appears to lower morbidity and mortality. Rate responsiveness is critically important for increasing cardiac output and work capacity during higher levels of activity (Figure 15). Therefore, a reasonable conclusion is that the ideal pacing system should provide and/or allow AV synchrony and rate responsiveness (Figure 16). In the chronotropically competent patient with AV block, a DDD pacemaker will fill this criterion. Conversely, the chronotropically incompetent patient with AV block requires a DDDR pacemaker to provide both AV synchrony and rate responsiveness.

HEMODYNAMIC CONSIDERATIONS OF UPPER RATE BEHAVIOR IN DUAL-CHAMBER PACING

With DDD pacing an upper rate limit must be programmed to prevent tracking rapid atrial rhythms resulting in undesirably fast ventricular rates. Programming an upper rate imposes a point at which the pacemaker will create some ventricular response to the atrial rate other than 1:1 pacing. The response may be pseudo-Wenckebach, 2:1, or some less commonly used upper rate mechanism. The details of upper rate response are discussed in Chapter 4, Comprehension of Pacemaker Timing Cycles. Since Wenckebach upper rate behavior results in the loss of a stable AV relationship and 2:1 block may result in a sudden decrement of ventricular rate, some patients may become symptomatic when the upper rate limit is reached. The hemodynamic disadvantage of upper rate behaviors may be minimized by optimal programming of the PVARP, AVI (using rate variable AVI when an option), and mode. There are potential hemodynamic advantages of the upper rate mechanisms of DDDR pacing. For patients with DDD pacing who have demonstrated hemodynamic compromise at the upper rate limit, DDDR pacing should be considered at the time of pulse generator change. The mechanisms of upper rate behavior in DDDR pacing are discussed in Chapter 4, Comprehension of Pacemaker Timing Cycles and Chapter 9, Pacemaker Electrocardiography.

HEMODYNAMIC ADVANTAGE OF PERMANENT PACING IN THE ABSENCE OF USUAL INDICATIONS FOR PACING

There are several conditions where controversy exists as to whether permanent pacing should be considered for the possible hemodynamic advantage that it may confer even in the absence of symptomatic bradycardia. Clinical situations where permanent pacing may be considered include paroxysmal atrial fibrillation, dilated cardiomyopathy, hypertrophic cardiomyopathy, and chronotropic incompetence in the elderly. These are discussed in Chapter 1, Indications for Permanent Pacing.

BIBLIOGRAPHY

Alpert MA, Curtis JJ, Sanfelippo JF, et al: Comparative survival after permanent ventricular and dual chamber pacing for patients with chronic high degree atrioventricular block with and without preexistent congestive heart failure. J Am Coll Cardiol 1986; 7:925–932.

Alpert MA, Curtis JJ, Sanfelippo JF, et al: Comparative survival following permanent ventricular and dual-chamber pacing for patients with chronic symptomatic sinus node dysfunction with and without congestive heart failure. Am Heart J 1987; 13: 958–965.

Ausubel K, Furman S: The pacemaker syndrome. Ann Int Med 1985; 103:420–429.

Baig MW, Perrins EJ: The hemodynamics of cardiac pacing: Clinical and physiological aspects. Prog Cardiovasc Dis 1991; 33:283–298.

Barbieri D, Percoco GF, Toselli T, et al: AV delay and exercise stress tests: Behavior in normal subjects. PACE 13 (Part II); 1990:1724–1727.

Blanc JJ, Mansourati J, Ritter P, et al: Atrial natriuretic factorrelease during exercise in patients successively paced in DDD and rate matched ventricular pacing. PACE 1992; 15:397–402.

Camm J, Katritsis D: Ventricular pacing for sick sinus syndrome—A risky business? PACE 1990; 13:695–699.

Daubert C, Ritter P, Mabo P, et al: Rate modulation of the AV delay in DDD pacing. In M Santini, M Pistolese, A Alliegro (eds.): Progress In Clinical Pacing 1990. New York, Elsevier Science Publishing Company, Inc, 1990, pp. 415–430.

Ebagosti A, Gueunoun M, Saadjian A, et al: Long-term follow-up of patients treated with VVI pacing and sequential pacing with special reference to VA retrograde conduction. PACE 1989; 11:1929–1934.

Fananapazir L, Srinivas V, Bennet DF: Comparison of resting hemodynamic indices and exercise performance during atrial synchronized and asynchronous ventricular pacing. PACE 1983; 6:202–209.

Fananapazir L, Bennett DH, Monks P: Atrial synchronized ventricular pacing: Contribution of the chronotropic response to improved exercise performance. PACE 1983; 6:601–608.

Feuer JM, Shandling AH, Messenger JC: Influence of cardiac pacing mode on the long-term development of atrial fibrillation. Am J Cardiol 1989; 64:1376–1379.

Greenberg B, Chatterjee K, Parmley WW, et al: The influence of left ventricular filling pressure on atrial contribution to cardiac output. Am Heart J 1979; 98:742–751.

Gross J, Moser S, Benedek AM, et al: Clinical predictors and natural history of atrial fibrillation in patients with DDD pacemakers. PACE 1990; 12(II):1828–1831.

Hartzler GO, Maloney JD, Curtis JJ, et al: Hemodynamic benefits of atrioventricular sequential pacing after cardiac surgery. Am J Cardiol 1977; 40:232–236.

Haskell, RJ, French WJ: Optimum AV interval in dual chamber pacemakers. PACE 1986; 9:670–675.

Hayes DL, Neubauer SA: Incidence of atrial fibrillation after DDD pacing. (abstract) PACE 1990; 13:501.

Heldman D, Mulvhill D, Nguyen H, et al: True incidence of pacemaker syndrome. PACE 1990; 13:1742–1750.

Hochleitner M, Hortnagl H, Ng CK, et al: Usefulness of physiologic dual-chamber pacing in drug-resistant idiopathic dilated cardiomyopathy. Am J Cardiol 1990; 66:198–202.

Janosik DL, Pearson AC, Buckingham TA, et al: The hemodynamic benefit of differential atrioventricular delay intervals for sensed and paced atrial events during physiologic pacing. J Am Coll Cardiol 1989; 14:499–507.

Kappenberger L, Gloor HO, Babotai I, et al: Hemodynamic effects of atrial synchronization in acute and long term ventricular pacing. PACE 1982; 5:639–645.

Karlof I: Hemodynamic effect of atrial triggered versus fixed rate pacing at rest and during exercise in complete heart block. Acta Med Scand 1975; 197:195–210.

Karpawich P, Stokes K, Gates J, et al: Septal His-Purkinje pacing: A new concept to improve paced ventricular function. (abstract) J Am Coll Cardiol 1992; 19:149A.

Kruse I, Arnman K, Conradson T-B, et al: A comparison of acute and long-term hemodynamic effects of ventricular inhibited and atrial synchronous ventricular inhibited and atrial synchronous ventricular pacing. Circulation 1982; 65:846–855.

Lau CP, Wong CK, Leung WH, et al: Superior cardiac hemodynamics ofatrioventricular synchrony over rate responsive pacing at submaximal exercise: Observations in activity sensing DDDR pacemakers. PACE 1990; 13:1832–1837.

Leclercq C, Mabo P, Le Helloco A, et al: Hemodynamic interest of preserving a normal sequence of ventricular activation in permanent cardiac pacing. (abstract) J Am Coll Cardiol 1992; 19:150A.

Linde-Edelstam C, Nordlander R, Pehrsson SK, et al: A double-blind study of submaximal exercise tolerance and variation in paced rate in atrial synchronous compared to activity-sensor modulated ventricular pacing. PACE 1992; 15:905–915.

Linde-Edelstam C, Hjemdahl P, Pehrsson SK, et al: Is DDD pacing superior to VVI,R? A study on cardiac sympathetic nerve activity and myocardial oxygen consumption at rest and during exercise. 1992; 15:425–434.

Linde-Edelstam C, Gullberg B, Nordlander R, et al: Longevity in patients with high degree atrioventricular block paced in the atrial synchronous or the fixed rate ventricular inhibited mode. PACE 1992; 15: 304–313.

Luceri RM, Brownstein SL, Vardeman L, et al: PR interval behavior during exercise: Implications for physiological pacemakers. PACE 1990; 13(Part II):1719–1723.

McDonald KM, Maurer B: Permanent pacing as treatment for hypertrophic cardiomyopathy. Am J Cardiol 1991; 68:108–110.

Markewitz A, Schad N, Hemmer W, et al: What is the most appropriate stimulation mode in patients with sinus node dysfunction. PACE 1986; 9:1115–1120.

Mehta D, Gilmour S, Ward DE, et al: Optimal atrioventricular delay at rest and during exercise in patients with dual chamber pacemakers: a non-invasive assessment by continuous wave Doppler. Br Heart J 1989; 61:161–166.

Mukharji J, Rehr RB, Hastillo A, et al: Comparison of atrial contribution to cardiac hemodynamics in patients with normal and severely compromised cardiac function. Clin Cardiol 1990; 13:639–643.

Noll B, Krappe J, Goke B, et al: Atrial natriuretic peptide levelsreflect hemodynamic changes under pacemaker stimulation. PACE 1990; 13:970–975.

Noll B, Krappe J, Goke B, et al: Influence of pacing mode and rateon peripheral levels of atrial natriuretic peptide (ANP). PACE 1989; 12:1763–1768.

Nordlander R, Pehrsson SK, Astrom H, et al: Myocardial demands of atrial-triggered versus fixed-rate ventricular pacing in patients with complete heart block. PACE 1987; 10:1154–1159.

Nordlander R, Hedman A, Pehrsson SK: Rate responsive pacing and exercise capacity— a comment. PACE 1989; 12:749–751.

Oldroyd KG, Rae AP, Carter R, et al: Double blind crossover comparison of the effects of dual chamber pacing (DDD) and ventricular rate adaptive (VVIR) pacing on neuroendocrine variables, exercise performance, and symptoms in complete heart block. Br Heart J 1991; 65:188–193.

Pearson AC, Janosik DL, Redd RR, et al: Doppler echocardiographic assessment of the effect of varying atrioventricular delay and pacemaker mode on left ventricular filling. Am Heart J 1988; 115:611–621.

Pehrsson SK, Hjemdahl P, Nordlander R, et al: A comparison of sympathoadrenal activity and cardiac performance at rest and during exercise in patients with ventricular demand or atrial synchronous pacing. Br Heart J 1988; 60:212–220.

Rediker DE, Eagle KA, Homma S, et al: Clinical and hemodynamic comparison of VVI versus DDD pacing in patients with DDD pacemaker. Am J Cardiol 1988; 61:323–329.

Rees M, Haennel RG, Black WR, et al: Effect of rate-adapting atrioventricular delay on stroke volume and cardiac output during atrial synchronous pacing. Can J Cardiol 1990; 6:445–452.

Ritter P, Daubert C, Mabo P, et al: Haemodynamic benefit of a rate-adapted A-V delay in dual chamber pacing. Eur Heart J 1989; 10:636–646.

Ronaszeki A, Ector H, Denef B, et al: Effect of short atrioventricular delay on cardiac output. PACE 1990; 13(Part II):1728–1731.

Rosenqvist M, Brandt J, Schuller H: Atrial versus ventricular pacing in sinus node disease: A treatment comparison study. Am Heart J 1986; 111(2):292–297.

Rosenqvist M, Brandt J, Schuller H: Long-term pacing in sinus node disease: Effects of stimulation mode on cardiovascular morbidity and mortality. Am Heart J 1988; 116: 16–22.

Ryden L, Karlsson O, Kristensson BE: The importance of different atrioventricular intervals for exercise capacity. PACE 1988; 11:1051–1062.

Santini M, Alexidou G, Ansalone G, et al: Relation of prognosis in sick sinus syndrome to age, conduction defects and modes of permanent cardiac pacing. Am J Cardiol 1990; 65:729–735.

Sasaki Y, Shimotori M, Akahane K, et al: Long-term follow-up of patients with sick sinus syndrome: A comparison of clinical aspects among unpaced, ventricular inhibited paced, and physiologically paced groups. PACE 1988; 11:1575–1583.

Sasaki Y, Furihata A, Suyama K, et al: Comparison between ventricular inhibited pacing and physiologic pacing in sick sinus syndrome. Am J Cardiol 1991; 67:771–774.

Schuller H, Brandt J: The pacemaker syndrome: Old and new causes. Clin Cardiol 1991; 14:336–340.

Stangl K, Seitz A, Wirtzfeld A, et al: Differences between atrial single chamber pacing (AAI) and ventricular single chamber pacing (VVI) with respect to prognosis and antiarrhythmic effect in patients with sick sinus syndrome. PACE 1990; 13:2080–2085.

Stangl K, Weil J, Seitz K, et al: Influence of AV synchrony on theplasma levels of atrial natriuretic peptide (ANP) in patients with total AV block. PACE 1988; 11:1176–1181.

Wirtzfeld A, Schmidt G, Himmler FC, et al: Physiological pacing: Present status and future developments. PACE 1987; 10:41–56.

Zanini R, Facchinetti A, Gallo G, et al: Morbidity and mortality of patients with sinus node disease: Comparative effects of atrial and ventricular pacing. Pace 1990; 13: 2076–2079.

Zanini R, Facchinetti A, Gallo G, et al: Survival rates afterpacemaker implantation: A study of patients paced for sick sinus syndrome and atrioventricular block. PACE 1989; 12:1065–1069.

Chapter 6

PACEMAKER CODES

Seymour Furman

ICHD CODE

Implantable pacemakers have a variety of different modes of operation. They may pace atrium or ventricle and be insensitive to the chambers paced. They may sense and pace one chamber, sense one chamber and pace the other, sense one and pace both, or pace and sense both. Pacemaker codes were designed to indicate pacemaker function so that, despite the model pacemaker or pacemaker name, the mode of operation will be known. The first pacemaker code was published in 1974 by the pacemaker committee of the Intersociety Commission for Heart Disease Resources and has been widely adopted and used internationally for pulse generator designation. It is well understood and has been adopted by regulation in some jurisdictions. The code is so widely used that some know what the three-position describes about a specific generator without being aware of the meaning of each letter of the three positions. The code was modified in 1981 by the members of the original committee under NASPE auspices and extended to five positions. The revised code was then reemphasized in a second ICHD report in 1983. The first three positions are basic to the code and constituted a complete designation. The latest revision, i.e., the 1987 NBG code, requires four positions for completeness (Table I).

NBG CODE

The rapid evolution in bradycardia and tachycardia pacing has necessitated a revision in the existing ICHD/NASPE five-position code. To maintain its usefulness, the code has undergone three revisions since its introduction in 1974. The initial revision was an expansion from three to five positions to represent programmability in position IV and tachycardia management in position V. The latest revision (1987) expands its utility into rate-modulated pacemakers and refines the description of techniques of tachycardia management in position V.

The basic grammar of the code has remained unchanged since its introduction. Letters have been added to each of the positions and some letters have been removed in order to increase the utility of the code as needs have changed. In the instance of tachycardia management, the letter "R" had been placed in position III to indicate a pacemaker that was inhibited at normal or slow cardiac rates but functions in a "reverse" mode in response to a tachycardia. As no such

219

Table I
The Five-Position ICHD Code

Position	I	II	III	IV	V
Category	Chamber(s) paced	Chamber(s) sensed	Modes of response(s)	Programmable functions	Special antitachyarrhythmia functions
Letters used	V—ventricle	V—ventricle	T—triggered	P—programmable (rate and/or output)	B—bursts
	A—atrium	A—atrium	I—inhibited	M—multiprogrammable	N—normal rate competition
	D—double	D—double	D—double* O—none	C—communicating	S—scanning
		O—none	R—reverse	O—none	E—external A—active antitachycardia fixation otherwise undefined
Manufacturer's designation only	S—single chamber	S—single chamber		Comma optional here	

* Triggered and inhibited response.

Modified and reprinted with permission of Futura Publishing Company from Bernstein et al: Report of the NASPE Mode Code Committee. *PACE* 7:396, 1984.

pacing mode now exists, and as all tachycardia management is now in position V, "R" was removed from position III and the letter has been used once again, now in position IV, to indicate the function of adaptive rate pacing or rate modulation.

Position V has been troublesome since its introduction, largely because of uncertainty and evolution in the field of tachycardia management. While the earlier version of the code allowed description of various modes of antitachycardia pacing, all have now been consolidated into an indication of stimulation output levels. The letter "O" indicates the absence of any antitachycardia function. The second letter "P" is for output at the microjoule or traditional pacing level and the third letter "S" is for output of one or more joules, and is an abbreviation of "shock." The fourth letter "D" is a combination of pacing and shock, i.e., P + S, in anticipation of devices soon to be available.

It is hoped that this simplification will increase the utility of the code while avoiding attempts at specific description of techniques that may soon be obsolete. In order to provide a code for a pacemaker that has been programmed to the OFF mode, i.e., entirely inactive, the letter "O" has been allowed in each of the five positions. As each position must have a letter, just as a multidigit number requires a digit in each position, i.e., 150 differs from 1050, the placement of "O" in each of the five positions allows a meaningful sixth position when it becomes necessary.

POSITION I—designates the chamber(s) paced. Five letters are possible: "A" for atrium, "V" for ventricle, "D" if both atrium and ventricle are paced, and

"O" if the unit is shut down and no pacing is to occur. The letter "S" is for manufacturer's use only and indicates that the device paces a single chamber only, but that the chamber may be either atrium or ventricle.

POSITION II—designates the chamber(s) sensed. Five possibilities exist and consequently five letters. If the atrium alone is sensed, the letter "A" is used, if the ventricle, "V." If both atrium and ventricle are sensed, the letter "D" is used, and if the pacemaker is used in either atrium or ventricle, but only in a single chamber at a time, a manufacturer may use the letter "S." "O" indicates that the pacemaker is insensitive to incoming signals. This may be used as part of the totally inactive state with an "O" in position I or a unit may be insensitive while pacing.

POSITION III—designates the response to a sensed signal. "I" indicates that pacemaker output is inhibited by a sensed event, "T" that a stimulus is triggered by a sensed event, and "D" that a stimulus may be triggered by a sensed event in one chamber and inhibited by a sensed event in the other. In practice this means ventricular inhibited and atrial triggered. The letter "O" in this position indicates that there is no mode of response to the lack of sensitivity indicated by the "O" in position II.

The three-position code is often used by manufacturers to indicate the intended use of the pulse generator. Programmable pulse generators commonly have sensitivity and refractory periods that allow use of the same generator in the atrium or the ventricle as a single-chamber device. Dual-chamber devices are, of course, used in both atrium and ventricle. To allow manufacturers to designate a pulse generator as single-chamber pacing and sensing as opposed to one that is designed for use in the atrium or the ventricle but should not be used in both chambers, the letter "S" exists in positions I and II. "S" in either position indicates that a single chamber is being paced (position I) and sensed (position II). The mode of response to sensing in position II, as the pacemaker is delivered, is designated in position III. As positions IV and V are used to indicate programmability and antitachycardia functions, the same letters available to physicians are used by manufacturers.

The increasing complexity of pacemakers has necessitated the addition and then the modification of two additional positions, IV and V.

POSITION IV—describes two different device characteristics: the degree of programmability and the presence or absence of a rate modulation mechanism. The letters are hierarchal, from the absence of function in this channel to the most complex. The assumption is that the next higher level will incorporate all of the features of all lower levels. Five letters are possible in this position. The letter "O" in this position indicates that the device is not programmable and does not provide rate modulation. The letter "P" indicates simple programmability, almost always, in practice, change in rate or output or both. "M" indicates multiprogrammability, i.e., more than two functions. The presence of sensitivity programmability will make a "P" device into an "M" device. The addition of telemetry (in practice telemetry is always added to multiprogrammable capability) allows the use of the letter "C" which is the abbreviation for "communicating." The obvious letter "T" was avoided as it had been previously used for "triggered function" in position III. The degree of programmability refers to antitachycardia features as well as (and even in the absence of) antibradycardia pacing. The last letter in this position is "R" (rate modulation) which indicates sensor-driven variation of the antibradycardia escape interval in response to a physiological or nonphysiological stimulus other than the atrium. Such stimuli include the interval from pacemaker emission to repolarization (i.e., the QT interval), respiratory rate, central venous temperature, right ventricular dP/dt, and others. Excluded are all means of upper rate limitation including AV block, Wenckebach, rate smoothing, etc.

POSITION V—indicates the presence of one or two antitachycardia functions activated manually or automatically in an implanted device when a tachycardia is anticipated or has occurred. "O" once again indicates the absence of any such capability; "P" indicates a pacing modality and includes underdrive, burst, and scanning, but at a level of electrical output of a cardiac pacemaker, i.e., in the microjoule range. "S" indicates a shock to terminate the tachyarrhythmia, i.e., at the level of joules or several orders of magnitude above pacer output. The letter "S," used previously to indicate "single chamber," has been redefined for position V but this should offer little confusion. If the device is capable of pacing level and shock level output either simultaneously and/or successively, the letter "D" indicates both pacing and sensing (i.e., P + S).

Position V has been devised to allow its use for any electrical stimulating device that provides either bradycardia or tachycardia management or both. Unlike the earlier versions of the code, position V may be used for a bradycardia pacemaker, or for a simple, i.e., nonprogrammable defibrillator or cardioverter incapable of pacing, or for an antitachycardia device with bradycardia and tachycardia pacing functions, multiprogrammability, and the capability of emitting a shock to terminate a tachycardia (Table II).

It is important when using the code that each letter be properly positioned. The position is as important as it is in a number. The "O" designation is thus as critical as in the number system. A comma may be used (optional) after the first three positions, much as in a long number. A complete code consists of four or five positions. Fewer than four positions is incomplete. Examples of the new code are given in Table III.

Some who write about or design pacemakers are anxious to use the code with additional letters, such as an "X" in one position or another. As the "X" is an undefined letter in this system, little clarity is added and obscurity may be caused. Because many pulse generators now being introduced have a maximum capability of pacing and sensing in both chambers, such a multiprogrammable unit may be designated as DDD,M but may be used in a lesser mode after implant, i.e., AAI, VVI, DVI, VDD, etc. The practice of designating the pacemaker maximum capability as well as its actual operation is useful.

Table II
The NASPE/BPEG Generic (NBG) Pacemaker Code

Position	I	II	III	IV	V
Category	Chamber(s) paced	Chamber(s) sensed	Response to sensing	Programmability, rate modulation	Antitachyarrhythmia function(s)
	O = None	O = None	O = None	O = None	O = None
	A = Atrium	A = Atrium	T = triggered	P = Simple Programmable	P = Pacing (antitachyarrhythmia)
	V = Ventricle	V = Ventricle	I = Inhibited	M = Multiprogrammable	S = Shock
	D = Dual (A + V)	D = Dual (A + V)	D = Dual (D +I)	C = Communicating	D = Dual (P + S)
				R = Rate modulation	
Manufacturer's designation only	S = single (A or V)	S = single (A or V)		Comma optional here	

Note: Positions I through III are used exclusively for antibradyarrhythmia function.

Table III
Examples of the NASPE/BPEG Generic (NBG) Code

Code	Meaning
VOOO or VOOOO	Asynchronous ventricular pacing. No adaptive rate control or antitachyarrhythmia functions (also VOO in clinical use but not in device labelling)
DDDM or DDDMO	Multiprogrammable "physiological" dual-chamber pacing. No adaptive rate control or antitachyarrhythmia capability
VVIPP	Simple-programmable VVI pacemaker with antitachyarrhythmia-pacing capability
DDDCP	DDD pacemaker with telemetry and antitachyarrhythmia-pacing capability
OOOPS	Simple-programmable cardioverter, defibrillator, or cardioverter defibrillator
OOOPD	Simple-programmable cardioverter, defibrillator, or cardioverter defibrillator with antitachyarrhythmia-pacing capabilities
VVIMD	Multiprogrammable VVI pacemaker with defibrillation (or cardioversion), or cardioversion and defibrillation and antitachyarrhythmia-pacing capabilities
VVIR or VVIRO	VVI pacemaker with escape interval controlled adaptively by one or more unspecified variables
VVIRP	Programmable VVI pacemaker with escape interval controlled adaptively by one or more unspecified variables, also incorporating antitachyarrhythmia-pacing capability
DDDRD	Programmable DDD pacemaker with escape interval controlled adaptively by one or more unspecified variables, also incoroprating antitachyarrhythmia-pacing capability and cardioversion (or defibrillation, or cardioversion and defibrillation) functions

THE NASPE SPECIFIC CODE

While the ICHD code and the NBG modification have been very useful and have achieved widespread acceptance, the growing complexity of cardiac pacemakers and especially the increasing availability of dual-chamber devices have necessitated another code that will, more specifically, indicate pacemaker function in management of bradyarrhythmias. The NASPE specific code can deal with this complexity. A problem with the first three positions of the ICHD code is that they may be inadequately specific for dual-chamber modes. For example, there are four possible modes in which both atrium and ventricle are sensed and paced. In one mode, a spontaneous P wave inhibits the atrial channel and triggers the ventricle. It is referred to as DDD. In another mode, a spontaneous QRS complex produces triggered responses without delay, while the P wave also triggers a stimulus in the atrium and the ventricle after a delay. No pacemaker inhibition occurs at any time. The mode is DDT. The "T" in position III indicates that no inhibition of pacemaker function ever occurs. However, there are two additional modes, one in which the atrial channel is triggered and the ventricular channel is inhibited and the other in which the atrial channel is inhibited (although sensing a P wave triggers a ventricular response) and the ventricular channel is triggered. The ICHD code cannot accommodate these two modes. They can be described clearly with the NASPE specific code.

Atrial and ventricular channel functions are described in the numerator and denominator of a ratio or fraction format. If the code is limited to one printed line, a virgule (slash) separates the atrial (numerator) from the ventricular (denominator) designation. A letter code describes pacemaker activity.

O = No antibradycardia activity in the chamber
P = Pacing
S = Sensing
I = Inhibited in response to a sensed event

T = Triggered in response to a sensed event
A = Atrial activity
V = Ventricular activity

A subscript of the chamber affected is appended to indicate the chamber in which the activity is sensed and which causes the triggered or inhibited pacemaker response. By convention, pacing is indicated first, sensing next, followed by an inhibited response (I_v or I_a), and then a triggered response (T_a or T_v). Atrial activity is listed first. The omission of a letter designation in either chamber means that it does not apply. While the order of activity is maintained, the code would be equally comprehensible if the order were not maintained. For example, P, S, I_a, I_v (correct) is no more comprehensible than I_v, P, S, I_a (incorrect).

Antitachyarrhythmia functions also are readily specified by the chamber in which they occur. The function is indicated by an upper-case letter in the chamber in which it occurs. The subscript is the chamber that prompts the specific response, much as the bradycardia is inhibited (I) or triggered (T).

U = Underdrive—pacing at a rate lower than that of the tachyarrhythmia.

B = Burst—overdrive; fixed rate pacing of limited duration at a rate greater than that of the tachyarrhythmia.

R = Ramp—asynchronous pacing of limited duration and systematically varying rate, both chosen by the user

X = Extrastimulus—stimulus or stimuli synchronous with a previous event sensed by the device, with fixed or variable coupling and/or interstimulus intervals.

C = Cardioversion—delivery of a synchronized shock of preselected energy.

D = Defibrillation—delivery of an asynchronous shock of preselected energy.

The following lower-case modifiers may be applied as appropriate to any of the antitachyarrhythmia modes represented by U, B, R, X, C, and D;

a = atrial (initiated by sensing of an atrial event);
v = ventricular (initiated by sensing of a ventricular event);
e = external (activated by the user).

Each upper-case letter antitachyarrhythmia function or symbol or combination of symbols is followed by a subscript modifier. One example of combined antibradyarrhythmia and antitachyarrhythmia pacemakers can be described as follows in combined format.

A ventricular inhibited single-chamber pacemaker would be indicated as follows:

Bradyarrhythmia
atrial channel—no activity O
ventricular channel—P,S,I_v
The equivalent ICHD code is VVI;
the NASPE code $\dfrac{O}{P,S,I_v}$.

If this unit also has antitachycardia functions, only in the ventricle, and only prompted by external control, these would be added to the numerator. If burst (B) pacing were available under external control while defibrillator occurred automatically in response to ventricular sensed events, B_eD would be added to the denominator making this device. $\dfrac{0}{P,S,I_v(B_eD)}$ Antitachycardia symbols are in parentheses. Other designations are possible (Table IV).

Table IV
Examples

ICHD Code	Modified Generic Code	NBG Code	NASPE Specific Code	Description
VOO	VOO	VOO	$\dfrac{O}{P}$	Ventricular pacing, asynchronous
VVI,P	VVI,P	VVI,P	$\dfrac{O}{PSI_v}$	Ventricular pacing inhibited by sensing in ventricle, simple programmable
VVI,M	VVI,M	VVI,M	$\dfrac{O}{PSI_v}$	Ventricular pacing inhibited by sensing in ventricle, multiprogrammable
VVI,C	VVI,C	VVI,C	$\dfrac{O}{PSI_v}$	Ventricular pacing inhibited by sensing in ventricle, telemetry and multiprogrammable
VVI,M	VVI,M	VVI,R	$\dfrac{O}{PSI_v}$	Ventricular inhibited multiprogrammable pacing with rate modulation
AAI,M	AAI,M	AAI,R	$\dfrac{PSI_a}{O}$	Atrial inhibited multiprorammable pacing with rate modulation
DVI,M	DVI,M	DVI,M	$\dfrac{PI_v}{PSI_v}$	Atrial pacing inhibited by sensing in ventricle; ventricular pacing inhibited by sensing in ventricle
VDD,M	VDD,M	VDD,M	$\dfrac{S}{PSI_vT_a}$	Ventricular pacing trigered by sensing in atrium, inhibited by sensing in ventricle
DDD,M	DDD,M	DDD,M	$\dfrac{PSI_aI_v}{PSI_vT_a}$	Atrial pacing inhibited by sensing in atrium or ventricle; ventricular pacing triggered by sensing in atrium, inhibited by sensing in ventricle
DDD,M	DDD,M	DDD,M	$\dfrac{PST_aI_v}{PSI_vT_a}$	Atrial pacing triggered by sensing in atrium, inhibited by sensing in ventricle; ventricular pacing triggered by sensing in atrium, inhibited by sensing in ventricle
DDD,M	DDD,M	DDD,R	$\dfrac{PSI_aI_v}{PSI_vT_a}$	Atrial pacing inhibited by sensing in atrium or ventricle; ventricular pacing triggered by sensing in atrium inhibited by sensing in ventricle with rate modulation
DDD,M	DDD,M	DDD,MS	$\dfrac{PSI_aI_v}{PSI_vT_a}$	Atrial pacing inhibited by atrial or ventricular sensing; ventricular pacing triggered by atrial sensing, inhibited by ventricular sensing; shock termination of tachyarrhythmia

Table IV   *(Continued)*

ICHD Code	Modified Generic Code	NBG Code	NASPE Specific Code	Description
DDD,C	DDD,CB	DDD,CD	$\dfrac{PSI_aI_v}{PSI_vT_a(D)}$	Atrial pacing inhibited by atrial or ventricular sensing; ventricular pacing triggered by atrial sensing, pacing termination in atrium or ventricle of tachyarrhythmia followed by a high output shock to terminate a tachyarrhythmia if necessary
VVI,MB	VVI,MA	VVI,MP	$\dfrac{O}{PSI_v(B_v)}$	Ventricular pacing inhibited by sensing in ventricle; bursts in ventricle activated by tachycardia detection in ventricle
AAR,ON	OOO,OA	OOO,OP	$\dfrac{O(UA)}{O}$	Underdrive in atrium activated by tachycardia detection in atrium
VI,MB VVI,MN VVI,ME	VVI,MA		$\dfrac{O}{PSI_v(B_eU_eR_eBX_eX_e)}$	Pacing in ventricle inhibited by sensing in ventricle; burst, underdrive, ramp, burst plus extrastimulus, or extrastimulus in ventricle activated externally
DDD,CB DDD,CN	DDD,CA	DDD,CP	$\dfrac{PSI_aI_v(B_aB_vU_v)}{PSI_vT_a(U_v)}$	Atrial pacing inhibited by atrial or ventricular sensing; ventricular pacing triggered by atrial sensing, inhibited by ventricular sensing; bursts in atrium or ventricle; underdrive in atrium and ventricle activated by tachycardia detection in ventricle

IMPLANTABLE CARDIOVERTER DEFIBRILLATOR CODE

A code for a desciption of the implantable cardioverter defibrillator has been considered to be necessary and one has been introduced and approved by NASPE and the British Pacing and Electrophysiology Group (BPEG). This code is similar to the earlier ICHD and NBG codes and is termed the NASPE/BPEG Defibrillator (NBD) code. Because of its simplicity it is likely to be as widely used as the pacemaker code (Tables V, VI).

Table V
The NASPE/BPEG Defibrillator (NBD) Code

I	II	III	IV
Shock Chamber	Antitachycardia Pacing Chamber	Tachycardia Detection	Antibradycardia Pacing Chamber
O = None	O = None	E = Electrogram	O = None
A = Atrium	A = Atrium	H = Hemodynamic	A = Atrium
V = Ventricle	V = Ventricle		V = Ventricle
D = Dual (A + V)	D = Dual (A + V)		D = Dual (A + V)

In position III tachycardia detection may be by electrogram analysis (E) or with the addition of a hemodynamic (H) component to the electrogram. Detection of tachycardia is always presumed to involve electrogram analysis.

Table VI
The Short Form of the NASPE/BPEG Defibrillator (NBD) Code

ICD-S = ICD with shock capability only
ICD-B = ICD with bradycardia pacing as well as shock
ICD-T = ICD with tachycardia (and bradycardia) pacing as well as shock

ICD = Implanted cardioverter/defibrillator.

BIBLIOGRAPHY

Bernstein AD, Camm AJ, Fisher JD, et al: PACE 1993 (in press).

Bernstein AD, Brownlee RR, Fletcher R, et al: Report of the NASPE mode code committee. PACE 1984; 7:395–402.

Bernstein AD, Camm AJ, Fletcher R, et al: The NASPE/BPEG generic pacemaker code for antibradyarrhythmia and adaptive-rate pacing and antitachyarrhythmia devices. PACE 1987; 10:794–799.

Bernstein AD, Parsonnet V: Notation system and overlay diagrams for the analysis of paced electrocardiograms. PACE 1983; 6:73–80.

Bredikis JJ, Stirbys PP: A suggested code for permanent cardiac pacing leads. PACE 1985; 8:320–321.

Brownlee RR, Shimmel-Golden JB, DelMarco CJ, et al: A new symbolic language for diagramming pacemaker/heart interaction. PACE 1982; 5:700–709.

Brownlee RR, Shimmel JB, DelMarco CJ: A new code for pacemaker operating modes. PACE 1981; 4:396–399.

Furman S: Coding for pacemaker leads. (editorial) PACE 1985; 8:319.

Furman S: Pacemaker codes. (editorial) PACE 1981; 4:357.

Irnich W: Development of coding system for pacemakers. PACE 1984; 7:882–901.

Kruse I, Markowitz T, Ryden L: Timing markers showing pacemaker behavior to aid in the follow-up of a physiological pacemaker. PACE 1983; 6:801–805.

Olson WH, McConnell MV, Sah RL, et al: Pacemaker diagnostic diagrams. PACE 1985; 8:691–700.

Parsonnet V, Furman S, Smyth NPD, et al: Optimal resources for implantable cardiac pacemakers. Report of Inter-society Commission for Heart Disease Resources. Circulation 1983; 68:226a-244a.

Parsonnet V, Furman S, Smyth NPD: A revised code for pacemaker identification. Five-position pacemaker code (ICHD). PACE 1981; 4:400–403.

Parsonnet V, Furman S, Smyth NPD: Implantable cardiac pacemakers: Status report and resource guideline. A report of the Inter-society Commission for Heart Disease Resources. Am J Cardiol 1974; 34:487–500.

PART II.

CLINICAL CONSIDERATIONS

Chapter 7

Temporary Cardiac Pacing

David L. Hayes, David R. Holmes, Jr.

Familiarity with temporary cardiac pacing is essential for those involved in permanent cardiac pacing, and the treatment of patients in coronary care units and on postsurgical wards. Knowledge of the indications, techniques, and routes of implantation, post-insertion management, and risk/benefit ratio for each patient is required for safe, reliable pacing.

INDICATIONS (TABLE I)

Because temporary pacing is an invasive procedure with a potential, albeit minimal, risk for serious complications, it is essential to analyze the benefits and the risks. The indications for temporary pacing include both bradycardia and tachycardia. There are three general categories.

1. Patients with symptomatic bradycardia—the indication is clear.
2. Patients with asymptomatic bradycardia or conduction defects—the decision to proceed with temporary pacing depends upon assessment of the risk of development of symptomatic bradycardia. With the advent of reliable and readily available external temporary pacing it is less common to place a temporary transvenous pacemaker in patients with asymptomatic conduction disturbances.
3. Patients with tachycardia—in selected patients, temporary pacing may be used to terminate or prevent tachycardia. This is a temporary therapeutic maneuver until the tachycardia can be prevented with medications, ablation, surgery, or, in some patients, permanent pacing.

Symptomatic Bradycardia or Conduction Defects

Patients with symptomatic bradycardia and recurrent syncope or near syncope require temporary pacing. Patients in this category include those with second- or third-degree atrioventricular (AV) block. Block may occur in chronic conduction system disease or in acute myocardial infarction, drug intoxication, or electrolyte imbalance. Patients with sinus node dysfunction and symptomatic bradycardia also may require temporary pacing. In patients in these groups with fixed conduction system lesions, the temporary pacemaker may be placed before and discontinued after permanent cardiac pacing. In patients in whom symptomatic bradycardia is reversible, for example, by discontinuing administration of drugs, the temporary pacemaker is used until an acceptable rhythm returns.

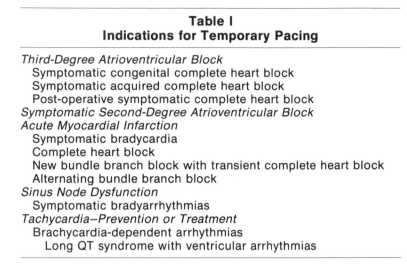

Table I
Indications for Temporary Pacing

Third-Degree Atrioventricular Block
    Symptomatic congenital complete heart block
    Symptomatic acquired complete heart block
    Post-operative symptomatic complete heart block
Symptomatic Second-Degree Atrioventricular Block
Acute Myocardial Infarction
    Symptomatic bradycardia
    Complete heart block
    New bundle branch block with transient complete heart block
    Alternating bundle branch block
Sinus Node Dysfunction
    Symptomatic bradyarrhythmias
Tachycardia–Prevention or Treatment
    Brachycardia-dependent arrhythmias
        Long QT syndrome with ventricular arrhythmias

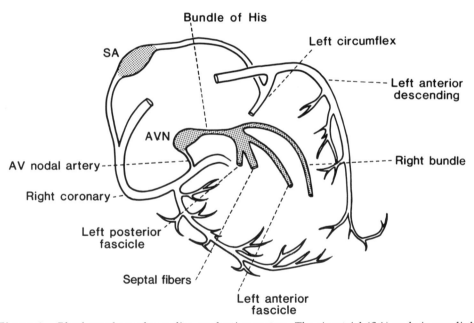

Figure 1. Blood supply to the cardiac conduction system. The sinoatrial (SA) node is supplied by a branch of the right coronary artery in 60% and the left circumflex coronary artery in 40% of patients. During inferior infarction, if the right coronary artery is occluded proximal to the origin of the SA nodal artery, sinus node dysfunction may occur. The atrioventricular (AV) node is supplied by a branch of right coronary artery in 90% of patients. During inferior infarction, occlusion of the right coronary artery may result in AV block that is usually at the level of AV node. Anterior infarctions may result in conduction defects that usually indicate more extensive infarction with involvement of the conduction system distal to the AV node.

Asymptomatic Bradycardia or Conduction Defects

In patients with asymptomatic bradycardia, assessment of the risk/benefit ratio is essential because the decision to proceed with pacing depends upon the risk of symptomatic bradycardia developing. Patients with asymptomatic acquired complete heart block that develops postoperatively should also undergo temporary cardiac pacing. (Because of the potential for developing AV block postoperatively most patients will have temporary epicardial pacing wires placed at the time of surgery.) In these persons, the reliability of the escape focus is often uncertain and the risk of symptomatic bradycardia developing outweighs the risk of temporary pacing.

Temporary pacing in patients with acute myocardial infarction is somewhat more controversial. In these patients, the decision to proceed with temporary pacing is based on knowledge of the blood supply of the conduction system, the location and extent of infarction, and the presence of preexisting conduction system disease (Figure 1). All of these factors influence the risk of symptomatic bradycardia developing. It is important to try to assess the level of the conduction abnormality as it has important implications for the need for permanent pacing and long-term outcome.

Conduction Abnormalities Proximal to the His Bundle (Table II)

Conduction disturbances proximal to the bundle of His are most commonly associated with an inferior infarction. The escape rhythms often have a narrow QRS complex, although they may be wide, and they tend to be faster and more stable than distal escape rhythms. If AV block develops, it is usually gradual in onset and transient. A typical clinical occurrence would be Wenckebach AV block followed by higher grades of block in a patient with inferior myocardial infarction. In patients with inferior infarction and high grade block, the indication for pacing is a rate persistently less than approximately 40 bpm or the development of symptoms such as a low output state or recurrent bradycardia associated with angina or ventricular irritability. In other asymptomatic patients

---

Table II
Atrioventricular Conduction Abnormalities Associated with Acute Myocardial Infarction

	Anterior MI	Inferior MI
Conduction abnormality proximal to His bundle	–	Yes
Conduction abnormality distal to His bundle	Yes	–
Degree of necrosis	Extensive	Less extensive
Escape rhythm	Wide QRS	Narrow QRS
	Rate <40 bpm	Rate 40–50 bpm
	Less stable	Stable
Progression of AV block	Rapid	Gradual

with conduction abnormalities proximal to the His bundle, temporary pacemakers need not be inserted prophylactically.

Conduction Abnormalities Distal to the His Bundle

Distal conduction system abnormalities usually occur in association with anterior infarctions. A wide spectrum of electrocardiographic patterns can be seen, including bundle branch block and high-grade AV block. The escape rhythms usually have a wider QRS morphology, are slower, and are less stable than the proximal escape rhythms. In addition, unlike proximal conduction abnormalities, distal conduction abnormalities often progress rapidly to complete AV block. If the patient has anterior infarction and significant conduction abnormalities, the degree of myocardial damage usually is extensive and often is associated with pump failure. The progression to complete heart block, however, contributes independently to morbidity and mortality in some patients. In patients with high-grade AV block, the decision to proceed with temporary pacing is straightforward. In patients with only bundle branch block, the decision to proceed is based on the risk of AV block developing. In patients at high risk, placement of a temporary pacemaker is recommended.

Tachycardia

The placement of temporary pacemakers in patients with tachycardia can be useful in selected cases. The ability to simultaneously record atrial deflections and the surface electrocardiogram on a two-channel monitor facilitates analysis of the relationship between the atrial and the ventricular electrograms (Figure 2). Documenting ventriculoatrial (VA) block or VA dissociation in this situation is often helpful in the differential diagnosis of supraventricular and ventricular tachycardias. It is also helpful in patients with supraventricular tachycardia, for example, recording atrial rates of 300 bpm establishes the diagnosis of atrial flutter. In addition to diagnostic uses, pacing can also be used to prevent or treat arrhythmias. The principles and rationale for pacing for tachycardia are more fully outlined in Chapter 13. In patients with bradycardia-dependent arrhythmias, for example, sinus node dysfunction and recurrent supraventricular tachycardia after a sinus pause, treatment of the bradycardia prevents the tachycardia. If the bradycardia is related to acute infarction, or drug or electrolyte abnormality, temporary pacing can be used until normal rhythm returns. If the bradycardia is related to underlying conduction system disease, pacing can be used on a temporary basis until a permanent unit is implanted. In selected patients with re-entrant tachycardia (either supraventricular or ventricular), burst pacing can be used to terminate tachycardia (See Chapter 13, "Pacing For Tachycardia"). In these patients, temporary pacing can be used until an effective drug regimen is instituted or until the clinical factors responsible for the arrhythmia have been controlled, as in patients with drug- or electrolyte-induced arrhythmias. In occasional patients, overdrive pacing can be very useful in the prevention of arrhythmias. For overdrive pacing, the rate required varies with

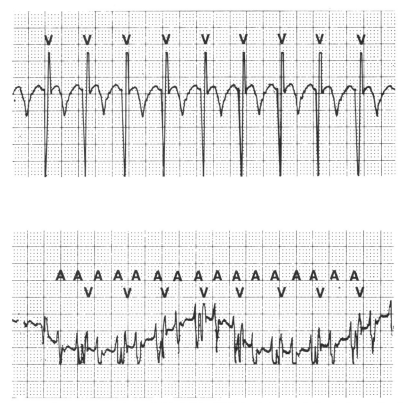

Figure 2. *A simultaneous two-channel ECG. The ECG (top) demonstrates tachycardia at a 480 ms coupling interval (125 bpm). No clear-cut atrial activity is seen. The simultaneous atrial recording (bottom) documents atrial activity at a rate of 250 bpm (240 ms) and 2:1 atrioventricular block. V = ventricular depolarization; A = atrial depolarization.*

the underlying rhythm. It must exceed the spontaneous rate by approximately 10% to 25% to effect complete capture. As the arrhythmia subsides or responds to drug therapy, the overdrive rate is reduced or pacing is discontinued. Such pacing is usually a temporizing maneuver. A special circumstance in which pacing can be very effective is in the patient with a prolonged QT interval and recurrent ventricular tachycardia. In these patients, rapid atrial pacing shortens the QT interval, decreases the temporal dispersion of refractoriness, and is often very effective for preventing ventricular tachycardia. This approach can be used in a temporary fashion if the QT prolongation is transient or, if effective, this approach can be used for permanent pacing.

TEMPORARY PACING MODE

Atrial Pacing

Atrial pacing is used in selected patients, including some with sinus node dysfunction without AV block. In these patients, pacing can be used for overdrive suppression of supraventricular tachycardia, overdrive burst pacing for treatment of tachycardia, or treatment of symptomatic bradycardia. In this clinical setting, permanent pacing often is required eventually, but temporary pacing may be very helpful in the interim. In addition, in patients with possible drug-induced symptomatic sinus bradycardia, temporary atrial pacing may be used until the specific need for the drug in question is determined. Finally, in some patients with prolonged QT syndromes (either drug-induced or spontaneous) and recurrent ventricular tachycardia, temporary atrial pacing may help to prevent the arrhythmia by decreasing the QT interval and suppressing ventricular ectopy.

Dual-Chamber Pacing

Advances in technology have occurred along with our increased knowledge about the hemodynamics of pacing. These two factors have been responsible for the increased use of temporary dual-chamber pacing. Both temporary AV sequential and temporary DDD units are available. These are particularly useful in patients with noncompliant ventricles in whom the atrial contribution to ventricular filling is essential. In patients with AV block and acute myocardial infarction, dual-chamber pacing may maintain optimal hemodynamics. It may be especially helpful in patients with an acute right ventricular infarction. Another use of temporary dual-chamber pacing is to assess the need for a permanent dual-chamber system or upgrade of a ventricular demand system. Measurement of blood pressure and cardiac output with different temporary pacing modes may help to document the need for a specific permanent pacing mode in equivocal cases.

TEMPORARY PACEMAKER PLACEMENT

Temporary pacing usually is performed by a transvenous approach. The clinical setting determines the urgency with which pacing is required and, to a certain extent, the venous access chosen. The basic equipment required for temporary transvenous pacing includes a surgical pack with instruments to obtain venous access, a pacing catheter, an external pulse generator, and under usual circumstances, a procedure room for placement.

Catheters

Several types of temporary pacing catheters are available (Figure 3), each of which has advantages and disadvantages. The mode of pacing selected determines, in part, the catheter system used. Although both unipolar and bipolar catheters are available, the overwhelming majority of temporary pacing systems are bipolar.

There are two major types of catheter design (Figure 3). The first is a more rigid, firm catheter, usually made of woven Dacron, that requires fluoroscopic

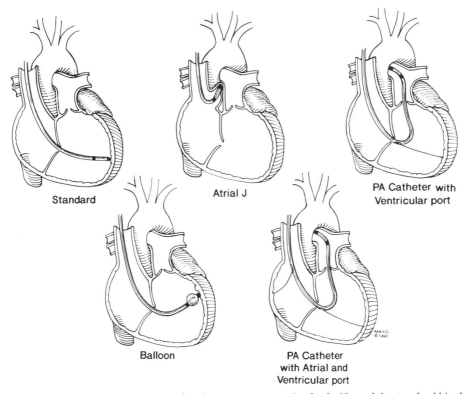

Standard

Atrial J

PA Catheter with
Ventricular port

Balloon

PA Catheter
with Atrial and
Ventricular port

Figure 3. *Schematic representation of various temporary pacing leads. Upper left: standard bipolar pacing catheter positioned along the free wall of the right ventricle. Lower left: balloon tipped flotation catheter positioned near the ventricular outflow tract. Upper center: bipolar atrial "J" lead. Upper right: Pulmonary artery catheter with ventricular pacing port. Lower right: Pulmonary artery catheter with atrial and ventricular pacing ports.*

imaging during the procedure for safe and proper placement. Because this catheter remains somewhat firmer after placement, it is more reliable in maintaining temporary pacing. The other major type of catheter is more flexible and may have a balloon tip. Balloon flotation catheters do not require fluoroscopy for insertion and are particularly useful during emergencies. For placement of these catheters, the balloon is inflated after it enters the central circulation. A steerable balloon flotation catheter is also available. In addition, there is a flexible pacing catheter without a balloon that can be positioned with or without fluoroscopy. This catheter is called a "semi-floating"™ catheter because it is flexible enough that placement is flow assisted.

If fluoroscopy is not available or not used at the time of placement, intracardiac electrograms can be used to position the leads. Intracardiac electrograms are strikingly different from surface electrocardiograms. When the lead enters the right atrium, large P waves are seen. Passage of the lead across the tricuspid valve into the right ventricle is associated with recording of large QRS complexes that indicate ventricular position. Contact with the endocardium is manifested by elevation of ST segments with a current of injury (Figure 4). Because they

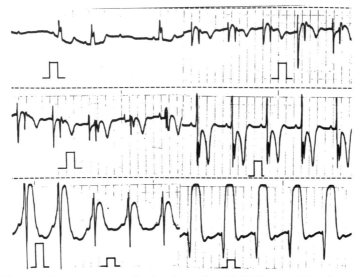

Figure 4. *Passage of a transvenous bipolar electrode with ECG control involves recognition of the electrograms of different intracardiac positions. Upper left: intermittent AV block. Upper right: the electrode is in the right atrium with P waves larger than the QRS complexes. Middle left: the electrode is moved into the inferior vena cava where the P waves are reduced in size, now smaller than the QRS complexes. Middle right: within the right ventricle, past the tricuspid valve, the QRS complexes are enlarged, the P waves small, and the T waves inverted. Lower left: the P waves virtually disappear, the ventricular electrogram is 6 mV in amplitude. (The standardization has been reduced by half.) Lower right: increase in pressure on the endocardium increases electrogram amplitude and the elevation of the ST segment.*

are so flexible, balloon flotation and semi-floating pacing catheters may not maintain stable pacing positions as well as more rigid catheters.

Pulmonary artery catheters are available that allow ventricular or AV sequential temporary pacing (Figure 3). The catheter is designed with a special channel(s) to direct a small pacing wire into the right ventricle and/or right atrium. In addition to catheters for ventricular placement, there are atrial J catheters that can be used for right atrial appendage placement. The original pulmonary artery catheter capable of AV sequential pacing was hexapolar. Any of the four proximal electrodes that were within the atrium could be used to pace the atrium, and the distal pair of electrodes could be used to pace the right ventricle. It was difficult to position the pulmonary artery catheter such that reliable atrial and ventricular pacing could be achieved and maintained and, at the same time, to adequately monitor PA pressures reliably.

External Generators

There are several external pulse generators. The most commonly used are single-chamber, constant current devices with variable output up to 20 mA, variable rate up to approximately 180 bpm, and variable sensitivity. In addition to these single-chamber units, AV sequential pacemakers and DDD temporary pacemakers are available. Finally, programmable stimulators can be used for burst pacing and the introduction of one or multiple extrastimuli when the indication for temporary pacing is termination of tachycardia.

Venous Access and Placement

Access to the venous system for placement of temporary pacing catheters is possible from several sites including the subclavian, external and internal jugular, brachial, and femoral veins (Figure 5). Selection of the specific approach

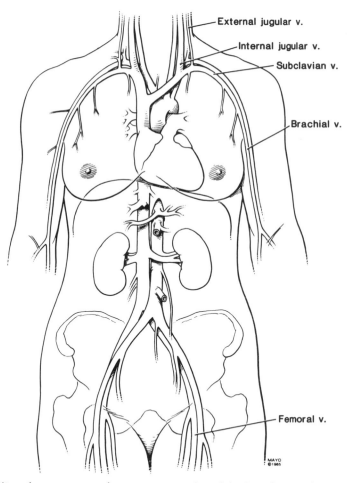

Figure 5. *Sites of venous access for temporary pacing. Selection of a specific approach depends upon clinical conditions and the experience of the operator. (Reproduced by permission of the Mayo Foundation.)*

depends upon the clinical conditions and the experience of the operator. At our institutions, a central venous approach is preferred because of ease of insertion, percutaneous placement, and stability. Insertion should be done under sterile, aseptic conditions. Electrocardiographic monitoring and emergency equipment, including a defibrillator, are essential. If a rigid transvenous catheter is to be used, the catheter must be positioned with fluoroscopy. The insertion site should be thoroughly prepared and draped, and an instrument pack with equipment for percutaneous entry or venous cutdown should be available.

Selection of the specific vein (subclavian, jugular, brachial, or femoral) depends upon the patient's condition and the operator's experience. Usually, the subclavian or internal jugular vein is used because the catheter is more stable and the incidence of dislodgment is lower. There are risks with each approach that must be balanced against the benefits.

Whenever possible, a percutaneous technique is used. Local anesthesia is administered to the subcutaneous and deeper structures and a small puncture is made with a scalpel blade. With the use of a hemostat, the subcutaneous tissues are dissected bluntly in the direction the introducer will follow. A thin-walled needle, usually 18 gauge, is used to enter the vein. Blood is aspirated after venous entry to document placement within the lumen. A guide wire is then advanced through the needle into the venous circulation, and the needle is removed. The dilator and venous sheath are then advanced over the wire. Several introducer kits of different sizes are available commercially; they include the needle, guide wire and syringe, and dilator-introducer. We prefer to use sheaths that have a sidearm for fluid administration and a diaphragm to prevent back-bleeding. The pacing catheter can be advanced into the central circulation through this sheath.

If two central lines are needed, for example, a pulmonary artery catheter and a temporary pacing wire, two sheaths can be placed with a single central venous puncture. After placing a single sheath, two guide wires can be placed through the diaphragm of the sheath, advanced into the central vein, and the sheath removed. Two separate sheaths can then be placed over the two indwelling guide wires. Alternatively, a pulmonary arterial catheter with a pacing port can be used.

Rarely, a cutdown is necessary to identify and cannulate the venous entry site. The cutdown approach was most commonly used for the brachial veins. We prefer to avoid this approach if possible, because it is difficult to immobilize the arm to assure a stable lead position and it is uncomfortable for the patient.

Subclavian Approach

The techniques for subclavian venous entry for temporary pacing are identical to those for permanent pacing (See Chapter 8, ''Permanent Pacemaker Implantation''). The vein is entered at the junction of the middle and inner thirds.

Placing the patient in the reverse Trendelenburg position or positioning a towel between the scapulae often helps to facilitate venous entry. Infiltration of the subcutaneous and deeper tissues, particularly the ligament between the clavicle and the first rib, and the periosteum, is important for patient comfort. If permanent pacemaker implantation is anticipated, use of a vein other than the subclavian, for example, the internal or external jugular, is preferred. After placement of a sheath with a sidearm and diaphragm, the pacing lead can be advanced into the central venous circulation.

Internal Jugular Approach

The internal jugular venous approach also allows easy access to the central circulation (Figure 6). The patient's head is turned away from the side of venipuncture. There are several approaches to the internal jugular vein. We prefer to infiltrate the apex of the triangle formed by the medial and lateral borders of the sternocleidomastoid muscle with a local anesthetic. A small incision is made with a scalpel blade, and the subcutaneous tissue is dissected bluntly in the direction of the vein that lies lateral to the carotid artery. A 23-gauge needle can

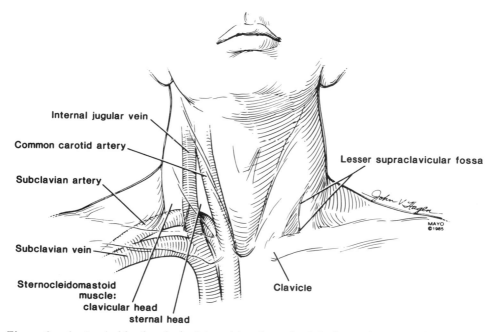

Figure 6. *Anatomical landmarks for internal jugular and subclavian venipuncture. (Reproduced by permission of Mayo Foundation.)*

be used to identify the location of the vein. After the vein has been identified with the smaller needle, a short 18-gauge needle is used for venipuncture. Care should be taken to avoid puncture of the apical pleura or carotid artery. The guide wire and introducer and venous sheath are placed successively. The pacing lead then can be advanced into the right side of the heart.

External Jugular Venous Approach

Either external jugular vein can provide easy access for temporary pacing, although the right external jugular vein is the more direct approach. The vessels often can be seen, particularly in patients with elevated venous pressure or during a Valsalva maneuver. The external jugular veins course downward toward the middle third of the clavicle, just beneath the platysma muscle. Their position and course can be marked with an indelible pen, and then the area is prepared and draped for venipuncture. After infiltration with a local anesthetic, a small incision is made over the vein with a scalpel. The vein often is very superficial, and care must be taken to avoid laceration. The vein is then entered, and a venous sheath is placed.

Femoral Venous Approach

Temporary pacing through the femoral vein is less common because more immobilization of the patient usually is required than with a jugular or subclavian approach. The vein is medial to the femoral artery (Figure 7). It is entered 1 to 2 cm distal to the inguinal ligament. This ligament runs along a line between the anterosuperior iliac crest and the superior pubic tubercle. The inguinal crease is often a rough approximation of the ligament. After infiltration of the site with a local anesthetic, the vein is entered with a long 18-gauge needle (Figure 8). Care must be taken to avoid arterial damage, since in some patients the vein is very close to the artery. In patients who have had femoral arterial or venous punctures, femoral arterial surgery, or cannulation of the femoral artery for bypass, there may be considerable fibrous tissue impeding entry into the femoral vein. After placement of the venous sheath, the pacing lead can be introduced. In some patients, the lead enters a small parallel vein and buckles, causing local low back or pelvic pain. Withdrawing the lead and rotation usually allows passage up the femoral vein into the inferior vena cava. In patients who require temporary pacing immediately before implantation of a permanent pacemaker, we may avoid a central venous approach and use the femoral vein. This route allows easy access to the central circulation and optimal flexibility in selection of a site for placement of the permanent pacing lead.

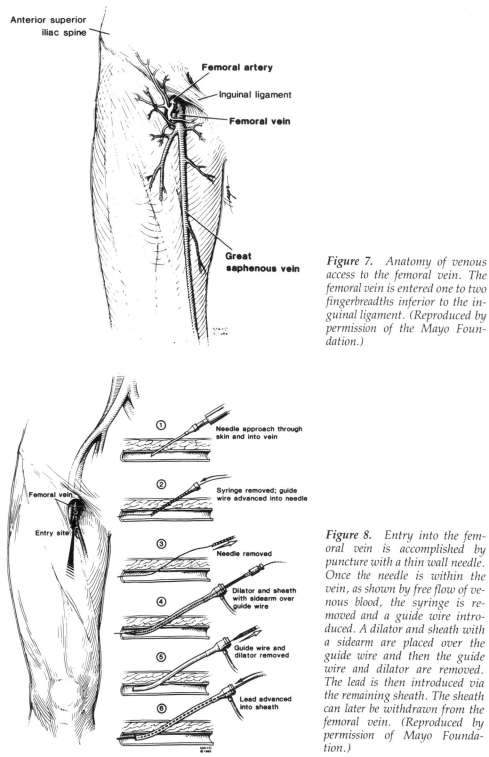

Figure 7. Anatomy of venous access to the femoral vein. The femoral vein is entered one to two fingerbreadths inferior to the inguinal ligament. (Reproduced by permission of the Mayo Foundation.)

Figure 8. Entry into the femoral vein is accomplished by puncture with a thin wall needle. Once the needle is within the vein, as shown by free flow of venous blood, the syringe is removed and a guide wire introduced. A dilator and sheath with a sidearm are placed over the guide wire and then the guide wire and dilator are removed. The lead is then introduced via the remaining sheath. The sheath can later be withdrawn from the femoral vein. (Reproduced by permission of Mayo Foundation.)

Brachial Venous Approach

A brachial venous approach usually is avoided because of the problems of immobilization and dislodgment; in some instances, however, it may be necessary. If possible, the percutaneous approach is used to enter the brachial vein. If a cutdown is required, the area should be prepared and draped as it would be for percutaneous insertion. After infiltration of the subcutaneous and deeper tissues with a short-acting local anesthetic, an incision is made over the antebrachial crease. A tourniquet may be placed proximally to distend the veins. Superficial veins are used if possible. If none are identified, blunt dissection must be carried deeper toward the brachial artery which lies beneath the bicipital aponeurosis. Care must be taken to avoid injury to arterial or neural structures. Adequate veins usually are located in this region. The vein is isolated with ligatures and the distal vein is tied. A venotomy is made, and the pacing lead is introduced. Upper extremity veins draining into the cephalic system should be avoided if possible because it may be difficult to pass the catheter through the angle where the cephalic vein enters the subclavian vein.

If the left arm is used for venous access, it is important to remember that the catheter may enter the coronary sinus rather than the right ventricle. This must be recognized to avoid damage to the coronary sinus itself. Ventricular pacing can be achieved with coronary sinus placement but it is left ventricular in origin and will result in a right bundle branch block configuration. It is important to remember this because an electrocardiogram documenting right bundle branch block with right ventricular placement may also indicate perforation or placement of the temporary catheter across an atrial or ventricular septal defect into the left side of the heart.

CATHETER PLACEMENT

Ventricular Placement

Placement of a temporary ventricular pacing lead involves consideration of the type of lead selected, the venous access used, and specific patient factors, for example, right atrial enlargement and tricuspid insufficiency. For placement from the subclavian or jugular vein, the more rigid woven Dacron catheters can be passed with a gentle curve through the tricuspid valve into the right ventricular apex. In some patients, a loop is fashioned within the right atrium and then is rotated counterclockwise across the tricuspid valve. In some patients, a loop may be made within the right atrium and backed across the tricuspid valve (See Chapter 8, Permanent Pacemaker Implantation.) For placement from the femoral venous approach, a gently curved lead can be passed toward the tricuspid valve and may cross and be easily positioned in the right ventricular apex. In other patients, a loop must be fashioned in the right atrium and then rotated anteriorly across the tricuspid valve. Avoiding undue pressure on the right atrium is important because it is thin and may be perforated. For balloon flotation leads, the balloon is inflated in the superior vena cava, inferior vena cava, or right atrium, and the catheter then is flow-directed across the tricuspid valve into the right ventricle. Occasionally, rotation of a loop of catheter may be required. Once the lead is within the right ventricle, the balloon is advanced to a stable ventricular position and is deflated.

The most stable position is the right ventricular apex. This usually provides adequate pacing and sensing thresholds. Pacing thresholds should be less than 1 mA, and the position should be stable despite deep breaths and coughing.

Atrial Placement

For dual-chamber or atrial pacing, several options are available. The atrial lead usually is placed in the right atrial appendage because this position allows for stable, reliable pacing. The currently available temporary J leads can be easily inserted from the subclavian or jugular vein. Advancing the lead from the superior vena cava into the right atrium with medial rotation allows the J to form and facilitates right atrial appendage intubation. Right atrial appendage placement from the femoral vein is accomplished by a straight passage through the right atrium and rotation toward the spine. Slow advancement with medial rotation usually results in right atrial intubation, which is characterized by the typical medial and lateral movement during atrial systole.

Dual-chamber temporary pacing can be accomplished in several ways (Table III). Most commonly, two separate catheters are placed (Figure 9). Alternatively, a multipolar catheter can be used with electrodes that can be placed against the right ventricle and lateral border of the right atrium. There are also pulmonary artery catheters with both atrial and ventricular pacing ports.

Table III
Modes of Temporary Pacing

Mode	Methods
Atrial	Atrial "J" lead
Ventricular	Balloon-tipped lead
	Woven dacron bipolar lead
	PA catheter with ventricular pacing port
Dual-chamber	Separate atrial and ventricular catheters
	PA catheter with atrial and ventricular pacing ports
	Single multielectrode catheter for atrial and ventricular pacing

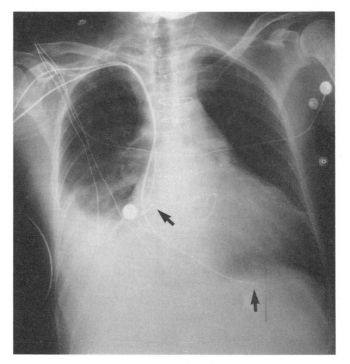

Figure 9. *Chest radiograph of patient with temporary dual-chamber pacing system. The "J" lead is in right atrial appendage (arrow), and the ventricular lead is in right ventricular apex (arrow).*

CATHETER FIXATION

After placement of the catheter and documentation of satisfactory pacing thresholds, the catheter is fixed to the skin at the entry site with secure non-absorbable sutures. If the sidearm of the sheath is to be used for drug admin-istration, the sheath is also sutured; if not, the sheath is withdrawn to the lead bifurcation. The site is covered with a self-adhesive semi-permeable transparent dressing after application of antiseptic or antibiotic ointment. Sterility of the system can also be enhanced by placed a sterile plastic sleeve over the pacing catheter before positioning (Figure 10). Once the catheter is positioned, the sleeve can be connected to the end of the indwelling venous sheath.

The pacing lead is connected to the external pulse generator, and the pacing rate and mode are selected. The maintenance stimulation current is set at two or three times the threshold (usually 3 to 5 mA). The rate selected depends upon the clinical setting. The patient's bed and other equipment must be properly grounded because the pacing lead provides a low resistance circuit through which current can flow to the heart and produce significant arrhythmias. If the ends of the pacing wires are exposed, i.e., the pacing lead is not connected to the external pulse generator, the exposed connector should be placed in an insulating cover.

After placement of the catheter, a chest radiograph should be obtained to

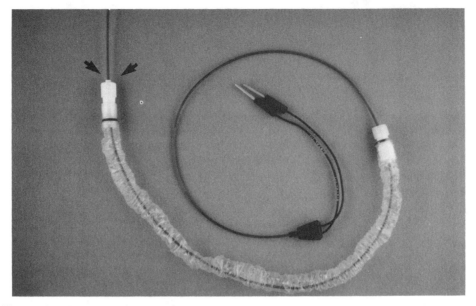

Figure 10. *Temporary pacing catheter covered by a protective sleeve. The sleeve can be connected to the indwelling venous sheath (arrow notes portion of sleeve that would connect to the venous sheath) to provide sterility at the connection and the exterior portion of the pacing catheter.*

document catheter position. The chest radiograph must also be evaluated for complications related to the procedure, such as pneumothorax. An electrocardiogram should also be obtained to document the paced QRS complex and adequate pacing and sensing. The baseline chest radiograph and electrocardiogram are essential for follow-up after placement so that any changes in pacing can be assessed.

CARE AFTER PACEMAKER PLACEMENT

For continued safe and reliable temporary pacing, meticulous attention must be paid to the insertion site and the pacing system itself. It must be kept in mind that the more prolonged the period of temporary pacing, the greater the risk of complication. Temporary pacing from a single site usually can be maintained for up to 7 days if meticulous attention is paid to detail.

Monitoring

All patients with transvenous temporary pacemakers have continuous electrocardiographic monitoring to ensure continued reliable pacing and to detect any other significant arrhythmias.

The underlying cardiac rhythm should be evaluated during the course of temporary pacing. Discontinuance may present a problem in patients who have become dependent on the temporary pacemaker. In these patients, the intrinsic rhythm usually can be evaluated if the paced rate gradually is reduced. A spon-

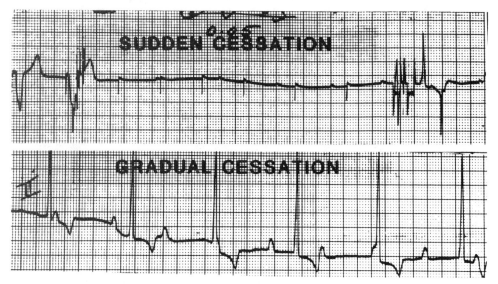

Figure 11.   *Upper:Temporary pacemaker at a rate of 80 bpm is turned off abruptly resulting in ventricular asystole. Lower: In the same patient the rate of the temporary pacemaker gradually is lowered and the patient displays a ventricular escape rhythm at a rate of 50 bpm.*

taneous rhythm may be slow to appear and may begin at a very slow rate, but if sustained, it usually will rise to 30 to 40 bpm. If the temporary pacemaker is abruptly turned off, ventricular asystole may occur (Figure 11).

Pacing and sensing thresholds must be checked daily. Changing thresholds may be the first manifestation of lead dislodgment. Chest radiographs and electrocardiograms should be obtained periodically and physical examination should be performed daily to identify any complications or change in pacing function. If the patient's intrinsic rate is dominant, the pacemaker rate is increased to approximately 10 beats above the intrinsic rate so that the paced activity can be evaluated. The stimulation current is then slowly decreased until capture is lost. The point at which capture is lost is noted in the chart. The output is then increased to at least three times the threshold value, usually at least 3 to 5 mA.

Nursing Care

Meticulous nursing care is essential for patients with temporary transvenous pacemakers. As previously noted, the patient is monitored constantly and notation is made of the status of intrinsic rhythm, clinical condition, and on/off status of the temporary pacemaker. The external pulse generator is pinned to the patient's gown or to the bed so that it cannot be inadvertently moved away from the patient. Even though the temporary pacing wire is secured to the skin, any undue pressure placed on the pacing wire, for example, application of pressure to the external pulse generator connected to the temporary pacemaker, could result in dislodgment. All connections are checked daily to be certain that they are secure.

The entry site should be assessed on a regular basis. Our protocol requires redressing the site every 48 hours. The old dressings are removed, the exposed site is cleansed with alcohol, swabbed with iodine, and an ointment such as povidone-iodine is applied. The area is again covered with a self-adhesive semipermeable transparent dressing. Careful attention to site care significantly reduces the potential for infection. The pacing catheter should be immobilized as much as possible at the skin entry site. With femoral or brachial vein placement, immobilization of the extremity usually is required. With jugular or subclavian vein placement, the patient is less restricted. The junction between the temporary lead and the pulse generator should be protected with insulation, and the noninsulated connecting tip of the lead must be shielded.

Post-insertion Practices

If possible, the patient should not receive anticoagulants at the time the temporary pacing lead is placed. If a temporary pacing procedure is performed as an emergency in a patient known to be receiving anticoagulants, a femoral or antecubital site may be safer because any bleeding may be easier to control. After the temporary pacemaker is in place, anticoagulation, if indicated, can be carried out cautiously. The insertion site should be watched closely for evidence of bleeding.

Antibiotics are not used prophylactically when a temporary pacemaker is placed. Antibiotic solutions and ointments may be used locally in site care.

EPICARDIAL SYSTEMS

Epicardial temporary pacing systems are used exclusively in patients undergoing cardiac surgery. In some institutions, these systems are placed prophylactically in all patients undergoing cardiac surgery. In other institutions, epicardial electrodes are placed only in patients in whom AV block develops during the procedure. Temporary epicardial pacing systems can be used for the treatment of symptomatic bradycardia. With atrial or ventricular wires, or both, any combination of pacing, including VVI, AAI, DVI, or DDD, can be used as described for temporary transvenous systems. The selection of the specific mode depends upon the clinical setting. In addition to pacing for bradycardia, temporary epicardial systems are of particular use in the evaluation and even treatment of tachycardia. Electrograms can be recorded to document the relationship between atrial and ventricular depolarizations. Recording rapid atrial rates with 2:1 or greater AV block allows ready documentation of atrial flutter (Figure 2).

The electrodes used for temporary epicardial pacing are stainless steel teflon-coated wires that are sutured loosely onto the epicardium and brought out through the chest wall. Usually, pairs are put on the atrium and the ventricles and one or more skin ground wires may be placed. The atrial and ventricular wires should be carefully distinguished, either by marking or distinctive placement, for example, atrial leads may be brought out to the right side of the chest and ventricular leads to the left side. The leads should be fixed to the skin to prevent inadvertent traction or displacement. As is true with transvenous pacing, maintaining an insulating cover over the exposed ends of the pacing wires is very important.

Care of Temporary Epicardial Wires

Patients who have temporary epicardial wires in the postoperative period are monitored for the duration the pacing leads are connected to an external pulse generator. If the pulse generator is disconnected before the temporary pacing wires are removed, the patient does not need continued monitoring. The exit sites for the epicardial wires should be redressed daily with an antiseptic or antibiotic ointment to avoid infection. Stimulation thresholds with epicardial wires tend to increase rapidly, and the result may be failure to pace. Thresholds, both pacing and sensing, should be checked daily, particularly in patients who are pacemaker-dependent. In pacemaker-dependent patients, early conversion to temporary or permanent transvenous pacing systems should be considered. During atrial pacing, a ventricular wire should never be used as the anodal ground.

The only significant difference in care between patients with temporary epicardial wires and those with temporary transvenous pacing systems is that the former are allowed to ambulate normally without restrictions on movement.

ESOPHAGEAL PACING AND RECORDING

The esophagus can also be used as a route for obtaining cardiac electrograms as well as for cardiac pacing. It has been used primarily in children but can also be useful in adults. A conventional coronary sinus lead can be placed via the nares. Alternatively, a small 4-Fr quadripolar catheter or a pill electrode catheter have also been used. The catheter is advanced and positioned to record the largest and most distinct atrial electrogram. Fluoroscopy is not required. Recording the electrogram is helpful in the diagnosis of the mechanism of arrhythmias, for example, atrial flutter when flutter waves are not seen on the standard electrocardiogram. In addition, the timing of the relationship of atrial and ventricular potentials can be helpful in analyzing the underlying electrophysiological substrate. The same catheter can also be used for stimulation for attempts at supraventricular tachycardia induction or termination to assess antiarrhythmic therapy. Complications with transesophageal pacing are uncommon, however, a wide pulse width of 10 ms must be used to avoid patient discomfort.

EMERGENCY PACING TECHNIQUES

In patients in whom the need for temporary pacing is an emergency because of severe bradycardia with hemodynamic instability or asystole, cardiopulmonary resuscitation should be carried out until some type of emergency temporary pacing can be established. External/transcutaneous pacing is now the technique of choice in the emergency situation. In the past, balloon flotation pacing catheters or transmyocardial pacing (placement of an intracardiac cannula through the chest wall into the ventricle) have been used in the emergency situation until a standard pacing catheter could be placed with fluoroscopic guidance. Transmyocardial pacing should no longer be used. The technique was rarely successful and carried with it significant potential risks, for example, laceration of a coronary artery. Balloon flotation pacing catheters are still used by some physicians, but external/transcutaneous pacing is the technique of choice.

External Transcutaneous Pacing

External cardiac pacing devices have become accepted as necessary emergency equipment after having been introduced by Zoll more than 25 years ago. For patients in whom cardiac arrest is precipitated by bradycardia, external cardiac pacing can be lifesaving.

External cardiac pacing devices are designed for easy and rapid application and are especially helpful in the following situations: (1) to support symptomatic bradyarrhythmias until a transvenous pacemaker can be placed; (2) on a standby basis for patients at an increased risk for developing ventricular asystole (that is, patients with a myocardial infarction and a new conduction abnormality); and (3) for potential backup pacing during cardioversion of atrial tachyarrhythmias.

External pacing can be uncomfortable for the conscious, alert patient. However, it usually can be tolerated until a temporary transvenous pacemaker can be placed.

COMPLICATIONS

Complications of temporary cardiac pacing usually are minor and not associated with either major morbidity or mortality. The complication rate depends upon the skill of the physician, the duration of temporary pacing, and the attention given to the care of the system.

Intracardiac Lead Dislodgment

The most common complication with temporary pacing is lead dislodgement. Temporary pacing leads are not as reliable as permanent leads. They cannot always be placed as accurately as permanent leads and do not have active or passive fixation mechanisms. Movement of the electrode tip may cause failure to pace and/or sense. In other instances, pacing may continue but stimulation thresholds may rise or there may be changes in the configuration of the QRS complex. In some cases, maintenance of pacing, despite significant intraventricular motion, can be achieved with a greater output of current. This increase can be continued without danger in most patients; however, if there is evidence of significant movement of the electrode, repositioning of the electrode or a change in the system usually is required (Figure 12 A,B,C).

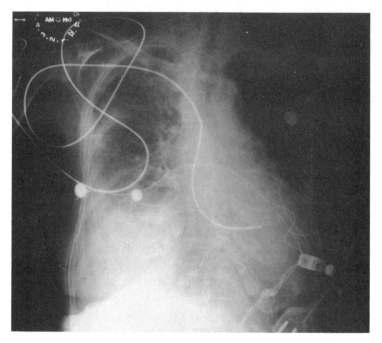

Figure 12A.   *Portable AP chest x-ray showing a temporary pacing wire positioned in the vicinity of the right ventricular apex.*

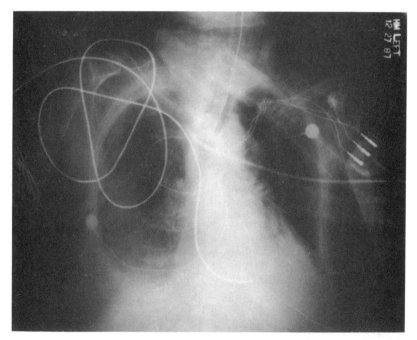

Figure 12B.   *A subsequent chest x-ray shows slight but definite movement of the temporary wire.*

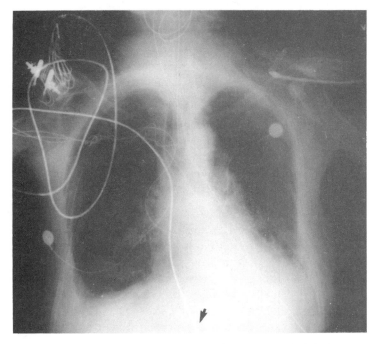

Figure 12C. *A third chest x-ray shows displacement of the lead into the inferior vena cava (arrow).*

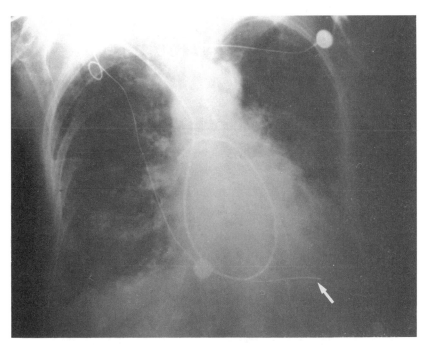

Figure 12D. *A final chest x-ray is obtained after placing a pulmonary artery catheter that has a port for a ventricular pacing wire (arrow) to be passed into the ventricle.*

If the electrode tip moves toward the tricuspid or pulmonary valve area or to the free cavity of a large right ventricle, extremely high currents may be required to maintain pacing. Displacement to the pulmonary artery or right atrium results in loss of ventricular capture, or occasionally, fluctuating atrial and ventricular capture.

If one suspects that the temporary pacing lead has moved, a chest radiograph should be obtained. This radiograph can then be compared with the one obtained immediately after temporary pacemaker placement. If dislodgment has occurred, the lead is repositioned.

Perforation

Perforation of the right ventricle is a well-recognized complication of temporary pacing (Figure 13). If perforation is suspected during placement of the lead, the lead usually can be immediately withdrawn into the right ventricular cavity without significant consequences. Late perforation results from continuous or intermittent pressure of the catheter on a thin right ventricular apex or the right ventricular free wall. Although the overall incidence of perforation is low, the incidence is higher with the standard woven Dacron temporary lead than with a floating temporary lead that is more flexible. If the brachial or femoral

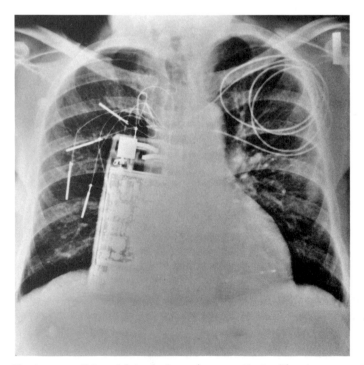

Figure 13. Chest x-rays, PA and lateral views, from a patient with a temporary transvenous pacemaker. **A.** On the PA film the lead tip appears to be near the right ventricular apex.

route is used, excessive motion of the extremity may increase the incidence of perforation.

Perforation may become evident clinically because of a friction rub, loss of pacing and/or sensing, diaphragmatic stimulation, a change in the QRS complex (specifically, ventricular pacing continued but development of a right bundle branch block pattern), and, rarely, by pericardial tamponade. When perforation is suspected, the lead should be repositioned.

Pneumothorax

Pneumothorax most commonly occurs when the subclavian or internal jugular vein is used. This complication is directly related to the experience of the operator. If pneumothorax occurs, one should proceed as outlined in Chapter 8, "Permanent Pacemaker Implantation."

Arterial Entry

Inadvertent entry into an adjacent artery may occur with the subclavian, internal jugular, or femoral venous approach. If it occurs, the needle should be

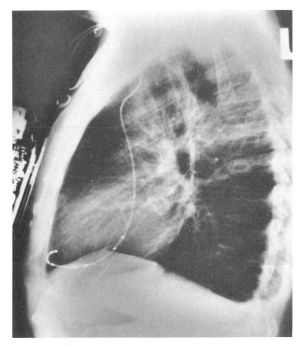

Figure 13B. *On the lateral film the lead tip appears to curve around the heart. The lead has perforated.*

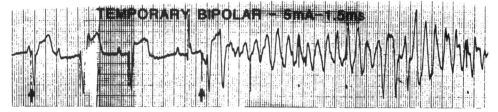

Figure 14. *Temporary bipolar pacing with failure to sense a native QRS complex. The pacing stimulus occurred during repolarization and induced ventricular tachycardia.*

withdrawn promptly and pressure placed over the puncture site to control bleeding. This complication also depends upon the experience of the operator. After local hemostasis, entry into the same venous site can be attempted.

Arrhythmias

As with placement of any intracardiac catheter, a temporary pacing lead may induce certain arrhythmias, the most common of which is ventricular ectopy. Ventricular ectopy is of most concern in the patient with a recent myocardial infarction in whom there may be significant myocardial irritability. If sustained ventricular ectopy occurs during placement of a temporary pacing lead in a patient with an acute infarction, it should be treated by moving the lead to a different, more stable position. An intravenous antiarrhythmic agent, i.e., lidocaine, may be necessary.

In patients with left bundle branch block in whom a temporary pacing catheter is being placed, mechanical trauma to the right bundle branch may result in complete heart block. The incidence is very low. If block does occur, rapid passage of the intracardiac electrode into the right ventricle should establish effective ventricular pacing.

A patient with a malfunctioning permanent pacemaker may require temporary pacemaker placement until the permanent system can be corrected. If the malfunctioning permanent pacemaker is not sensing appropriately, competition between the temporary and permanent pacemakers could result in ventricular rhythm disturbances. Similarly, if the temporary pacemaker is not sensing appropriately, a pacemaker stimulus delivered during the repolarization phase of a native QRS complex could induce ventricular tachycardia or fibrillation (Figure 14). A rare but reported arrhythmia with temporary pacing is that of "runaway pacemaker." Runaway can occur if there is a component failure of the temporary pacemaker.

In patients with temporary atrial pacing, as in patients with permanent atrial pacing, if stimulation occurs during the vulnerable period after intrinsic atrial depolarization, atrial fibrillation may result.

Local Skin or Suture Area Infection

Skin or suture area infection of clinical importance rarely occurs in patients with temporary pacing if attention is paid to skin care as described above. A small amount of purulence at the site of skin suture is rarely important, and usually heals as soon as the sutures are removed.

Bacteremia

If sterile conditions are not maintained during placement of a temporary pacing lead or if the temporary pacing lead is left in place for prolonged periods without adequate care of the system, bacteremia may result. We prefer not to leave a transvenous temporary pacing lead in for longer than 1 week.

If bacteremia does occur, it is treated by identification of the responsible organism and then the appropriate antibiotics. The pacing leads should be removed as soon as possible, and a culture of the lead and sheath should be obtained at the time of removal. If temporary pacing is still required, a new temporary pacing lead may be inserted by another venous route during antibiotic therapy.

Lyme Disease

Lyme disease is a specific entity that may require temporary pacing. Lyme disease is a tick-borne spirochetal infection that causes an acute systemic infection, a skin eruption, erythema chronicum migrans (ECM), myalgias, arthritis, fever, and in 4%–10% of those infected, carditis. The intermediate vector of the causative organism, Borrelia burgdorferi, is the deer tick, Ixodes dammini, although other tick and spirochete are carried by the common deer, small mammals, and some birds. Infection usually occurs in summer months during outdoor activities.

Without antibiotic treatment over half the patients develop further complications, the most common of which are arthritis and neurological manifestations such as meningoencephalitis. The carditis, when it occurs, manifests as a transient myocarditis with varying degrees of atrioventricular block, nonspecific ECG changes, arrhythmias, and left ventricular dysfunction. Rarely, complete heart block with asystole (Figure 15) may occur. In that case, temporary cardiac pacing is appropriate but implanted pacing is unnecessary. All patients with reported Lyme disease and myocarditis with high-degree AV block have returned to normal sinus rhythm, sometimes even without of antibiotic treatment.

The diagnosis of Lyme disease is clinical including the presence of ECM which is pathognomonic, but may have gone unnoticed, unrecognized as to significance, or misdiagnosed. Serological confirmation, provided by many public health services in endemic areas is helpful but is often delayed, may be insensitive, and is affected by antibiotic treatment if that has been given before a specific diagnosis has been reached. Further, a positive serological diagnosis can occur after the onset of carditis and AV block.

AV block of varying severity is the most common manifestation of carditis and occurs in 88% (43 of 49 reported cases). Sinoatrial block has been reported once. In the presence of high-grade AV block, a wide QRS morphology is present

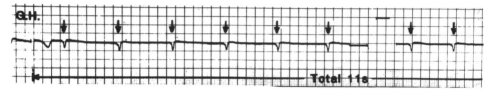

Figure 15.   *A recording of ventricular asystole with normal atrial activity during complete heart block caused by Lyme disease. The P waves are marked by arrows, and while the full duration of the asystole is not shown, it was 11 seconds.*

in about one third of patients and fluctuating right and left bundle branch block may exist as well as a ventricular rate below 40 beats per minute. In the few patients who have had electrophysiological assessment, the block usually has been proximal to the His bundle. AV block has an excellent prognosis for return to normal sinus rhythm despite the inconsistency of therapy. The block resolves within several days to 2 weeks, rarely remaining for 6 weeks at lesser levels of block. Other evidences of carditis with reduced ejection fraction, ST segment depression, and T wave flattening also resolve.

Should carditis occur with AV block, hospitalization with continuous ECG monitoring is appropriate, and temporary cardiac pacing may be necessary if the cardiac rate is slow or is complicated by prolonged asystole. Implantation of a cardiac pacemaker is not indicated. Three patients have been reported who have had a pacemaker implanted. In each case, the procedure was, almost certainly, unnecessary. It is especially important to be alert to the possibility of Lyme disease usually in a young male in whom the possibility of complete heart block is otherwise remote, who is in or from an endemic area, and who has the sudden onset of complete heart block, possibly with profound asystole but who seems not to have any reason for the AV block. If the block vanishes within several days of its onset, the level of suspicion of Lyme disease should be very high.

BIBLIOGRAPHY

Austin JL, Preis LK, Cramptom RS, et al: Analysis of pacemaker malfunction and complications of temporary pacing in the coronary care unit. Am J Cardiol 1982; 49:301–306.

Billhardt RA: Temporary Pacing. Clin Prog Pacing Electrophysiol 1984; 2:305–324.

Ferguson TB Jr, Cox JL: Temporary external DDD pacing after cardiac operations. Ann Thorac Surg 1991; 51:723–732.

Gould BA, Marshall AJ: Noninvasive temporary pacemakers. PACE 1988; 11:1331–1335.

Guzy P: Emergency cardiac pacing. Emerg Med Clin North Am 1986;4:745–759.

Haffajee CI: Temporary cardiac pacing: Modes, evaluation of function, equipment and troubleshooting. Cardiol Clin 1985; 3:515–526.

Hartzler GO, Maloney JD, Curtis JJ, et al: Hemodynamic benefits of atrioventricular sequential pacing after cardiac surgery. Am J Cardiol 1977; 40:232–236.

Hauser RG, Vicari RM: Temporary pacing: Indications modes and techniques. Med Clin N Am 1986; 70:813–827.

Hedges JR, Feero S, Shultz B, et al: Prehospital transcutaneous cardiac pacing for symptomatic bradycardia. PACE 1991; 14:1473–1478.

Hindman MC, Wagner GS, JaRo M, et al: The clinical significance of bundle branch block complicating acute myocardial infarction. 2. Indications for temporary and permanent pacemaker insertion. Circulation 1978; 58:689–699.

Hynes JK, Holmes DR Jr, Harrison CE: Five-year experience with temporary pacemaker therapy in the coronary care unit. Mayo Clin Proc 1983; 58:122–126.

Jacob AS, Schweiger MJ: A method for inserting two catheters, pulmonary arterial and temporary pacing, through a single puncture into a subclavian vein. Cathet Cardiovasc Diagn 1983; 9:611–615.

Janosik D, Stratmann HG, Walter KE, et al: Torsade de Pointes: A rare complication of temporary pacing for permanent ventricular pacemaker failure. PACE 1985; 8:558–561.

Jowett NI, Thompson DR, Pohl JEF: Temporary transvenous cardiac pacing: 6 years experience in one coronary care unit. Postgrad Med J 1989; 65:211–215.

Klein RC, Zakauddin V, Mason DT: Intraventricular conduction defects in acute myocardial infarction: Incidence, prognosis, and therapy. Am Heart J 1984; 108:1007–1013.

Lang R, David D, Klein HO, et al: The use of the balloon-tipped floating catheter in temporary transvenous cardiac pacing. PACE 1981; 4:491–496.

Lau CP, Cheung KL, Mok CK: Biventricular perforation by a temporary pacing electrode: Recognition from the lateral chest radiograph. Int J Cardiol 1989; 24:368–371.

Littleford PO: Physiologic temporary pacing: Techniques and indications. Clin Prog Pacing Electrophysiol 1984; 2:236–254.

Luck JC, Markel ML: Clinical applications of external pacing: A renaissance? PACE 1991; 14:1299–1316.

Lumia FJ, Rios JC: Temporary transvenous pacemaker therapy: An analysis of complications. Chest 1973; 64:604–608.

Morris D, Mulvihill D, Lew WYW: Risk of developing complete heart block during bedside pulmonary artery catheterization in patients with left bundle branch block. Arch Intern Med 1987; 147:2005–2010.

Murphy P, Morton P, Murtagh JG, et al: Hemodynamic effects of different temporary pacing modes for the management of bradycardias complicating acute myocardial infarction. PACE 1992; 15:391–396.

Noe R, Cockrell W, Moses HW, et al: Transcutaneous pacemaker use in a large hospital. PACE 1986; 9:101–104.

Rosenfeld LE: Bradyarrhythmias, abnormalities of conduction, and indications for pacing in acute myocardial infarction. Cardiol Clin 1988; 6:49–61.

Rosenthal E, Thomas N, Quinn E, et al: Transcutaneous pacing for cardiac emergencies. PACE 1988; 11:2160–2167.

Rubin DA, Sorbera C, Baum S, et al: Acute reversible diffuse conduction system disease due to Lyme Disease. PACE 1990; 13:1367–1373.

Rubio PA: Simplified suture technique for implanting temporary pacemaker electrodes. J Cardiovasc Surg 1989; 30:998–999.

Scheinman MM: Treatment of cardiac arrhythmias in patients with acute myocardial infarction. Am J Surg 1983; 145:707–710.

Sharkey SW, Chaffee V, Kapsner S: Prophylactic external pacing during cardioversion of atrial tachyarrhythmias. Am J Cardiol 1985; 55:1632–1634.

Simoons ML, Demey HE, Bossaert LL, et al: The Paceport catheter: A new pacemaker system introduced through a Swan-Ganz catheter. Cathet Cardiovasc Diagn 1988; 15:66–70.

Stefanadis C, Gavaliatsis I, Stratos C, et al: Temporary cardiac pacing using a new, steerable, balloon-tipped pacing catheter. Cathet Cardiovasc Diagn 1990; 21:198–202.

Sulzbach LM, Lansdowne LM: Temporary atrial pacing after cardiac surgery. Focus Crit Care 1991; 18:65, 68–74.

Syverud SA, Dalsey WC, Hedges JR: Transcutaneous and transvenous cardiac pacing for early bradyasystolic cardiac arrest. Ann Emerg Med 1986; 15:121–124.

Tilden SJ, Koopot R, Sansbury D, et al: Runaway temporary pacemaker caused by a component defect. Crit Care Med 1989; 17: 1231–1232.

Trankina MF, White RD: Perioperative cardiac pacing using an atrio-ventricular pacing pulmonary artery catheter. J Cardiothoracic Anesth 1989; 3:154–162.

Waldo AL, Henthorn RW, Epstein AE, et al: Diagnosis and treatment of arrhythmias during and following open heart surgery. Med Clin North Am 1984; 68:1153–1169.

Wallenhaupt SL, Rogers AT: Intraoperative use of dual chamber demand pacemakers for open heart operations. Ann Thorac Surg 1989; 48:579–581.

Weinstein J, Gnoj J, Mazzara JT, et al: Temporary transvenous pacing via the percutaneous femoral vein approach: A prospective study of 100 cases. Am Heart J 1973; 85:695–705.

Winner SJ, Boon NA: Transvenous pacemaker electrodes placed unintentionally in the left ventricle: three cases. Postgrad Med J 1989; 65:98–102.

Winner S, Boon N: Clinical problems with temporary pacemakers prior to permanent pacing. J R Coll Physicians 1989; 23:161–163.

Wirtz St, Schulte HD, Winter J, et al: Reliability of different temporary myocardial pacing leads. Thorac Cardiovasc Surg 1989; 37: 163–168.

Wood M, Ellenbogen KA: Bradyarrhythmias, emergency pacing, and implantable defibrillation devices. Crit Care Clin 1989; 5:551–568.

Zoll PM: Resuscitation of the heart in ventricular standstill by external electric stimulation. N Engl J Med 1952; 247:768–771.

Zoll PM, Zoll RH, Falk RH, et al: External noninvasive temporary cardiac pacing: Clinical trials. Circulation 1985; 71:937–944.

Chapter 8

PERMANENT PACEMAKER IMPLANTATION

David L. Hayes, David R. Holmes, Jr., Seymour Furman

The transthoracic approach for the placement of epimyocardial pacing electrodes dominated pacemaker implantation until the introduction of implantable transvenous systems in 1965. Increased experience with the transvenous approach, coupled with the development of active and passive fixation leads that greatly decrease the frequency of dislodgment has resulted in the current approach to cardiac pacing in which transvenous systems account for approximately 95% of all pacemaker implants. For the most part, thoracotomy implantation is now limited to patients needing permanent pacing who are undergoing thoracotomy for other reasons, for example, bypass graft surgery.

IMPLANT FACILITY

Requirements for the rooms, personnel, and equipment for cardiac pacemaker implantation were described in the 1983 InterSociety Commission for Heart Disease Resources report. Pacemakers should be implanted in a surgical environment, whether a specially equipped operating room or a catheterization suite. Requirements include excellent fluoroscopy, electrocardiographic monitoring, oxygen saturation monitoring (via finger plethysmography), and standby defibrillator and life-support equipment. Additional desirable features are facilities for lateral and anteroposterior fluoroscopy projection, fluoroscopy table capable of tilting, and equipment to measure intra-arterial pressure and conduction intervals.

ANESTHESIA

Local anesthesia is used for all patients unless contraindicated. Special circumstances including, but not limited to, pediatric patients, uncooperative patients, or confused patients undergoing permanent pacing may require general anesthesia. Supplemental parenteral sedatives are used as needed for patient comfort.

ANATOMICAL APPROACH

Before 1979, transvenous pacing leads were almost always placed through a cephalic vein cutdown in the deltopectoral groove. If the cephalic vein was too small or friable or had previously been used for implantation or if a second lead was required, the ipsilateral external or internal jugular vein was used. Rarely, subclavian or axillary vein cutdowns were performed. Deep dissection demanded precise surgical techniques, a disadvantage for medical cardiologists who implanted pacemakers. Each approach has its own particular advantages and disadvantages. The subclavian puncture and cephalic cutdown approaches are most commonly used today. Placement through the external or internal jugular veins, in addition to more local dissection, requires the operator to tunnel the lead over or under the clavicle to the pulse generator. Techniques for permanent lead placement via the iliac vein has also been described but is not used.

Subclavian Approach

The introducer approach for subclavian venipuncture has become well known. Because this technique is fast, usually causes minimal trauma, is useful when the cephalic vein is absent, and facilitates placement of multiple leads, it has become the procedure of choice in many institutions. The basic procedure, a modification of the Seldinger technique, requires detailed knowledge about the route of the subclavian vein and the relationship of the vein to the clavicle, first rib, subclavian artery, and apex of the lung (Figure 1). The ease, efficacy, and safety of the technique are directly related to adherence to specific guidelines (Table I) and the expertise of the physician performing the venipuncture.

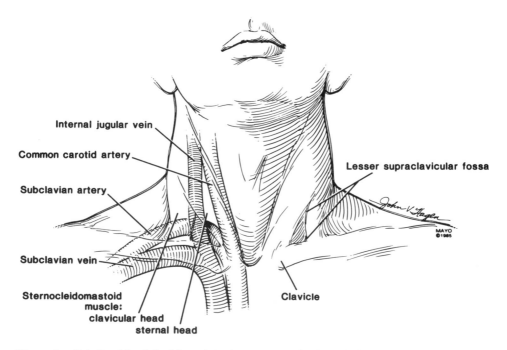

Figure 1.   *Relationship of clavicle, subclavian artery, and vein and of carotid artery and internal jugular vein. (Reproduced by permission of the Mayo Foundation.)*

Table I
Principles of Subclavian Puncture

Know the anatomy
Distend the subclavian vein
  Hydration
  Trendelenburg's position
Use as small a needle as possible (18 gauge)
Approach the vein as medially as possible:
  Start at junction of middle & lateral thirds of the clavicle
Avoid repeated punctures

After infiltration with a local anesthetic agent, a 4- to 6-cm incision is made approximately 2 cm below and parallel to the clavicle, beginning at the junction of its middle and inner thirds. This incision is carried down to the pectoralis fascia. By use of blunt and sharp dissection, a prepectoralis fascial pocket is fashioned for the pulse generator. This pocket should be large enough to allow an adequate fit of the pulse generator and the leads selected. It should be placed medially rather than laterally near the axilla to prevent migration of the pulse generator and impingement on the anterior axillary fold. Care should be taken to avoid either an excessively tight pocket, which may result in erosion, or an excessively large pocket, which may permit pacemaker migration. After dissection and development of the pocket, a sponge soaked with antibiotic solution may be kept within it during placement of the leads, but its removal is mandatory before wound closure.

Prepackaged kits containing a needle, guide wire, dilator, and peel-away sheath are available (Figure 2). The subclavian vein is entered through the infraclavicular incision with an 18-gauge needle (Figure 3A). Placing the patient in the Trendelenburg position may facilitate entry because the subclavian vein may be less distended in the recumbent patient with normal venous pressure. This is even more of a problem if the patient has been fasting for several hours prior to the procedure and is volume depleted. The vein usually is entered at the junction of the middle and inner thirds of the clavicle; more lateral veni-

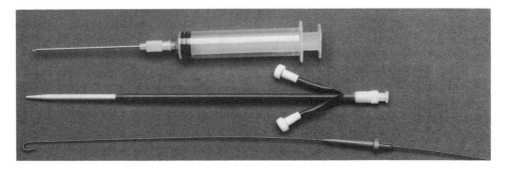

Figure 2. Prepackaged kit for subclavian venipuncture; contains needle, guide wire, dilator, and peel-away sheath.

puncture has greater potential for damage to the apex of the pleural space. More recently, however, some have advocated very medial puncture of the subclavian vein. Using an extreme medial approach for subclavian venipuncture has been referred to as the "safe introducer technique." The landmarks for venipuncture have been defined as the region between the first rib and clavicle at the lateral edge of the sternum in a 40° arc.

The subclavian venipuncture should be performed with a syringe with saline or 1% xylocaine attached to the needle. As the puncture is performed, a slight vacuum should be maintained on the syringe. The syringe should be observed constantly for the aspiration of air, blood, or other fluids.

Once the vein is punctured successfully, the introducer guide wire is advanced through the needle and into the right side of the heart under fluoroscopic control (Figure 3B). On occasion, this guide wire enters the jugular system and ascends. This error can be corrected by manipulation under fluoroscopy. After removal of the needle, the introducer, dilator, and peel-away sheath are advanced over the guide wire into the superior vena cava (Figure 3C). Selection of the appropriate size introducer (ranging from 8 Fr to 14 Fr) is based on the size of the lead or leads to be used. After removal of the dilator and guide, the pacing lead or leads are advanced through the sheath into the right side of the heart. One should take care to avoid air embolism during this procedure by pinching the sheath ends closed and by having the patient hold respiration until passage of the lead into the right side of the heart. The sheath is then peeled away (Figure 3D).

In some patients, the space between the clavicle and the first rib is tight or the costoclavicular ligament is fibrotic and calcified. This can be recognized by problems with needle entry into the vein or problems with advancement of the dilator. (This can often be a problem when the extreme medial approach to subclavian puncture is used.) Although lead placement can be achieved, it may be suboptimal. Insulation defects and conductor coil fractures have been identified at this site. These defects may be due to crush injury or continued pressure on the lead or traction because the lead is fixed in the right ventricle and also at the space between the clavicle and first rib. When such a tight space is identified during implantation, consideration should be given to repositioning the venous entry laterally or using a cephalic approach. Potential complications of subclavian vein puncture that have been described include pneumothorax, hemopneumothorax, lung laceration, inadvertent arterial puncture, air embolism, arteriovenous fistula, thoracic duct injury, and brachial plexus injury. Meticulous attention is required to minimize these risks.

Subclavian puncture may also be facilitated and complications minimized by the use of contrast venography. This requires no additional preparation with the exception of being certain that the patient does not have a contrast allergy and placement of an intravenous line (20 gauge or larger) in the arm on the side of the pacemaker implantation. The intravenous line should be checked for patency before injection of contrast media. Two strategies have evolved for the use of contrast venography. In patients with normal costoclavicular relationships, no prior permanent pacing leads, and no venous thrombosis, a "blind" venipuncture is first attempted as previously described. If the subclavian vein

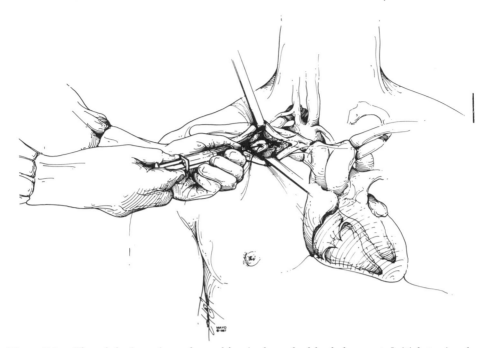

Figure 3A. *The subclavian vein can be used for single- or dual-lead placement. Initial step involves puncturing the vein with an 18-gauge needle. Blood is aspirated to ensure proper positioning in venous structure.*

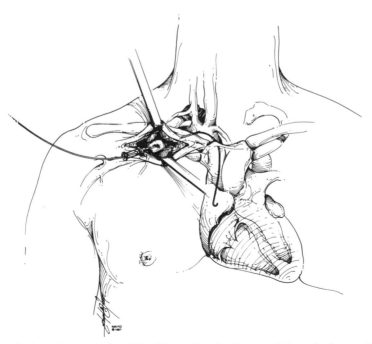

Figure 3B. *Syringe is removed and flexible guide wire is passed through the needle, passing proximal end of the wire into the region of right atrium.*

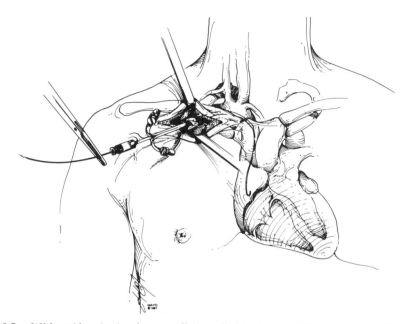

Figure 3C.   *With guide wire in place, needle is pulled back and off the guide wire. Dilator and peel-away sheath are then placed over the guide wire and passed into the subclavian vein. Sizes of dilator and peel-away sheath depend on size of lead(s) to be used. As dilator and sheath are being passed into the vein, a hemostat is placed on the guide wire to prevent the guide wire from being lost into the venous circulation.*

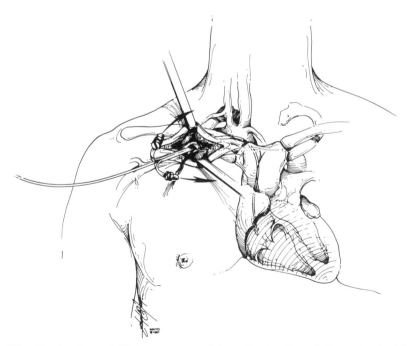

Figure 3D.   *Guide wire and dilator are removed from the sheath, and the pacing lead is passed quickly through the sheath into the right atrium. Arrows indicate pulling of the peel-away introducer away from the lead.*

is not punctured during the initial attempts, possibly with the use of fluoroscopy, then a contrast agent is used to assist in localizing the subclavian vein. In patients who may have unusual venous anatomy, it may be desirable to use contrast venography before the initial attempt to ensure venous patency and location. Such patients might include those with kyphoscoliosis or prior clavicular fracture or permanent pacemaker lead implantation.

The contrast injection usually is performed by a nonsterile assistant. Approximately 14 to 20 mL of either ionic or nonionic iodinated contrast is rapidly injected through the intravenous line in the forearm. A saline bolus is then used to flush the contrast into the venous system. At this time, the arm can be massaged to assist in venous return and venous visualization. This can be performed either under the sterile drapes by an assistant or over the sterile drapes by the implanter. The subclavicular area is monitored with fluoroscopy for the appearance of contrast, which usually takes approximately 5 to 20 seconds (Figure 4).

With contrast in the vein, the venipuncture needle can then be positioned directly into the subclavian vein with fluoroscopic guidance (Figure 5). The anteroposterior location of the subclavian vein is not appreciated with anteroposterior fluoroscopy. Needle passes occasionally may be too anterior or posterior despite appearing to be within the column of contrast. Repeat injections are given as needed. Alternatively, if the contrast venogram demonstrates a non-

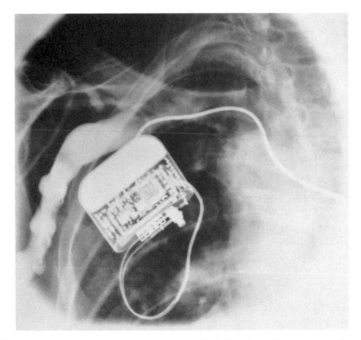

Figure 4. *Contrast venogram demonstrating an occluded right subclavian vein in a patient with a chronic pacing lead in the subclavian vein. The venogram was obtained prior to attempted placement of an atrial lead and a dual-chamber pacemaker. The image was obtained approximately 15 to 20 seconds after contrast injection.*

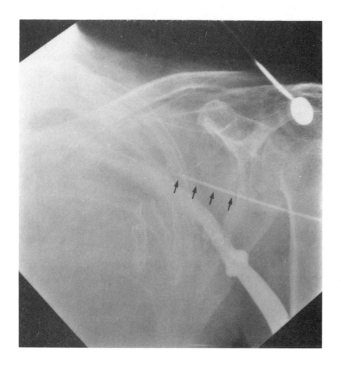

Figure 5. *Contrast venogram obtained during subclavian venipuncture. With contrast in the vein, the venipuncture needle, denoted by arrows, can be positioned directly into the subclavian vein with fluoroscopic guidance.*

patent or small subclavian vein, the implanting physician may choose a different venous access site.

Cephalic Approach

Some physicians, including one of the authors of this text [SF], prefer the cephalic or jugular approach, which avoids the risks of subclavian venipuncture. The cephalic vein always lies within the deltopectoral groove. The deltopectoral groove is a constant anatomical site and lies between the deltoid and pectoralis major muscles. The cephalic vein is commonly sufficiently large for a single bipolar lead and often large enough for two unipolar or even two bipolar leads. The operative skills required for the cephalic approach are modest and can be readily taught to anyone sufficiently skilled to perform subclavian puncture or other invasive cardiovascular procedures. Cannulation of the cephalic vein is free of significant complications. If damaged, it can be ligated with prompt cessation of bleeding. In addition, the normal venous pressure and the venous valves prevent aspiration of air into the central circulation.

If the cephalic vein is too small to accommodate even a single lead, a guide wire technique may be useful. To perform the guide wire technique the cephalic vein is opened in the usual manner, but instead of attempting to pass the lead,

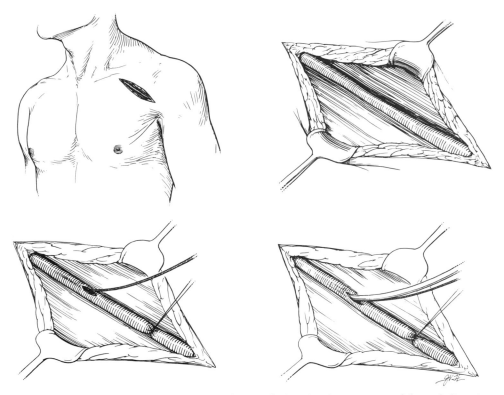

Figure 6. *A partial cephalic cutdown, introducer technique involves exposure of the cephalic vein in the delto-pectoral groove (upper left, upper right). If the vein is too small to accept a lead, a guide wire is placed (lower left) and the introducer over it (lower right).*

a guide wire is placed through the opening into the superior vena cava or right atrium. The introducer is then placed over the guide wire, as in a conventional subclavian approach, and a lead or leads introduced. A modification of this technique can be used if a single lead is passed into the cephalic vein and the vein will not accommodate a second lead necessary for dual-chamber pacing. In this case, the guide wire is passed into the subclavian vein alongside the initially placed lead. An introducer can then be placed over the guide wire and a second lead introduced (Figure 6).

Jugular Approach

If the external or internal jugular vein is selected, two incisions are required. An incision is made immediately above the clavicle, over the area between the posterior border of the sternocleidomastoid muscle and the anterior border of the trapezius muscle. External jugular access to the heart usually is easier by the right external jugular vein than by the left because the vessel is often less tortuous. If no satisfactory external jugular vessel is found, the incision is extended to a point anterior to the sternal head of the sternocleidomastoid muscle.

The carotid sheath is exposed after the superficial fascia is opened behind the posterior border of the sternocleidomastoid muscle. The muscle is then elevated to visualize the carotid sheath optimally. On occasion, the clavicular head of the sternocleidomastoid muscle must be divided to expose the carotid sheath (Figure 7). The carotid sheath is then opened; the internal jugular vein is identified and isolated with nonabsorbable ligatures. After venotomy, the lead or leads can be introduced. Use of either the external or the internal jugular vein requires that the lead be tunneled down to the pulse generator site, either superficial or deep to the clavicle. In addition, the internal jugular procedure requires more extensive dissection with the possibility of damage to the subclavian artery and vein and the recurrent laryngeal nerve. Should the cutdown route be attempted before subclavian puncture, use of the cephalic and external jugular veins for introduction of lead systems remains consistent and reliable. Of all primary dual-chamber implants by one of the authors [SF], the cephalic vein was used for two unipolar leads in 61% of instances, the external jugular and cephalic veins in 8%, while subclavian puncture alone was required for only 16% of implants. During dual-chamber bipolar implant, the cephalic vein alone was used 43% of the time, the external jugular 14% of the time, and subclavian puncture for 7% of implants. For unipolar lead systems, the cephalic and external jugular venous routes alone were used in 78% of implants, for bipolar leads, 72%.

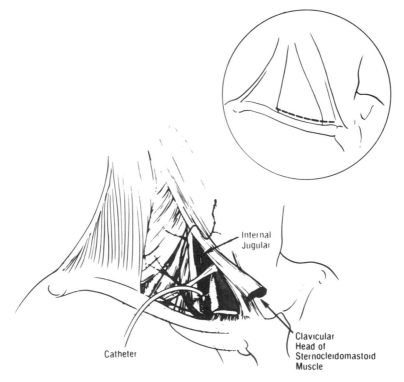

Figure 7.   *Approach to the internal jugular vein. Incision (insert) is made immediately above the clavicle. The carotid sheath is exposed and then opened (see text for details). (Reproduced with permission from Annals of Thoracic Surgery).*

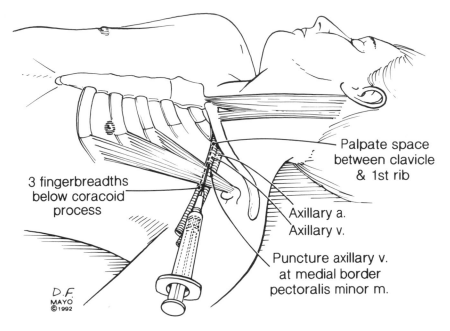

3 fingerbreadths
below coracoid
process

Palpate space
between clavicle
& 1st rib

Axillary a.
Axillary v.

Puncture axillary v.
at medial border
pectoralis minor m.

D.F.
MAYO
©1992

Figure 8. *Anatomical landmarks used for axillary venipuncture.*

Axillary Approach

Axillary vein puncture recently has been advocated as a safe approach to lead placement. If the needle is kept anterior to the thoracic cavity the potential for pneumothorax and hemopneumothorax is eliminated. The landmarks for the infraclavicular course of the axillary vein are shown in Figure 8. The axillary vein can be located medially at a point below the medial aspect of the clavicle where a space becomes palpable between the first rib and clavicle. The vein extends to a point approximately three fingerbreadths below the inferior aspect of the coracoid process. It has been recommended that the arm be abducted 45° for the venipuncture. The skin is punctured at the medial border of the pectoralis minor muscle at a point above the vein as defined by the surface landmarks. The needle is passed anterior to the first rib, aiming posteriorly and medially along the lateral-to-medial course of the vein. The needle never passes between the first rib and clavicle.

VENTRICULAR LEAD PLACEMENT

Successful placement of a reliable right ventricular pacing system requires knowledge of and experience with the specific lead used as well as knowledge of right heart anatomy and catheterization techniques. Great care must be taken during implantation to avoid damage to the lead. The lead stylet, in particular, should not be forced, as this may result in perforation of the stylet through the conductor coil and into the insulation. Keeping the stylet clean and free of blood and moistened with saline will help avoid trauma to the lead during multiple stylet changes. Several placement techniques are used; all must result in stable right ventricular catheter position with adequate pacing and sensing thresholds. Usually, the right ventricular apex is selected. Other sites, e.g., the right ventricular outflow tract, occasionally are used because of local myocardial problems, such as prior inferior-apical infarction.

Once the ventricular lead is in the superior vena cava it should move freely. The stylet should be withdrawn about 5 cm and the lead moved inferiorly. It will often catch in the right atrium and be deflected towards the tricuspid valve (Figure 9). If it passes the tricuspid valve it will be in the inflow tract of the right ventricle. It may cause several premature ventricular contractions as it passes through the outflow tract, but these usually cease as the catheter passes into the main pulmonary artery. All of this is readily visible fluoroscopically and, if seen, assures that the lead has traversed the right ventricle. The lead occasionally will enter the coronary sinus from the right atrium. A lead within the coronary sinus may appear to be within the right ventricle, but the passage will not be superiorly but rather more laterally toward the left cardiac border. Should the lead begin to curl about the left cardiac border, then it is certainly in the coronary sinus. In addition, there will be no ventricular ectopy if the lead is in the coronary sinus. Attempts at entering the pulmonary artery will be unsuccessful, but the most important clue will be in the lateral fluoroscopic view. The outflow tract of the right ventricle is an anterior structure, and a lead in it will be seen in the retrosternal position. The coronary sinus is on the posterior wall of the heart, and a lead within it will be visualized on the posterior cardiac border.

If the lead cannot be deflected across the tricuspid valve, the straight stylet should be removed and a curved stylet inserted into the lead. (A curved stylet is accomplished by wetting the stylet and the gloved index finger and thumb and pulling the stylet through the apposed fingers while rotating the fingers to

---

Figure 9 (Opposite page). *Intracardiac manipulation is basic to successful pacemaker implantation. Implantation of a dual-chamber pacemaker involves placement of an atrial lead and a ventricular lead. (1) Both leads may be introduced via the subclavian, cephalic, or external jugular veins. Initially both will be in the superior vena cava or the right atrial appendage. (2) As ventricular stimulation is more important than atrial stimulation, the atrial lead guide wire, which makes it a straight catheter, should be placed into the upper inferior vena cava. The ventricular lead can then be directed through the tricuspid valve. (3) Once past the valve and in the mid-right ventricle it should be advanced into the pulmonary artery to insure that is has not entered the coronary sinus (Panel 6). (4) If the lead tip will not pass the tricuspid valve, entry via curve, deflected from the lateral atrial wall, may be successful. (5) Advancing the bowed lead in the right ventricle and then the guide wire within the bow can flip the lead tip into the right ventricular outflow tract. Note that during this entire maneuver the atrial lead is "parked" in the inferior vena cava. (6) As above, the lead is passed into the pulmonary artery. (7) Once there, the lead is slowly withdrawn so that it falls toward the right ventricular apex. 8) Once at the diaphragmatic surface of the ventricle, it is advanced into the apex. A deep breath is a useful maneuver as it angulates the apex downward and allows easier access. (9) When the ventricular lead has been positioned properly, the guide wire is allowed to remain withdrawn about one inch from the tip to hold it in position while the atrial lead is being manipulated. (10) As the two leads often will adhere lightly one to the other, when manipulating one lead the other should be held so that it is not inadvertently displaced. The lead should be pulled into the low right atrium and the guide wire withdrawn about 7 cm. The "J" will form. (11) The atrial lead should then be pulled upward slowly. Entry into the base of the atrial appendage will be recognized by straightening of the "J" with pull on the lead. (12) Additional pulling is stopped and the lead advanced into the tip of the atrial appendage.*

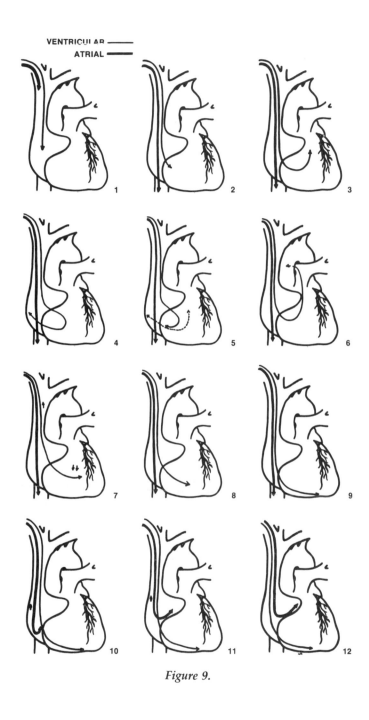

Figure 9.

impart a curve to the wire.) The curved stylet will be helpful in introducing the lead through the tricuspid valve. Alternatively, the lead tip can be projected against the lateral atrial wall and the curved portion of the lead backed into the tricuspid valve. This technique works best with the leads that have fins or a fixation mechanism as part of the electrode, as opposed to tined leads, which tend to catch on the chordae tendineae and impede entry of the tip into the right ventricular outflow tract. Once the lead tip is in the outflow tract, the curved guide wire should be replaced by a straight stylet. The stylet is not passed completely into the lead initially. Slow withdrawal of the lead will then cause the lead tip to fall toward the right ventricular apex. The stylet should be advanced as the lead is slowly withdrawn allowing the straightened lead to fall toward the apex. Once the lead falls from the outflow tract and is directed towards the apex, the lead, with stylet in place, should be advanced toward the apex. This maneuver may be assisted by asking the patient to breathe deeply which causes the right ventricular apex to descend with the diaphragm. At that point the lead can be advanced. If an atrial lead is not to be implanted, the guide wire can be removed from the ventricular lead and the lead can be checked for stability with deep breathing and/or coughing.

SECURING THE LEAD

If pacing and sensing thresholds are satisfactory and there is no diaphragmatic stimulation measured with pacing at 10 V, the silicone rubber sleeve pro-

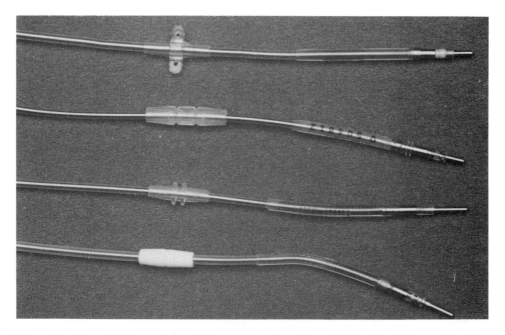

Figure 10.   *Several different types of sleeves are used to fix the lead to adjacent tissue. The sleeve protects the lead from damage that could be induced by placing the ligature directly on the lead.*

vided on the lead is positioned over the lead at the point of entry into the vein (Figure 10). Synthetic nonabsorbable ligature is used to fix the sleeve to the lead and to the muscle or the vein itself. It is essential to use the sleeve and not affix the lead directly to the adjacent tissue. Ligatures applied directly to the lead may damage the insulation and act as a fulcrum, and lead fracture at the fixation site may eventually result.

DUAL-CHAMBER PACEMAKER IMPLANTATION

The subclavian introducer technique can be used for placement of two leads. With this technique, two thin leads (one for atrial and one for ventricular placement) can be advanced through the same introducer sheath into the right side of the heart (Figure 11). (A #14 introducer can accommodate two bipolar leads simultaneously.) The atrial lead is held in a stable position in the right atrium, while the ventricular lead is positioned in the right ventricular apex. After stable ventricular placement is achieved to allow ventricular pacing during the remainder of the procedure, the right atrial catheter is positioned. Alternatively, two subclavian venipunctures can be used, one for each catheter to be inserted, the ventricular lead being placed first (Figure 12). This technique reduces the problem of displacement of one lead while the other is being positioned (as sometimes occurs with the single cannulation technique) but does require two

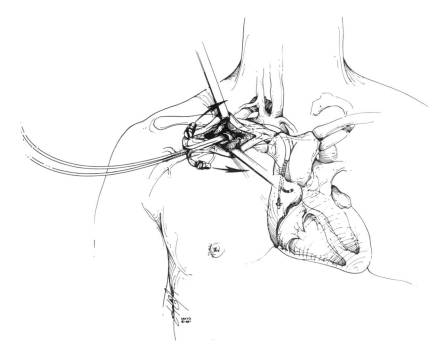

Figure 11. *If two pacing leads are necessary, both leads can be inserted simultaneously if a peel-away introducer large enough to accommodate both leads is used. With straight stylets in place, one lead is staggered 1–2 cm behind the other lead, and they are passed simultaneously into the right heart and the introducer is then peeled away.*

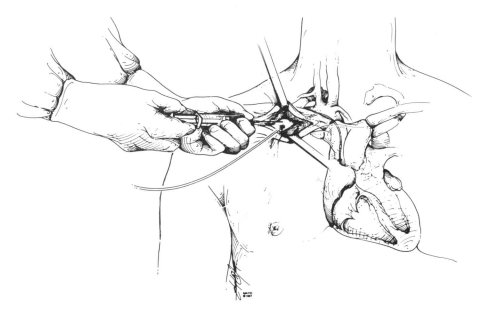

Figure 12.   *If a second lead is to be used, a second subclavian puncture can be performed parallel to the already placed pacing lead or the second puncture can be performed after the first guide wire is in place but before the first pacing lead is inserted. If the second puncture is performed after the initial lead is already in place, care should be taken to avoid puncturing the indwelling lead. The potential for damage can be minimized by performing the puncture medial to the existing lead.*

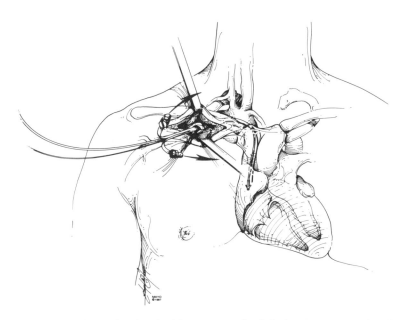

Figure 13A.   *Two leads can be placed without a second subclavian puncture and without simultaneously passing the leads. As the dilator and guide wire are removed and the initial pacing lead is passed into right heart, the guide wire is reinserted through the peel-away introducer alongside the pacing lead. The introducer is then peeled away and the pacing lead and guide wire are left in place.*

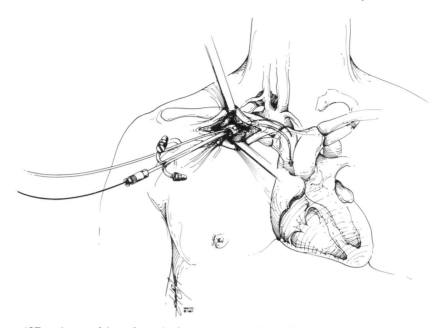

Figure 13B. *A second introducer is then passed over the guide wire that has been reintroduced and the second lead is placed. (Reproduced by permission of the Mayo Foundation.)*

separate venipunctures. In a third variation, one venipuncture is performed and one lead is introduced, and the guide wire is reintroduced or retained before peeling away the sheath (Figure 13A); a new introducer is placed over the retained guide wire to accommodate the second lead (Figure 13B).

Atrial Lead Placement

Placement of the atrial lead is identical for either single-chamber or dual-chamber pacemakers. Although the atrial lead most commonly is positioned in the right atrial appendage, satisfactory pacing can be achieved from multiple positions within the right atrium. In patients with previous cardiac surgery in whom the appendage has been cannulated or amputated, finding a stable position in the atrial appendage may be more difficult but is usually still possible.

The usual technique for atrial lead placement is to straighten the atrial lead with a straight stylet and pass the lead into the mid-right atrium. The atrial lead may have passive fixation in which case it will be "J" in shape when the guide wire is removed. The tip of the lead should be placed into the low right atrium (Figure 14A) and the straight guide wire withdrawn about 10 cm (Figure 14B). The "J" will be formed spontaneously and the entire lead can be drawn upward into the right atrial appendage (Figure 14C). Entry into the appendage is indicated by a rhythmic to and fro, medial and lateral motion of the "J" portion of the lead (Figure 14D). The PA fluoroscopic projection may show the lead medial or lateral, and a lateral projection will show the lead to be anterior at approximately the same level as a lead in the right ventricular apex. If the atrial lead is being placed as part of a dual-chamber procedure, the ventricular lead should be carefully observed so that it is not inadvertently displaced.

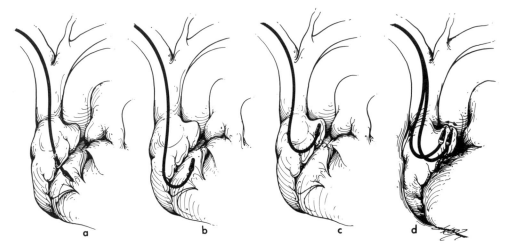

Figure 14A-D. *A. Atrial "J" lead at middle of right atrium with straight stylet in place. B. Straight stylet is removed; removal allows catheter to assume the preformed "J" configuration. C. Entire lead is pulled back and the tip of the electrode is allowed to enter the right atrial appendage. D. Characteristic to-and-fro motion of lead when positioned in the right atrial appendage. (Reproduced by permission of the Mayo Foundation.)*

Active fixation atrial leads may be "straight" or in a "preformed J" configuration. If a lead of the "preformed J" variety is used, the screw mechanism can be advanced with the straight stylet fully extended or with the stylet pulled back into the body of the lead, i.e., withdrawn from the "J" portion of the lead. If a straight active fixation lead is used, a "J" curved stylet will be needed to enter the atrial appendage. The stylet is introduced into the atrial lead in the low right atrium and the assembly pulled into the right atrial appendage. The active fixation lead is fixed in place by releasing the screw mechanism. Once fixed, the "J" guide wire is gently withdrawn so as not to displace from the point of attachment. Sensing and pacing thresholds should be checked. If adequate, the lead should be secured with the sleeve provided as previously described.

As noted above, locations other than the right atrial appendage may be used for atrial lead positioning. The right atrium can be explored, particularly when lateral fluoroscopy is available, to find optimal positioning for lead placement. With active fixation leads, the lead can be placed in the atrial septum or in the free atrial wall (Figures 15A and 15B). Coronary sinus placement rarely is used (Figures 16A and 16B). Specific problems with coronary sinus pacing include entry into the ostium itself, accurate positioning within the coronary sinus, and ventricular pacing or inappropriate sensing of ventricular potentials due to proximity to the ventricle. In addition, coronary sinus leads are not fixed but move freely within the coronary sinus.

Special circumstances may call for innovative placement of the atrial lead. Placement of an atrial endocardial lead through the atrial wall at the time of open heart surgery has been described with stable atrial pacing being maintained without complication (Figure 17).

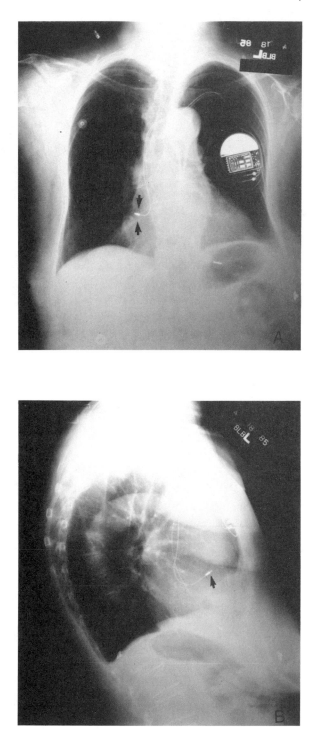

Figure 15. *Active fixation atrial lead placement in the lateral wall of the atrium. Posteroanterior (A) and lateral (B).*

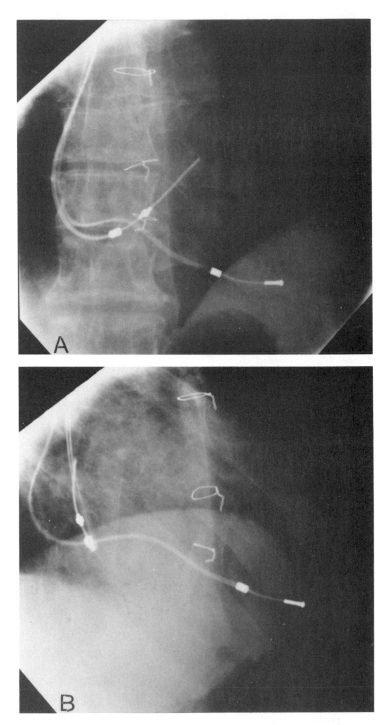

Figure 16. Posteroanterior (A) and oblique (B) radiographs in a patient with previous cardiac surgery and an atrioventricular sequential pacemaker. Atrial lead is positioned in the coronary sinus.

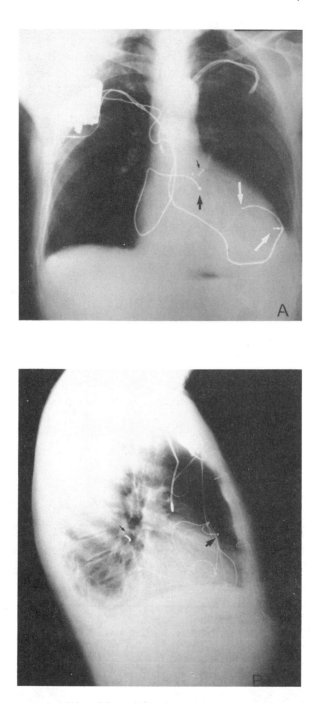

Figure 17. *Posteroanterior (**A**) and lateral (**B**) chest x-ray demonstrating ventricular epicardial leads (noted by white arrows) and an atrial endocardial lead that has been passed through the atrial wall (larger black arrow). (There is also a retained lead tip, noted by the smaller black arrow and a portion of an abandoned transvenous lead that has been pulled into the superior vena cava.)*

MEASUREMENT OF PACING AND SENSING THRESHOLDS

Knowledge and measurement of pacing and sensing thresholds are integral parts in the placement of permanent pacemakers. The equipment used and measurements made vary from laboratory to laboratory. In many institutions, pacing systems analyzers (PSA) are used. These are available from the pacemaker manufacturers (Figure 18). Ideally, the PSA used should be matched with the pulse generator manufacturer. (Using mismatched PSA and pulse generator manufacturers rarely, if ever, results in any clinical problem.) In some laboratories, physiological recorders with bandwidths of 0.1–2,000 Hz are used to assess intracardiac electrograms.

Determination of Pacing Threshold

The pacing threshold is the minimal electrical stimulus required to produce consistent cardiac depolarization. It should be measured with the same electrode configuration (unipolar or bipolar) as the lead and pulse generator that are to be used. During pacing, the output of the PSA gradually is decreased from 5 V down to the point at which loss of capture is documented. The pacing rate selected during this measurement is important. The rate should be just fast enough (approximately 10 bpm faster) to override the intrinsic rhythm. In some patients, pacing during measurement of thresholds suppresses intrinsic rhythm and results in the lack of a stable ventricular escape focus, or even asystole, when pacing is discontinued. The implanting physician may decide to position a temporary pacemaker in these patients. The lower the stimulation threshold, the better. Acceptable acute thresholds are less than 1 V for both ventricular

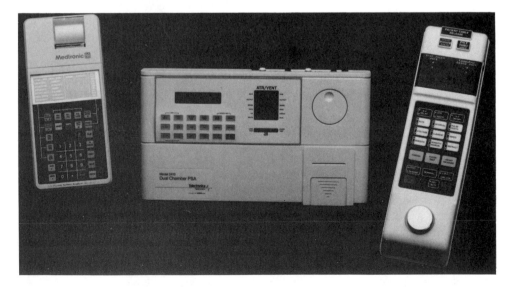

Figure 18.   Representative pacing systems analyzers from various manufacturers.

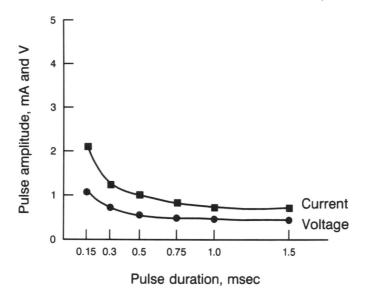

Figure 19. *Sample strength-duration curve plotted at time of implantation. This allows selection of optimal stimulation parameters (pulse duration, output voltage) that result in safe pacing but conserve battery life.*

and atrial leads at 0.5 ms pulse duration. Typical acute thresholds for ventricular leads at 0.5 ms pulse duration would be approximately 0.5 V and 1.4 mA, and typical thresholds for atrial leads would be 0.9 V and 1.8 mA.

Pacing threshold is determined by a combination of pulse duration and output voltage. "Strength-duration" curves may be helpful to determine appropriate stimulation parameters. Such curves can be plotted at the time of implantation (Figure 19). Two approaches exist. The output voltage is fixed and the pulse duration is varied; the pulse duration is fixed and the output is varied. The two techniques are equivalent and allow derivation of the current and voltage thresholds at a specific pulse duration. (Most centers no longer perform strength-duration curves routinely at the time of pacemaker implant. With the telemetric functions provided in many pulse generators, strength-duration thresholds can be performed noninvasively if needed.)

The impedance of the pacing electrode is also measured, usually by Ohm's law, in which volts equal current times resistance. Measurement of volts and current allows calculation of the lead resistance, which is usually 300–1000 ohms. Impedances should always be measured under standardized conditions of output and pulse duration. The finding of unsuspected low impedance raises the possibility of an insulation failure in the lead, that of a high impedance raises the possibility of a poor connection or lead fracture.

Determination of Sensing Threshold

Measurement of sensing thresholds is equally important. If a PSA is used, it is again ideal, but not absolutely necessary, to measure the electrogram with the analyzer made by the manufacturer of the pulse generator to be used, since there is no standardization of the sensitivity of pacemaker circuits. Adequate sensing thresholds are essential to avoid the problem of undersensing or oversensing after implantation. The pacemaker senses intracardiac events, not the events seen on the surface electrocardiogram (Figure 20). The intrinsic deflection is that component of the intracardiac electrogram that is sensed. It is the amplitude of this intracardiac signal in the chamber to be paced that is measured. The result is expressed as a voltage. The ventricular electrogram sensed for adequate long-term sensing should be more than 4 mV. More commonly, the ventricular signal is 6–10 mV, a range that provides excellent sensing. For atrial sensing, a signal of at least 2 mV is needed for stable, acceptable atrial sensing; often 2–3 mV is the range with an adequate atrial position.

In addition to peak amplitude, other aspects of sensing should be considered. The change in voltage with time (dV/dt), the slew rate, of the intrinsic deflection is also important. Usually, this is most important in patients with borderline sensing voltages. If an R wave of 10 mV is measured, the result almost always will be accurate sensing. In patients with low voltages (3–6 mV), the slew rate measurement is very important. Some patients with a QRS of 3 mV but a slow slew rate may have undersensing, whereas other patients with a QRS of 3 mV but a normal slew rate will have normal sensing. Some PSAs now offer the capacity to measure electrograms and slew rates. In the past, a physiological recording system was required.

If electrograms are assessed, an added feature is evaluation of current of injury at the time of pacemaker placement. The current, appearing as an elevation in the electrical potential that immediately follows the intrinsic deflection, represents a small area of damaged endocardium (Figure 21). This finding indicates adequate contact with the endocardium.

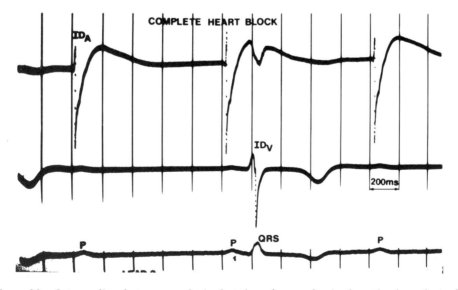

Figure 20. *Intracardiac electrograms obtained at time of pacemaker implantation in patient with complete heart block. Pacemakers sense intracardiac electrograms, specifically intrinsic deflection of either ventricle (IDV) or atrium (IDA). Slew rate is a measure of dV/dt (see text for details).*

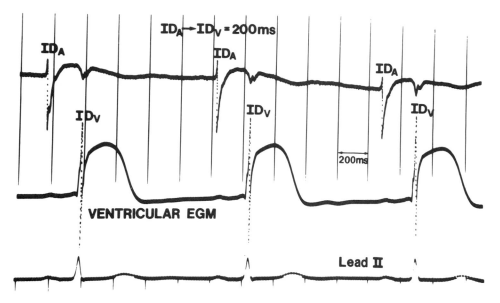

Figure 21. *Intracardiac electrograms at time of pacemaker implantation. In addition to assessment of magnitude and relationship of intrinsic deflection of atrium and ventricle (ID$_A$, ID$_V$), a current of injury is identified. This current of injury, which is manifested as an elevation in electrical potential after intrinsic deflection, indicates adequate endocardial contact. EGM = electrogram.*

Additional Measurements

At the time of dual-chamber implantation, measurements in addition to pacing and sensing thresholds and electrograms for both atrium and ventricle may be helpful (Table II), although some of these measurements can be made

---

Table II
Studies during Dual-Chamber Implantation

Threshold of stimulation
  Atrium
  Ventricle
Measurement of electrogram*
  Atrium
  Ventricle
Measurement of antegrade conduction*
  AV conduction interval (St$_A$ ID$_V$)
  Coupling interval for onset of AV block
Measurement of retrograde conduction*
  VA conduction interval (St$_V$ ID$_V$)
  Coupling interval for onset of VA block

ID$_A$ = intrinsic deflection of atrial depolarization; ID$_V$ = intrinsic deflection of ventricular depolarization; St$_A$ = atrial pacing stimulus; St$_V$ = ventricular pacing stimulus

* With pacemakers with the appropriate telemetric functions these measurements may be accomplished noninvasively

noninvasively post-implant if the pulse generator has the appropriate telemetric functions. Assessment of atrioventricular (AV) nodal conduction may be helpful in programming the pacemaker AV interval and upper rate. If this is performed during the implant procedure, the atrium is paced at rates nearly equal to the sinus rate and then at incremental rates up to approximately 150 bpm. A typical sequence might be 80, 100, 120, 140, and 160 bpm. The rate at which Wenckebach or higher grade AV block occurs is recorded, as is the AV interval.

THE PACEMAKER POCKET

Design of the pacemaker pocket is an integral part of pacemaker implantation. The pocket is commonly developed in the prepectoralis fascia (Figure 22). It should be placed medially, rather than laterally, and be large enough to allow for easy placement of the pulse generator and leads. It is important to avoid a tight pocket, which can cause erosion, or a loose pocket, which can permit excessive movement and migration. One of our centers routinely uses a snugly fitting polyester pouch (Parsonnet Pouch, CR Bard, Inc., Billerica, MA) to encase the pulse generator and leads within the pocket to reduce migration and prevent torsion of the pacing system (Figure 23).

The site of placement of the pulse generator is extremely important in providing long-term comfort and complete mobility for the adjacent shoulder. The

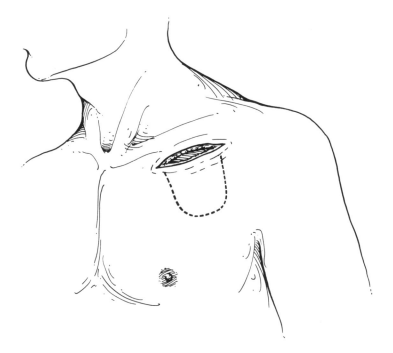

Figure 22.   *Location of pacemaker pocket in upper left aspect of chest. Note that the incision is made parallel to and several centimeters below lower clavicular margin. (Reproduced with permission from the Mayo Foundation.)*

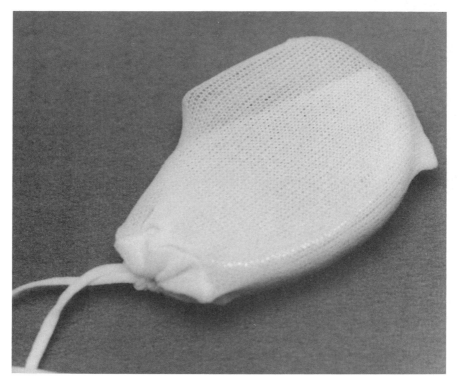

Figure 23. *Polyester pouch (Parsonnet pouch) used to reduce migration of pulse generator.*

pulse generator should be implanted in the subcutaneous tissue, deep to the fatty layer of the pectoral region. The inexperienced operator may not find the plane between the subcutaneous tissue and the pectoral fascia. Occasionally the space developed may be subcuticular with the subcutaneous fatty layer deep to the pulse generator. In that case the pulse generator will press on the under-surface of the skin and the wound will be continually painful. Characteristically, light touch of the overlying skin will produce exquisite pain. The equally in-experienced evaluator of this circumstance may not recognize the nature of the problem, which can be solved by repositioning the pulse generator to a sub-cutaneous site.

The pulse generator should be sufficiently inferior to the clavicle so that a full range of shoulder motion is not restricted by its impingement against the clavicle. It should be sufficiently medial so that it does not approach the anterior axillary fold. If it does, each anterior movement of the arm will be uncomfortable as it brushes past the pulse generator.

Postoperatively a patient may want to restrict the movement of the ipsi-lateral shoulder. Movement should be encouraged as immobility may cause later pain when full mobilization is attempted with consequent further restriction of movement. The authors actively encourage movement of the shoulder on the first postoperative day. A well-placed and secured lead system will not be dis-placed by early movement.

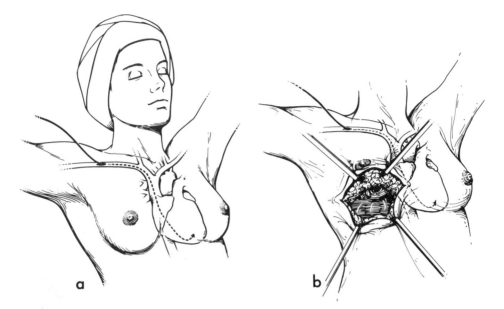

Figure 24.   *Placement of pacemaker in retromammary position. **A.** Subclavian puncture and lead placement performed through limited (2–3 mm) incision. **B.** Inframammary incision is made and dissected to the pectoral fascia. Breast is then lifted from the fascia.*

In general, the smallest pulse generator appropriate for the patient should be selected. This is of particular importance in pediatric patients, young adults, and thin patients. If the prepectoral position is not suitable because the optimal pulse generator is too large or because there are cosmetic or other considerations, there are other choices. Although rarely necessary, the pacemaker can be placed deep to the pectoral muscle. This location may result in a higher incidence of pectoral muscle stimulation or muscle inhibition with a unipolar system; therefore, in this situation, a bipolar system is preferred.

Another option is retromammary implantation, which may be used for cosmetic purposes or, in a thin woman, for protection of the implant site by the fatty layer of the breast. Implantation of the modern small pulse generator of a 20- to 30-mL volume can be accomplished with no deformity of the breast. Often there is so little difference in breast size that it is barely visible. There is no interference with lactation or other breast function.

For retromammary placement, implantation should be done under light general anesthesia (Figures 24A-D). Complete relaxation is not required. Subclavian puncture or approach to the cephalic vein is accomplished routinely. Puncture may be preferable because the incision adjacent to the clavicle may be limited to a length of 1–2 cm. Once the leads are in place, they are fastened to the pectoralis fascia with nonabsorbable ligature about the sleeve. An incision is then made in the inframammary fold, which is clearly visible when the breast is elevated. The incision is carried down to the pectoral fascia behind the breast, and the breast is lifted from the fascia. After a long instrument is introduced deep to the breast and brought through the upper small incision, the lead (or

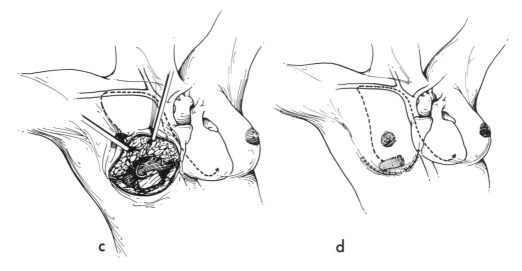

Figure 24C. *Pacing lead or leads are tunneled deep to the breast and connected to pulse generator.* **D.** *Skin is closed routinely.*

leads) are brought to the retromammary incision and are connected to the pulse generator. It is wise to use a polyester pouch and to suture it lightly to the pectoral fascia with two or three sutures. Mammary tissue is resutured anatomically inferior to the pulse generator to provide an additional cushion, and the skin is closed routinely. Hemostasis is especially important. The pulse generator will be barely palpable and probably not visible. The inframammary incision is invisible when the patient is standing. The pulse generator can be readily replaced through reopening of the inframammary incision.

PULSE GENERATOR CHANGE

The pulse generator obviously must be replaced when it displays replacement, or end-of-life, indicators that indicate battery depletion. Pulse generator replacement is usually a straightforward procedure.

When a patient presents for pulse generator replacement there are several questions that must be assessed. The physician responsible for the replacement must know the patient's underlying rhythm disturbance that led to permanent pacing and whether or not the patient is pacemaker-dependent. It is also important to know whether the patient is anticoagulated or receiving antiplatelet agents that may lead to complications during or after the surgical procedure. The implanting physician must also assess the patient's general medical condition. Even though the procedure is straightforward and usually brief, it may be complicated by an associated illness, i.e., if the patient were in congestive heart failure, had resting hypoxia, etc.

Once the patient is in the procedure room, the site of the previous pacemaker should be prepped and draped as it would be for an initial pacemaker implantation. Sterile technique is as important for a pulse generator replacement as it is for the initial implant. There are two approaches that can be used for incising and removing the depleted pulse generator. After infiltration with local anesthetic the prior incision can be carefully reincised taking great care to protect the underlying leads. The advantage of this technique is cosmetic in that the patient is left with a single surgical scar. The disadvantage is the increased chance of inadvertently damaging the pacing leads that are probably located, at least in part, in the vicinity of the original incision. If this technique is used, the risk of lead damage can be minimized by pushing the inferior edge of the pulse generator in a cephalad direction. This is done in an attempt to displace the pacing leads superior to the old incision and the pulse generator below the old incision. Even with the use of this technique, the dissection must be made with great care, palpating the tissues carefully before cutting.

Alternatively, a new incision can be made directly over the pulse generator. With the exception of the obese patient, it usually is easy to determine that the leads are not overlying the pulse generator. If the dissection is directly over the pulse generator there is minimal risk to the pacing leads. The disadvantage is cosmetic in that the patient will have a second incision. The options can be discussed with the patient, and if there are no cosmetic concerns, the safer technique should be used.

Once the pulse generator is exposed it can be grasped and removed from the pocket. If the pacemaker is operating in a bipolar configuration, pacing will continue after it is removed from the pocket. If the pacemaker is in the unipolar configuration, pacing will cease when it is removed from the pocket. If unipolar, the patient's degree of pacemaker dependency should be determined prior to removal of the pulse generator from the pocket. If the pacemaker is bipolar, then pacemaker dependency should be known prior to disconnecting the pulse generator from the leads. The best way of determining pacemaker dependency is controversial. If the patient continues to pace when the pacemaker is programmed to the lowest programmable rate, the patient may be pacemaker-dependent. However, it is certainly possible that the patient will have a ventricular escape rate that is less than the lowest programmable rate of the pacemaker. If the patient has not displayed any escape rate prior to or during the procedure there are several potential approaches. A temporary pacemaker can be placed via the ipsilateral internal jugular vein or via the femoral vein. With an adequately functioning temporary pacemaker in place the permanent pacemaker can be disconnected without fear of asystole. There are arguments that the expense and potential morbidity of a temporary pacemaker are not justified.

If the pacemaker being explanted is in the unipolar mode it can be removed briefly from the pocket while watching the rhythm to determine if a slow ventricular escape focus is present. If there is no escape rhythm, the pulse generator, still connected to the pacing lead(s), can be placed back in the pocket. There are other techniques to maintain pacing in the unipolar configuration once the pacemaker is out of the pocket. An anodal clip can be used. This is a metal clip that fits onto the outside of the pulse generator with a wire to an alligator clip. With the clip on the pulse generator and the alligator clip connected to the exposed tissues, unipolar pacing will continue when the pacemaker is removed from the pocket. Alternatively, a thoroughly wet towel can be placed over the operating field with one end of the wet towel in the incision. If a pulse generator in the unipolar configuration is placed on the wet towel, pacing will continue.

If the escape rhythm is insufficient, an infusion of isoproterenol (Isuprel) may be used. The solution used at Montefiore Medical Center is 0.4 mg of isoproterenol in 250 cc of 5% dextrose and water. The infusion is started at approximately 0.5 to 1 cc per minute and the rhythm closely observed. The infusion is increased as necessary to achieve an escape rhythm that is hemo-dynamically stable.

Even in the absence of an adequate escape rhythm, the experienced operator may elect to proceed by removing the pulse generator from the pocket and rapidly releasing the set screw or connector apparatus. The cable to the PSA should be ready to connect immediately to the pacing lead and the "ground" or "+" terminal should already be connected so that pacing can resume im-mediately upon contact of the "−" terminal to the cable. The experienced op-erator can perform such a maneuver in a few seconds without compromising patient safety. However, for the less experienced operator or in the event of a problem with the cable, a delay could be catastrophic for the patient. This risk could be minimized by having the patient connected to an external pacing device in the event the asystole occurs. This is a reasonable approach, but it must be determined that ventricular depolarization is possible with the external device.

For the patient with a bipolar pacemaker, the same techniques can be used. Once the bipolar ventricular lead is disconnected from the pulse generator it must be rapidly connected to the cable. Time can be shortened if the pulse generator is programmed to the unipolar configuration ahead of time, if it is polarity programmable. If not, prior to unscrewing the set screws, grounding the "+" end of the cable to the PSA and initially pacing in a unipolar mode via the PSA may be faster than connecting both "+" and "−" terminals of the lead to the cable. Once pacing is re-established in the unipolar configuration, the "+" end of the cable can be connected to the "+" terminal of the pacing lead to allow bipolar pacing and threshold measurement. For the inexperienced op-erator use of this two-step method may minimize ventricular asystole. When a dual-chamber pacemaker is being replaced the atrial lead can be disconnected leisurely.

Once pacing is established via the PSA, chronic thresholds should be de-termined. This should include capture threshold, amplitude of the sensed car-diac signal, i.e., measurement of the P wave on the atrial lead and/or R wave on the ventricular lead, and impedance. (If the patient is pacemaker-dependent it will not be possible to measure an R wave.) There is no absolute acceptable value for chronic thresholds. Acceptable chronic thresholds are to some degree related to the age of the pacing lead. Contemporary leads, i.e., pacing leads manufactured in the 1980s, would, in general, be expected to have lower chronic thresholds than older leads. In other words, the lead is expected to have an acceptable stable threshold for it's era. Ideally, we prefer to accept only a chronic ventricular capture threshold of less than or equal to 2.5 to 3.0 V at a pulse width of 0.5 ms and an impedance greater than 300 ohms. If the impedance value or capture threshold fails to meet these criteria, consideration should be given to removing the lead from service. If the patient has a low R wave value, i.e., <5 mV, it is of concern only if failure to sense has been documented clinically. Thresholds should be performed in the pacing configuration that will be used with the new pulse generator. For example, if the pacemaker will be in the bipolar configuration thresholds should be measured in a bipolar configuration.

After thresholds are measured and found to be acceptable, the new pulse generator must be connected to the chronic lead(s). In the pacemaker-dependent patient the same concerns during disconnection of the chronic pulse generator apply during connection of the new pulse generator. As previously described for the initial implantation, care should be taken to be certain that the lead is securely in the connector apparatus. The incision should then be closed as previously described.

Because the leads have not been manipulated, the patient could be allowed to ambulate as soon as any sedatives have worn off. Hospital discharge may be the evening of pulse generator replacement or the next day.

HOSPITAL STAY POST-IMPLANT

The length of time the patient should be kept in the hospital following pacemaker implantation is controversial and varies significantly among institutions. In the past we have kept patients hospitalized for 2 nights post-implant. Patients were kept at bedrest the day of the procedure, ambulated the following day, and were dismissed the following morning. The Mayo Clinic practice has evolved such that patients who are not pacemaker-dependent are allowed to be ambulated the evening of the procedure and are dismissed the following morning. The patient is monitored during the overnight stay. Prior to dismissal, thresholds are documented and the pacemaker is programmed to its final settings. If a rate adaptive pacemaker has been implanted, informal exercise is performed the morning after implant and the rate responsive parameters are adjusted to fit the needs of the patient. Pacemaker-dependent patients may be kept in the hospital for 1 or 2 nights but the practice is moving toward a single night stay. When the patient's pulse generator reaches end-of-life, the pulse generator replacement is performed as an outpatient procedure.

There are a number of implanting physicians who now perform initial pacemaker implantation as an outpatient procedure. Large series of ambulatory implants have been reported from the United States and Europe. Some physicians implant only nonpacemaker-dependent patients as outpatients while others perform outpatient procedures regardless of dependency status. The results are encouraging, and it is possible that ambulatory pacemaker implantation with outpatient follow-up the following day may become the norm.

At Montefiore Medical Center most initial implants are performed in the morning. Ambulation is allowed, whether the patient is pacemaker-dependent or not, about 4 hours later, i.e., by mid-afternoon. On the first postoperative day a Holter monitor is placed until the second postoperative day. The patient then undergoes careful testing of pacemaker function, including determination of atrial (when present) and ventricular pacing and sensing thresholds and setting of pacemaker programmable functions as indicated by the thresholds. Informal exercise testing is used to set rate modulation functions. The patient is discharged the following morning. For routine pulse generator replacement the procedure is often done in early afternoon and the patient is retained a single night. The following morning the patient is evaluated, as above, and discharged.

COMPLICATIONS

Complications of the transvenous approach to permanent pacing include two major groups: (1) those related to venous access and entry and (2) those related to placement of the lead. Both groups of complications are minimized by meticulous attention to detail.

Venous Access and Entry

Complications of entry, inherent in any approach to venous structures, include damage to associated arterial or neural structures, extensive bleeding, air embolism, and thrombosis. In the subclavian approach, the potential of pneumothorax also exists; it can be minimized by knowledge of the patient's anatomy and attention to details. Recent experience indicates that fewer than 0.5% of introducer implantations are associated with serious complications. In some patients, the subclavian vein may be difficult to locate. Contrast material infused through the ipsilateral arm during the search for the vein, as previously described, may be helpful (Figures 4 and 5).

Lead Placement

Complications of lead placement result from catheterization of the heart and from placement of a permanent lead itself.

Dislodgment

In the past, the most common complication of transvenous pacing was lead dislodgment. Extensive use of active and passive fixation leads has significantly reduced this complication both for atrial and ventricular pacing. Secondary intervention rates for all reasons should be well below 2% for ventricular leads and below 5% for atrial leads.

Perforation

Perforation carries with it the potential for cardiac tamponade. Ventricular perforation is caused by improper force on the lead. It may be a particular problem in elderly patients with a thin-walled right ventricle. It usually presents only as diaphragmatic, anterior chest, or abdominal wall stimulation and high thresholds, although tamponade may result rarely. Perforation of the atrium and coronary sinus also has been described. In the former, tamponade may be more frequent. Again, meticulous attention to detail minimizes these risks.

Arrhythmias

A frequent complication is development of supraventricular or ventricular arrhythmia related to lead manipulation. These effects usually are transient, stopping promptly when the lead position is changed. Rarely are they sustained. Atrial manipulation may result in sustained atrial tachycardia, fibrillation, or flutter, which complicates placement of a permanent atrial system. Atrial tachycardia may revert to normal sinus rhythm with gentle manipulation of the electrode against the atrial wall or by overdrive pacing. Management of atrial flutter or fibrillation is more difficult and may require intravenous administration of a drug, such as procainamide hydrochloride (Pronestyl), or cardioversion to restore normal sinus rhythm. Brief ventricular arrhythmias are more common, particularly during ventricular lead manipulation. They are usually easily controlled. However, patients with a history of spontaneous sustained ventricular tachycardia may experience these during lead manipulation. For this reason, all patients are monitored and life-support equipment and a defibrillator are immediately available.

In addition to tachycardia, bradyarrhythmias may occur. In patients with intermittent AV block and left bundle branch block, catheter trauma to the right bundle may result in an AV block. More commonly bradycardia results from overdrive suppression of an escape ventricular focus during threshold testing. In a patient at high risk for development of asystole or complete heart block during the procedure, a temporary pacemaker may be placed prior to implantation at the discretion of the implanter.

Pacemaker Pocket

Complications of the pacemaker pocket can be grouped into early and late. Local hematoma formation is common but usually is minor. It occurs particularly in patients receiving anticoagulants or antiplatelet agents. Aspirin is a major, and often unrecognized, offender. Careful local hemostasis is essential. In patients requiring oral anticoagulants, the prothrombin time should be normal before implantation. Administration of anticoagulants can be resumed 24 to 48 hours after implantation if there is no evidence of significant hematoma formation. Should a significant hematoma occur, local conservative treatment is preferred. If at all possible, needle aspiration or placement of a drain should be avoided so that the risk of infection is minimized. If evacuation of the hematoma is required to manage local pain or stop progression, it should be undertaken as a thoroughly sterile procedure.

Late complications, including erosion and migration, are often the result of suboptimal initial surgery. These can be minimized by careful technique at the time of initial pacemaker implantation and by the formation of an adequate pocket.

EPIMYOCARDIAL SYSTEMS

Epimyocardial systems account for no more than 5% of pacemaker implantation procedures. This shift from implantation by thoracotomy to the transvenous route occurred because of the higher morbidity and mortality with epicardial lead systems, the higher incidence of wire fracture, a lack of reliable atrial leads, and the increasing reliability of transvenous pacing systems with active and passive fixation leads. Three groups of patients still undergo placement of epicardial systems.

1. Patients undergoing cardiac surgery for another indication. In these patients, permanent epicardial leads may be placed at the time of surgery. Alternatively, some of these patients have temporary pacing until recovery from open-heart surgery. Before dismissal from the hospital, they may undergo placement of a transvenous pacing system. This latter approach is preferable, since transvenous leads have proven to be more reliable than epimyocardial leads.
2. Patients with recurrent dislodgment of transvenous system. The number of these patients has declined greatly with the use of active and new passive fixation leads, and it is now rare to see patients with recurrent dislodgment of a transvenous system.
3. Patients with a prosthetic tricuspid valve, a congenital anomaly, or atresia of the tricuspid valve. In these patients, epimyocardial ventricular leads usually are required. Prosthetic porcine valves are, however, compatible with transvenous implant.
4. Patients with ventricular septal defects or patients with right-to-left shunts in whom the possibility for systemic embolization exists.

Several surgical procedures have been described: (1) a subxiphoid or left costal approach and (2) left lateral thoracotomy.

Subxiphoid and Subcostal Approaches

These approaches allow epimyocardial pacing without the need for a formal thoracotomy. Through an upper abdominal incision with xiphoid resection, the diaphragmatic surface of the heart can be approached. With this approach, electrodes can be placed on the diaphragmatic surface of the heart, that is, the right ventricle and some portion of the left ventricle. The amount of left ventricle exposed depends on the anatomy of the patient. Left ventricular placement is preferred for improved sensing. Because of the small and unpredictable portion of the left ventricle available with the subxiphoid approach, some surgeons favor the use of a left subcostal incision, which allows better exposure of the left ventricle. Great care must be taken with these approaches to avoid laceration of the right or left ventricle, which requires emergency full thoracotomy for control of bleeding and treatment. Deaths have occurred from this complication. Atrial lead placement is almost impossible with these approaches.

Left Lateral Thoracotomy

With left lateral thoracotomy (Figure 25), left ventricular implantation is favored. The heart usually is approached through the fifth left intercostal space.

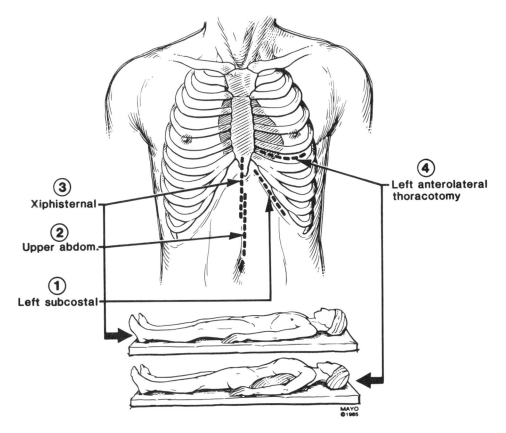

Figure 25. *Incisions and positions of patient used for placement of epimyocardial pacing systems (see text for details). (Reproduced with permission from the Mayo Foundation.)*

An incision is made from the left parasternal border to the left anterior axillary line. Sutureless electrodes can be placed into the left ventricular myocardium through the incision. Care must be taken to implant these at a distance from the phrenic nerve to avoid phrenic stimulation.

Both of these epimyocardial approaches require general anesthesia. Because of the potential surgical complications with these techniques as well as the higher historical incidence of system malfunction, the frequency with which epimyocardial pacing is used has declined significantly. The overwhelming majority of epimyocardial implants are performed in patients undergoing heart surgery at which time the leads are placed.

HARDWARE ADAPTATIONS

Connectors

The connector is the portion of the lead and the pulse generator header that provides the permanent but reversible connection between the two. The portion of the connector on the header holds that portion which is the extra-vascular end of lead. The connector has undergone substantial evolution since the earliest pulse generators. The first generators introduced had an integral lead system. The presumption was that the patient would not outlive the implanted pulse generator, predicted to have a longevity of 5 years. Pulse generators had a longevity of only several months and it was not until the era of lithium-powered pulse generators that a longevity of 5 years or more was achieved. It quickly became apparent that despite frequent lead fracture, the lead was a relatively more permanent element than the pulse generator. The need for the ability to disconnect the generator from the lead became clear and was soon introduced.

In Europe, the first connector type was the bare proximal end of the conductor wire. The receptacle, part of the pulse generator, was a set screw overlying a metal or plastic slot for the wire. The wire was inserted, the screw tightened, and the lead held. Pulse generator replacement was accomplished by transecting the lead adjacent to the connector and replacing the freshly cut end into the receptacle.

In the United States, the earliest connectors consisted of a pin (1.6 mm in diameter) to fit into the receptacle in the pulse generator and a silicone rubber plug immediately distal to the pin, which was 4.5 mm in diameter (referred to as 5 mm). The lead system was bipolar and two such connectors (one for each limb of the lead) were required. A second variety was a unipolar system in which a plug with two pins could be placed into the header. It was designed for an atrial synchronous system in which two connections were required, one for the atrium, the other for the ventricle, and correct placement of each was necessary. With the introduction of transvenous leads, the plug connector became progressively more unwieldly, and bipolar transvenous leads required a bifurcation, each limb of which fit into each of the pulse generator receptacles. The receptacle was replaced with a pin and plug combination. The plug was 5.5 mm in diameter (commonly referred to as 6 mm) and the diameter of the pin was somewhat greater (2.25 mm) than that associated with the 5 mm connector. These two varieties have come to dominate all connectors of all other manufacturers.

With the advent of lead systems for dual-chamber pacemakers and especially bipolar leads, the size of the header (now requiring 4 plugs for a dual-bipolar system) became as large or potentially larger than the electronic battery portion of the generator. The need for smaller connectors became obvious and unipolar and bipolar coaxial (or "inline") leads were introduced with a plug diameter of 3.2 mm. This new size was incompatible with the two earlier "standards" and the connectors introduced were incompatible with each other. Following a brief era during which lead systems had largely become compatible and interchangeable, incompatibility was again present. Urging from the physician community led manufacturers to cooperate in creating a standard for universal pacemaker and lead compatibility. Representatives of major pacemaker/lead manufacturers developed "ad hoc" specifications for a "voluntary standard" or VS-1 design to standardize all connectors, unipolar and in-line bipolar, to a single size, i.e., 3.2 mm. A formal, international pacing connector standard, the "international standard" or IS-1 design, was then jointly endorsed

Table III

VS-1/IS-1	Accepts only VS-1/IS-1 leads.
VS-1A/IS-1A	Accepts VS-1/IS-1 leads and Cordis style 3.2 mm in-line leads (incorporates a longer bore pin).
VS-1B/IS-1B	Accepts VS-1/IS-1 leads. Cordis, Medtronic, CPI and Telectronics style 3.2 mm in-line leads (incorporates a longer pin bore and sealing rings) (Figure 26).

by the International Standards Organization (ISO) and the International Electrotechnical Commission (IEC) after including additional performance requirements to the VS-1 standards.

VS-1/IS-1 pacing leads are 3.2 mm in diameter, have sealing rings on the lead, and a short (0.508 cm) terminal pin. They will fit all 3.2 mm pacemakers. VS-1/IS-1 pacemaker headers are 3.2 mm in diameter, have no sealing rings, a short (0.508 cm) receptacle for lead terminal and will accept only VS-1/IS-1 pacing leads. Table III provides an abbreviated compatibility guide for various pacing leads and pacemaker headers. It should be noted that pacemaker headers with the designation VS-1A and VS-1B still exist, which is a point of confusion. Pacemakers designated VS-1A are 3.2 mm in diameter, have no sealing rings, and a long (0.851 cm) receptacle for the lead terminal. Pacemakers with the VS-1B designation do have sealing rings in the header but are otherwise like the VS-1A designation (Figure 26). This terminology need not be confusing. Dimensions are the same for both unipolar and bipolar VS-1/IS-1 leads and pacers. There is only one configuration for VS-1 and IS-1 lead connectors. The VS-1 and IS-1 designs have provisions within the pacer connector for 3 functional opinions. These are listed in Table III.

Although the total conversion to VS-1/IS-1 pacing leads and pacemaker headers will take years, it will eventually eliminate the issue of incompatibility.

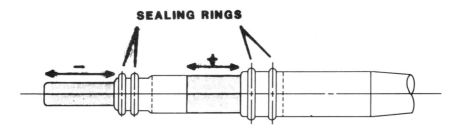

SEALING RINGS

Figure 26. *The VS-1/IS-1 connectors are intended to restore universal interconnection of all leads and pulse generators via the newly standardized 3.2-mm connectors. The pin is connected to the negative output, and the ring is connected to the positive terminal in the pulse generator header. Unipolar leads of similar configuration exist but without a positive terminal. These leads are the same size as and are interchangeable with a bipolar receptacle. The four ridges represent the sealing rings that prevent the ingress of fluid into the header.*

Many older connector leads remain in use; therefore, as pulse generator replacement is required, adapters will be necessary. Some pulse generators are now made specifically to accommodate pulse generator replacement. Some of the newest model generators are available only in a VS-1 or IS-1 connector format, and use with an older lead will require adaptation and often considerable ingenuity. The only technological advance that currently poses a threat to such compatibility is the introduction of "special" leads for rate adaptive pacing where an alteration in lead design and connector is necessary to incorporate all or part of the sensor.

Many new pulse generators are now made available in a variety of connector formats: (1) I-line bipolar, i.e., 3.2 mm; (2) 3.2 mm IS-1 unipolar; (3) unipolar to accept an older 5-mm lead only; (4) unipolar to accept a 5- or 6-mm lead.

An attempt should be made to match polarity and design of the pacing lead and pulse generator, i.e., a bipolar in-line lead to a bipolar in-line pulse generator; a bifurcated bipolar lead to a bipolar pulse generator, etc. It is increasingly necessary to use mismatched hardware. Special adaptors are necessary to allow use of polarity-mismatched lead and pulse generator. Table IV outlines possible combinations and adaptors necessary. Each adaptor is numbered and the numbers correspond to the numbers in Figure 27, which pictures the adaptors. Again, every attempt should be made to match lead and pulse generator hardware.

Table IV
Specific Adapter for Specific Combination

Pulse generator \ Lead	Unipolar	In-line bipolar	Bifurcated bipolar
Unipolar	ō	Low profile adaptor sleeve[1]	End cap[2]
In-line bipolar	Low profile lead to bifurcated pulse generator and an indifferent electrode[5][4]	ō	Bifurcated lead to in-line generator adaptor[3]
Bipolar with bifurcated connector	Indifferent electrode[4]	Low profile lead to bifurcated pulse generator adaptor[5]	ō

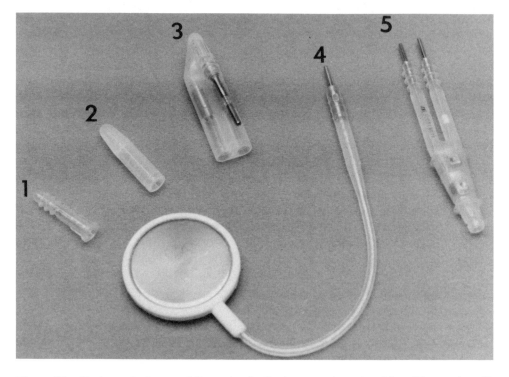

Figure 27. *Various adaptors used for pacing lead/pulse generator mismatches. The numbers (1 to 5) correspond to Table IV, which outlines specific adaptors needed for specific combinations. 1 = bipolar in-line sleeve adaptor; 2 = end cap; 3 = bifurcated lead to in-line connector; 4 = indifferent electrode; and 5 = in-line lead to bifurcated connector.*

SPECIAL CONSIDERATIONS IN PEDIATRIC PATIENTS

Permanent pacing in the pediatric population raises specific issues including the size of the patient, expected growth, presence of associated congenital heart disease, need for long-term pacing, and often a need for dual-chambered pacing systems.

Transvenous systems are used most frequently and have been shown to be superior to epicardial systems. Previous studies have shown that survival of endocardial leads in the pediatric pacemaker population is superior to that of myoepicardial leads.

In the pediatric patient undergoing permanent pacing, it is helpful to know prior to the implant if a persistent left superior vena cava is present. This usually can be determined echocardiographically. If concern exists, angiography is diagnostic (Figure 28). Advancing the pacing lead into a persistent left superior vena cava will result in traversing the coronary sinus to the right ventricle. While pacing has been accomplished from this position, it is often unstable and generally not reliable for permanent pacing. To avoid the problems associated with a persistent left superior vena cava, the right subclavian vein should be used if

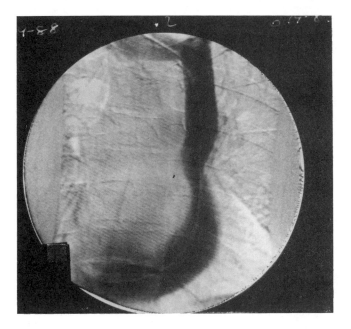

Figure 28.   *Contrast injection into the right side shows absence of the right superior vena cava and presence of a left superior vena cava. The dye enters the coronary sinus and then the right atrium.*

there is any doubt about the presence of a persistent left superior vena cava. Even in the presence of a left superior vena cava, the right superior vena cava usually is present.

In placement of the leads there are two potential approaches. The first is to allow more lead redundancy than would usually be left in an adult patient but to otherwise use standard techniques to place the lead, including securing the lead with the sleeve provided. The additional redundancy is left to allow for growth of the pediatric patient (Figure 29). If this approach is taken, the leads must be evaluated periodically during follow-up. If the child "outgrows" the lead, i.e., there is radiographic evidence of straightening of the lead, it will be necessary to place a new lead. Because of entrapment of the lead in the vein (subclavian or cephalic depending on the venous route used), it may not be possible to advance a lead that has been in place for a long period of time. Although a variety of clinical situations may occur when the patient truly "outgrows" the pacing system, most commonly, intermittent sensing abnormalities occur as tension develops on the lead at the electrode/tissue interface.

The second approach is to place the lead with the usual amount of redundancy but not to secure the lead to the underlying tissues with the sleeve provided. It is then possible that as the child grows the lead will advance as necessary to accommodate the child's growth. Lead advancement is not possible if the sleeve has been secured. It is of particular importance to select the smallest pulse generator that allows the desired pacing mode for the pediatric patient. Current pacemakers are now available that are as small as 22 g. The small weight

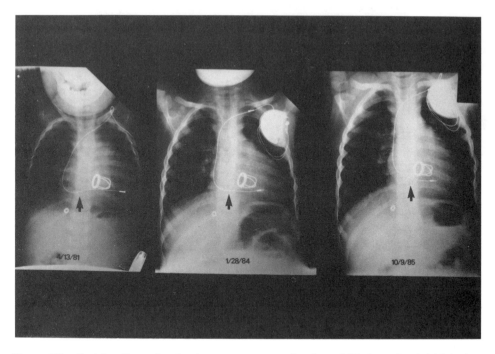

Figure 29. *Serial radiographs of a transvenous pacemaker in a child show that initial lead redundancy decreases with growth.*

and dimension of these pacemakers will allow implantation in a prepectoral position in almost any size patient. In very small infants in whom there is a concern that there is not enough subcutaneous tissue to protect the pacemaker, consideration may be given to placing the pacemaker in a subpectoral position. In our experience this is not often necessary. Prior to the advent of very small pulse generators, the transvenous lead occasionally was tunneled subcutaneously from the pectoral entry site to an area in the abdomen or flank where the pulse generator could be placed more easily. This, too, is rarely necessary with the small size of currently available pulse generators.

Traditional venous routes can be used in the pediatric patient. That is, the subclavian puncture technique with placement of one or two leads via the subclavian vein usually is possible. Two leads can often be placed via the cephalic vein as well.

Although any standard pacing lead can be used in the pediatric patient, many implanting physicians prefer the use of active fixation leads in the pediatric population for the following specific reasons. An active fixation lead may allow additional stability of the lead in the immediate post-implant period when it is difficult to control the activities of a pediatric patient as compared to the adult patient. The pediatric patient may require several pacing systems during the growth years. While a noninfected lead may be abandoned and left in place, it is reasonable to attempt removal of abandoned leads in the pediatric patient so that the patient will not accumulate an excessive amount of hardware throughout a lifetime. Some preference has therefore been given to active fixation leads because they may be potentially easier to remove than a chronic passive fixation (tined) lead.

Finally, active fixation leads can be placed in a greater variety of positions than passive fixation leads. This is important in the patient with associated congenital heart disease whose anatomy may be quite distorted. An active fixation lead allows placement in all portions of the atrium, not the atrial appendage alone. Active fixation leads have been used in patients following a Mustard procedure, placing the leads across the intra-atrial baffle and pacing the left atrium (Chapter 10, Pacemaker Radiography).

A specific problem in pediatric pacing involves cardiac pacing after the Fontan procedure. As postoperative anatomy precludes transvenous endocardial ventricular pacing, dual-chamber pacing in these patients has been accomplished by placing a ventricular epicardial lead at the time of surgery and subsequently placing an atrial endocardial lead and tunneling the two leads to a common prepectoral position to be attached to a dual-chamber pacemaker (Figure 30).

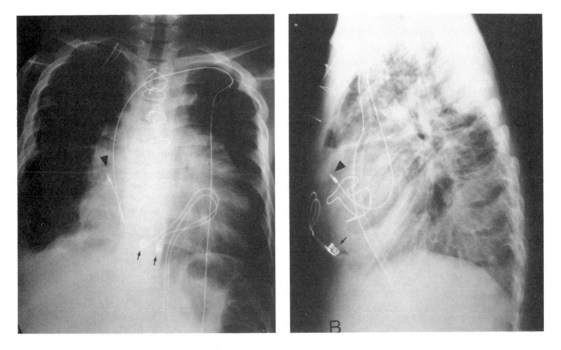

Figure 30. *Posteroanterior (A) and lateral (B) x-rays from a patient with a dual-chamber pacemaker. The ventricle is paced from the epimyocardial position, noted by small black arrows, and the atrium is paced from the endocardial position, noted by the black arrowhead. The atrial lead is then tunneled subcutaneously to the site of the pulse generator.*

PERMANENT PACING AFTER CARDIAC TRANSPLANTATION

As increasing numbers of cardiac transplantations are performed, information is emerging regarding special considerations in pacing this population. Following cardiac transplantation, the donor atrium (the one which is implanted with the donor ventricle) may have excessive bradycardia. This may result from the fact that it is denervated and minimally responsive to the usual stimuli to which the atrium is responsive. The donor atrium can no longer receive stimuli from the sinoatrial node. The sinoatrial node remains in continuity with the recipient atrium and may drive the recipient atrium at a normal rate or one more rapid than normal. The suture line between the free wall of the donor atrium and posterior recipient atrial wall, which becomes the posterior wall of the newly reconstituted atrium, is a complete barrier to the passage of stimuli that normally traverse the atrium to reach the AV node and bundle of His. Following transplantation, the patient has two atrial rhythms, that of the donor atrium and another of the recipient atrium, both of which may be visible on the ECG (Figure 31). If required, an increase in the atrial and ventricular rates of the graft may be achieved in several ways (Figure 32).

As normal AV conduction usually exists between the donor atrium and ventricle, atrial pacing can be used to preserve both the AV sequence and modulate the rate appropriately.

I. One approach, assuming a normal rate for the recipient atrium (but not the donor atrium) and normal AV conduction in the graft, is to implant a VDD or DDD unit. The recipient atrium is sensed and the donor atrium is paced. As the AA delay between sensing the recipient atrium and pacing the donor atrium will be added to the PR interval between the donor atrium and donor ventricle, the total delay may reduce the possible cardiac rate. Therefore, it is important

CARDIAC TRANSPLANT
TWO ATRIAL RHYTHMS

RECIPIENT ATRIUM

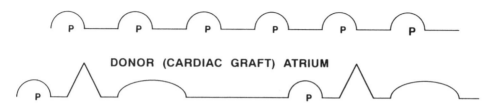

DONOR (CARDIAC GRAFT) ATRIUM

Figure 31. *Following cardiac transplantation, the donor atrium, i.e., part of the cardiac graft, will have been denervated from normal body stimuli so that the atrium may be both slow and substantially unresponsive to body stimuli. The recipient atrial rate is likely to be normal as the sinoatrial node remains with the recipient atrium, but it's impulses will be unable to cross the suture line to drive the donor atrium or ventricle. Two different atrial rates are likely to be visible, one more rapid (above) of the recipient atrium and a slower (below) of the donor atrium.*

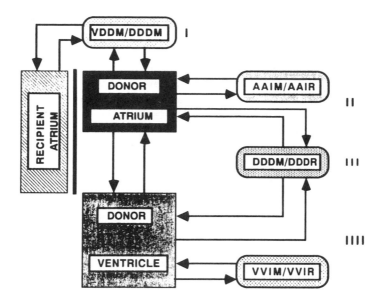

CARDIAC PACING FOR CARDIAC TRANSPLANT

Figure 32. *A variety of different approaches are possible for pacing the donor heart following cardiac transplantation. The cardiac graft is attached via its atrium to the recipient atrium, so that two atria are present. The recipient atrium may be normal and have a normal sinus node so that its rate of contraction will be responsive to the usual body stimuli. It cannot, however, transmit its atrial rate past the suture line to the donor atrium, which may be bradycardic. Usually, the donor AV conduction system is normal so that a normal donor atrial rate will be transmitted to the donor ventricle. Diagrammatically the simplest approach is ventricular (VVI,M or VVI,R) pacing, disregarding the atrium that may be driven retrograde. A better approach is to stimulate the atrium at a single rate or by a rate-modulated pacer (AAI,M OR AAI,R). Still, a better pacing mode is a DDD,M or DDD,R dual-chamber pacemaker sensing and pacing the donor atrium and ventricle with the DDD,R providing both atrial synchrony and rate modulation. Another possibility is a dual-chamber pacemaker either "VDD or DDD" in configuration that senses the recipient atrium and stimulates the donor atrium at the recipient atrium's normal rate. Another possibility is the VDD or DDD mode to sense the recipient atrium and drive the donor ventricle.*

to keep the programmed AA delay as short as possible, so that the ventricular rate can be as high as is necessary.

I(a). An alternative approach to pacing the atrium is the use of an atrial triggered pacemaker with a bifurcated lead. Two unipolar leads may be combined in a bipolar adapter with one lead to the recipient and the other to the donor atrium. In this approach, one lead senses and stimulates the recipient atrium and the second lead senses and stimulates the donor atrium. As the recipient atrium will have a normal rate, the stimuli will fall into the refractory period of the atrium, but since the donor atrium is likely to be bradycardic, these stimuli will be a shorter coupling interval. Pacemaker output is set sufficiently high so that the physiologically ineffective stimulus to the recipient atrium and the output delivered to the donor atrium are sufficient to stimulate the graft effectively.

II. The donor atrium may be stimulated directly with a single-chamber AAIM/ AAIR pulse generator. In this instance, the piezoelectric activity sensor may be most effective as others require sensing some atrial mechanical or physiological function, which may not be adequately large to drive the sensor. Since the activity sensor is independent of body function it may be most suitable. This approach too depends on intact AV conduction in the cardiac graft.

III. The recipient atrium may be disregarded and the donor atrium and ventricle paced by a DDD or preferably DDDR pacemaker. In the former instance, the pulse generator rate is set and, in the presence of sinus bradycardia, the atrium and ventricle will be paced at that rate, increasing if the sinus rate increases, but not decreasing. If a DDDR pacemaker is implanted then the atrial paced rate can increase and the ventricular rate will follow either by AV conduction or stimulation of the ventricle.

IV. Probably the least physiological mode is that of direct pacing of the ventricle with disregard of the atrium. Retrograde conduction can be anticipated and may have a deleterious effect on the hemodynamics as in a nontransplant patient. A VVI or VVIR pulse generator can be connected to the ventricle for conventional ventricular pacing. Use of a rate-modulated unit will allow the ventricular rate to change as the sensor deems is appropriate (Figure 32).

Few specific complications can be anticipated. Cyclosporine, a mainstay of immunosuppressive therapy in the transplant patient, may cause tremors. Such tremors have been reported to cause myopotential inhibition in paced transplanted patients. This may favor pacing transplanted patients in a bipolar configuration, which is less susceptible to myopotential interference.

Rejection episodes in the transplanted patient can alter the intracardiac electrogram and could potentially cause sensing abnormalities.

BIBLIOGRAPHY

Barin ES, Jones SM, Ward DE, et al: The right ventricular outflowtract as an alternative permanent pacing site: Long-term follow-up. PACE 1991; 14:3–6.

Belott PH: A variation of the introducer technique for unlimited access to the subclavian vein. PACE 1981; 4:43–48.

Belott PH, Byrd CL: Recent developments in pacemaker implantation and lead retrieval. In SS Barold, J Mugica (eds.): New Perspectives in Cardiac Pacing.2. Mount Kisco, NY, Futura Publishing Co. Inc., 1991, pp 105–131.

Belott PH: Outpatient pacemaker procedures. Int J Cardiol 1987; 17:169–176.

Byrd CL: Safe introducer technique. (abstract) PACE 1990; 13:50.

Byrd CL: Safe introducer technique for pacemaker leadimplantation. PACE 1992; 15:262–267.

Calfee RV, Saulson SH: A voluntary standard for 3.2 mm unipolar and bipolar pacemaker leads and connectors. PACE 1986; 9:1181–1185.

Costeas XF, Schoenfeld MH: Undersensing as a consequence of leadincompatibility: Case report and a plea for universality. PACE 1991; 14:1681–1683.

Dalvi B: Insertion of permanent pacemakers as a day case procedure. Br Med J 1990; 300: 119.

Dosios T, Gorgogiannis D, Sakorafas G, et al: Persistent leftsuperior vena cava: A problem in the transvenous pacing of the heart. PACE 1991; 14:389–390.

Draft International Standards (ISO/DIS 5841–5843).

Ellestad MH, French J:. Iliac vein approach to permanent pacemaker implantation. PACE 1989; 12:1030–1033.

Furman S: Venous cutdown for pacemaker implantation. Ann Thorac Surg 1986; 41:438–439.

Furman S, Hurzeler P, DeCaprio V: The ventricular endocardial electrogram and pacemaker sensing. J Thorac Cardiovasc Surg 1977; 73:258–266.

Fyke FE III: Simultaneous insulation deterioration associated with side-by-side subclavian placement of two polyurethane leads. PACE 1988; 11:1571–1574.

Hayes DL, Furman S: Atrioventricular and ventriculoatrial conduction times in patients undergoing pacemaker implant. PACE 1983;6:38–46.

Hayes DL, Holmes DR Jr, Maloney JD, et al: Permanent endocardial pacing in pediatric patients. J Thorac Cardiovasc Surg 1983; 85:618–624.

Hayes DL, Vlietstra RE, Puga FJ, et al: A novel approach to atrial endocardial pacing. PACE 1989; 12:125–130.

Hayes DL, Vlietstra RE, Trusty JM, et al: A shorter hospital stay after cardiac pacemaker implantation. Mayo Clin Proc 1988; 63:236–240.

Haywood GA, Jones SM, Camm AJ, et al: Day case permanent pacing. PACE 1991; 14:773–777.

Heinz G, Hirschl M, Buxbaum P, et al: Sinus node dysfunction afterorthotopic cardiac transplantation: Postoperative incidence and long-term implications. PACE 1992; 15:731–737.

Higano ST, Hayes DL, Spittell PC: Facilitation of the subclavian-introducer technique with contrast venography. PACE 1990; 13:681–684.

Markewitz A, Kemkes BM, Reble B, et al: Particularities of dual chamber pacemaker therapy in patients after orthotopic heart transplantation. PACE 1987; 10:326–332.

Markewitz A, Osterholzer G, Weinhold C, et al: Recipient P wavesynchronized pacing of the donor atrium in a heart-transplanted patient: A case study. PACE 1988; 11:1402–1404.

Messenger JC, Castellanet MJ, Stephenson NL: New permanent endocardial atrial J lead: Implantation techniques and clinical performance. PACE 1982; 5:767–772.

Miller FA Jr, Holmes DR Jr, Gersh BJ, et al: Permanent transvenous pacemaker implantation via the subclavian vein. Mayo Clin Proc 1980; 55:309–314.

Nichalls RWD: A new percutaneous infraclavicular approach to the axillary vein. Anesthesia 1987; 42:151–154.

Ong LS, Barold SS, Lederman, et al: Cephalic vein guide wire technique for implantation of permanent pacemakers. Am Heart J 1987; 114(4 Part 1):753–756.

Parsonnet V: A stretch fabric pouch for implanted pacemakers. Arch Surg 1972; 105:654–656.

Parsonnet V, Werres R, Atherley T: Transvenous insertion of double sets of permanent electrodes: Atraumatic technique for atrial synchronous and atrioventricular sequential pacemakers. J Am Med Assoc 1980; 243:62–64.

Smyth NPD: Pacemaker implantation: Surgical techniques. Cardiovasc Clin 1983; 14:31–44.

Smyth NPD: Techniques of implantation: Atrial and ventricular thoracotomy and transvenous. Prog Cardiovasc Dis 1981; 23:435–450.

Taylor BL, Yellowlees I: Central venous cannulation using the infraclavicular axillary vein. Anesthesiology 1990; 72:55–58.

Ward DE, Jones S, Shinebourne EA: Long-term transvenous pacing in children weighing 10 kg or less. Int J Cardiol 1987; 15:112–115.

Zegelman M, Kreyzer J, Wagner R: Ambulatory pacemaker surgery—medical and economical advantages. PACE 1986; 9:1299–1303.

Chapter 9

PACEMAKER ELECTROCARDIOGRAPHY

David L. Hayes, M.D.

An understanding of "Basic Concepts" of cardiac pacing and "Comprehension of Pacemaker Timing Cycles" of cardiac pacing (Chapters 2 and 4) is fundamental before approaching the paced electrocardiogram. The paced electrocardiogram must be approached in a systematic fashion, much as a nonpaced electrocardiogram, chest x-ray, or other diagnostic procedure. Knowing the type of pacemaker, the programmed parameters, and the underlying rhythm necessitating pacing are important factors in interpreting the paced electrocardiogram. Obviously, this information makes the interpretation much easier, but it frequently is not available.

INITIAL ECG INTERPRETATION

In reviewing an electrocardiogram of a patient with an implanted pacemaker, the underlying rhythm should be assessed carefully as well as its relationship to the pacemaker artifact(s). The first step is to find any portion of the electrocardiogram during which the heart is not paced, i.e., identify the intrinsic cardiac rhythm. That portion of the electrocardiogram should be interpreted as any electrocardiogram: PR, QRS, and QT intervals; rate; axis; voltage, etc. If no intrinsic rhythm is apparent, then the patient may be pacemaker-dependent or the pacemaker may be programmed to stimulate faster (i.e., at a shorter cycle length) than the intrinsic rhythm. **After determining both the spontaneous atrial and ventricular rhythms, one should look for any relationship between the two, i.e., does a P wave result in a QRS complex indicating intact AV conduction?** After the intrinsic rhythm has been carefully scrutinized, pacemaker activity should be assessed. **If pacemaker activity is present, is there one stimulus or two (Figures 1 and 2)? If only one stimulus is present, does it result in atrial (Figure 3) or ventricular depolarization (Figure 1)? Is there an apparent relationship between pacemaker activity and atrial activity, ventricular activity, or both?** If there is no relationship between the pacemaker stimulus and a preceding P wave and the pacemaker stimulus follows the intrinsic QRS complex at a consistent cycle length, then ventricular sensing as part of ventricular inhibited (VVI) pacing is present (Figure 1). If a pacemaker artifact is consistently found within intrinsic P or QRS complexes, then a triggered pacing mode (AAT or VVT) exists (Figure 4).

Usually, it is not possible to determine from the ECG whether the pacemaker is operating in a bipolar or unipolar configuration. At one time it was possible to assess the height of the pacemaker stimulus in an effort to determine polarity, i.e., if the pacemaker artifact was large, then it was most likely of the unipolar configuration (Figure 5), and if a very small pacemaker artifact was present it

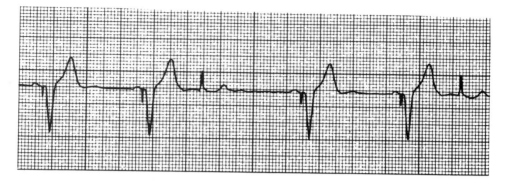

Figure 1.   *Normal ventricular demand pacing (VVI). The programmed rate is 50 bpm. Following the second and fourth paced complex an intrinsic ventricular complex occurs and appropriately inhibits the pacemaker.*

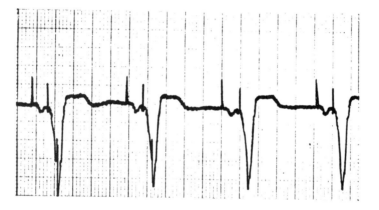

Figure 2.   *AV sequential pacing at a rate of 60 bpm. No intrinsic P or QRS activity occurs. It is impossible to distinguish whether the patient is pacing in the DVI, DDD, or DOO mode.*

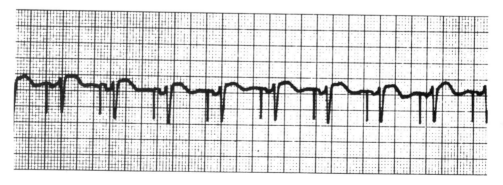

Figure 3.   *Normal AAI pacing in which no intrinsic P wave activity is seen. The programmed rate is 85 bpm. The paced atrial depolarization is followed by a conducted QRS complex. Without any intrinsic P wave activity, it is impossible to distinguish between AAI, DVI noncommitted, or DDD modes of pacing.*

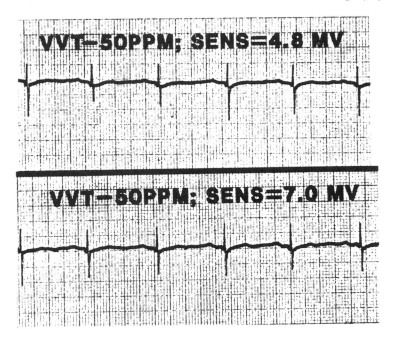

Figure 4. *Normal ventricular triggered pacing (VVT) with the pacemaker programmed at a rate of 60 bpm. The intrinsic rate is approximately 68 bpm so that the pacemaker is triggered and a stimulus artifact can be seen during the terminal portion of each QRS complex. If ventricular activity had not been sensed within 1000 ms (60 bpm) following a previous ventricular depolarization, a stimulus would have been emitted. The ventricular sensitivity is programmed to 4.8 mV in the upper panel and 7.0 mV in the lower panel. In addition to normal VVT operation the ECGs also demonstrate a ventricular sensing threshold of greater than 7.0 mV.*

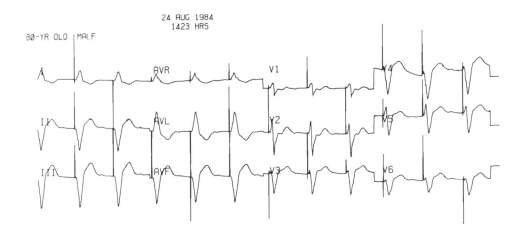

Figure 5. *A 12-lead electrocardiogram from a patient with a VVI pacemaker. Note the large pacemaker artifacts. Large artifacts are suggestive of unipolar pacing as contrasted to the smaller artifacts usually seen in patients with bipolar pacing system. However, with some types of monitoring and/or recording systems, the artifact size may have no relationship to polarity configuration.*

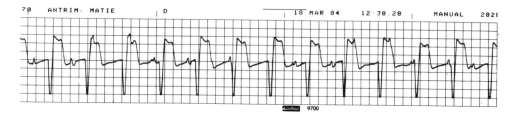

Figure 6.   *Lead II ECG of bipolar ventricular pacing. The pacemaker artifact is very small and not easily identified on this ECG. However, each QRS complex present is paced, and because there is no intrinsic activity, it is impossible to know whether the patient is being paced in the asynchronous (VOO) or demand (VVI) mode. Clearly, the P waves bear no relationship to the QRS complex.*

was most likely of the bipolar configuration (Figure 6). The ability to make this determination depends on the monitoring system used. In monitoring or ECG systems, such as the digital electrocardiograph, which artificially simulate the pacemaker artifact, this analysis cannot be used.

RESPONSE TO MAGNET APPLICATION

Assessing the magnet response of the pacemaker will provide additional information regarding pacemaker function and may be helpful in interpretation of the paced electrocardiogram. Magnet response may also be helpful in identification of the pacing mode and often the specific pulse generator and is equally useful for single- and dual-chamber pacing.

Application of a magnet to a single-chamber pacemaker always results in asynchronous pacing (Figure 7). In dual-chamber pacemakers, magnet application usually, but not always, results in asynchronous pacing in both the atrial and ventricular chambers (DOO mode) (Figure 8). Exceptions do exist. At least one dual-chamber pulse generator does not have a magnet mode, and in others the magnet mode may be programmed "off." There are dual-chamber pacemakers available in which magnet application will result in atrial asynchronous pacing but with retention of ventricular sensing (Figure 9). While in the magnet mode, the paced rate should be determined. Is the magnet rate faster or slower or the same as the programmed pacemaker rate? **If the pacemaker is a single-chamber pacemaker, does it result in atrial or ventricular depolarization?** Having determined what chamber is being paced, one can assess the pacemaker artifact and subsequent depolarization to assure proper capture. It should be remembered that pacemakers of different manufacturers respond differently to magnet application. Some will continue to pace asynchronously for a specific number of beats following magnet removal and may do so at more than one rate. The magnet response of a particular pacemaker may vary depending on the programmed parameters, i.e., the mode, of the pacemaker (Figure 10). The

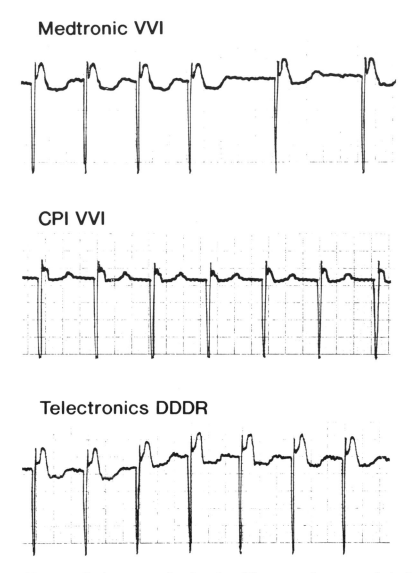

Figure 7. *Magnet application to pacemakers from three different manufacturers results in different responses. In the upper panel, magnet application to a Medtronic VVI pulse generator results in asynchronous pacing at a rate of 100 bpm for 3 beats followed by asynchronous pacing at the programmed rate. In the middle panel, magnet application to a CPI VVI pulse generator results in asynchronous pacing at 90 bpm. In the lower panel, magnet application to a Telectronics DDDR pacemaker results in VOO pacing.*

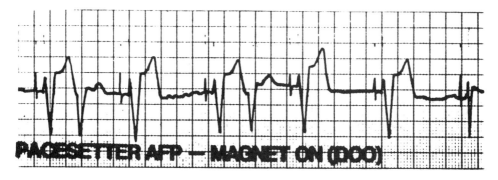

Figure 8. *Typical DDD magnet response. In this DDD pacemaker magnet application results in DOO pacing at the programmed lower rate limit and shortening of the AVI to 85 ms. The last ventricular pacing artifact occurs simultaneously with a native ventricular complex (pseudofusion).*

individual specifics of magnet application must be known for each pacemaker in order to determine that behavior is normal during magnet application and following removal.

When a single cardiac chamber is being paced, the effect of the paced chamber on the remaining chamber should be ascertained. For example, **if an atrial pacemaker is present, does atrial depolarization result in AV conduction and an intrinsic QRS complex, demonstrating intact AV conduction (Figure 11)? Alternatively, if a ventricular pacemaker is present, is there retrograde activation of the atrium, resulting in retrograde P wave activity following the paced ventricular complex (Figure 12)?** For dual-chamber pacemakers operating in the DOO mode, the AV interval should be measured during magnet application.

It is important that few assumptions be made concerning the details of the magnet mode of operation and to be aware of the specifics of the magnet re-

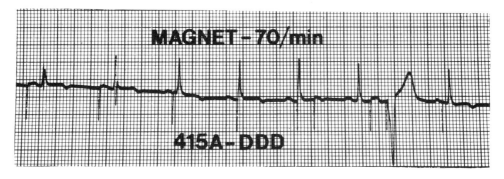

Figure 9. *Magnet application to an early DDD pacemaker, the Cordis 415A, resulted in asynchronous pacing from the atrial channel. Ventricular activity could be sensed following the atrial depolarization, and no ventricular output could be seen during magnet application. This is seen with the third and fourth pacing artifacts as well as the last pacing artifact in this example. In contrast to most current DDD pacemakers that pace asynchronously in both channels, ventricular sensing is retained during magnet application with this device.*

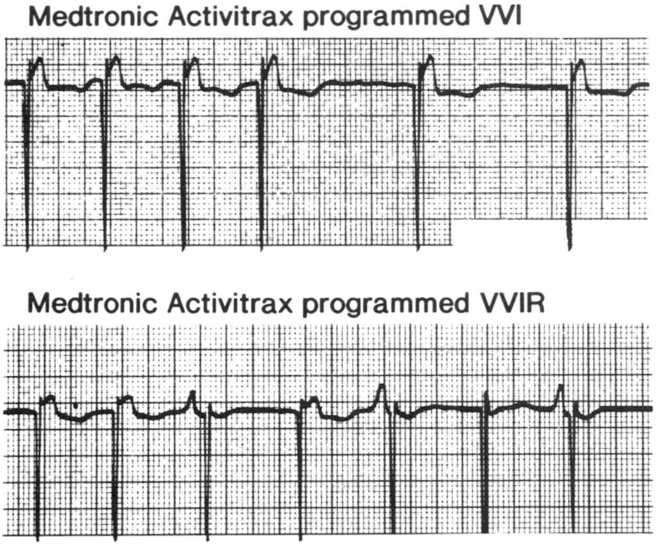

Medtronic Activitrax programmed VVI

Medtronic Activitrax programmed VVIR

Figure 10. *Magnet response may be dependent on the programmed mode of the pulse generator. In the upper panel, programmed to the VVI mode, the pacemaker paces asynchronously for 3 beats at 100 bpm followed by asynchronous pacing at the programmed rate. When the same pacemaker is programmed to the VVIR mode, magnet application results in asynchronous pacing at 85 bpm.*

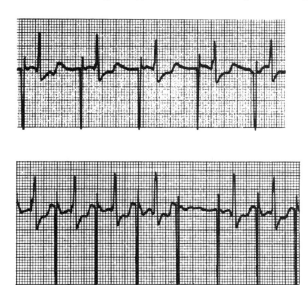

Figure 11. *Electrocardiogram demonstrating normal AAI pacing in the upper panel with the pacemaker programmed to 70 bpm. Normal AV conduction is present with each paced atrial depolarization resulting in an intrinsic ventricular depolarization. In the lower panel the magnet has been applied. The magnet rate is 100 bpm. At the faster rate the AR interval, atrial pacing artifact to intrinsic R wave, is longer than in the upper panel. The fourth pacing artifact results in atrial depolarization but AV block occurs with a single dropped ventricular beat. Retrograde atrial activation can occur readily.*

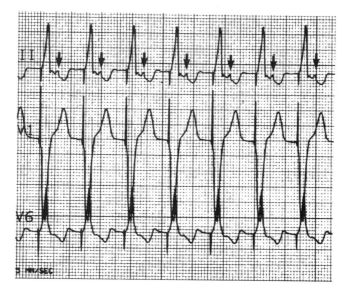

Figure 12. *VVI pacemaker with magnet application results in VOO pacing with definite retrograde conduction. Retrograde P waves are best appreciated in lead II (arrows). The three leads are recorded simultaneously.*

sponse in a particular unit or an erroneous interpretation of inappropriate operation may be made. The magnet mode is usually (but not always) free of sensing any events, and is often at a specific rate independent of the programmed rate and sensitivity settings. It allows determination, in the presence of a puzzling or unusual ECG, of whether the pulse generator is capable of operating normally.

SINGLE-CHAMBER PACEMAKERS

By following the preceding steps, determination will have been made as to whether a single- or dual-chamber pacemaker is present and whether the pacemaker stimuli result in atrial and/or ventricular depolarization. If a single-chamber atrial pacemaker is present, stimulation produces atrial capture, and if the pacemaker artifact is inhibited by intrinsic P waves, the pacemaker is in the atrial inhibited (AAI) mode (Figure 3). Paced ventricular activity will never be seen, with or without magnet application, and a pacemaker artifact will never occur within the intrinsic P waves. If one stimulus is seen that results in ventricular capture with inhibition by QRS complexes, the pacemaker is in the ventricular inhibited mode (VVI) (Figure 1). If the pacemaker is pacing asynchronously without sensing or capture of either the atrium or the ventricle, the mode cannot be determined. Similarly, with either a single-chamber atrial or ventricular pacemaker, if intrinsic activity is never seen and every complex is paced, the patient is either pacemaker-dependent or the pacemaker has been programmed faster than the intrinsic cardiac rate. If a single stimulus falls consistently into the spontaneous P wave or QRS complex, then the mode is of the triggered variety (AAT/VVT) (Figure 4). Although this mode of pacing is available in many multimodal programmable pacemakers, it rarely is utilized as a chronic pacing mode. Programming a pacemaker to the triggered mode is sometimes helpful to determine exactly where on the surface electrocardiogram sensing occurs (Figure 13).

An exception to the rule of the timing cycles in AAI and VVI pacing and a source of confusion is hysteresis. This programmable feature allows the escape interval for the initial paced beat to be at a longer cycle length than subsequent paced intervals (Figure 14). For example, if a patient has sinus node dysfunction with episodes of sinus bradycardia or sinus arrest, the pacemaker can be programmed to pace continuously at an interval of 1000 ms (rate of 60), but if hysteresis takes place at a rate of 40 bpm, 1500 ms without a paced event will be allowed before initiating pacing. If it is unknown that hysteresis is present, it may appear that there are two different functioning intervals. If these intervals are repetitive, hysteresis is the most likely explanation.

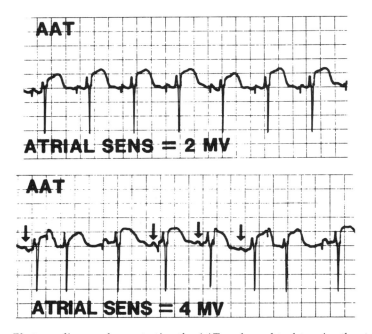

Figure 13. *Electrocardiogram demonstrating the AAT mode used to determine the atrial sensing threshold. At a programmed rate of 75 bpm and a sensitivity of 2 mV (upper panel), a pacing artifact can be seen within each intrinsic P wave. This documents normal sensing at a sensitivity level of 2 mV. In the lower panel with the pacemaker programmed to a sensitivity of 4 mV, P waves are no longer being sensed, and pacing occurs at the programmed rate of 75 bpm. At a sensitivity level of 4 mV, there is failure to sense in the atrium. (Arrows denote intrinsic P waves that are not sensed.)*

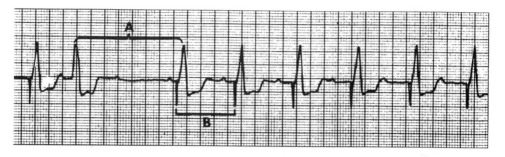

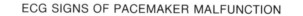

Figure 14. *Ventricular demand (VVI) pacing at a programmed rate of 72 bpm (833 ms, interval B). The preceding interval (interval A) is approximately 1550 ms in duration and represents normal VVI pacing with hysteresis. The prolonged cycle following a sensed ventricular event allows a longer period for the patient's intrinsic conduction system to escape before pacing at the programmed rate.*

Abnormalities of Single-Chamber Pacing

Abnormalities of pacing that can be recognized electrocardiographically can be simplistically divided into the categories that follow.

ECG SIGNS OF PACEMAKER MALFUNCTION

Inappropriate lack of pacemaker artifacts
(failure to output)

Failure to capture

Inappropriate pacemaker artifacts
(undersensing)

Inappropriate pacemaker rate

If each pacemaker stimulus is not followed by a QRS or P wave complex, failure to capture may exist (Figure 15). When considering the possible etiologies of failure to capture both true malfunctions and pseudomalfunctions should be considered. Potential etiologies are listed below.

CAUSES OF FAILURE TO CAPTURE

True Malfunction	Pseudomalfunction
Lead dislodgment	Inappropriately low-energy output
Lead insulation break	settings
Exit block	Pacemaker artifact in the myocardial
Metabolic abnormalities	refractory period
Battery depletion	

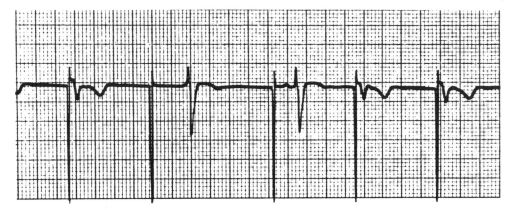

Figure 15. *VVI pacing at a rate of 70 bpm. The second and third pacing artifacts fail to capture the ventricle. The intrinsic QRS complex that occurs after the second pacing artifact is sensed normally, i.e., the next pacing artifact occurs approximately 850 ms later (70 bpm). The next intrinsic QRS complex is not sensed as demonstrated by the fourth pacing artifact which occurs approximately 600 ms later.*

It is sometimes difficult during magnet application to determine with certainty whether the myocardium is refractory at the time of the pacemaker artifact. However, if it is a nonmagnet electrocardiogram that is being evaluated, any failure to capture should be scrutinized carefully because if the pacemaker artifact is occurring early enough to raise the question of myocardial refractoriness as the cause for noncapture, failure to sense may also be present (Figure 16). (Figure 16 demonstrates fusion and pseudofusion beats.)

If the surface QRS represents elements of two depolarizations, it is a fusion beat. If the surface QRS is not altered by the pacing stimulus that is superimposed, it is a pseudofusion beat.)

The occurrence of pacemaker artifacts at an unexplained time suggests abnormal sensing. If the interval between the preceding QRS complex and the paced beat is shorter than the programmed paced cycle length, undersensing is likely (Figure 17). Potential malfunctions, true and pseudomalfunctions, that may result in undersensing are listed below.

CAUSES OF UNDERSENSING	
True Malfunction	**Pseudomalfunction**
Lead dislodgment	Magnet application
Poor lead position	Environmental electrical noise
Lead insulation defect	Pacemaker refractory period
Low-amplitude intracardiac signal	Monitor artifact

Failure to sense is often seen in combination with failure to capture (Figure 18), but the functions are separate and malfunctions may occur independently. The pacemaker senses the intracardiac electrogram. (See Chapter 4, "Comprehension of Pacemaker Timing Cycles.") It is not possible to know from the surface

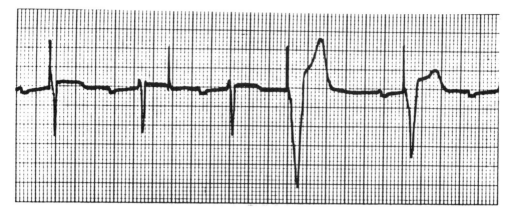

Figure 16. *VVI pacing at a rate of 50 bpm. Failure to sense is demonstrated by the second and third pacing artifacts which occur at intervals significantly less than 1200 ms, 50 bpm. The second pacing artifact does not result in ventricular capture. This is not true failure to capture but failure to depolarize the ventricle because the ventricular myocardium is still refractory from the preceding intrinsic QRS. Varying degrees of fusion are represented. The first pacing artifact occurs almost simultaneously and there is no significant alteration of the native QRS complex, i.e., pseudofusion. The third pacing artifact results in a ventricular depolarization that is totally paced and the fourth pacing artifact results in a fusion beat.*

ECG exactly where in relation to the ECG the intrinsic deflection exists, and thus where sensing occurs. The pacemaker artifact may fall within the QRS complex (Figure 19). This does not necessarily represent failure to sense, but instead an electrogram that occurs after the onset of the QRS as noted on the surface electrocardiogram. The stimulus may appear to be late when analyzed from the surface electrocardiogram, but reflects only pacemaker sensing after the onset of the surface QRS complex or P wave.

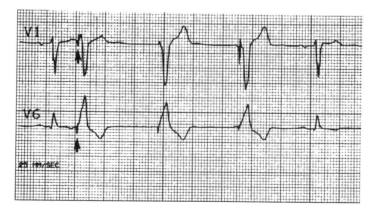

Figure 17. *VVI pacing at a rate of 55 bpm. The first complex is an intrinsic QRS complex which the pacemaker fails to sense, as evidenced by delivery of a pacemaker artifact approximately 400 ms later (arrow).*

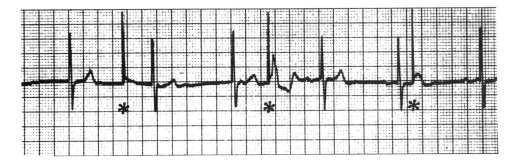

Figure 18. *Ventricular inhibited pacing (VVI) with failure to sense and intermittent failure to capture. Of the three pacemaker stimuli (*), ventricular depolarization occurs only after the second; the third probably falls during partial ventricular refractoriness.*

It is not uncommon for an otherwise normally functioning pacing system to fail to sense premature ventricular contractions. The amplitude and frequency content of each ventricular focus differs, and all possible foci may not be sensed by the pacemaker (Figure 20).

In contrast to the electrocardiographic manifestation of undersensing, events may occur that result in inappropriately long intervals on the paced ECG. Although failure to output may be due to oversensing, there are other true malfunctions and pseudomalfunctions that may result in failure to output. These are listed below.

CAUSES OF FAILURE TO OUTPUT

True Malfunction	Pseudomalfunction
Oversensing	Crosstalk
Total battery depletion	Invisible pacemaker artifact
Lead fracture	
Lead disconnection	
Oversensing	
Component failure (rare)	

Oversensing is the most common cause of failure to output. In this case the pacemaker interval is reset by inappropriate sensed events so that the interval between the pacemaker stimulus or intrinsic QRS activity and the subsequent paced beat is greater than the programmed pacemaker cycle. T waves, P waves (Figure 21), muscle activity (Figure 22), electromagnetic interference, and, rarely, afterpotentials from pacemaker discharge may result in oversensing (Figure 23). Ventricular activity may arise from different foci within the ventricle and will appear with different configurations or even appear isoelectric on the

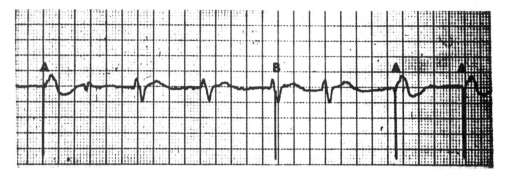

Figure 19.   *Ventricular inhibited pacing (VVI) in which the first, third, and fourth pacing artifacts result in ventricular depolarization. The second pacing artifact (B) occurs within the native QRS complex. This does not represent failure to sense. The surface electrocardiographic finding reflects a difference in actual electrogram sensing and sensing apparent on the electrocardiogram. This may be particularly apparent in patients with right bundle branch block.*

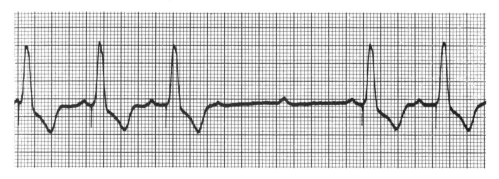

Figure 20.   *Ventricular inhibited pacing (VVI) at a programmed rate of 71 bpm and multifocal PVCs. The first PVC is sensed appropriately. The second PVC is not sensed (arrow). A paced ventricular beat follows approximately 230 ms after the PVC. The amplitude and frequency content of each ventricular focus differs, and all possible foci may not be sensed by the pacemaker.*

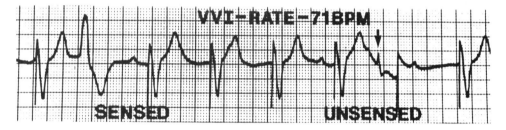

Figure 21.   *Ventricular inhibited (VVI) pacing with a delay between the third and fourth paced complexes caused by P wave sensing and recycle. Note the paced rate with calipers and measure back from the fourth paced complex. The escape interval falls within the P wave, which is sensed by the pacemaker.*

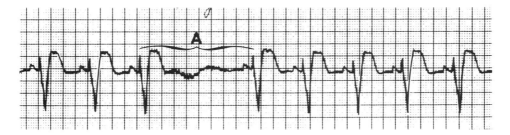

Figure 22. *An electrocardiogram of atrial synchronous (VDD) pacing with electromyographic interference. During the interference (irregular baseline) the ventricular channel senses muscle activity and inhibits ventricular output.*

surface electrocardiogram. An isoelectric QRS complex can cause an apparent "pause" that gives the impression of oversensing. Multichannel electrocardiograms are helpful in evaluating that possibility as it is unlikely that a QRS will be isoelectric in all leads (Figure 24). Alternatively, if an isoelectric event occurs simultaneously with a pacemaker artifact, a fusion beat may result and may appear as failure to capture. Pacemaker capture can be confirmed by noting the T wave or repolarization activity that follows the pacing artifact (Figure 19).

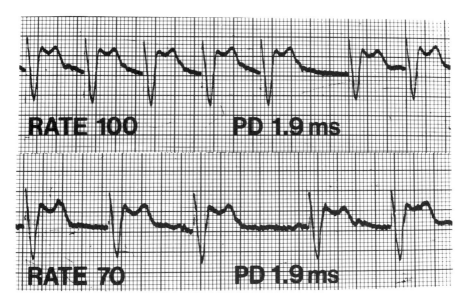

Figure 23. *Ventricular inhibited (VVI) pacing with a pause longer than the programmed cycle length in both the upper and lower panels. This prolonged cycle is caused by sensing of the afterpotential following a high output stimulus, i.e., a pulse duration of 1.9 ms. Note the escape cycle length and measure backward from the QRS complex following the prolonged cycle. It will be noted that the event sensed is the afterpotential. Decreasing the pulse duration, prolonging the refractory period, or making the ventricular channel less sensitive may correct the problem.*

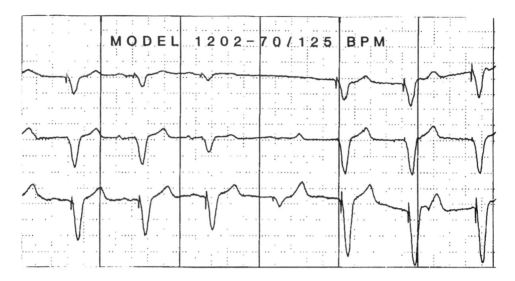

Figure 24. *Simultaneously recorded three-lead electrocardiogram of a patient with a DDD pace-maker programmed to a lower rate of 70 bpm and an upper rate of 125 bpm. In the top lead there appears to be an inappropriate pause. In the middle lead some electrical activity is present but there still appears to be a pause greater than the programmed lower rate limit, i.e., greater than 850 ms. It is only in the lower lead that normal function can be verified by the presence of a fusion beat. Without the multichannel recording this could easily have been misinterpreted as oversensing or failure to output.*

Dual-Chamber Pacemakers

If it has been determined that a dual-chamber pacemaker is present, the steps already outlined should be followed including determination of the AV interval and the status of AV and VA conduction.

When interpreting an electrocardiogram with dual-chamber pacing, the next step should be to determine the pacing mode. **During the free-running (non-magnet) pacemaker mode it should be determined whether P waves consistently are unsensed, i.e., does the pacemaker always recycle from the ventricular stimulus?** If so, the pacemaker may be in the DVI mode (ventricular sensing only) or there may be atrial failure to sense in the DDD mode. If in the DVI mode, QRS complexes that occur during the AV interval may be sensed or unsensed. A QRS complex that occurs following an atrial stimulus may inhibit the ventricular channel of the pacemaker. If the ventricular channel is inhibited, then the pacemaker is of the DVI noncommitted variety (Figure 25). If following paced atrial activity, intrinsic QRS activity occurs, but a ventricular artifact follows the atrial pacing artifact at the preset AV delay, falling during or after the intrinsic QRS complex, the pacemaker is of the DVI committed variety (Figure 26). Alternatively, the DVI pacemaker may be noncommitted but with failure of ventricular sensing. Regardless of whether the DVI pacemaker is committed or noncommitted, lack of atrial sensing allows competition between the intrinsic

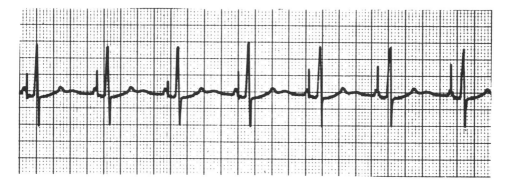

Figure 25. *Normal noncommitted DVI pacing in which the lower rate limit is 70 bpm (850 ms). The intrinsic sinus rate also is approximately 70 bpm, and there is competition between the atrial stimuli and intrinsic P wave activity. As this is a noncommitted unit, QRS activity occurs following the atrial stimulus and inhibits the ventricular channel.*

atrial activity and paced atrial activity. This competition may result in atrial rhythm disturbances (Figure 27). Although pacemakers capable of DVI pacing as the only dual-chamber pacing mode are no longer implanted, familiarity with DVI operation is important because most current dual-chamber pacemakers can be programmed to the DVI mode.

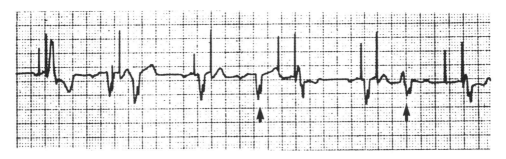

Figure 26. *DVI committed pacing programmed to a rate of 50 ppm. At the beginning of the tracing a native P wave occurs, but because atrial activity is not sensed in a DVI system, an atrial pacing artifact occurs and is followed at an abbreviated AVI by a ventricular pacing artifact. The shortened AVI is due to "safety pacing," and the AVI is approximately 110 ms as opposed to the programmed AVI of 250 ms. The second atrial pacing artifact is delivered simultaneously with a native QRS (2nd QRS complex). Had the native QRS occurred slightly earlier the pacemaker would have been inhibited and no atrial pacing artifact would have been delivered. The subsequent AVI is again abbreviated because of safety pacing, and the delivered ventricular pacing artifact fails to result in ventricular depolarization because the ventricular is still refractory. This is followed by a native ventricular event (3rd QRS complex) that resets the timing cycle. This is determined by the subsequent ventricular pacing artifact that occurs 1200 ms (50 ppm) after the intrinsic event. Because the 4th QRS complex does not occur early enough to reset the timing cycle and prevent delivery of an atrial pacing artifact, once delivered, the pacemaker is committed to delivering a ventricular pacing artifact even though it occurs after the QRS complex. The 5th and 8th QRS complexes (arrows) are not sensed appropriately because they fail to reset the timing cycle.*

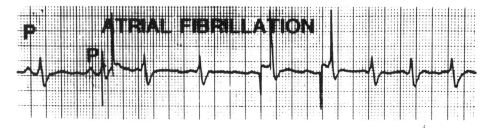

Figure 27. *A committed DVI pacemaker is inhibited by intrinsic activity during the first P-QRS complex. A normally unsensed P wave occurs, and the atrial stimulus is emitted during the vulnerable period of atrial depolarization and causes atrial fibrillation.*

If P wave activity is being sensed, does each P wave begin a pacemaker cycle? If each spontaneous P wave results in a paced ventricular complex at a consistent preset AV delay, the pacemaker is P synchronous and may be in the DDD or VDD mode (Figure 28). One can distinguish VDD from DDD pacing only if intermittent atrial pacing is present (Figure 29) in the magnet test mode, in the absence of intrinsic atrial activity, and when atrial undersensing is present. In the absence of intrinsic atrial activity or the presence of atrial undersensing, a VDD pacemaker will escape at the lower rate limit with ventricular pacing (Figure 30), and a DDD pacemaker will escape at the lower rate limit with AV

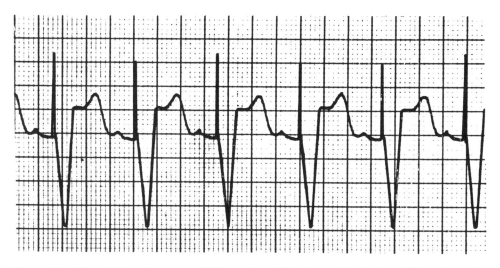

Figure 28. *Normal P synchronous or VDD pacing. Following each intrinsic atrial depolarization, the ventricle is paced at a preset AV delay. In this example, spontaneous ventricular activity does not occur. Without additional information, it is impossible to know whether the pacemaker is of the VDD, VAT, or DDD variety. One can only conclude that atrial sensing and ventricular pacing exist.*

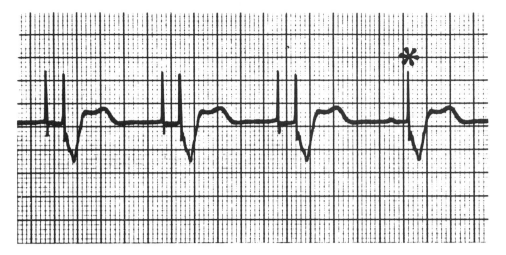

Figure 29. DDD pacing in which the first three complexes are of continuous pacing of atrium and ventricle. From this portion of the ECG, DVI pacing cannot be distinguished from DDD. There is sensing of the intrinsic atrial activity with the fourth beat and paced ventricular activity follows after the preset AV delay. Because there is pacing of both chambers and sensing of the atrium the pacing mode is either DDD or DDDR.

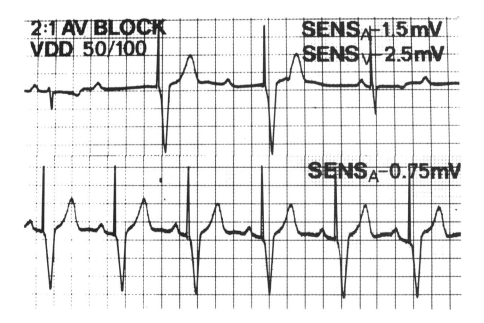

Figure 30. Upper panel: VDD pacing at an atrial sensitivity of 1.5 mV with failure to sense atrial activity. Ventricular escape or VVI pacing results at a preset rate of 50 bpm (1200 ms, cycle length). Lower panel: With atrial sensitivity increased to 0.75 mV, normal P synchronous pacing is restored, and paced ventricular activity follows each intrinsic atrial depolarization at a preset AV delay.

sequential pacing (Figure 31). In the VDD mode, if a P wave falls so late that the lower rate interval and the programmed AV interval cannot both be preserved, then the lower rate (or ventricular escape) interval will be preserved and the programmed duration of the AV interval will be sacrificed.

If each sensed P wave inhibits pacemaker output but does not start a pacemaker cycle, the pacemaker is in the DDI mode (Figures 32 and 33). Sensed atrial activity inhibits atrial output but does not result in a ventricular stimulus following the AV delay. This is a refinement of the DVI mode in that it prevents competitive atrial pacing caused by a lack of atrial sensing. As with the DVI mode, AV sequential pacing at the programmed rate will be provided in the absence of intrinsic activity. Intrinsic ventricular activity occurring during the atrial escape interval or AV delay will inhibit the pacemaker and reset the timing cycle.

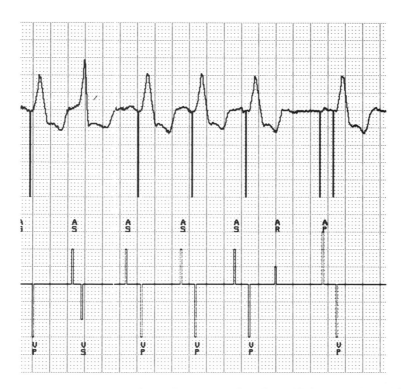

Figure 31. *Electrocardiogram with simultaneous Marker Channel™ from a patient with a DDD pacemaker. The ECG demonstrates atrial sensed events (AS) followed by paced ventricular events with two exceptions. The second ventricular event is a premature ventricular contraction that is sensed (VS) and inhibits ventricular output. Following the fifth ventricular event there is an atrial event that occurs in the PVARP (AR) and is therefore not sensed. The pacemaker escapes at the lower rate interval of 60 bpm. The pacing mode must be either DDD or DDDR since there are both atrial sensed and paced events and tracking of atrial events.*

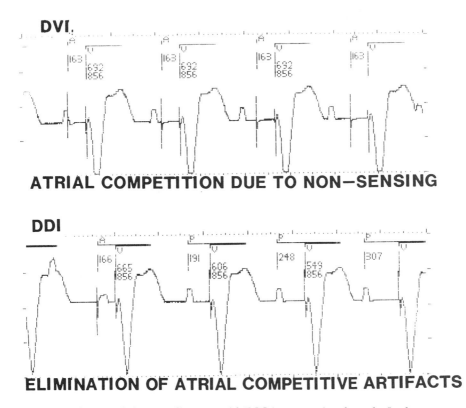

Figure 32. *Telemetered electrocardiograms with ECG interpretation channels. In the upper panel, the patient is programmed to a noncommitted DVI mode. Atrial competition occurs in the absence of atrial sensing. In the lower panel, the same patient has been programmed to the DDI mode with resultant elimination of atrial competition. Variation in the AV interval occurs because the atrial and ventricular events are no longer separated by a fixed AV interval.*

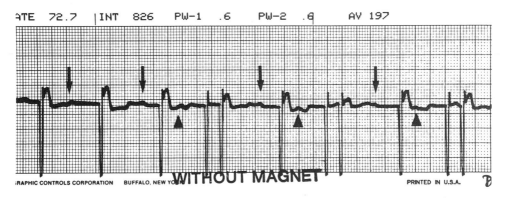

Figure 33. *Electrocardiographic recording from a patient with a DDI pacemaker programmed to a rate of 72 bpm. Arrows pointing down note sensed P waves. The P waves are not tracked but they do inhibit atrial output. The PV interval, intrinsic P wave to ventricular pacing artifact, varies because the rate of 70 bpm cannot be violated. Arrowheads pointing up note P waves that occur in the PVARP and are not sensed.*

ABNORMALITIES OF DUAL-CHAMBER PACING

Failure to capture and sense in the atrium and/or ventricle can occur with dual-chamber pacing as it does with single-chamber pacing. Intermittent failure to capture in the atrium is shown in Figure 34, atrial undersensing in Figure 30, intermittent failure to capture in the ventricle in Figure 35, and failure to output due to crosstalk in Figure 36. It must be remembered that failure to capture or sense in one chamber will most likely affect the function of the other chamber. Because of the complexity of the timing cycles of dual-chamber devices, it is sometimes difficult to determine from the surface electrocardiogram whether normal sensing and pacing are present (Figure 37).

When interpreting electrocardiograms of DDD pacemakers, all pacemaker intervals must be considered. A frequent source of confusion is the appearance of atrial undersensing caused by the occurrence of a P wave during the PVARP,

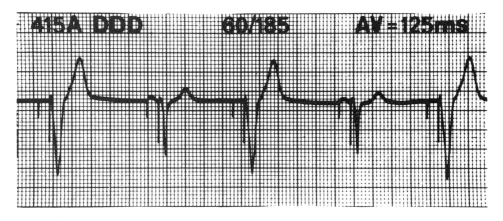

Figure 34.   *DDD pacing with intermittent failure to capture the atrium in the first, third, and fifth paced complexes. The ventricle is paced in each. The second and fourth ventricular depolarizations represent fusion complexes between conducted intrinsic QRS activity and the pacemaker stimulus.*

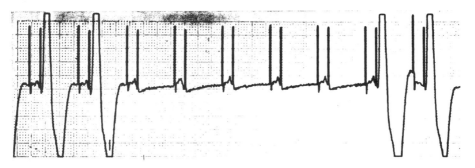

Figure 35.   *AV sequential pacing, DDD mode, with consistent atrial capture. There is failure to capture the ventricle with the third through seventh ventricular pacing artifacts. The cause of the intermittent failure to capture was dislodgment of the ventricular lead.*

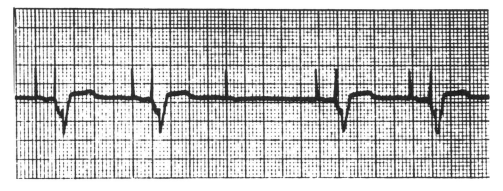

Figure 36. *AV sequential pacing, DDD mode, with consistent atrial and ventricular capture. However, following the third atrial pacing artifact and atrial depolarization there is no ventricular output resulting in a 2-second pause. Failure to output was due to crosstalk.*

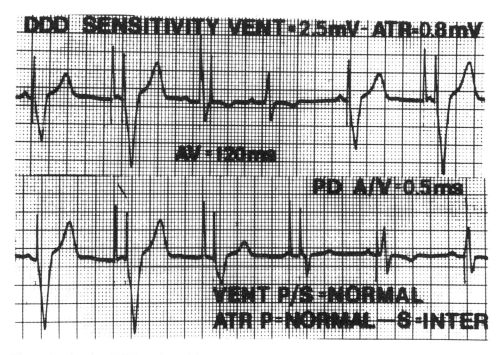

Figure 37. (Top): *DDD pacing with programmed parameters as indicated. The first complex is started by an intrinsic atrial depolarization with paced ventricular activity following a preset AV delay of 120 ms. The second complex demonstrates pacing of atrium and ventricle when atrial activity fails to appear before the end of the lower rate limit followed by ventricular pacing at the preset AV delay. The third QRS complex is of a P wave followed by a normal QRS fused with two pacer artifacts. This represents failure to sense atrial activity followed by an unsensed QRS that falls into the ventricular blanking period. This is followed by an intrinsic P QRS complex that is sensed. The fifth P wave is sensed properly. (Bottom): The first complex is started by normal atrial sensing, the second complex by atrial pacing. The third and fourth complexes are fused in atrium and ventricle, and determination of whether these complexes would have been sensed properly is impossible. The fifth and sixth complexes show atrial undersensing, but QRS occurs after the blanking period and inhibits the ventricular channel.*

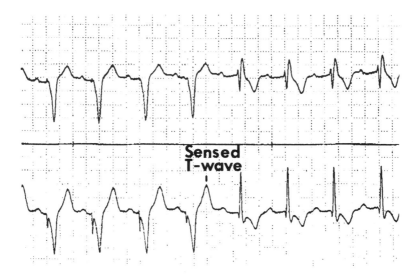

Figure 38. *Simultaneous electrocardiographic tracings from a patient with a DDD pacemaker. In the initial portion of the tracing there is P-synchronous pacing with a ventricular paced beat that occurs at the programmed AV interval of 200 ms after the P wave. The last 4 ventricular depolarizations are intrinsic QRS complexes that are preceded by a P wave, but not at the programmed AV interval of 200 ms, but instead at approximately 300 ms. This is not atrial undersensing. Intermittently a T wave of a paced ventricular depolarization is sensed by the ventricular lead. Having sensed what are interpreted as two consecutive ventricular events, the paced ventricular beat and the T wave, without an intervening atrial event, the pacemaker presumes that a premature ventricular event has occurred and the PVARP is extended. In this particular example the PVARP is extended from the programmed value of 300 ms to 480 ms. When the next true ventricular event occurs, the first of the four intrinsic QRS complexes, the pacemaker has still not sensed an atrial event so the PVARP is extended again. This will continue until the cycle is once again interrupted by a P wave occurring outside the extended PVARP.*

so called "functional atrial undersensing." When DDD pacemaker operation includes a PVARP that is extended after an event that the pacemaker identifies as a PVC, there is even more opportunity for P waves to occur in the extended PVARP. This possibility should be considered before concluding that there is atrial undersensing (Figure 38).

AV INTERVAL

To understand the potential inconsistencies of the AV interval, one must first understand the components of a normal AV interval (Figure 39). (See Chapter 4, Comprehension of Pacemaker Timing Cycles.) In current DDD and DDDR pulse generators, there may be several variations of the AV interval resulting in variable durations of the AV interval throughout the ECG. The electrocardiogram should be analyzed to see if AV intervals are consistent throughout. The differential for explaining a variant AV interval is discussed in the following paragraphs.

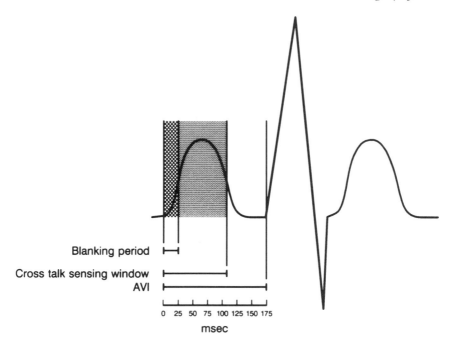

Figure 39. *The AV interval should be considered a single interval with two subportions. The entire AV interval corresponds to the programmed value. The initial portion of the AV interval is the blanking period (crosshatched shading). This interval is followed by the crosstalk sensing window (dot shading).*

Ventricular Safety Pacing

AV interval inconsistencies can occur in the presence of crosstalk or in an attempt to prevent crosstalk. Crosstalk is the sensing of the output of one pacemaker channel in the other. (Other "noise" sensed on the ventricular lead could also result in the appearance of crosstalk.) The major concern is the sensing of an atrial stimulus in the ventricular channel (Figure 36). To prevent crosstalk ventricular inhibition a blanking period begins simultaneously in the ventricular channel with the atrial stimulus. During this period the sensing circuits are insensitive. This interval is most commonly of 12- to 50-ms duration, depending on the pulse generator, and is programmable in many pulse generators. If the blanking period is too long, a spontaneous R wave, occurring soon after the atrial stimulus, will be unsensed and a competitive ventricular stimulus will be emitted. This situation is of greater concern with longer blanking periods. Any blanking period in excess of 100-ms duration has a greater potential of competing with a ventricular premature contraction and exaggerating ventricular competition in the presence of episodic atrial undersensing (Figures 37 and 40). If the blanking period is too short, the possibility exists that crosstalk and ventricular inhibition may result (Figures 36 and 41). Crosstalk occurs more frequently as the voltage output of the atrial stimulus increases or, less commonly, as pulse

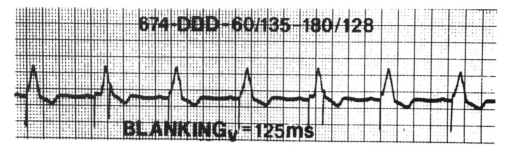

Figure 40. *The second and fifth P waves are unsensed, and the atrial stimulus (the first of the pair) falls during the AV interval. The blanking period in the ventricular channel begins with the atrial stimulus and extends 125 ms. As the intrinsic deflection of the ventricular depolarization occurs during the blanking period, it is unsensed and the ventricular stimulus is emitted.*

duration increases. The potential for crosstalk should be evaluated carefully and the blanking period appropriately lengthened.

In an effort to create the safest situation possible while retaining a relatively short blanking period, it is followed in many pacemakers by another portion of the AV interval during which activity sensed in the ventricular channel results in ventricular pacing (Figure 39). This has been referred to as *ventricular safety pacing* or the *nonphysiological AV delay*. Both terms are descriptive, as the paced interval is often shorter than the programmed AV interval and is present to assure ventricular pacing when crosstalk or other "noise" is sensed early in the AV interval. Since the "safety" stimulus occurs at a fixed delay after the begin-

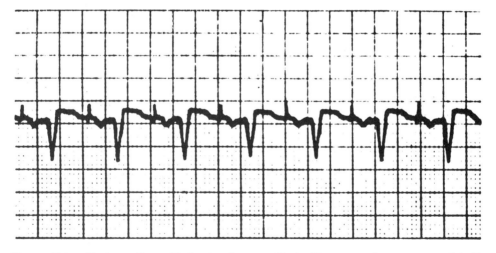

Figure 41A. *Electrocardiographic tracing from a patient with a pacemaker programmed to the DDI mode at a rate of 86 bpm, AV delay 165 ms, blanking period 13 ms. The AR interval, atrial pacing artifact to intrinsic QRS complex, is approximately 220 ms, 55 ms longer than the programmed AV delay. This abnormality can be explained by crosstalk. The short blanking period of 13 ms does not prevent crosstalk. Therefore, the ventricular output is inhibited and there is conduction through the AV node with a first-degree AV block.*

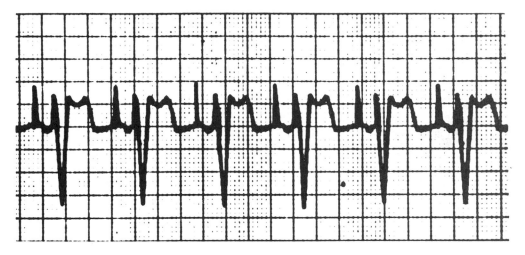

Figure 41B.   *When the blanking period is lengthened to 40 ms, crosstalk from the atrial channel is effectively blanked and the ventricular pacing artifact occurs at the expected interval of 165 ms, as programmed.*

ning of the "safety pacing" interval, the total AV interval is likely to be abbreviated. Because several early pulse generators had a ventricular safety pacing interval of 110 ms, this has also been referred to as the *110-ms phenomenon* (Figure 42).

Differential AV Interval or AV Interval Hysteresis

If there is a consistent difference between AV intervals initiated by a sensed event versus a paced event, then the likely explanation is that of a differential

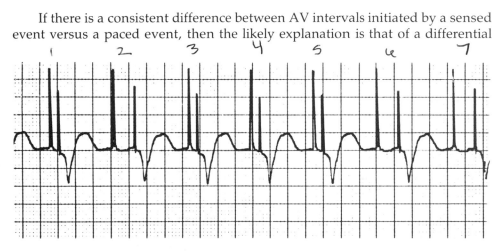

Figure 42.   *Crosstalk is the sensing of the output of one channel in the other. "Safety pacing" is one means of dealing with crosstalk. In this instance, the atrial stimulus has been sensed in the ventricular channel after the end of the blanking period. The ventricular channel response is not inhibition but emission of a ventricular stimulus at a short AV interval. The first and fourth paced pairs are at the programmed AV interval. The second and third are at a short AV interval as a result of the safety pacing response to crosstalk.*

1,3,4,5 show safety pacing   2,6,7
after A pace, test window 110ms,
if activity in window, commit to pace V @ 110 ms

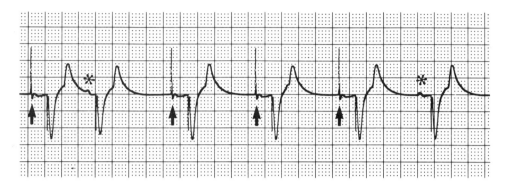

Figure 43. *Electrocardiographic recording from a patient with a DDD pacemaker with differential AV delay. The AV delay following the paced atrial artifacts (arrows) is 200 ms. The AV delay following the sensed atrial events (*) is 150 ms.*

AV interval. This is an attempt to provide a PR interval, i.e., the hemodynamic interval, which is of equal duration whether the atrial contraction is paced or sensed. The AV interval following a sensed atrial event will be shorter than that following a paced atrial event (Figure 43). In some pacemakers the differential is programmable, and in others a preset differential is used when the differential AV interval is programmed "on."

Rate Variable or Rate Adaptive AV Interval

Some DDDR pacemakers may have the capability of shortening the AV interval during AV sequential sensor-driven pacing. The rate adaptive or rate variable AV interval is intended to optimize the cardiac output by mimicking the normal physiological decrease in the PR interval that occurs in the normal heart as the atrial rate increases (Figure 44). The rate-related shortening of the AV interval may also improve atrial sensing by shortening the total atrial refractory period, thereby giving more time for the atrial sensing window.

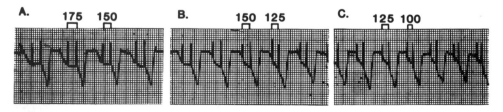

Figure 44. *Electrocardiogram demonstrating progressive AV delay shortening as the pacing rates exceed 90, 110, and 130 ppm. The AV delay was programmed to 175 ms and progressively shortened to 150 ms (A), 125 ms (B), and 100 ms (C) during exercise.*

DDD OPERATION AT THE UPPER RATE LIMIT

Pseudo-Wenckebach Upper Rate Behavior

It is unlikely that P-synchronous pacing will be sustained at exactly the upper rate limit for prolonged periods (Figures 45A and B). When the sinus rate exceeds the upper rate limit, pseudo-Wenckebach behavior is initiated. The appearance is that of patterned beating, progressive lengthening of the PV interval, and intermittent pauses on the ECG when the intrinsic atrial rate exceeds the programmed upper rate interval (Figures 45C and 46). In DDD pacemakers, the AVI and the upper rate interval must be completed before a ventricular stimulus can be released. A sensed P wave initiates the AVI. Upon completion of the AVI, if the upper rate interval has been completed, or timed out, a pacemaker stimulus will be released. If the upper rate interval has not yet been completed upon completion of the AVI, the release of the ventricular output pulse will be delayed until the upper rate interval has timed out. This has the functional effect of lengthening the PV interval. It also places the ensuing ventricular paced beat

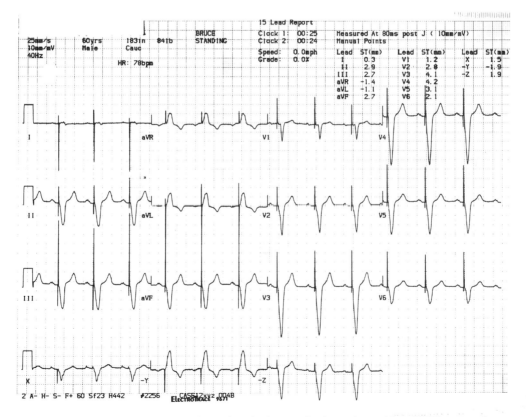

Figure 45A. *Electrocardiogram obtained early in exercise in patient with a DDD pacemaker. Normal DDD pacing is seen.*

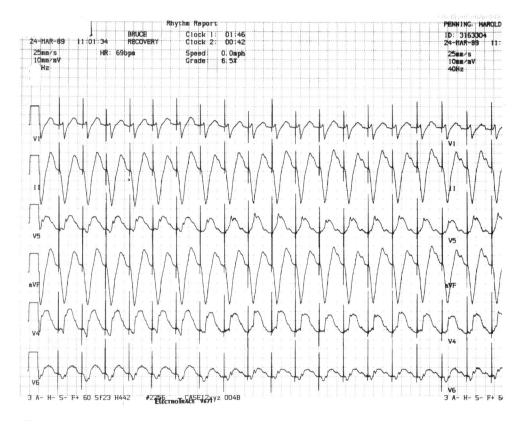

Figure 45B. *At a later stage of exercise the patient has almost reached the programmed upper rate limit of 120 bpm and is tracking every P wave with a paced ventricular beat.*

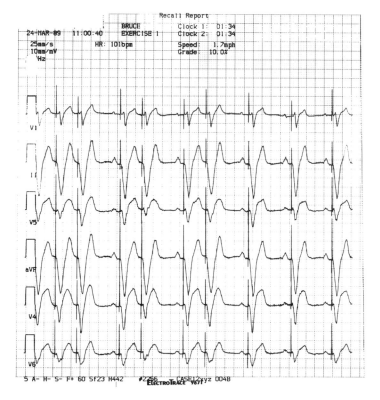

Figure 45C. *As exercise continues, the sinus rate exceeds the programmed upper rate limit. In the initial portion of the electrocardiogram there is pseudo-Wenckebach behavior. Every third P wave falls in the PVARP and is not sensed. At the end of the tracing, the sinus rate is faster and every other P wave falls in the PVARP resulting in 2:1 block and a significantly slower ventricular rate.*

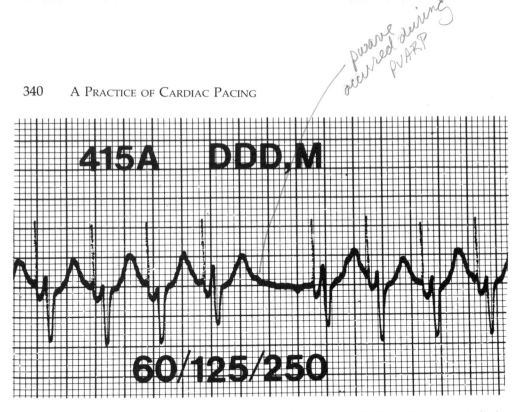

Handwritten margin note, top right: p wave occurred during PVARP

Figure 46. *DDD pacing in which the upper rate limit response is AV block. The lower rate limit is set at 60 and the upper rate limit at 125 with an AV delay of 250 ms. When the upper rate limit has been exceeded after the first four complexes, a P wave falls in the atrial refractory interval and AV block occurs, with a pause of 760 ms until the next P wave starts a new cycle.*

Handwritten margin note, left side (rotated): Pseudo-Wenckebach — due to electronics

closer to the next P wave. The PVARP and upper rate interval are each initiated by a paced or sensed ventricular event. During Wenckebach upper rate behavior, a P wave eventually coincides with the PVARP, is not sensed, and therefore, is ignored by the pacemaker. This results in a relative pause. The upper rate interval can then be completed and, depending upon the atrial rate and programmed lower rate, one of two events may occur. Either the P wave that follows the unsensed P wave is tracked, restarting the cycle at the programmed AVI or the pause is terminated by AV sequential pacing. If the native atrial rate is fast enough that every other P wave occurs in the PVARP, each P wave occurring in the PVARP would not be sensed and hence would not be tracked resulting in an effective paced rate of approximately half the atrial rate (Figure 45C).

There are still some pacemakers with a programmable option of 2:1 block as the upper rate mechanism (Figure 46). Depending on the patient's atrial rate, the pseudo-Wenckebach period may be very brief before 2:1 block occurs. In general, pseudo-Wenckebach is felt to be preferable to sudden 2:1 block to minimize sudden changes in the effective ventricular rate.

Fallback

While operating in the basic pseudo-Wenckebach or AV block upper rate mechanism, some DDD generators avoid marked variation in the RR interval during sinus or atrial tachycardia by using a gradual fallback method. Instead of blocking the atrial event or prolonging the AV interval, rate fallback involves decoupling of atrial and ventricular events at the upper rate limit. The ventricular inhibited pacing rate then gradually decrements to a programmed lower or fallback rate over a programmable duration. When the fallback rate is reached, atrial synchrony is resumed. Although AV synchrony is lost temporarily, the gradual transition to a lower pacing rate may moderate the hemodynamic consequences of sudden shifts in RR intervals, which can occur with the AV block mechanism.

Rate Smoothing

"Rate smoothing" was introduced as an option in a dual-chamber pacemaker manufactured by Cardiac Pacemakers Inc. (CPI, St. Paul, Minnesota). It is intended to eliminate large cycle-to-cycle variations in rate by preventing the paced rate from changing more than a certain percentage from one paced VV interval to the next (Figure 47). (Rate smoothing is programmable at a fixed percentage, i.e., 3%, 6%, 12%, etc.) This option would eliminate large fluctuations in rate during fixed-ratio or pseudo-Wenckebach block that may occur at the upper rate limit.

6 minutes – Postexercise

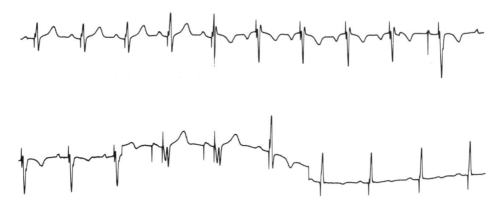

Continuous strip

Figure 47. A continuous ECG strip (changing leads) taken 6 minutes post-exercise from a patient with a CPI 0925 DDD pacing device. The pacemaker was programmed with "rate smoothing" at 3%. All ventricular activity is paced. In an effort to "smooth" the decrease in heart rate, an atrial stimulus can be seen to occur on three occasions to prevent the RR interval from slowing by more than allowed of the previous RR cycle.

Sensor-Driven Rate Smoothing In DDDR Pacing

See DDDR Electrocardiography below.

DDDR ELECTROCARDIOGRAPHY

DDDR pacing is designed to restore rate responsiveness while maintaining atrioventricular (AV) synchrony. DDDR, by definition, indicates that there is pacing and sensing in both the atrial and the ventricular chambers, that the response to sensing includes triggered pacing and inhibition by intrinsic activity in each chamber, and that the device has rate adaptive capability. As with any DDD pacemaker, a DDDR pacemaker must have a programmed lower rate as well as an upper rate. All the basic rules that apply to DDD upper rate behavior must still be considered when the upper rate behavior of a DDDR pacemaker is interpreted. The major difference lies in understanding the interplay between P-tracking and sensor-driven pacing, either or both of which may determine upper rate behavior. Understanding this interplay allows optimal programming of rate response parameters to achieve the upper rate response that is subjectively and objectively best for the patient. The type of lower rate timing system in a particular DDDR pacemaker, that is, atrial, ventricular, or a hybrid of both, may also have a direct effect on the upper rate behavior of the pacemaker. (For the purpose of this chapter, the term "upper rate limit" represents the maximum achievable paced ventricular rate regardless of whether it is accomplished by P-tracking or by sensor activation.)

At the upper rate limit, a DDDR device may display several behaviors: pseudo-Wenckebach block, 2:1 AV block, AV sequential pacing, P-synchronous pacing, or a combination of these. In some DDDR devices, the maximum rate at which the sensor can drive the pacemaker is programmed independently from the maximum tracking rate, that is, the maximum rate at which there is 1:1 response between intrinsic atrial activity and paced ventricular activity. In other DDDR pacemakers, a single programmable value limits the upper rate regardless of whether it is reached by tracking of intrinsic atrial activity or by sensor-indicated activity. In addition, there are other upper rate behaviors unique to individual DDDR models.

Pseudo-Wenckebach Behavior

If the rate response parameters of a DDDR pacemaker are programmed such that the sensor consistently indicates a slower rate than the intrinsic atrial rate, it is possible that sensor-driven pacing may never be seen, so that only DDD operation is seen. This would include P-synchronous pacing, pseudo-Wenckebach behavior, and 2:1 block response as previously described for DDD pacemakers. However, pseudo-Wenckebach or 2:1 upper rate behavior (or both) is seen in a DDDR pacemaker only if the sensor-driven rate is slower than the patient's intrinsic atrial rate.

AV Sequential Pacing

Sensor-directed pacing predominates if the patient is chronotropically incompetent or if the sensor is programmed to indicate a faster rate than the intrinsic atrial rate. In a DDDR pacemaker, AV sequential pacing can be seen at any rate between the programmed lower and upper rate limits. If the pacemaker reaches the programmed upper rate limit via the sensor, AV sequential pacing continues at the upper rate limit even if the patient's exercise intensity increases.

In DDDR pacemakers that require independent programming of the maximum tracking and maximum sensor rates, it is possible to program these upper rates discrepantly. For example, the maximum tracking rate could be programmed to 100 ppm and the maximum sensor rate to 150 ppm, in which case P wave tracking should not occur at sinus rates of greater than 100 bpm. It is possible, however, to see what appears to be P wave tracking above the maximum tracking rate. The mechanism for this apparent P wave tracking is inhibition of the atrial output because of precise timing of the intrinsic atrial beat. The atrial sensing window (ASW) is the period during which the atrial sensing channel is alert. The ASW can be defined as that portion of the pacing cycle other than the PVARP and AVI, because during both of these intervals there is no atrial sensing. If the PVARP or AVI (or both) is extended, there may effectively be no ASW. For example, at a programmed upper rate limit of 150 ppm, the minimum VV cycle length is 400 ms. If the PVARP is 250 ms and the AVI is 150 ms, there is no ASW; that is, 250 + 150 = 400 ms, which is the same as the upper rate limit. However, if a DDDR pacemaker has exceeded the programmed maximum tracking rate and is pacing at faster rates on the basis of sensor activation, an appropriately timed intrinsic P wave can still inhibit sensor-driven atrial pacing artifacts and give the appearance of P wave tracking at rates greater than the maximum tracking rate (Figure 48). The maximum tracking rate appears to be variable and equal to the sensor-driven rate when the sensor-driven rate exceeds the programmed maximum tracking rate if a P wave occurs during the ASW to inhibit output of an atrial pacing artifact. Although this behavior has the appearance of variable maximum tracking, the same behavior could theoretically be seen with DDIR pacing. In the DDIR mode, sensed atrial activity can only inhibit atrial pacing and not trigger ventricular pacing. Appropriately timed P waves could occur within the ASW and inhibit the subsequent A spike. Again, although this pacing mode is incapable of atrial tracking, this event would make it appear that the P wave were tracked at a rate equal to the current sensor rate.

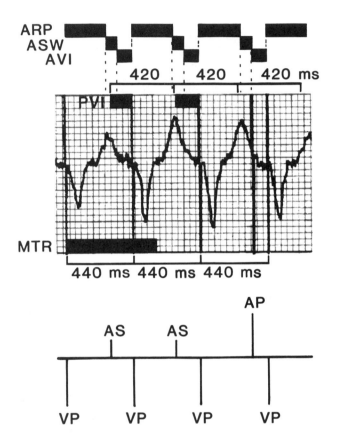

Figure 48. *Diagram showing how an appropriately timed P wave can inhibit the sensor-driven atrial pacing artifact and result in apparent P wave tracking above the maximum tracking rate (MTR). In this example, the MTR is 100 ppm (upper rate interval = 600 ms) and the sensor rate is 136 ppm (sensor-driven interval = 440 ms). The intrinsic rate is 143 bpm (PP interval = 420 ms). The second and third complexes are preceded by an intrinsic P wave that occurred during the atrial sensing window (ASW). This resulted in inhibition of the atrial pacing artifact, or P wave tracking above the MTR. The fourth complex was initiated by atrial pacing, because the preceding native P wave occurred outside the ASW in the atrial refractory period (ARP, 275 ms). Note the short P stimulus interval produced by the subsequent atrial pacing artifact. Also shown are the ASW, 65 ms, atrioventricular interval (AVI, 100 ms), and variable PV (intrinsic P wave followed by paced ventricular complex) interval (PVI). A diagram in Marker Channel™ (Medtronic, Inc., Minneapolis, MN) fashion demonstrates the electrocardiographic findings. AP = atrial paced event; AS = atrial sensed event; VP = ventricular paced event. (From Hayes DL, Higano ST. DDDR pacing: Follow-up and complications. In SS Barold, J Mugica (eds.): New Perspectives in Cardiac Pacing. 2. Mount Kisco, NY, Futura Publishing Company, 1991, p. 486, with permission.)*

Sensor-Driven Rate Smoothing

For an understanding of the combination of upper rate behaviors that can be observed with DDDR pacing, the fundamental difference between DDD and DDDR pacing must be emphasized (Figure 5). In DDD pacing, two potential mechanisms achieve ventricular pacing. The first is the lower rate interval; for example, if the lower rate of the DDD pacemaker is programmed to 70 ppm (857 ms) and the AVI is 150 ms, the atrial pacing stimulus occurs at 707 ms after the previous ventricular event (857–150 ms) and the paced ventricular event occurs after the programmed AVI of 150 ms to maintain a lower rate limit of 70 ppm. The second mechanism of driving the ventricle is in 1:1 synchronization with the sinus rate; that is, if the sinus rate is greater than the programmed lower rate limit, 1:1 P-synchronous pacing occurs until the upper rate limit is reached and DDD upper rate behavior is imposed. However, a third mechanism is possible with DDDR pacing (Figure 49). The ventricle can be paced in an AV sequential fashion in response to sensor input (Figure 50). For example, if the sensor input at a given point of exercise corresponds to an appropriate heart rate of 100 bpm, the DDDR pacemaker paces AV sequentially at 100 ppm. The only exception is that if the sinus rate at that time is greater than 100 bpm, the sinus rate predominates and P-synchronous pacing occurs. If the sinus rate is less than 100 bpm, the sensor predominates. Either the sinus or the sensor may be wholly predominant at any point in time. It is possible, however, for control to be mixed: sensor-driven AV sequential pacing is seen for a few cycles and is followed by emergence of the sinus rate with P-synchronous pacing. This interplay between sinus and sensor must be appreciated to understand DDDR behavior.

Establishing an optimal interplay between sinus and sensor should be the goal of programming in an effort to maximize hemodynamic benefits of DDDR pacing. This is accomplished by achieving a smooth transition between sinus- and sensor-driven pacing. The transition has been designated "sensor-driven rate smoothing," after true "rate smoothing" as described earlier in this chapter. With DDDR pacemakers, fluctuations in cycle length can be prevented or significantly minimized by optimal programming of the pacemaker, resulting in sensor-mediated rate smoothing. If the rate responsive parameters are programmed to mimic the native atrial rate, the paced ventricular rate should not demonstrate 2:1 behavior and would demonstrate pseudo-Wenckebach behavior for only short periods or not at all. Conversely, if the rate responsive circuitry is programmed to very low levels of sensor-driven pacing, little or no rate smoothing takes place. This rate response is illustrated in Figure 51. The upper panel in Figure 52 shows the DDD response, that is, sensor "off," or "passive," to exercise-induced increases in atrial rate with the maximum tracking rate limited to 110 bpm. The lower panel in Figure 52 shows the response that occurs with the sensor "on" (DDDR) and a maximum sensor rate of 140 bpm. Below the maximum P wave tracking rate, the ventricle is paced in a P-synchronous fashion, similar to DDD function. However, with the sensor "on" (DDDR), there is a transition from P-synchronous to AV sequential pacing through a period of

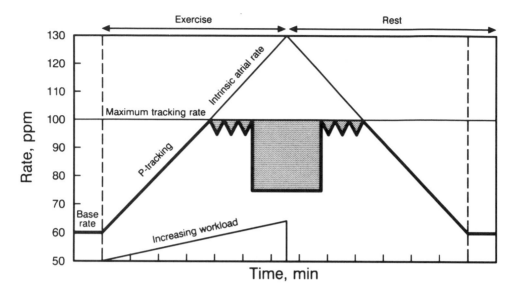

Figure 49A. *Diagram illustrating the rate response of a DDD pacemaker with Wenckebach-type block at the upper rate limit (100 ppm). The heavy black line represents the ventricular paced rate, assuming complete heart block. Note the varying RR intervals during Wenckebach-type block as the atrial rate exceeds the maximum tracking rate. (The shaded area is meant to represent potential paced ventricular rates that may occur during DDD upper rate behavior.) After termination of exercise, if the patient's atrial rate had increased to the point that the pacemaker was responding to every other P wave, that is, 2:1 block, the paced ventricular rate will actually increase to the maximum tracking rate as the atrial rate slows and fewer P waves fall within the PVARP.*

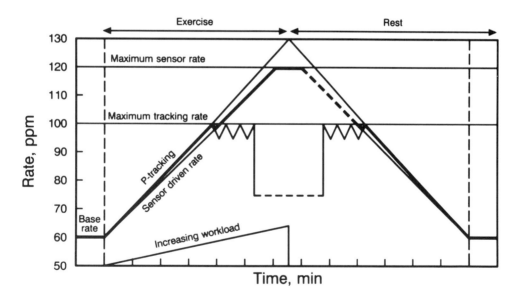

Figure 49B. *Diagram illustrating the rate response of the DDDR pacemaker and its behavior at both the maximum tracking and the maximum sensor rates. The heavy black line shows the ventricular paced rate, assuming complete heart block, as it progresses from the P-tracking mode to atrioventricular sequential pacing through a period of Wenckebach-type block. The rate may increase to the programmed maximum sensor rate. At termination of exercise, the ventricular paced rate gradually decreases to the base rate or lower rate limit unless activity resumes. Pseudo-Wenckebach activity can be minimized by optimal programming of the sensor rate response parameters.*

346

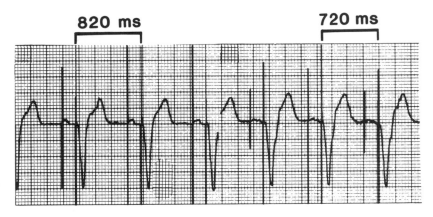

Figure 50. *Electrocardiogram obtained during exercise. The patient was exercising at 1.5 mph, 6% grade. At the beginning of the tracing, the paced RR cycle length is 820 ms; at the end of the tracing, the cycle length has shortened to 720 ms.*

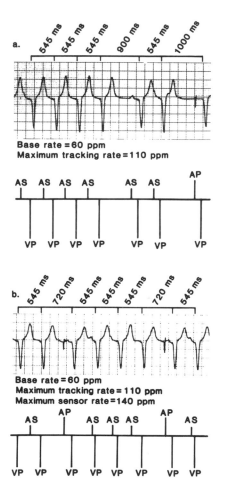

Figure 51A. *Electrocardiogram showing DDD pacing (sensor is programmed "passive") with Wenckebach-type block at the maximum tracking rate of 110 ppm. RR cycle length alternates from 545 to 1000 ms. Under the electrocardiogram is a diagram done in "ECG interpretation channel" (Medtronic, Inc.) fashion. Normal DDD function is represented by an atrial sensed event (AS) followed by a ventricular paced event (VP) in the absence of a sensed ventricular event. In the absence of an atrial sensed event, an atrial pacing stimuli (AP) is emitted, followed by VP. In this tracing, it is difficult to be certain that AP stimuli result in atrial depolarization.*
B. *Electrocardiogram showing DDDR pacing in the same patient with the same maximum tracking rate (110 ppm) and a maximum sensor rate of 140 ppm. With the sensor "on," there is less variation in cycle length, 545 to 720 ms. In the diagram under the tracing, it can be seen that an AP is emitted twice even though the escape interval is less than the programmed base rate. The decrease in cycle length variation occurs because the sensor level at that point in exercise indicates that the pacing rate should be 83 ppm (720 ms cycle length).*

pseudo-Wenckebach block as the atrial rate exceeds the maximum tracking rate. The cycle containing the unsensed P wave at the end of a Wenckebach sequence is shortened by sensor-driven pacing. Sensor-driven rate smoothing requires optimal programming of rate response parameters. (When true "rate smoothing" is an option in DDDR pacing, other manifestations are possible; see below.) Examples of sensor-driven rate smoothing are demonstrated in Figures 52 and 53.

If the sensor-indicated rate and the intrinsic rates are not well matched, there will be greater cycle-to-cycle variation, that may result in suboptimal hemodynamics. Figure 54 demonstrates the electrocardiographic manifestations of programming that results in a slight difference between sensor-indicated and intrinsic rates. In this example, the pacemaker is in the DDDR mode with a lower rate of 60 ppm, maximum tracking rate of 100 ppm, maximum sensor rate of 150 ppm, AV interval of 175 ms, and PVARP of 250 ms. When the intervals are carefully measured, it is apparent that all but one of the VV cycles are either 600 ms or 630 ms. Each of the VV cycles that is P-synchronous, that is, without a sensor-driven atrial pacing artifact, is 600 ms, which is equivalent to a paced rate of 100 ppm. As noted before, the maximum tracking rate was programmed to 100 ppm, so that these cycles demonstrate normal behavior. The other predominant cycle length of 630 ms occurs when the intrinsic P wave occurs within the PVARP. The P wave, therefore, is not sensed, and before another intrinsic P wave occurs, the sensor-indicated interval of 630 ms, or a rate of 95 ppm, occurs. This is normal function in a DDDR pacemaker when the atrial rate exceeds the maximum tracking rate and there is concomitant sensor-driven pacing.

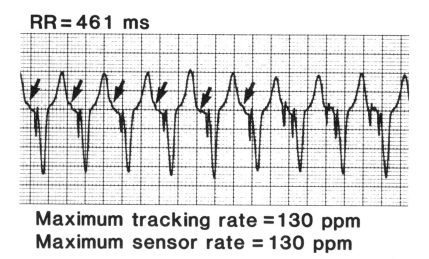

RR = 461 ms

Maximum tracking rate = 130 ppm
Maximum sensor rate = 130 ppm

Figure 52. *Electrocardiographic tracing from a patient with a DDDR pacemaker programmed to a maximum tracking rate of 130 ppm and a maximum sensor rate of 130 ppm. There is essentially no difference in VV cycle length between P-synchronous pacing (arrows) and sensor-driven atrioventricular sequential pacing (the last three complexes).*

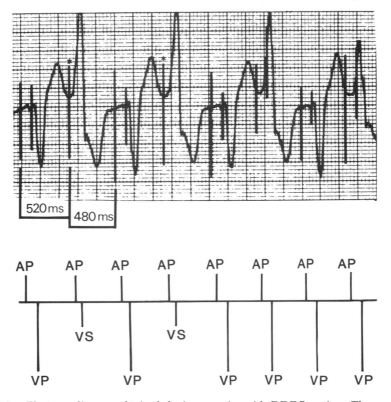

Figure 53. *Electrocardiogram obtained during exercise with DDDR pacing. The pacemaker is programmed to a base rate of 60 ppm, maximum tracking rate of 155, and maximum sensor rate of 150. Ventricular ectopy in a bigeminal pattern occurs during exercise. At times, the ventricular ectopic beat occurs early enough after the atrial pacing stimulus to inhibit ventricular output (asterisks), and at times the ventricular stimulus occurs during the early portion of the ectopic beat. Despite the ectopic beats, there is very little variation in cycle length, approximately 480 to 520 ms (measurements are made from atrial pacing stimulus to atrial pacing stimulus). A diagram in "ECG interpretation channel" (Medtronic, Inc.) fashion is used to further illustrate this electrocardiogram. AP = atrial paced event; VP = ventricular paced event; VS = ventricular sensed event.*

Slowing of the rate from 100 to 95 ppm is a function of sensor programming. This minimal difference, 5 ppm, between atrial rate and sensor-indicated rate would not be clinically significant. The actual sensor input signal to the pacemaker cannot be ascertained from the electrocardiogram. Although the pacemaker is capable of a maximum sensor rate, 150 ppm, its actual sensor-controlled rate is based on the actual input signal. (Programming in this manner, a maximum tracking rate significantly lower than the maximum sensor rate, is somewhat unusual in a patient capable of achieving faster sinus rates. It may occasionally be useful in patients with paroxysmal supraventricular rhythm disturbances; see below.)

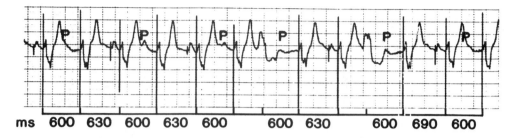

Figure 54. *Electrocardiographic tracing from a patient with a DDDR pacemaker programmed to a maximum tracking rate (MTR) of 100 ppm and a maximum sensor rate of 150 ppm. Two VV cycle lengths are seen, 600 ms and 630 ms. The 600-ms cycle length corresponds to the MTR of 100 ppm. However, when the P wave occurs within the postventricular atrial refractory period, the pacemaker escapes by the sensor-driven rate, a sensed P wave, or the lower rate limit. In this example, the escape after the 600-ms cycle length is sensor-driven. The sensor indicates that the appropriate rate is 95 ppm (630 ms) at a time when the corresponding sinus rate is approximately 115 bpm. (From Barold SS, Mugica J: New Perspectives in Cardiac Pacing. 3. Futura, Mount Kisco, NY, 1993, with permission.)*

Variations of DDDR Upper Rate Behavior

DDDR upper rate behavior may differ among devices from different manufacturers because of the lower rate timing system used, that is, ventricular-based, atrial-based, or a combination of ventricular- and atrial-based timing behaviors as well as other design-specific characteristics. Because upper rate behavior may be device-specific, it is necessary to refer to the specific pacemaker.

In a ventricular-based timing system, the VA interval, or atrial escape interval (AEI), which is the interval from a ventricular sensed or paced event to an atrial paced event, is fixed (Figure 55, upper panel). A ventricular sensed event occurring during the AEI would reset this timer, causing it to start all over again. A ventricular sensed event occurring during the AVI would terminate the AVI and initiate an AEI. If AV conduction is intact and the time from atrial pacing to intrinsic QRS (AR interval) is shorter than the programmed AVI, the AEI would be reset by the intrinsic ventricular event. The atrial cycle length therefore is slightly shorter than if the programmed AVI had been completed, resulting in a slight acceleration of the atrial pacing rate. By contrast, if a DDDR pacemaker operated on an atrial-based timing system, the AA interval would be fixed (Figure 55, lower panel).

Although acceleration of the ventricular rate in ventricular-based timing systems is minimal at the lower rate limit, it may become more significant as sensor-driven rates increase. In a ventricular-based timing system, the effective atrial paced rate could theoretically be significantly higher than the programmed upper rate limit if AR conduction were present (Figure 56, top panel). If it is assumed that the maximum sensor-controlled rate is 150 ppm (a cycle length of 400 ms), with a programmed AVI of 200 ms, the AEI is also 200 ms. If there is intact AV conduction such that the AR interval is 150 ms, the actual pacing interval is the AR interval + AEI, or 150 ms + 200 ms, or 350 ms.

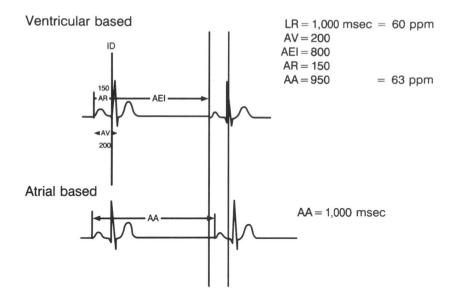

Ventricular based

LR = 1,000 msec = 60 ppm
AV = 200
AEI = 800
AR = 150
AA = 950   = 63 ppm

Atrial based

AA = 1,000 msec

Figure 55. *(Upper panel): With ventricular-based timing in patients with intact atrioventricular (AV) nodal conduction after atrial pacing (AR pacing), the sensed R wave resets the atrial escape interval (AEI) (the term "VA interval" could be used interchangeably with AEI). Because the base pacing interval is the sum of the AR and AEI, it is shorter than the programmed minimum rate interval. (Lower panel): With a true atrial-based timing in patients with intact AV nodal conduction after AR pacing, the sensed R wave would inhibit the ventricular output but would not reset the basic timing of the pacemaker. There would be AR pacing at the programmed base rate. ID = intrinsic deflection; LR = lower rate. (Modified from Levine, Hayes, Wilkoff, et al.)*

A cycle length of 350 ms is equal to 171 ppm, which is significantly higher than the programmed upper rate limit of 150 ppm.

If a DDDR pacemaker had a true atrial-based timing system, sensor-driven pacing could not exceed the programmed maximum pacing rate because the AA interval would be maintained (Figure 56, middle panel). Therefore, intact AR conduction would not alter the basic timing. At present, there are no pure atrial-based DDDR pacemakers.

Rate acceleration can be minimized in a ventricular-based timing system with a rate responsive AV delay (RRAVD). As the sinus- or sensor-driven rate progressively increases, RRAVD causes the PV and AV intervals to progressively shorten (Figure 56, bottom panel). Shortening the AVI with RRAVD results in a shorter TARP (shorter AVI + PVARP). This increases the intrinsic atrial rate that can be sensed, reducing the likelihood of both a fixed block upper rate response and functional atrial undersensing; that is, fewer P waves occur in the PVARP. It also minimizes the chance of an inappropriately long PV interval at higher rates that may occur with a fixed AVI when the fixed AVI is programmed appropriately for lower rate behavior. When the Synchrony II DDDR pacemaker by Pacesetter Systems, Inc., is operating under sensor control with RRAVD programmed "on," as the AVI shortens, the ventricular rate is held to that governed by the sensor. The time subtracted from the AVI due to RRAVD is

Ventricular-based timing--fixed AV delay

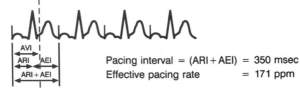

Pacing interval = (ARI + AEI) = 350 msec
Effective pacing rate   = 171 ppm

Atrial-based timing

Pacing interval (AA) = 400 msec
Effective pacing rate = 150 ppm

Ventricular-based timing--rate responsive AV delay

Pacing interval = ARI + AEI (AVI =   125 msec)
                 = 120 + 275 msec = 395 msec
Pacing rate   = 152 ppm

Figure 56. *Effect of different timing systems on maximum sensor rate with intact, stable atrioventricular (AV) nodal conduction (AR [atrial paced event followed by intrinsic R wave] pacing). (Top panel): In a ventricular-based timing system, in which the programmed AV interval remains constant at all rates, a significant increase in the paced atrial rate could exceed the programmed upper rate limit. In the example shown, even though the maximum sensor rate programmed is 150 ppm (upper rate interval of 400 ms, which is equal to the AV interval at 200 ms and the atrial escape interval of 200 ms), the effective pacing rate achieved is 171 ppm, because the effective pacing rate is a function of the AR interval (ARI) and the atrial escape interval (AEI), which remains constant in a ventricular-based timing system; that is, 150 + 200 = 350 ms (171 ppm). (Middle panel): In a true atrial-based system, the R wave sensed during the AV interval (AVI) would not alter the basic timing during stable AR pacing. This would result in atrial pacing at the sensor-indicated rate. (At present, there are no DDDR pacemakers that have pure atrial-based timing.) (Bottom panel): The addition of rate responsive AV delay to a ventricular-based timing system compensates for the difference between the AVI and the ARI and minimizes the increase in the paced atrial rate above the programmed sensor-indicated rate. In this example, the pacemaker is operating at the maximum sensor rate, and the rate responsive AV delay shortens the AVI by 75 ms (AVI of 200 ms at lower rate interval. 75 ms = AVI of 125 ms). With an AR interval of 120 ms, there is now only a minimal difference between the AVI and the ARI. The 75 ms subtracted from the AVI is effectively added to the AEI (200 ms + 75 ms = 275 ms). (Modified from Levine PA, Hayes DL, Wilkoff BL, et al: Electrocardiography of Rate-Modulated Pacemaker Rhythms. Siemens-Pacesetter, Inc., Sylmar, CA, 1990, with permission.)*

added to the AEI. Thus, if the programmed upper rate is 150 ppm, the pacing interval is 400 ms, and the RRAVD results in shortening of the AVI by 75 ms from an initially programmed AVI of 200 ms, the AVI shortens to 125 ms. Since the overall ventricular timing is held constant, the 75 ms subtracted from the AVI is added to the AEI, increasing it to 275 ms. In this example, the upper rate interval is 275 ms (AEI) + 125 ms (AVI), or 400 ms, corresponding to an upper rate limit of 150 ppm.

The RRAVD provides a more physiological AVI at the faster rate, and if there is intact AR conduction, it minimizes the degree of rate increase over the programmed maximum sensor rate. Assuming that the upper rate limit is 150 ppm and the initial AVI is 200 ms, the RRAVD results in an AVI of 125 ms at the upper rate limit. If intact AR conduction is present at 120 ms, the overall shortening of the pacing interval is only 5 ms above that seen at 150 ppm, a rate of 152 ppm (Figure 56, bottom panel).

The META (Telectronics, Inc., Englewood, CO) DDDR pacemaker uses a conventional ventricular-based timing cycle and determines the sensor-driven rate and metabolic-indicated rate (MIR) by minute ventilation. The META DDDR allows the programming of a baseline PVARP, which is the PVARP that exists when the MIR is indicating a resting or minimum rate. As the MIR increases because of an increase in workload or emotional stress, the pacemaker has the capability of not only an RRAVD but also a rate adaptive PVARP. The PVARP shortens in a linear fashion so that at maximum rate the AVI plus the PVARP is equal to the maximum rate interval. The shortening of the AVI and the PVARP prevents the upper rate limit from being restricted by fixed values of the AVI and PVARP. The pacemaker monitors the atrial rate or, more specifically, the PP interval. When the PP interval is less than the operational TARP, the atrial rate is considered to be a nonphysiological atrial tachyarrhythmia, for example, atrial fibrillation, atrial flutter, or paroxysmal atrial tachycardia. If what the pacemaker has determined to be a nonphysiological atrial rhythm is present, the pacing mode automatically changes to VVIR until the criteria for nonphysiological atrial rhythms are no longer met, at which time DDDR pacing resumes (Figure 57). This feature can obviously affect the upper rate limit behavior. The upper rate response during a physiological atrial rate increase is based on the Automatic Mode Switching mechanism described. During a physiological in-

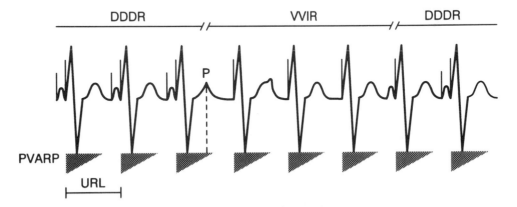

Figure 57. Electrocardiographic appearance of Automatic Mode Switching (AMS) when the pacemaker is programmed to an upper rate limit (URL) of 150 ppm. The first three cardiac cycles are due to sensor-driven atrioventricular (AV) sequential pacing, that is, DDDR pacing. After the third paced ventricular complex, a P wave occurs during the postventricular atrial refractory period (PVARP) (triangles) and initiates AMS to the VVIR mode because the atrial rate has exceeded the URL. The pacing mode reverts to DDDR when the atrial rate falls below the programmed URL; that is, P waves fall outside the PVARP. (From Barold SS, Mugica J: New Perspectives in Cardiac Pacing. 3. Futura, Mount Kisco, NY, 1993, with permission.)

crease in the atrial rate, that is, increased sinus rates based on increasing work-load or stress, the TARP shortens as the MIR increases to the programmed upper rate limit at which TARP equals the maximum rate interval. When the atrial rate exceeds the programmed maximum rate, the PP interval is less than the TARP and the device reverts to VVIR pacing.

To overcome the potential rate variability of ventricular-based DDDR devices already described, modified AA timing regimens have been developed for several DDDR pacemakers. The Relay (Intermedics, Inc., Angleton, TX) DDDR pacemaker is considered atrial-based, but it incorporates some features of ventricular-based timing. Whenever the time from the atrial event, whether sensed or paced, to the ventricular event, whether sensed or paced, is less than the programmed AVI, AA timing exists. Whenever the time from an atrial sensed event to the ventricular event, be it sensed or paced, is greater than the programmed AVI, ventriculoatrial timing (ventricular-based) occurs. (This would also include a ventricular sensed event not preceded by an atrial event, for example, premature ventricular contractions.)

The Relay pacemaker also incorporates a modified tracking limit scheme to prevent inappropriate upper rate ventricular pacing in response to atrial tachyarrhythmias (Figure 58). In this device, a programmable option exists that allows the sensor output to be cross-checked against the sensed atrial rate. A

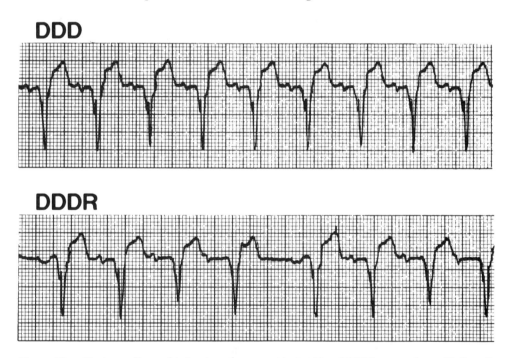

DDD

DDDR

Figure 58.   *Electrocardiographic tracings from a patient with a DDDR pacemaker with "conditional tracking limit™." In both tracings, the patient is at rest despite the rapid sinus rate. In the upper panel, P wave tracking occurs with a sinus rate of 100. In the lower panel, the pacemaker is programmed DDDR, lower rate 70 ppm. Because the patient is resting, the sensor indicates that a slower ventricular rate is appropriate. Because the atrial sensed events are more than 35 bpm faster than the lower rate limit, the pacemaker operates in pseudo-Wenckebach behavior. (An artifact is present during the fifth T wave.) (From Barold SS, Mugica J: New Perspectives in Cardiac Pacing. 3. Futura, Mount Kisco, NY, 1993, with permission.)*

"conditional tracking limit" set to 35 ppm above the lower pacing rate is in effect if the sensor output indicates that the patient is at rest. This limits the ventricular pacing rate if any atrial sensed events occur faster than 35 ppm above the lower pacing rate. This "conditional tracking limit" is deactivated when the sensor detects a period of exercise, or it can be programmed off.

In the PRECEPT DR and VIGOR DR (Cardiac Pacemakers, Inc., St. Paul, MN), the upper rate behavior may be altered by rate smoothing. Rate smoothing is designed to minimize cycle-to-cycle rate variations and is programmable to a fixed percentage value of the cycle-to-cycle pacing interval. This value defines for the pulse generator what is a physiological rather than a pathological change for the patient; rate changes less than the programmed percentage are considered physiological and changes greater than the percentage are considered pathological. When a sensed event exceeds this percentage of the previous cycle's interval, either faster or slower, the subsequent cycle is allowed to increase or decrease up to the programmed percentage for each cycle. As always, if a P wave is not sensed by the end of the calculated rate-smoothing window, atrial pacing occurs. This prevents sudden changes in cycle length while maintaining AV synchronous operation.

In a DDDR pacemaker with rate smoothing programmed "on," even if rate-response parameters are suboptimally programmed, that is, "sensor-driven rate smoothing" is suboptimal or minimal, there should not be any sudden alterations in cycle length, because they are prevented by rate smoothing (Figure 59).

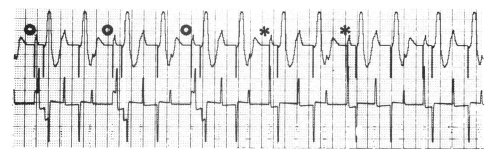

Figure 59. *Electrocardiographic tracing from a DDDR pacemaker (VIGOR DR, Cardiac Pacemakers, Inc., St. Paul, MN) with rate smoothing as a programmable option. In this example, the pacemaker is programmed to 60 ppm, upper rate limit of 100 ppm, and maximum sensor rate of 150 ppm with rate smoothing "on" at 21%. The electrocardiogram (ECG) is shown in the upper portion of the tracing, and the event markers immediately below the ECG identify the various electrocardiographic events. (On the event marker, atrial events are noted by upward deflections and ventricular events by downward deflections.) For the atrial events noted, there are three different sizes of upward deflections. The largest deflection, approximately 15 mV, represents a paced atrial event, the 10 mV deflection represents a sensed atrial event, and the 5 mV deflection represents an atrial event that has occurred in the postventricular atrial refractory period. If the deflection representing a paced atrial event has a step-shaped deformity, the paced atrial event occurred because of rate smoothing, denoted by the circles above the ECG. If there is no indicator of rate smoothing, denoted by the asterisks, the paced atrial event was sensor-driven. Without the event marker, it may be very difficult to determine which paced atrial events are sensor-driven and which are the result of rate smoothing. Had rate smoothing not been programmed "on" in this example, there would have been greater variation in paced ventricular cycle length because the pacemaker would have responded with pseudo-Wenckebach behavior until the time that enough activity was present to activate the sensor. (From Barold SS, Mugica J: New Perspectives in Cardiac Pacing. 3. Futura, Mount Kisco, NY, 1993, with permission.)*

Rate smoothing will continue to prevent RR or VV cycle interval alterations until a steady state is reached with the sinus rate or until the workload has increased to the point at which sensor-driven pacing predominates.

DDDR Upper Rate Behavior With Paroxysmal Supraventricular Tachyarrhythmia

As with DDD pacing, if a paroxysmal supraventricular tachyarrhythmia (PSVT) occurs in a patient with a DDDR pacemaker, the pacemaker may track the supraventricular rhythm. Tracking may be irregular and may result in paced ventricular rates that remain at the upper rate limit or vary between the lower and upper rate limits. The sensor will most likely not come into play, because the PSVT controls the rate and inhibits sensor activity. In a discussion of DDDR upper rate behavior, this subject warrants inclusion because tracking of PSVT while maintaining the capability of rate responsiveness is possible in a DDDR pacemaker. Several DDDR pacemakers currently available can be programmed to the DDIR mode. In this mode, "tracking" of the atrial rate is not possible.

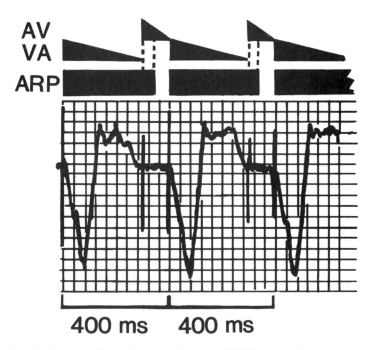

Figure 60. *In this electrocardiographic example from a DDDR pacemaker, the maximum sensor rate is 150 bpm (400 ms), the PVARP is 350 ms, and the AV interval is 100 ms. As illustrated in the block diagrams above the ECG, the two sensor-driven atrial pacing artifacts both occur during the terminal portion of the PVARP. Even though no atrial sensing can occur during the PVARP (as can be seen in this example by the intrinsic P wave that occurs immediately after the first paced ventricular depolarization), a sensor-driven atrial pacing artifact is not prevented by the PVARP. Whether a sensor-driven atrial pacing artifact is delivered depends on the sensor-indicated rate at that time and not the PVARP. (Reproduced by permission of Futura Publishing Company, Inc.)*

Therefore, whether the patient has normal sinus rhythm or PSVT, atrial activity is not tracked. However, in the DDIR mode, rate responsiveness can still be achieved by the sensor. If the DDIR pacing mode is not available, there are alternatives. If the maximum tracking rate and maximum sensor rate are independently programmable, the maximum tracking rate can be programmed to a lower rate, for example, 100 ppm, and the maximum sensor rate can be programmed to a higher rate, such as 150 ppm. If PSVT occurs, tracking is limited to a rate of 100 ppm. During exertion, rates to 150 ppm can be achieved through the sensor. If the upper rate limit is a single programmable value, the maximum rate desired through the sensor can be programmed as the upper rate limit. Tracking can in turn be limited by programming of the TARP (AVI + PVARP). If the AVI is 150 ms and the PVARP is 350 ms, the TARP is 500 ms and tracking is limited to 120 ppm. This outcome is possible because even though the PVARP prevents sensing of atrial activity, it does not prevent pacing the atrium on the basis of sensor activation (Figure 60).

DDDR upper rate behavior is more complex than upper rate behavior with any other pacing mode. The additional complexity is justified by the potential clinical advantages of DDDR pacing, the greatest of which is the avoidance of large cycle-to-cycle variations at the upper rate limit. Design-specific differences that exist among DDDR pacemakers from various manufacturers make it necessary to know the capabilities of the specific DDDR pacemaker to understand its upper rate behavior.

The analysis of a paced electrocardiogram using these guidelines should allow one to determine if pacemaker function is normal. As variations are certain to occur, anyone interpreting a paced electrocardiogram must be aware of the specifics of the operation of each pulse generator.

BIBLIOGRAPHY

Ajiki K, Sagara K, Namiki T, et al: A case of a pseudomalfunction of a DDD pacemaker. PACE 1991; 14:1456–1460.

Alt EV, von Bibra HV, Blamer H: Different beneficial AV intervals with DDD pacing after sensed or paced atrial events. J Electrophysiol 1987; 1:255–256.

Barold SS: Upper rate of DDD pacemakers. The view from the atrial side. PACE 1988; 11:2149–2159.

Barold SS, Falkoff MD, Ong LS, et al: Upper rate response of DDD pacemakers. In SS Barold, J Mugica (eds.): New Perspectives in Cardiac Pacing. Mount Kisco, New York, Futura Publishing Company, 1988, pp. 121–172.

Barold SS, Falkoff MD, Ong LS, et al: Timing cycles of DDD pacemakers. In SS Barold, L Mugica (eds.): New Perspectives in Cardiac Pacing. Mount Kisco, NY, Futura Publishing Company, 1988, pp. 69–119.

Barold SS: Management of patients with dual chamber pulse generators: Central role of the pacemaker atrial refractory period. Learning Center Highlights, American College of Cardiology 5:8–16, Summer 1990.

Barold SS, Falkoff MD, Ong LS, et al: A-A and V-V lower rate timing of DDD and DDDR pulse generators. In SS Barold, J Mugica (eds): New Perspectives in Cardiac Pacing. 2. Mount Kisco, NY, Futura Publishing Company, 1991, pp 203–247.

Barold SS, Levine PA: Autointerference of demand pulse generators. PACE 1981; 4:274–280.

Brandt J, Fahraeus T, Schuller H: Far-field QRS complex sensing via the atrial pacemaker lead. I. Mechanism, consequences, differential diagnosis and countermeasures in AAI and VDD/DDD pacing. PACE 1988; 11:1432–1438.

Brandt J, Fahraeus T, Schuller H: Far-field QRS complex sensingvia the atrial pacemaker lead. II. Prevalence, clinical significance and possibility of intraoperative prediction in DDD pacing. PACE 1988; 11:1540–1544.

Calfee RV: Pacemaker-mediated tachycardia: Engineering solutions. PACE 1988; 11:1917–1928.

Combs WJ, Reynolds DW, Sharma AD, et al: Cross-Talk in bipolar pacemakers. PACE 1989; 12:1613–1621.

Den Dulk K, Lindemans FW, Wellens HJJ: Noninvasive evaluation of pacemaker circus movement tachycardias. Am J Cardiol 1984; 53:537–543.

Falkoff M, Ong LS, Heinle RA, et al: The noise sampling period: A new cause of apparent sensing malfunction of demand pacemakers. PACE 1978; 1:250–253.

Frumin H, Furman S: Endless loop tachycardia started by an atrial premature complex in a patient with a dual-chamber pacemaker. J Am Coll Cardiol 1985; 5:707–710.

Furman S: Dual chamber pacemakers: Upper rate behavior. PACE 1985; 8:197–214.

Hanich RF, Midei MG, McElroy BP, et al: Circumvention of maximum tracking limitations with a rate modulated dual chamber pacemaker. PACE 1989; 12:392–397.

Hayes DL, Higano ST, Eisinger G: Electrocardiographic manifestations of a dual-chamber, rate-modulated (DDDR) pacemaker. PACE 1989; 12:555–562.

Hayes DL, Higano ST. DDDR pacing: Follow-up and complications. In SS Barold, J Mugica (eds.): New Perspectives in Cardiac Pacing. 2. Mount Kisco, NY, Futura Publishing Company, 1991, pp. 473–491.

Hayes DL, Higano ST, Eisenger G: Electrocardiographic manifestations of a dual-chamber, rate modulated (DDDR) pacemaker. PACE 1989; 12:555–562.

Higano ST, Hayes DL, Eisinger G: Advantages of discrepant upper rate limit in a DDDR pacemaker. Mayo Clinic Proc 1989; 64:932–939.

Higano ST, Hayes DL, Eisinger G: Sensor-driven rate smoothing in a DDDR pacemaker. PACE 1989; 12:922–929.

Higano ST, Hayes DL: P Wave tracking above the maximum tracking rate in a DDDR pacemaker. PACE 1989; 12:1044–1048.

Janosik DL, Pearson AC, Buckingham TA, et al: The hemodynamic benefit of differential atrioventricular delay intervals during physiologic pacing. J Am Coll Cardiol 1989; 14:499–507.

Lau C-P, Tai Y-T, Fong P-C, et al: Clinical experience with a minute ventilation sensing DDDR pacemaker: Upper rate behavior and the adaptation of the PVARP (abstract). PACE 1990; 13:1201.

Lee MT, Adkins A, Woodson D, et al: A new feature for control of inappropriate high rate tracking in DDDR pacemakers. PACE 1990; 13:1852–1855.

Lesh MD, Langberg JJ, Griffin JC, et al: Pacemaker generatorpseudomalfunction: An artifact of Holter monitoring. PACE 1991; 14:854–857.

Levine PA: Normal and abnormal rhythms associated with dual-chamber pacemakers. Cardiol Clin 1985; 3:595–616.

Levine PA: Postventricular atrial refractory periods and pacemaker mediated tachycardias. Clin Prog Pacing Electrophysiol 1983; 1:394–401.

Levine PA, Hayes DL, Wilkoff BL, et al: Electrocardiography of Rate-Modulated Pacemaker Rhythms. Siemens-Pacesetter, Inc., Sylmar, CA, 1990, pp. 12–31.

Levine PA, Sholder JA: Interpretation of rate-modulated, dual-chamber rhythms: The effect of ventricular based and atrial based timing systems on DDD and DDDR rhythms. Pacesetter Systems, Inc., A Siemens Company, March 1990.

Levine PA, Sholder J, Duncan JL: Clinical benefits of telemetered electrograms in assessment of DDD function. PACE 1984; 7:1170–1177.

Markowitz HT: Dual chamber rate responsive pacing (DDDR) provides physiologic upper rate behavior. PhysioPace 1990; 4:1–4.

Papp MA, Mason T, Gallestegui J: Use of rate smoothing to treat pacemaker-mediated tachycardias and symptoms due to upper rate response of a DDD pacemaker. Clin Prog Pacing Electrophysiol 1984; 2:547–553.

Parsonnet V, Berstein AD: Pseudomalfunctions of dual-chamber pacemakers. PACE 1983; 6:376–381.

Perrins EJ, Sutton R: Arrhythmias in pacing. Med Clin North Am 1984; 68:1111–1138.

Rosenqvist M, Vallin HO, Edhag KO: Rate hysteresis pacing: How valuable is it? A comparison of the stimulation rates of 70 and 50 beats per minute and rate hysteresis in patients with sinus node disease. PACE 1984; 7:332–340.

Sutton R, Perrins EJ, Duffin E: Interpretation of dual chamber pacemaker electrocardiograms. PACE 1985; 8:6–16.

Van Gelder LM, Bracke FALE, El Gamal MIH: Fusion or confusion onHolter recording. PACE 1991; 14:760–763.

van Mechelen R, Ruiter J, De Boer H, et al: Pacemaker electrocardiography of rate smoothing during DDD pacing. PACE 1985; 8:684–690.

Vanerio G, Patel S, Ching E, et al: Early clinical experience with a minute ventilation sensor DDDR pacemaker. PACE 1991; 14:1815–1820.

Chapter 10

PACEMAKER RADIOGRAPHY

David L. Hayes

PACING SYSTEM RADIOGRAPHIC INSPECTION

Radiographic inspection of a pacing system should be performed in an organized manner, much as a routine chest x-ray. Without such an organized approach, essential information may go unobserved. The posteroanterior (PA) and lateral chest x-rays of any patient with a permanent pacemaker should be obtained and reviewed by the implanting or follow-up physician. Both views are essential, a single PA projection is inadequate. Oblique views do not commonly provide additional data. As lead systems often are faintly visible, use of thoracic spine exposures rather than the lung technique may occasionally be helpful in making the leads more visible. One systematic approach is to interpret the radiograph's components in the following order:

1. bony structures,
2. aorta,
3. cardiac shadow,
4. trachea,
5. diaphragm,
6. lung,
7. other.

Inspection of the pacing system falls into the final category. It can then be further subdivided into the categories that follow.

I. Overall View

Before radiographic abnormalities can be appreciated, the radiographic appearance of a normal pacing system should be understood. A radiographically normal pacing system will be reviewed in its entirety for reference throughout the remainder of this chapter. Carefully following a systematic approach it is possible to interpret almost all pacing systems radiographically (Figure 1).

Ventricular Lead

The ventricular lead usually is positioned in the right ventricular apex. Radiographically, the end of the ventricular lead appears on the PA projection to be between the left border of the vertebral column and the cardiac apex. The position of the heart, vertical or relatively more horizontal, largely determines the position of the lead in relation to the cardiac apex and varies among patients.

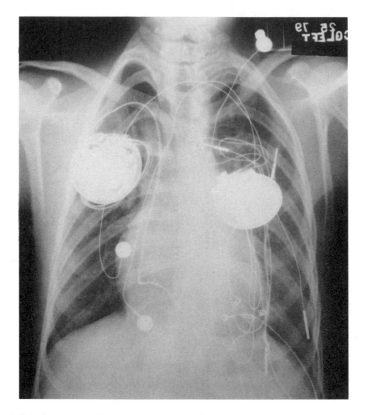

Figure 1. *A PA chest x-ray in a patient with multiple leads and two permanent pacemakers. It is impossible to determine from this x-ray whether one or both pulse generators are functional and which of the various leads are intact, functional, or abandoned.*

The lateral view is necessary to distinguish between an apical position in which the lead tip is anterior and caudally directed, directed posteriorly in the right ventricle, or on the posterior surface of the heart, i.e., within the coronary sinus. The ventricular lead should have a gentle curve along the lateral wall of the right atrium and cross the tricuspid valve to the ventricular apex (Figure 2). Redundancy of the lead within the cardiac chambers, which normally should be avoided, may be visible.

Atrial Lead

The atrial lead is most commonly positioned in the right atrial appendage (other atrial positions are considered later in this chapter). The "J" portion of the lead is slightly medial on the anteroposterior projection and anterior on the lateral projection. Optimally, the limits of the "J" should be no greater than approximately 80° apart. Redundancy proximal to the "J" within the atrium or superior vena cava should not be seen.

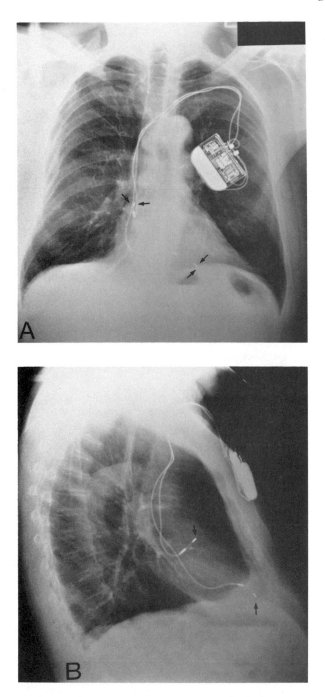

Figure 2. *An implanted bipolar dual-chamber pacing system. The atrial lead is well positioned in the right atrial appendage. Atrial position is more difficult to determine on the PA projection but is clearly anteriorly positioned on the lateral projection. The ventricular electrode lies well to the left of the vertebral column in the ventricular apex on the PA projection and anterior on the lateral projection.*

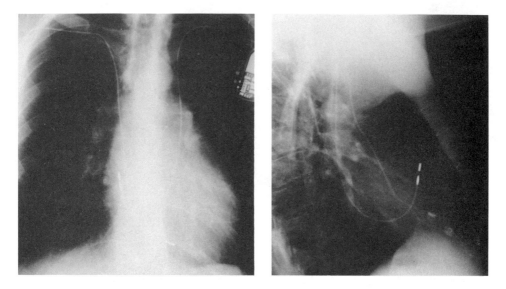

Figure 3. *Persistent left superior vena cava can cause unusual radiographic lead positions. The permanent lead descends on the right and assumes a conventional position. The temporary lead from the left traverses the left superior vena cava and enters the ventricle via the communication of the left superior vena cava and the coronary sinus. On the lateral projection, the temporary lead (within the coronary sinus) is on the posterior wall of the heart.*

Anatomical Variations

There are obviously innumerable anatomical variations that can alter the placement of the pacing system and therefore the radiographic appearance. Only a few of the more common anatomical variations will be discussed here.

It is possible to implant a permanent pacing system via a persistent left superior vena cava. (If this anatomical variation is noted prior to the pacemaker implant it is much easier to implant the system on the right side.) If pacing leads are implanted via a persistent left superior vena cava (Figures 3 and 4), the lead in the PA projection descends within the left side of the cardiac shadow and enters the atrium and then the ventricle via communication of the left superior vena cava and the coronary sinus. On the lateral projection, the ventricular lead will then be seen on the posterior cardiac wall within the coronary sinus.

Transposition of the great vessels can be diagnosed when the lead enters the superior vena cava, the right atrium, and the left or venous ventricle. In this instance, the lateral projection will show the lead anterior, and the PA projection will show it almost directly below the superior vena cava (Figure 5).

II. PULSE GENERATOR POSITION

For most transvenous implants, the pulse generator is visible on the chest radiograph and most are high in the pectoral region, away from the axilla, well inferior to the clavicle, and relatively medial (Figure 2).

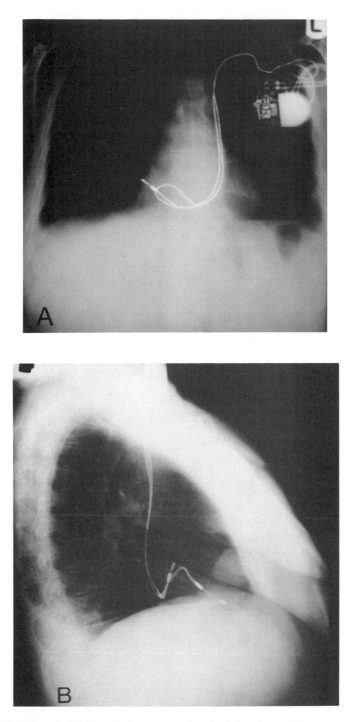

Figure 4. **(A)** PA and **(B)** lateral chest x-ray of a dual-chamber pacing system placed via a persistent left superior vena cava. (Figure courtesy of Dr. Neil G. Dewhurst, Mount Stuart Hospital, Torquay, Devan, United Kingdom.)

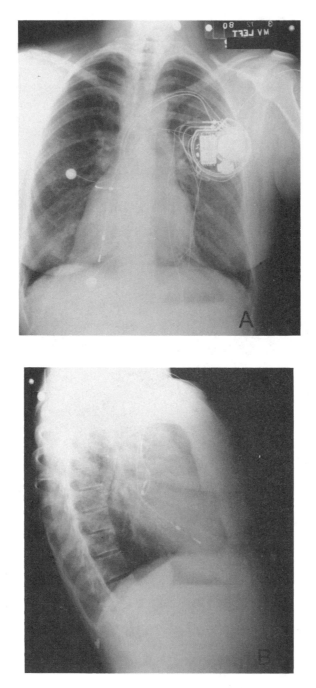

Figure 5.   PA **(A)** and lateral **(B)** chest x-rays in a patient with corrected transposition of the great vessels and dextrocardia. An AV sequential pacemaker is in the pectoral region, and the leads were placed via the subclavian vein. The atrial lead lies in the lateral aspect of the right atrium, and the ventricular lead lies in the apex of the venous ventricle, the morphological left ventricle. The lateral projection seems less bizarre than the PA projection with the ventricular lead well positioned in the apex of the left ventricle.

In many epicardial implantations, especially those performed more than a decade ago, the pulse generator was placed in a superficial position in the upper abdomen (Figures 6 and 7). If pacing leads are present on the standard chest x-ray and no pulse generator is seen (and the full chest is included on the chest radiograph), a flat film of the abdomen may verify pulse generator type and placement in the subcutaneous tissue of the abdominal wall. The other possibility is that a temporary pacemaker is being used, and the lead can be traced as it exits the body.

Other chest positions for pacemaker placement include the retromammary space (Figure 8) or intrapleural space (Figure 9).

It is now most common to place the pulse generator in either the right or left pectoral regions (Figure 2). In assessing pulse generator position, malposition may be readily noted. A pulse generator adjacent to or within the axilla is too far lateral, and placement within an excessively large pocket may allow its rotation with twisting or coiling of the lead (Figure 10), may be spontaneous or result from patient manipulation (Twiddler's syndrome—Figure 11).

III. Pulse Generator Identification

All pulse generators can be identified by their x-ray appearance. As the position of the cell or battery and the position of the radiopaque circuit components is unique to each model, identification of the individual model is often possible by the recognition of these components. Most current pulse generators contain some variety of radiographic identification code visible on x-ray within the generator shadow (Figure 12). These codes are unique to each manufacturer:

RADIOGRAPHIC IDENTIFICATION CODES

1. Manufacturer's name or initials
2. Model number only
3. Manufacturer's name and letter
4. Letter code for manufacturer and number

5. Manufacturer's logo and code for model number

All manufacturers and several independent sources provide tables, charts, and other printed material to assist in radiographic identification. Data for x-ray identification is published periodically in *PACE* as well as books and computer databases dedicated to the subject. For older devices still implanted that do not have a specific x-ray identification code, the overall shape of the pulse generator, its electronics, and battery provide an excellent identification, especially when compared to x-rays previously published for the purposes of such identification.

If there is no access to written pacemaker identification information, once the manufacturer is identified either by radiographic code or by can shape, etc., the technical service division of the manufacturer will be able to identify the device via the radiographic code.

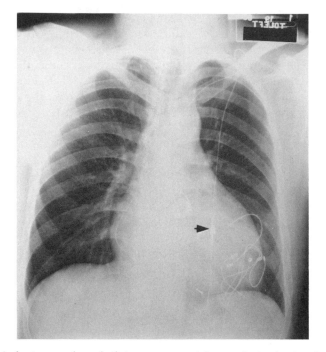

Figure 6A. *PA chest x-ray shows both transvenous, right ventricular (one) and epicardial (four) permanent pacing leads. No pulse generator is seen. The black arrow points to a connector that has been attached to the lead to allow abdominal positioning of the pacemaker.*

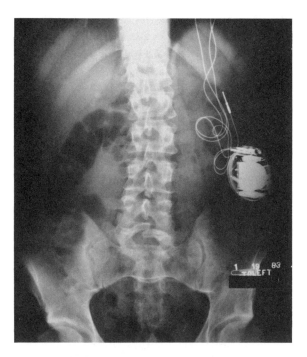

Figure 6B. *The transvenous lead has been tunneled to an abdominal site. An abdominal film documents the position of the pulse generator in the left upper quadrant.*

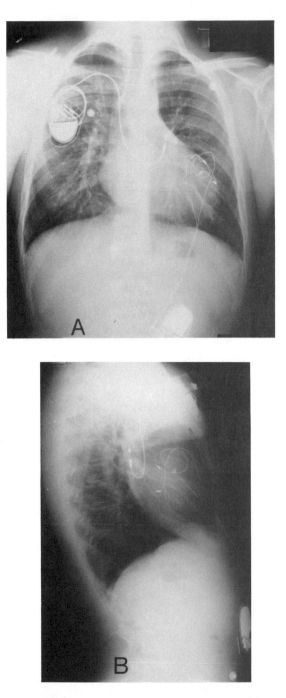

Figure 7. *PA chest x-ray of a pediatric patient with d-transposition of the great arteries following a Mustard procedure and requiring a ventricular epicardial pacemaker placed for symptomatic bradycardia. The pacemaker is positioned in the abdomen. The child subsequently developed supraventricular tachyarrhythmias that required an antitachycardia pacemaker. The antitachycardia pacemaker is placed in the right prepectoral region with an atrial endocardial lead.*

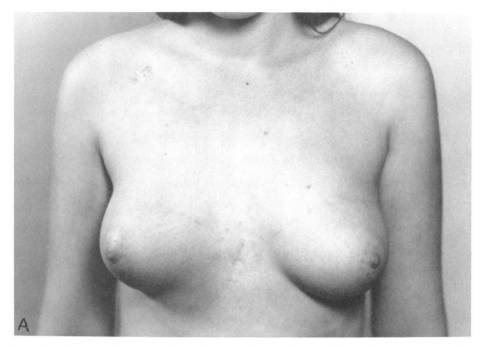

Figure 8.   *For cosmetic reasons the pulse generator may be placed in a retromammary position. In (A) the right inframammary incision is not noticeable.*

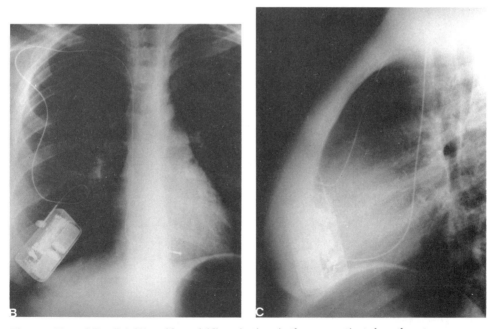

Figures 8B and C.   *PA (B) and lateral (C) projections in the same patient show the retromammary placement, which is directly behind the breast and is therefore inferior to the usual higher pectoral position.*

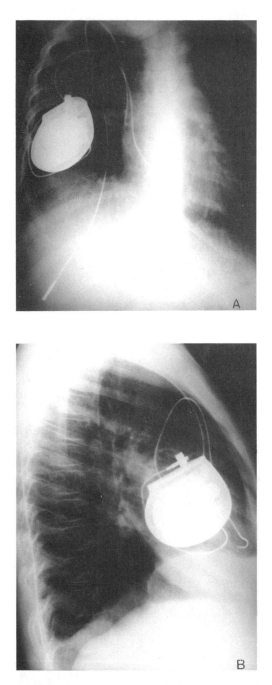

Figure 9. *Intrapleural placement is now primarily of historic interest. It was previously used as an alternative for patients with inadequate tissue for pectoral or retromammary placement. In this child, a single-chamber ventricular pacemaker was placed in a Dacron pouch and attached to the lateral pleura of the right pleural space. An atrial lead was implanted but unused and is seen in the right costophrenic sulcus unattached to a pulse generator. A. The generator size is substantially magnified in this oblique view. B. Lateral projection.*

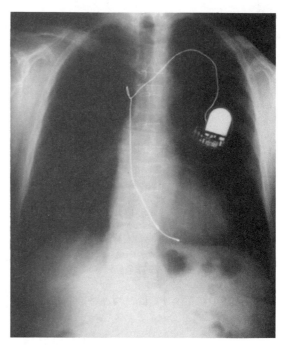

Figure 10. Torsion of the pacing lead, either by spontaneous twisting of the pulse generator in the subcutaneous pocket or by patient manipulation, has withdrawn the electrode from the right ventricular apex. The white arrowhead points to a portion of the lead in the superior vena cava that has twisted.

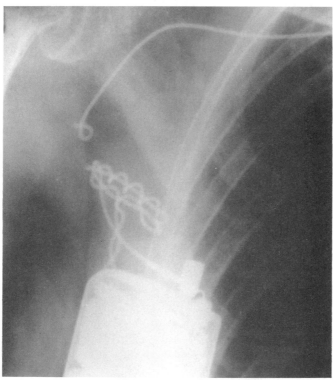

Figure 11. Patient manipulation of a pulse generator (Twiddler's syndrome) has resulted in sufficient tension to cause lead fracture.

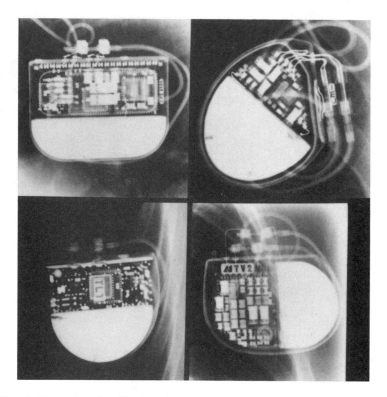

Figure 12. *Radiographic identification of pulse generators. Arrows note radiographic identification. Upper left: pacemaker manufactured by CPI, Inc., identified by CPI 0925; upper right: pacemaker by Intermedics, Inc., identified by IEJ; lower left: pacemaker by Telectronics Pacing Systems, identified by TLT; lower right: pacemaker by Medtronic, Inc., identified by company logo and TV2.*

IV. Polarity

The polarity of the pulse generator can be determined from the pacemaker profile and the number and type of connector pins. Unipolar, bifurcated bipolar, and coaxial (inline) bipolar pulse generators can be distinguished. Several coaxial bipolar pacemakers may be programmable for polarity, so that a coaxial bipolar lead connector does not necessarily imply bipolar pacemaker function. Other bipolar generators may accept either a bipolar inline or a unipolar lead. The connector assembly should be carefully scrutinized to ascertain which variety of lead is in use (Figure 13). A bifurcated bipolar lead may be unipolarized and connected to a unipolar pulse generator. The abandoned terminal usually can be found to be unattached to the pulse generator, lying free in the immediately adjacent subcutaneous tissue (Figure 14). Alternatively, a bipolar pulse generator can be connected to a unipolar lead, and an indifferent electrode connected to its positive terminal (Figure 14).

2 connection points for each lead
each point has set screw

1 connection point for lead

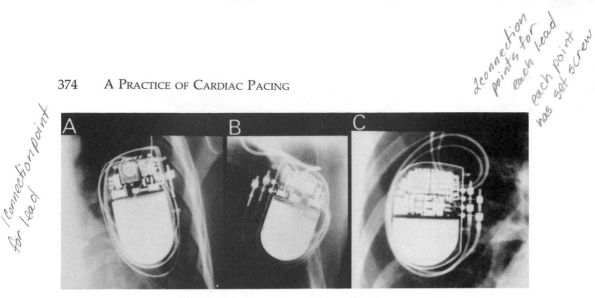

Figure 13. *Polarity of a pulse generator can be distinguished at the connector. A. Unipolar single-chamber pulse generator with a single connector; B. Dual-chamber unipolar pulse generator with two unipolar connectors; C. Bipolar dual-chamber pacemaker with a bipolar, coaxial in-line connector block accepting two bipolar leads.*

dual chamber devices have the connection points offset; 1 for V; 1 for A

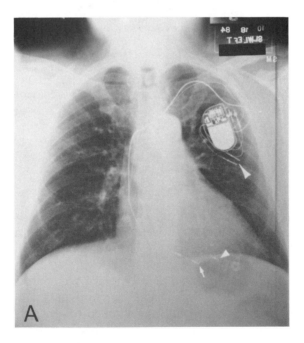

Figure 14. *A bipolar single-chamber pacing system. Because of rising thresholds, the system had been unipolarized with placement of an indifferent electrode and abandonment of the original bipolar lead. Its connector pins are seen lying unconnected, adjacent to the pulse generator.* ***A.*** *PA projection.*

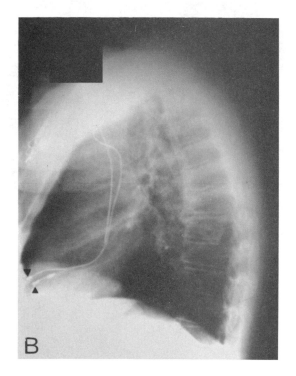

Figure 14B. *Lateral projection.*

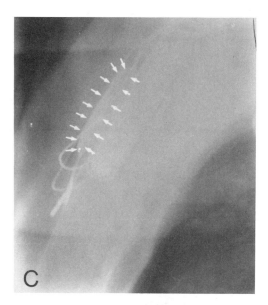

Figure 14C. *Close-up with arrows outlining the indifferent plate that has been used to unipolarize the pulse generator.*

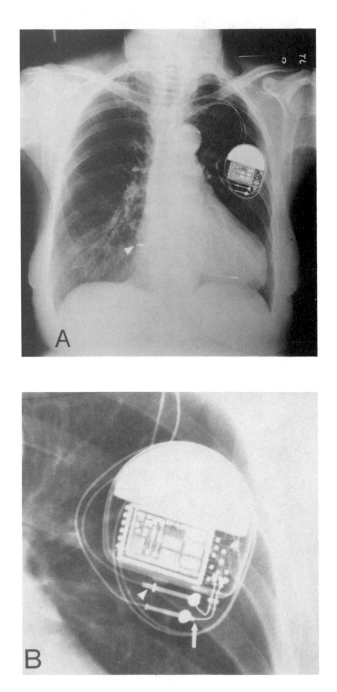

Figure 15. *PA **(A)** and close-up **(B)** of x-rays of a patient with a unipolar dual-chamber pacing system with radiographic evidence of a disparity in alignment of the connector pins. The patient presented with intermittent failure to pace. At operation, one pin was loose (arrowhead) because a set screw had not been tightened adequately.*

V. Connector Block

When the pulse generator has been located and identified, the connector block should be inspected to determine that connector and pin are firmly in contact. In a patient with intermittent complete pacemaker failure, an insecure connection may be present. Incomplete advancement of the pin into the connector receptacle or incomplete tightening of the screw, which also may be diagnosed radiographically, can produce similar findings (Figure 15).

VI. Lead Placement

The lead(s) may be transvenous or myocardial. If the lead is outside the cardiac shadow until the electrode enters the cardiac silhouette, then it is myocardial. If it courses within the heart, especially from the area of the neck or pectoral region, then it is transvenous. The vein of entry should be determined because different stresses on the lead system exist at different sites. However, the specific transvenous route may be difficult to determine. If lead placement is via subclavian puncture, it is difficult on the x-ray to distinguish radiographically from the cephalic venous route as both enter below the clavicle. If leads

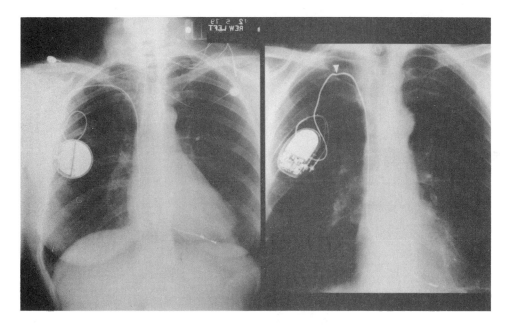

Figure 16. *Radiographically differentiating cephalic placement from a subclavian placement can be very difficult. In the PA chest x-ray on the left, the permanent pacing lead is in the cephalic vein. In the PA chest x-ray on the right, the permanent pacing lead is in the subclavian vein. A clue to subclavian vein placement is the slight bend in the lead as it crosses underneath the clavicle. (This bend, or crimp, in the lead where it passes between the clavicle and first rib has been shown to be a common site for lead damage.)*

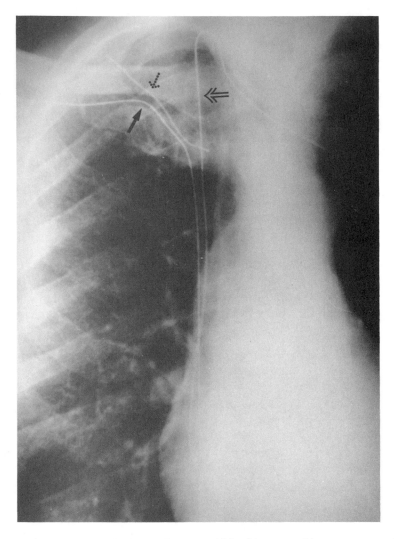

Figure 17. *Three venous positions can be compared in this x-ray with permanent pacing leads in: the right cephalic vein (solid arrow); right external jugular vein (dotted arrow); the internal jugular vein (open arrow). Jugular leads can be placed either deep or superficial to the clavicle.*

enter the venous system superior to the clavicle, a jugular venous cutdown approach has most likely been used. External versus internal jugular veins may be difficult to distinguish. If compared simultaneously, placement in the internal jugular is more medial than the external (Figures 16, 17, 18). If the lead is relatively close to the trachea, an internal jugular approach was likely used.

Intracardiac Position

1. Ventricular. The transvenous ventricular lead is almost universally placed in the right ventricular apex (Figure 2) but other positions such as the right

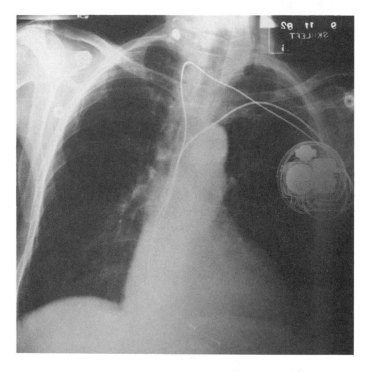

Figure 18. *Jugular and subclavian positions are seen in this x-ray with permanent pacing leads in the left subclavian vein and the right internal jugular vein.*

ventricular outflow tract may be used for permanent pacing (Figure 19). If a passive fixation lead is not in the right ventricular apex, comparison with earlier films is important to determine whether the lead has been displaced or was initially placed elsewhere. If an active fixation lead is used, i.e., screw-in fixation mechanism, it may be anywhere within the right ventricle, i.e., in the ventricular septum, or the pulmonary outflow tract (Figure 19).

A lead may be purposefully or inadvertently placed in the coronary sinus or posterior cardiac vein (Figure 20).

Undesirable positions for the ventricular lead would be in the left ventricular cavity, i.e., either via perforation of the ventricular septum, having inadvertently crossed a patent foramen ovale, atrial septal defect, or ventricular septal defect during transvenous placement, or in the pericardial space as a result of perforation (Figure 21).

2. Atrial. An atrial lead is most commonly placed in the right atrial appendage (Figure 2 and 22), less commonly in the lateral atrial wall (Figure 23), and infrequently in the coronary sinus (Figure 24). Pacing the left atrium via a transvenous approach is at times possible in certain congenital abnormalities (Figure 25). (The lateral projection is especially useful to discern the coronary sinus position, which is on the posterior cardiac wall, while the PA view alone may not allow distinction between the coronary sinus and a right ventricular position.)

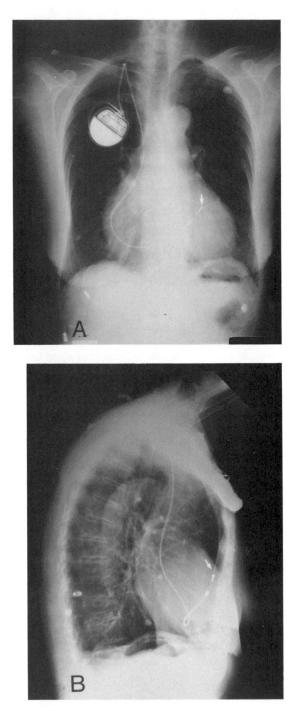

Figure 19. *PA (A) and lateral (B) chest x-rays in a patient in whom the best stimulation and sensing thresholds were found in the right ventricular free wall adjacent to the outflow tract. (The white arrow points to the tip of the pacing lead.) Although the PA projection is compatible with coronary sinus placement, the anterior direction of the lead on the lateral projection is incompatible with coronary sinus placement.*

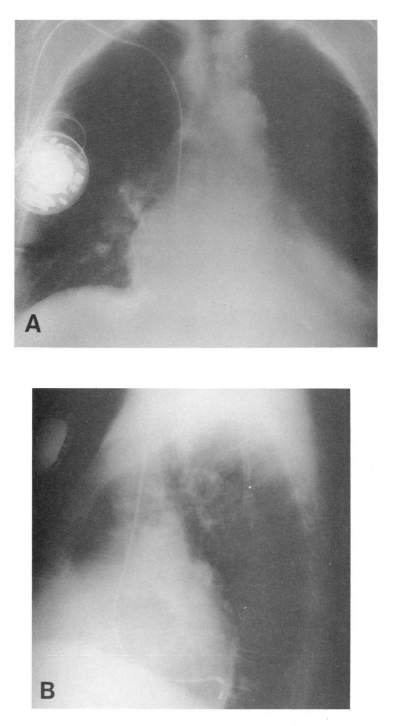

Figure 20. *PA (A) and lateral (B) chest x-ray demonstrating a pacing lead that inadvertently has been placed into a tributary of the coronary sinus. On the PA projection, the position appears to be satisfactory, but on the lateral projection the lead is clearly within the posterior cardiac vein.*

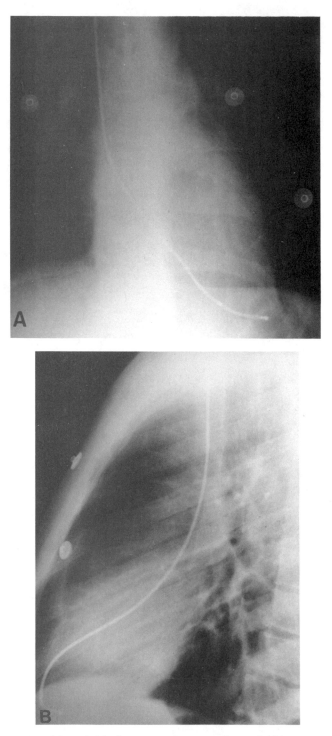

Figure 21.   *PA (A) and lateral (B) chest x-ray demonstrating a rigid temporary pacemaker lead that has perforated the right ventricle and lies with a gentle curve within the pericardium.*

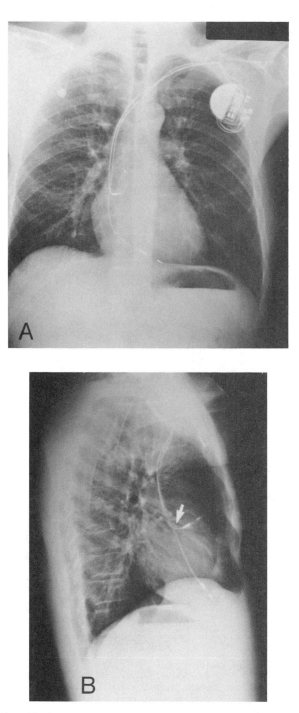

Figure 22. *PA **(A)** and lateral **(B)** chest x-rays demonstrating a dual-chamber pacing system with shallow placement of both leads. The atrial lead is most likely in the right atrial appendage. The atrial lead is not optimally positioned and is best appreciated on the lateral view. The white arrow points to the angle of the "J" of the atrial lead which in this case is about 90°. There is also inadequate redundancy of the ventricular lead.*

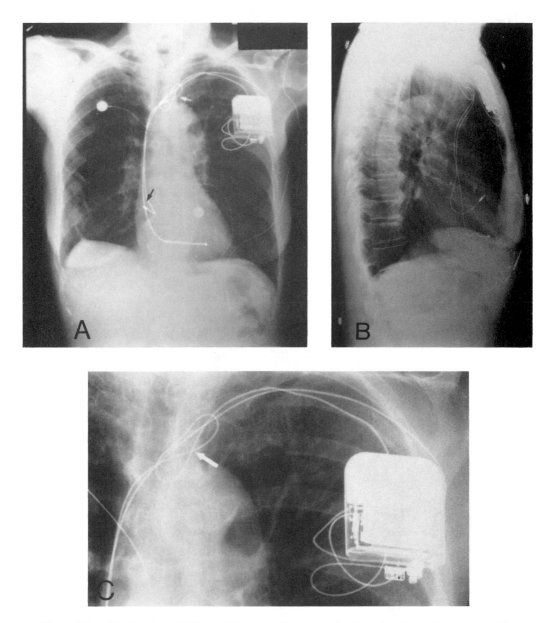

Figure 23.   PA **(A)**, lateral **(B)**, and close-up **(C)** x-rays of a dual-chamber pacing system. The atrial lead is positioned somewhat laterally, best appreciated on the PA (black arrow). The atrial lead is still oriented anteriorly as can be seen on the lateral x-ray. Incidentally noted is a knotting of the leads in the innominate vein (white arrow). This is best appreciated on a close-up **(C)**.

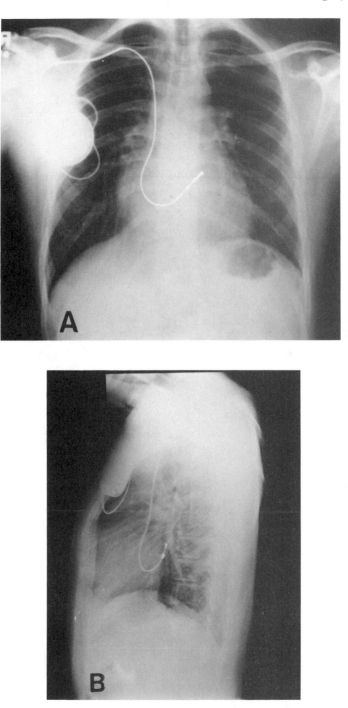

Figure 24. *PA (A) and lateral (B) chest x-rays demonstrating a pacing lead positioned in the coronary sinus for atrial pacing. Previous amputation of the right atrial appendage precluded the usual atrial position. On the PA projection the lead seems to be in the outflow tract of the right ventricle but on the lateral projection the lead is clearly on the posterior cardiac wall and not in the right ventricle.*

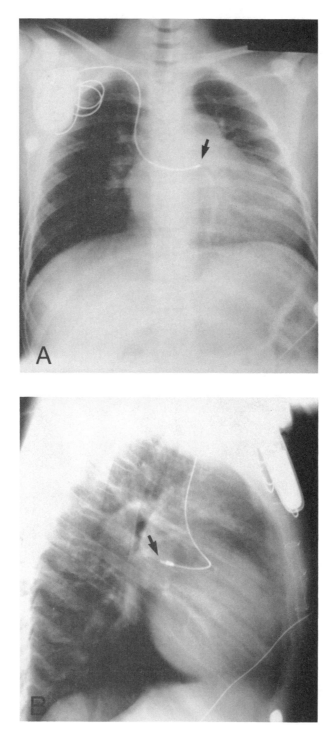

Figure 25. *PA* **(A)** *and lateral* **(B)** *chest x-rays of a patient with transposition of the great vessels and an active fixation lead in the left atrium.*

Epimyocardial Position

The location and type of leads should also be identified when pacing via the epimyocardium. Myocardial ventricular pacing usually is accomplished from the right ventricle by placing the lead(s) on the diaphragmatic cardiac surface (Figure 26). The left ventricle is commonly paced from the free wall via the left anterolateral thoracotomy or the subcostal route. Atrial epimyocardial leads may be placed on either the right or the left atrial appendage. Atrial epimyocardial pacing is relatively uncommon (Figure 27 and 28).

There are also reports of pacing the endocardial surface by placing an endocardial lead through the myocardium from the epicardial surface and placing a pursestring suture around the lead at the entry site. Figure 29 demonstrates such a lead. The patient had a prosthetic tricuspid valve that prevented usual endocardial lead placement. Epimyocardial pacing was attempted several times, and although acute thresholds were acceptable, chronic thresholds were high and pacing could not be maintained.

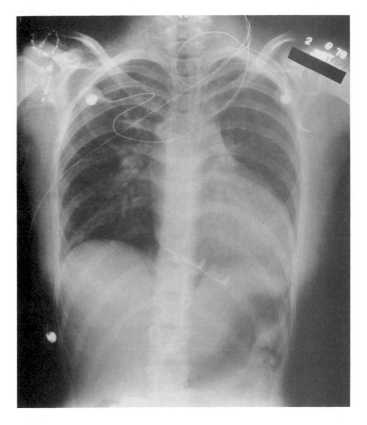

Figure 26. *A bipolar right ventricular epi/myocardial lead system. The sutureless myocardial lead is of the three-turn "screw-in" configuration. The leads have been placed on the diaphragmatic surface of the right ventricle.*

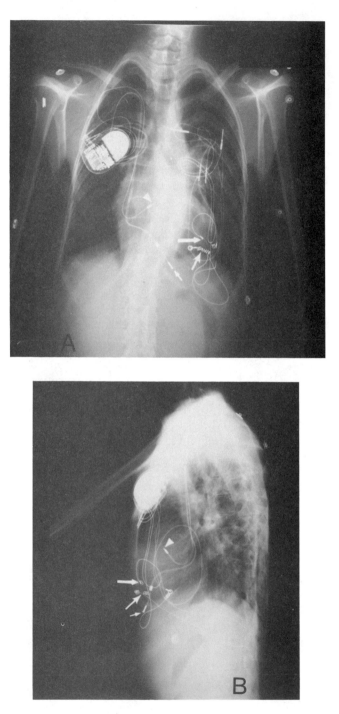

Figure 27.   *PA **(A)** and lateral **(B)** chest x-rays demonstrating a dual-chamber endocardial pacing system. In addition there are multiple abandoned epicardial leads. The largest white arrow points to an epicardial electrode of the "stab-in" variety. There are also multiple "screw-in" **(three-turn)** electrodes.*

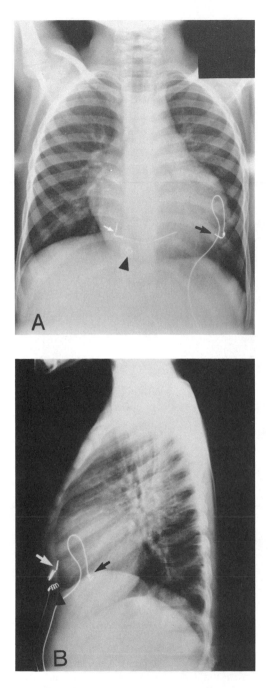

Figure 28. *PA (A) and lateral (B) chest x-rays in a child who had undergone multiple epicardial lead placements. Three different epicardial leads are seen: a fractured Medtronic 6913 lead of which only an abandoned remnant remains (white arrow), the lead had been placed on the right ventricular wall; a Medtronic 5815 "stab-in" epicardial lead (black arrow) placed on the wall of the left ventricle; a Medtronic 6917 sutureless "screw-in" three-turn electrode (black arrowhead) placed on the diaphragmatic surface of the right ventricle between the fractured 6913 and the right ventricular apex.*

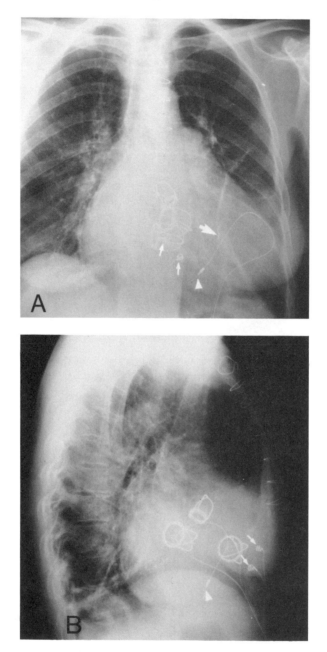

Figure 29. *PA **(A)** and lateral **(B)** chest x-rays demonstrating three pacing leads in a patient with three prosthetic heart valves. Two "screw-in" epicardial leads are seen near the midline on the PA view. A remnant of a "stab-in" epicardial lead is noted by the largest white arrow. The third lead is an endocardial screw-in lead that has been placed through the right ventricular free wall and screwed into the ventricular endocardial surface. This lead is indicated by the arrowhead. A pursestring suture is placed around the myocardium where the lead enters. Of the various polarity combinations possible, the best thresholds were obtained in a bipolar configuration with the endocardial (transmyocardial) lead as the negative and the screw-in epicardial lead as the positive terminal.*

VII. Lead Polarity

The lead should be radiographically identified as unipolar or bipolar. The cathode is always within the heart, and in the unipolar system, the anode is the metallic housing of the pulse generator; only the radiopaque catheter electrode is seen. In a bipolar system, both the radiographic electrode at the lead tip and a more proximal ring electrode can be seen. On occasion, a bipolar lead is converted to a unipolar configuration to accommodate a unipolar pulse generator or to take advantage of superior unipolar sensing or pacing. For this, the positive terminal of the lead is insulated by placing a radiolucent rubber cap over the lead connector pin (Figure 14).

More than two radiographically identifiable metallic poles may be present on the pacing lead. Figure 30 demonstrates a tripolar lead in which one pole is part of the sensor mechanism for a rate adaptive pacing system. Figure 31 demonstrates a unipolar tip and two poles in the region of the atrium. This lead is part of a single-lead VDD pacing system. There are two atrial poles for sensing and unipolar ventricular pacing and sensing.

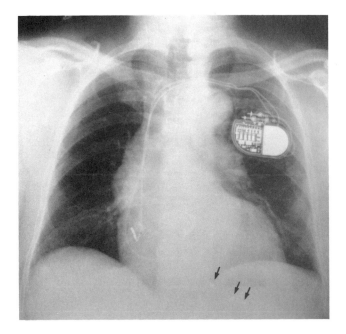

Figure 30.   *PA chest x-ray demonstrating a tripolar ventricular lead. The third pole is for impedance measurements as part of a rate adaptive pacing system. (Incidentally noted is a "crimp" in the lead as it passes between the clavicle and first rib. This patient subsequently developed an insulation failure of the ventricular lead.)*

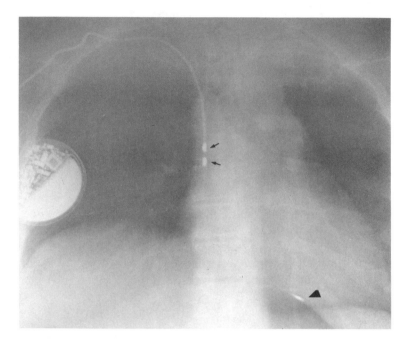

Figure 31. *PA chest x-ray demonstrating a pacing system with a single lead with three poles: one at the tip of the lead (black arrowhead) and two in the region of the right atrium (black arrows). The two atrial poles provide atrial sensing as part of a single-lead VDD pacing system.*

VIII. Lead Type

Although it is often not possible to accomplish, an attempt should be made to identify the specific type of transvenous lead. It can often be determined whether lead fixation is active or passive. Active fixation leads can be differentiated from passive fixation leads with certainty only if an active fixation device can be seen to penetrate the endocardium (Figure 25) or the epicardium-myocardium (Figure 26).

A variety of epicardial active fixation devices are available. In each instance the radiographic appearance of the active fixation mechanism will be different. Four different myocardial leads account for the vast majority of all epimyocardial pacing leads. These are the Medtronic 6917 (three-turn) and 6917A (two-turn) sutureless "screw-in" leads, the older so-called "cobra head" (Medtronic 6913), and the Medtronic 4951 stab-in lead (Figures 27, 28, 29).

IX. Lead Integrity

The lead should be inspected for integrity. An insulation break usually cannot be identified radiographically, but a lead fracture can often be identified (Figures 32, 33, 34, 35). Fractures often occur at positions where strain is applied

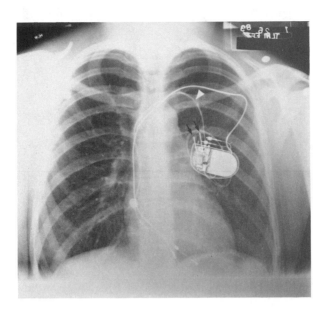

Figure 32A. *Two bipolar leads entering the left subclavian vein, one of which has clearly been abandoned. (Arrows note the proximal portion of the abandoned lead.)*

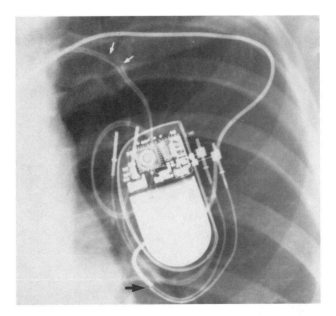

Figure 32B. *A close-up the pulse generator and leads as they enter the subclavian vein shows one lead to have a fracture of one of the conductors at the entry to the subclavian vein (white arrows). The intact lead shows discontinuity at the point of bifurcation (black arrow). This is not a fracture but normal x-ray appearance of this lead.*

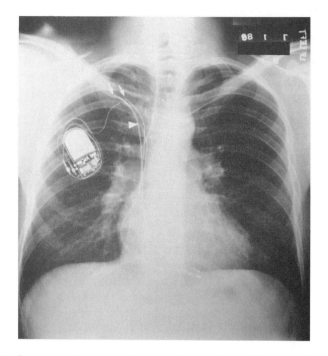

Figure 33. *PA chest x-ray demonstrating a fractured endocardial ventricular lead (arrowhead) and two abandoned and transected endocardial ventricular leads (white arrows).*

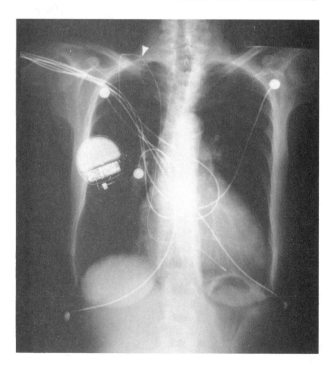

Figure 34. *PA chest x-ray demonstrating a fractured endocardial ventricular lead. The lead was positioned in the internal jugular and the lead fractured where it passed over the clavicle.*

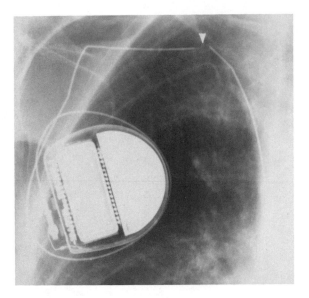

Figure 35A. *A portion of the PA projection of an x-ray of a patient in whom a stylet was left within a permanent pacing lead at the time of initial placement. A fracture occurred of both the lead and the stylet.*

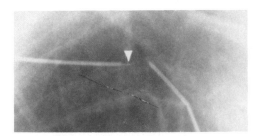

Figure 35B. *A close-up of the lead shows the fractured stylet within the coil of the lead. The fracture occurred at a sharp angulation.*

to the lead and, therefore, within the subcutaneous tissue at the point of fastening of the lead to the vein of entry or within the vein near the point of entry, especially as the lead passes under the clavicle when a subclavian puncture has been used. A fracture may occur near the pulse generator at the connector block (Figure 36) or (infrequently) within the central vein itself. In the first two instances, repair may be possible and easy; in the third instance repair may not be possible.

"Pseudofractures" are radiographic findings only. The term has been applied to two entirely different circumstances. It applies most aptly to the indentations caused by ligatures compressing the insulating material of a rubber or, more recently, polyurethane lead. Such a finding is of special concern because it has been associated with polyurethane deterioration. Use of a nonopaque

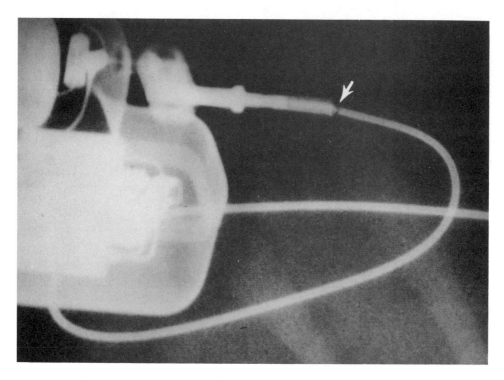

Figure 36.   Close-up of a PA projection of a lead fracture just beyond the connection of the lead and the connector pin.

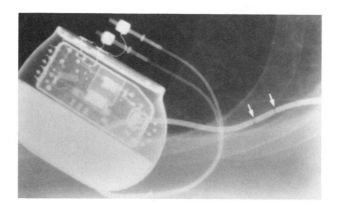

Figure 37.   Close-up of a PA projection of a pulse generator and a proximal portion of the implanted lead. Inspection of the lead clearly shows two areas of indentation caused by ligature compression of the lead unprotected by a rubber sleeve.

rubber "sleeve" for securing the lead may avoid the radiographic finding (Figure 37). The term "pseudofracture" has also been applied, incorrectly, to the normal radiographic appearance of some bipolar leads at the point of bifurcation. Discontinuity may be misinterpreted as a fracture; it is however, only a fine wire connection, which may not be recognized unless one anticipates its presence (Figure 32). Lead integrity of epimyocardial systems may be easier to evaluate. Earlier designs (e.g., Medtronic model #6913) resulted in an incidence of fracture that was greater than in modern leads and which usually occurred at the site of higher stress (Figure 28).

LEAD POSITIONING

Adequate radiographic placement for atrial or ventricular transvenous and myocardial lead positions should be documented. Lead dislodgment may occur and is a common cause of failure to pace and/or sense. Dislodgment may be obvious, i.e., macrodislodgment. Such dislodgement can be anywhere other than its original position, i.e., the pulmonary artery, coronary sinus, ventricular cavity, or superior or inferior vena cava. Dislodgment also can be nonidentifiable radiographically. This has been labeled "microdislodgment," but, in the absence of x-ray documentation, there is no evidence of its presence. It is, therefore, a presumptive diagnosis. It is imperative that when lead malposition or dislodgment is considered, the chest film be compared with previous radiographs (Figures 38 and 39).

X. Multiple Leads

When multiple leads or, uncommonly, multiple pacemakers are visible on the chest radiograph, an attempt should be made to trace each lead from its origin in the pacemaker to its intracardiac or intravascular position. An abandoned lead should be traced on the x-ray to prove that it is free-standing and not connected to the pulse generator. With multiple leads present, the radiographic appearance can become confusing and individual leads can be difficult to trace (Figure 1).

XI. Complications

Complications of the implant procedure itself (hemothorax, pneumothorax, and hemo-pneumothorax) may be identified radiographically (Figures 1 and 2, Chapter 9/Pacemaker Complications). Other complications, including lead perforation, a malpositioned pulse generator, and displaced leads, have been discussed previously in this chapter or in Chapter 9.

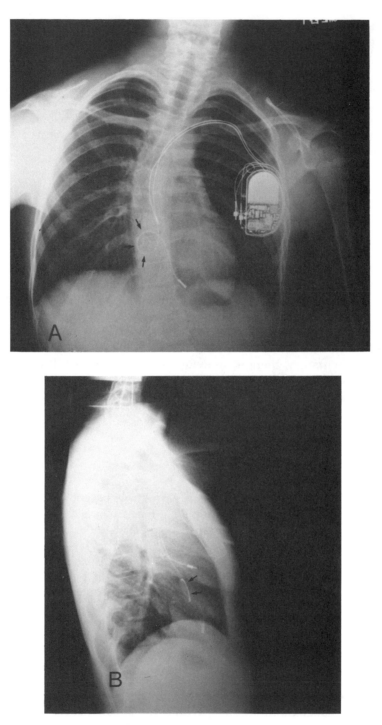

Figure 38. *PA **(A)** and lateral **(B)** chest x-rays demonstrating ventricular and atrial lead dislodgment. A large loop of ventricular lead is coiled in the right atrium and the ventricular lead tip is not in the ventricular apex. The atrial lead is shallow as well.*

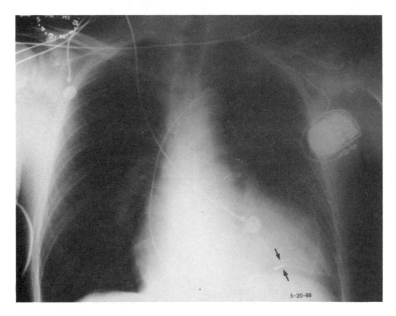

Figure 39A. *PA x-ray demonstrating a bipolar ventricular lead with the lead tip superiorly directed. This x-ray was obtained 24 hours after implant and the patient was displaying intermittent failure to pace and sense.*

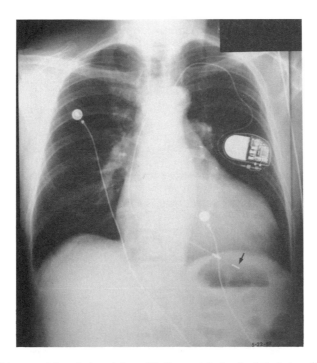

Figure 39B. *PA x-ray taken 2 days later with the ventricular lead tip being directed inferiorly. It appears to be in an apical position. The lead movement had occurred spontaneously, that is, the patient did not undergo invasive repositioning of the lead. Pacing and sensing function was normal.*

SUMMARY

A systematic approach to the interpretation of the radiographic appearance of the pacing system should follow a sequence.

INTERPRETATION OF RADIOGRAPHIC APPEARANCE OF THE PACING SYSTEM

1. Inspect the routine chest PA and lateral x-rays, ignoring the pacing system. Obtain overpenetrated, i.e., thoracic spine films, if necessary.
2. Identify the pulse generator location.
3. Identify the pulse generator model and polarity.
4. Inspect the connector block.
5. Determine the lead(s) position:

   a. transvenous or epimyocardial
   b. atrial or ventricular, or both
   c. if transvenous, its location within a cardiac chamber or the coronary sinus
6. Determine lead polarity and type of fixation.
7. Evaluate lead integrity.
8. Look for other specific complications.

BIBLIOGRAPHY

Austin SM: Pseudofracture of dual chamber pacemaker leads: Avoidance of surgical intervention. New Engl J Med 1987; 84:178–180.

Dunlap TE, Popat KD, Sorkin RP: Radiographic pseudofracture of the Medtronic bipolar polyurethane pacing lead. Am Heart J 1983; 106:167–168.

Grier D, Cook PG, Hartnell GG: Chest radiographs after permanent pacing. Are they really necessary? Clin Radiol 1990; 42:244–249.

Gyarmati J, Worum F, Barnak G, et al: Radiological diagnosis of complications in pacemaker treatments. Radiol Diagn (Berl) 1979; 20:666–675.

Hertzberg BS, Chiles C, Ravin CE: Right atrail appendage pacing: Radiographic considerations. Am J Roentgenol 1985; 145:31–33.

Steiner RM, Tegtmeyer CJ: The radiology of cardiac pacemakers. In D Morse, M Steiner, V Parsonnet (eds.): A Guide to Cardiac Pacemakers. Philadelphia, F.A. Davis Company, 1983, pp. 27–70.

Steiner RM, Tegtmeyer CJ, Morse D, et al: The radiology of cardiac pacemakers. Radiographics 1986; 6:373–399.

Weschler RJ, Steiner RM, Kinore I: Monitroing the monitors: The radiology of thoracic catheters, wires and tubes. Sem Roentgenol 1988; 23:61–84.

Zerbe F, Bornakowski J, Sarnowski W: Pacemaker electrode implantataion in patients with persistent left superior vena cava. Br Heart J 1992; 67:65–66.

Chapter 11

RATE MODULATED PACING

Seymour Furman

The initial approach to implanted ventricular pacing was to provide a stable, regular, reliably paced ventricular rate and rhythm more rapid than the idioventricular rate, which would eliminate the episodes of ventricular asystole and escape tachycardias that characterized the unprotected, atrially dissociated idioventricular rate and rhythm of complete heart block. It was recognized within several years that increased cardiac output resulted from an increase in the ventricular rate. Pacemakers responding to the atrial rate and producing atrial synchrony were evaluated as were ventricular asynchronous pacemakers with external rate control manually set to be slower at rest and more rapid for activity. What seemed to be less well understood was that some level of physiological need, usually exercise, was necessary to increase cardiac output further, as a result of a greater increase in rate. Many studies demonstrated that during a rise in paced ventricular rate, the absence of physiological need produced a brief increase in cardiac output that soon returned (at the higher rate) to the cardiac output at the lower rate (resulting from a decrease in stroke volume). As the increase in rate with constant cardiac output required a commensurate decrease in stroke volume it was then speculated that such a decrease in stroke volume always occurred when rate was increased. The need for the critical element, physiological requirement or exercise, was not clearly understood (Figure 1).

The past decade has demonstrated the central role that ventricular rate plays in cardiac output. The role of the atrial contraction, ventricular preload, the "atrial kick," and AV synchrony remains controversial as it has been for the past several hundred years. Present data seems to indicate that atrial synchrony may be more important at the lower end of the "normal" rate range, i.e., between 50 bpm and perhaps 90–100 bpm. At more rapid ventricular rates, i.e., 120–180 bpm, rate alone seems more important and AV synchrony less so. The normal atrium provides two functions, contraction to empty into and preload the ventricle for its contraction and the provision of a cardiac rate derived from the sensitivity of the sinoatrial node to body metabolic changes, including changes in blood pH, intra-atrial pressure, oxygen and carbon dioxide tension, temperature, reflex signals from the carotid body, and circulating catecholamines.

The four atrial functions relative to cardiac hemodynamics are, therefore, to:

1. propel blood into the ventricle;
2. set the ventricular rate appropriate for need;
3. separate the atrial and ventricular contractions by the most efficient AV interval;
4. avoid ventriculoatrial conduction.

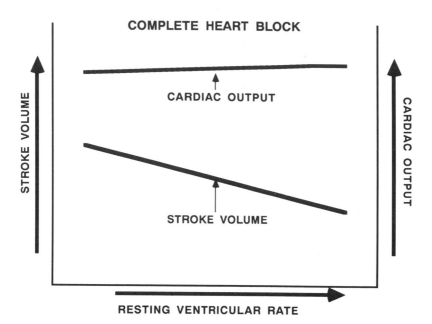

Figure 1. *An increase of resting cardiac rate increases cardiac output very little as stroke volume undergoes corresponding decrease. To increase cardiac output by rate increase, a physiological need must exist.*

The PR interval may have an important effect on cardiac output, although the overall effect may be subtle in many patients and even defy quantification in most patients. A short AV delay (approaching 50 ms) and prolonged AV delay (i.e., 250 ms) reduce cardiac output at rates between 50 and 100 bpm. At more rapid atrial rates the PR interval normally abbreviates, an effect which is reproduced in dual-chamber pulse generators now available. A prolonged PR interval, i.e., 250–400 ms may place atrial contraction after a preceding QRS complex producing the hemodynamic effect of retrograde conduction (Figure 2). Ventriculoatrial conduction can be of very great importance in some patients and in the absence of such VA conduction the ventricular rate is a major determinant of cardiac output (See Chapter 5). Specifically, body compensatory mechanisms reduce stroke volume at increased rates in the absence of need so that simply increasing rate at rest to determine the effect on cardiac output gives a result that if incorrectly extrapolated is erroneous.

The effect of rate modulated ventricular pacing differs, depending on the rhythm being paced. Pacing complete heart block may provide one result while ventricular pacing in the presence of sinus bradycardia with retained retrograde conduction may produce retrograde atrial contraction and the pacemaker syndrome. The consequences of making the right ventricular apex the most rapid "pacemaker" of the heart and the potential reversal of the cardiac contraction sequence remains uncertain. It is important to note that the incidence of retrograde conduction decreases with increases in ventricular rate. Dual-chamber rate modulated pacemakers are now widely available and modulate the normal AV sequence as well as the stimulation rate. Each circumstance, whether atrial,

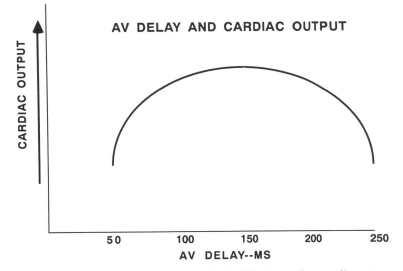

Figure 2. *The electronic analog of the PR interval, the AV delay, affects cardiac output especially at the lower range of atrial rates. While the exact change depends on many factors, maximum output seems to be at about 150 ms from the beginning of atrial depolarization. Efficiency falls at shorter and longer interval durations.*

ventricular, or dual-chamber pacing, each rhythm, AV nodal, or SA nodal disease, or combinations of both in the presence or absence of retrograde conduction, should be judged when selection of a pacing mode is made. It should also be remembered that comparisons should be cautious between single- and dual-chamber pacing whether or not it is rate modulated. The comparison between atrial driven ventricular pacing (VDD or DDD) and rate modulated ventricular pacing (VVIR) should be made cautiously.

With the passage of a quarter century the issues of the existence and duration of an AV delay, extensively discussed during the initial evaluation of atrioventricular sequential (DVI) pacing, have become better understood. The provision of an AV delay of physiological duration is important and the avoidance of retrograde conduction is critical in some patients, but a cardiac rate responsive to activity is probably the single most important factor for increase of cardiac output.

It has also been repeatedly demonstrated that in the presence of complete heart block with fixed antegrade and retrograde block, cardiac output during exercise is similar during atrial synchrony with a normal chronotropic response and ventricular pacing alone at a rate matched to the atrial rate but without atrial synchrony (Figure 3).

With the recognition of the importance of rate, several simultaneous approaches have been undertaken. The one earliest to fruition was the development of a device that would sense the atrium to drive the ventricle and sense the ventricle to avoid competition. VDD and DDD pacemakers provided this capability. In 1976 Cammilli implanted a pacemaker that drove only the ventricle but its rate was set, independently of the atrial rate, by the pH of the central

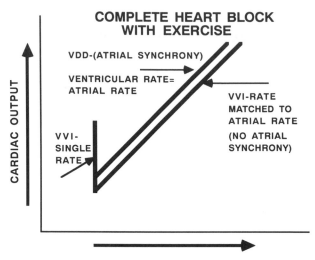

Figure 3.   *In patients with fixed antegrade and retrograde heart block, rate increase, with a normal AV delay, can occur during exercise by pacing with atrial synchrony (VDD), producing a ventricular rate equal to the atrial rate. The ventricular rate can also be paced at the atrial rate but without atrial synchrony. The cardiac output achieved will be similar for both. This realization is the basis for the use of single-chamber (VVI,R) rate modulated pacemakers. At a single rate, (VVI) exercise increases cardiac output far less.*

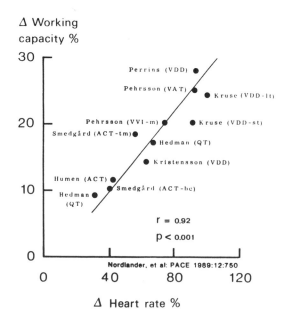

Figure 4.   *Working capacity as a function of increase in cardiac rate has been repeatedly demonstrated. Repeated studies with a variety of sensors including normal atrial activity have shown results that fall on a single regression line at a high level of reliability. The proper name is the first author of the study and the sensor is in parenthesis. ACT = activity; VDD/VAT = atrial synchrony; QT = the stimulus-T sensor) Courtesy of R. Nordlander.*

venous blood. This device, which never achieved acceptance, demonstrated the feasibility of sensing a function other than the atrial depolarization to set the ventricular rate. The increase in cardiac output follows the formula:

$$\text{Cardiac Output} = \text{Rate} \times \text{Stroke Volume}$$

In the normal, increase in cardiac output bears a linear relationship to oxygen consumption that can be increased in three ways. The cardiac rate may be increased in normals by about three-four times between rest and maximal activity. The stroke volume may increase by some 50% and the AV oxygen difference broadens. Oxygen consumption thus depends on:

$$\text{Rate} \times \text{Stroke Volume} \times \text{AV Oxygen Difference}$$

Other consequences such as changes in peripheral and central arterial pressures and in blood pH follow.

The relationship between cardiac rate and work capacity has been repeatedly demonstrated during evaluation of rate modulated pacing systems and is now an established feature of cardiovascular physiology (Figure 4). Rate increases rapidly at low- level exercise, then decreases its rate of increase, and finally reaches a plateau where further increases of rate do not occur even if increasing stroke volume may continue to increase cardiac output (Figure 5).

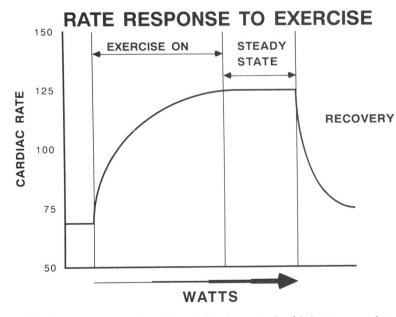

Figure 5. *Cardiac rate response to rest is a stable slow rate. In this instance, pacing at a rate of 70 bpm was selected. With increasing exercise the rate rises rapidly and then at maximum exercise a steady rate is achieved as progressive lactic acidosis occurs. With the cessation of exercise the cardiac rate returns rapidly to resting settings in the normal.*

PHYSIOLOGICAL RATIONALE

Several changes occur during exercise as the metabolic rate increases:

1. Arterial-venous oxygen difference is broadened, i.e., venous oxygen saturation decreases;
2. anaerobic metabolism can occur;
3. venous blood pH is reduced;
4. right-sided cardiac pressures are increased;
5. left-sided cardiac pressures are increased;
6. myocardial contractility is increased;
7. stroke volume increases;
8. body temperature rises;
9. pre-ejection interval changes;
10. changes occur in cardiac muscle electrophysiology.

With these mechanisms cardiac output can be increased several fold at a fixed ventricular rate in a patient with relatively normal myocardial function. Even those with congenital complete heart block can achieve relatively normal cardiac output by the ability to increase stroke volume, associated with the modest rate increase of which congenitals are capable.

But increase of cardiac output by anaerobic metabolism and broadening of the arteriovenous oxygen difference causes oxygen debt that, when sufficiently severe, is always symptomatic producing: (a) breathlessness, and at still more severe levels; (b) chest pain; (c) lightheadedness; (d) muscle cramps, and (e) ventricular ectopy. Reduction of anaerobic metabolism during exercise is desirable.

Sensors of physiological function, whether directly measuring metabolic effect such as central venous pH or oxygen consumption or indirectly by measuring activity can substitute for the normal atrial sensitivity to physiological need. The results of this measurement can then be used to trigger a pacemaker without sensing the atrium. Conditions for which sensor-driven single-chamber ventricular pacing is useful include:

1. large silent atrium;
2. fixed sinus bradycardia with or without nodal rhythm;
3. fixed atrial fibrillation or flutter with AV block;
4. post-ablation AV block with residual atrial arrhythmias;
5. frequent atrial arrhythmias with AV block;
6. chronotropic incompetence, in which the responsiveness of the atrium is not proportional to activity needs and in the absence of retrograde conduction;
7. atrial rate modulated pacing is useful in the presence of fixed sinus bradycardia or chronotropic incompetence with intact AV conduction.

Despite the more clear-cut indications listed above, implantation of a rate modulated single-chamber pacemaker may be used in the presence of intermittent, partial, or complete AV block and sinus node dysfunction to produce a rate variable ventricular pacemaker with a single ventricular lead. In the atrium, with satisfactory AV conduction, such a pacemaker can produce a variable ventricular rate by atrial drive. In the later instance both the normal AV sequence and rate response will result. A DVI or DDD pacemaker in a patient with atrial chronotropic incompetence restores the normal AV sequence but not the cardiac rate response. Dual-chamber rate modulated pacemakers are now widely available.

SENSOR REQUIREMENT

During exercise (i.e., muscle metabolism) various by-products are emitted. These are:

1. heat, producing body temperature;
2. electricity, producing the ECG and EMG (electromyogram);
3. carbon dioxide;
4. lactic acid, i.e., the blood pH will be reduced;
5. intracardiac pressure;
6. movement.

Other electrophysiological changes occur including changes in the duration of the electrocardiographic QT interval, in the ventricular depolarization gradient, i.e., the area under the curve of depolarization beginning with a stimulus and ending as the depolarization returns to baseline. The duration of the pre-ejection interval (PEI) from a stimulus to the resulting ventricular mechanical contraction also changes.

The sinus node responds by changes in rate to variation in carbon dioxide and oxygen tension, temperature, intra-atrial pressure, and hormonal stimuli. Some of these parameters can be measured directly to change pacemaker stimulation rate. Atrial sensing is the traditional measure of body need.

A sensor useful in cardiac pacing is a transducer that will measure one of the effects of by-products of increased metabolism and exercise and produce a signal (usually electrical) that can be sensed by the pacemaker electronic circuit to change the pacemaker automatic interval and therefore the escape rate. The response of the pacemaker to what the sensor detects is referred to as "rate responsiveness," "rate modulation," or "adaptive rate" pacing.

The sensor must respond to physiological or near physiological body activities and be proportional to and capable of mimicking the normal cardiac response. The rate of increase in cardiac rate should be similar to that of the normal human, as should the rate of cool down. The sensor response should parallel the normal response, i.e., it should neither be delayed until well into exercise nor persist after exercise has ended (Figure 6). The onset should be as rapid as the normal atrium, free of idiosyncrasies, i.e., smooth over the entire exercise range, stable over the decades, and reproducible from one time to the next. It should be suitable or adjustable for a wide range of patients, from young to old and from cardiovascular health to fragility. It should respond to nonphysical activity demands such as emotion and mental work. Finally, it should respond appropriately to three different states:

a. rest;
b. mild to moderate activity, i.e., the usual submaximal activity of normal life;
c. maximal activity.

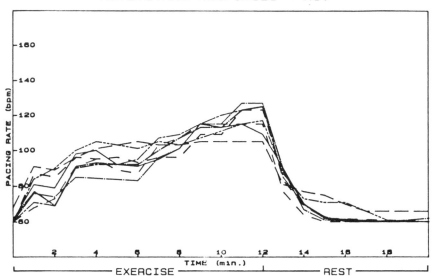

Figure 6. *A graph depicts the external activity responsive pulse generator pacing rate responses, on a treadmill, and at setting MEDIUM 6 of each of 8 healthy volunteers.*

If response is not equal in all three states, the most important is the response to submaximal activity.

Development of a sensor based rate modulated pacing system requires at least four components:

1. Selection of a physiological indicator, changes of which are associated with metabolic need;
2. A sensor that will detect these changes and respond reliably and reproducibly;
3. An algorithm that will translate the changes in the physiological function, detected by the sensor, into a change in pacemaker stimulation rate;
4. A single- or dual-chamber cardiac stimulator (Figure 7).

The opportunity exists to improve upon the atrium that responds to drugs, intercurrent illness, and the development of arrhythmias. It is difficult to stop atrial control of ventricular response in the presence of AV conduction and even in the presence of an arrhythmia. The artificial sensor should be self-monitoring, incapable of exceeding specific high and low rate limits, and should failure occur it must be in a safe manner. Its response should be similar to that of change in the physiological function, without nonlinear response introduced by the sensor itself.

The algorithm is certainly a most important element. The algorithm absorbs the information generated by the sensor and determines the response that will drive the pulse generator. An example of this effect is pacemaker response in a temperature driven system. Blood warmed by lower extremity activity is driven into the central venous system, but is preceded by cool (unwarmed) blood. The first blood to reach an intracardiac thermistor will reduce blood temperature.

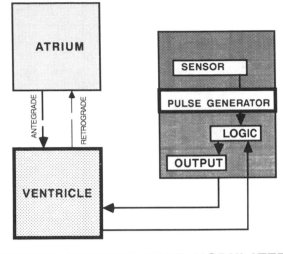

SINGLE CHAMBER-RATE MODULATED
(VVIR)

Figure 7. *A diagrammatic representation of a single-chamber rate modulated pacemaker shows one ventricular input and output channel as in a conventional single-chamber pacemaker. In addition a second input signal originates from the sensor and is directed to the logical system to achieve rate modulation.*

The algorithm should not reduce the cardiac rate in response to the flush of cool blood, rather in the usual algorithm, this flush will cause a step function INCREASE in cardiac pacing rate, perhaps by 15 bpm, i.e., from 70 to 85 bpm. If warm blood follows, the rate increase will be maintained and become proportional to temperature, if not, the rate will return to the preset level. The algorithm will determine the degree of rate change in response to a specific change in sensor activity. It will determine how long to consider a physiological function change as physiological or as artifactual.

Terminology to be understood is that of **OPEN LOOP** and **CLOSED LOOP** sensors. The open loop sensor may not respond to a specific physiological function. If it does, that physiological function is not modified by the pacemaker response, i.e., heart rate generated by the pacemaker. Activity, the most widely used sensor, responds to body motion, imposed extracorporeal movement (e.g., vehicular motion or that imposed directly on the pulse generator, i.e., by tapping the device in its subcutaneous position or by direct pressure on the pulse generator, neither circumstance a natural function), or by direct pressure on the pulse generator. It will not respond to fever or mental stress, both of which are associated with increased metabolic needs. A temperature sensor is partially open loop. An increase in body temperature may be pathological, but even that is associated with increased metabolic need and an increase in heart rate which is in response to the febrile state. The increased metabolism associated with normal vigorous exercise increases central venous temperature which will increase the rate of a temperature sensitive pacemaker, and in this instance, assist in returning temperature to normal. Respiration is also partially open loop. As oxygen is consumed with exercise, the respiratory rate increases, but respiratory rate is also under voluntary (and even involuntary, nonphysiological, e.g., psychiatric) control and to that extent the sensor is not closed loop. The closed loop system responds to physiological change, will increase or decrease rate as a response to such needs, measure the degree of effect on the sensed parameter, and modify its output to the pacemaker accordingly. In the ideal formulation of a closed loop sensor the pacing rate will be modulated by the effect of the pacing rate on the physiological parameter being sensed to establish the pacing rate in the first instance. Were a closed loop system to operate effectively and near perfectly no need would exist for adjustments of sensor sensitivity or responsiveness as presently exists with all sensors in clinical use or evaluation.

Sensors suited to closed loop function include those that measure myocardial mechanics such as the pre-ejection interval and the dP/dt of right ventricular contraction and the stimulus-T interval. For example, the stimulus-T sensor will increase the cardiac rate as the stimulus-T interval is abbreviated, presumably in response to exercise. As the stimulus-T interval is prolonged, the pacemaker-imposed cardiac rate will decline. The difference between the open and closed loop is responsiveness to a specific physiological function and the resultant pacemaker rate affecting the function being sensed. In practice, there may be little difference between the two approaches, and an open loop system may seem to function as well as or better than a closed loop system. Indeed, over 90% of all implanted rate modulated systems (1992) are open loop (activity), most of the remainder are combinations (respiratory rate and minute volume), while a few are closed loop (stimulus-T). Other closed loop systems that have been implanted in humans, i.e., oxygen saturation, pre-ejection interval, and right ventricular dP/dt remain in clinical evaluation.

Sensor utility is based on its response to physiological need resulting from muscular and mental function, the rapidity of onset of response, its smoothness and flexibility, and physiological return to the resting setting. Some responses may be physiological but slow in onset. Central venous temperature, for example, follows muscular activity very well, but its responsiveness is slow, and a brief burst of activity may be completed before a temperature response and a consequent cardiac rate response occurs. Imposed temperatures such as drinking warm or cold liquids will affect the central venous temperature and the pacemaker-imposed cardiac rate. Activity, temperature, and QT interval sensors do not respond proportionately to intellectual activity or to emotion.

Other idiosyncrasies include unequal responsiveness to activity needs. The activity sensor responds to motion, not really to body needs. The response, for example, to movement of the arm on the side of the implanted activity sensor is much greater than to movement of the contralateral arm. Descending a staircase produces a similar or greater rate response to ascending the same staircase, although the metabolic needs are quite different.

All of the single-chamber rate modulated devices suffer from the defect that the ventricle only is paced. This means that for these pacemakers the normal sequence of atrial and ventricular depolarization is lost, and in some patients the variation in cardiac output resulting from the change in position of the atrial contraction relative to the ventricular can produce distinct hemodynamic deterioration and symptomatic fluctuation of blood pressure. The change in the beginning of cardiac depolarization from the SA node to the right ventricular apex can have important hemodynamic effects.

MULTIPLE SENSORS

The era of multiple rate modulating sensors began with the dual-chamber rate modulated pulse generator, in which the atrium, sensitive to the usual mechanisms that increase the sinus rate, and an additional artificial sensor combine to set the ventricular stimulation rate. This mechanism introduces two data inputs, atrium and sensor with the adjudication indicated in Table I. At present, three different artificial sensors have been used in rate modulated dual-chamber pacing: activity, minute ventilation, and that for pre-ejection period and right ventricular pressure. Activity and minute ventilation rate modulated dual-chamber pacemakers are commercially available. Pre-ejection period remains in clinical evaluation. Progressively more sensors will be combined either in single- or dual-chamber pacemakers. Two needs will require the use of multiple sensors:

1. To overcome the limitations of the individual sensor: For example, the stimulus-T and temperature sensors respond well to long-term physiological need, but both respond slowly to onset of activity. "Sprint" activity may have ended before the stimulus-T sensor responds, and may not increase central venous temperature sufficiently to provide any temperature sensor response. Because of the rapid response of the piezoelectric crystal (activity sensor), an effect that most other sensors do not possess, its combination with other less rapidly responsive sensors is being pursued. The idiosyncratic responses of the activity sensor in increasing rate more descending a staircase than ascending and a greater response to upper extremity activity than lower (i.e., bicycle exercise, change in treadmill slope) may be ameliorated by a second sensor more responsive to sustained exercise.

Table I
Atrium and Artificial Sensor

	Atrial Rate		
Sensor Rate	*Below LRL*	*Between LRL & URL*	*Above URL*
Below LRL	Pace at lower rate limit	Track at atrial rate	Track atrial rate to URL
Between LRL & URL	Pace at sensor driven rate	Track or pace at higher rate-atrium/sensor	Pace at maximum sensor rate
Above URL	Pace at maximum sensor rate	Track or pace at higher rate-atrium/sensor	Pace at sensor rate

URL = upper rate limit for atrial tracking; LRL = lower rate limit for atrial tracking.

2. To evaluate the rate modulation function of those sensors setting the stimulation rate: A piezoelectric sensor may be used for its rapid response, while another, e.g., measuring myocardial mechanics, may be used to ascertain whether the most suitable rate had been achieved. It's data may then be used to modify the rate response, i.e., increase or decrease the response in order to achieve the most physiological state. These efforts remain in intensive evaluation and depend on the complexity available from microprocessors, which are progressively being introduced into implantable devices.

DUAL SENSORS

Many of the difficulties of sensors for rate modulation have been the slow response that occurs, sometimes resulting in a rate change after the end of a sprint activity. These sensors may be very responsive to sustained activity but slow in onset, wasting much of their responsiveness to sustained activity because of slow onset of rate modulation. The activity, i.e., piezoelectric sensor, which is not proportional to metabolic need, is nevertheless rapid in the onset of its response—far more rapid than other more metabolically sensitive sensors. Three single-chamber pulse generators with dual-sensor combinations that are (or will soon be) in clinical evaluation include the following:

1. Stimulus-T and piezoelectric (activity)—a combination of an evoked endocardial potential effect, the interval between the pacemaker stimulus and the subsequent T wave and a conventional piezoelectric sensor. The combination provides rapid onset and then sustained response.
2. Minute ventilation and piezoelectric (activity)—a combination of the demonstrated effective minute volume sensor and the piezoelectric sensor.
3. Minute ventilation and paced depolarization integral have been joined in a pulse generator combining the relatively rapid response of the ventricular depolarization gradient and the prolonged response of minute ventilation.

The most common dual-sensor combination is the atrium and another sensor. Four such combinations are commercially available in the form of the DDDR pacemaker. Two device series combine the piezoelectric activity sensor with the atrium, the third is the minute ventilation sensor with the atrium, and the fourth combines an accelerometer and the atrium as a DDDR pacemaker. In comparison with DDD (atrially responsive) pacemakers the activity-atrial dual-sensor combination has not demonstrated sufficient improvement to cause the US Food and Drug Administration (FDA) to allow a claim of improved work tolerance and duration in the device labeling. The minute ventilation-atrial DDDR combination has demonstrated improvement of work tolerance and duration and may so claim in device labeling.

PROGRAMMING

Programming the rate of a single-chamber, single rate pacemaker is generally not difficult as the options are few and the indications for the proper rate under all conditions of activity are even fewer. It has been traditional, and probably correct, to program the rate of a patient in fixed or intermittent complete heart block at 70 bpm, while for those with sinus node dysfunction another rate may be selected. For the dual-chamber, atrial sensing pacemaker, the atrium itself sets the pacemaker rate. The person programming sets a lower rate limit, i.e., that rate below which the heart beat was not allowed, and an upper rate, that above which the pacemaker will not stimulate the ventricle (or track the atrium). Between the two limits the atrium controls the ventricular stimulation rate, the rate of increase or decrease, and the responsiveness to specific activities (Figure 8).

For a rate modulated pacemaker the physician must set the lower and upper rates and the responsiveness of the pacing system, including the acceleration with which it increases and decreases rate and the threshold of physiological or imposed change necessary to produce a change in pacing rate. While the setting of the nonsensor-driven DDD pacemaker may be relatively simple because of the guide the atrium provides, that of the sensor-driven single- or dual-chamber pulse generator may be much more difficult. Programming the DDD pacemaker may be far less labor intensive than programming the rate modulated pacemaker. In the rate modulated device the SENSITIVITY setting determines when response begins and RESPONSIVENESS determines how much of a change will occur. Both settings are required. It is as yet unclear whether a stress or activity test will be routinely required. Should a stress test be performed, the most suitable is as yet unknown. The most widely used stress tests have been designed to evaluate coronary artery disease. It is likely that the majority of patients with implanted cardiac pacemakers have coronary artery disease and testing them will only prove that, but may not give an indication of how best

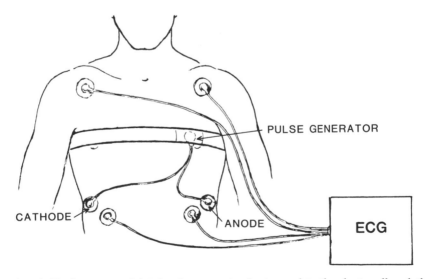

Figure 8. *A bipolar rate modulated pulse generator is strapped to the chest wall and the two outputs are placed as indicated. Pacemaker output is programmed to maximum and produces stimuli that can be detected on the ECG without being felt by the test subject. The response will mimic the implanted pulse generator response.*

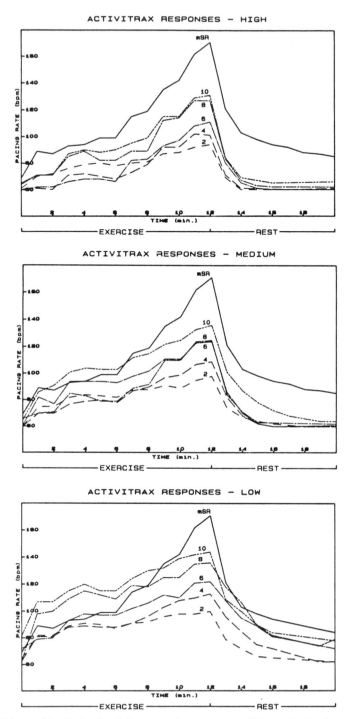

Figure 9.   *This graphic display is of the pacemaker rate set at different levels of responsiveness at the three levels of sensitivity, in each instance compared to the mean sinus rate (mSR) of a group of normal subjects. An external activity responsive pulse generator was used to determine its response.*

to program the implanted pacemaker. The performance of a stress test is a labor-intensive effort. If the test is done at a single setting which then proves to be "incorrect," one or more other tests must be done at other settings (Figure 9).

PROGRAMMING OF RATE MODULATED PACEMAKERS

Programming of the rate modulated parameters is essential to the pacemaker's proper function. Its sensitivity and responsiveness must be such that normal atrial function is approached. Upper and lower rates must also mimic the normal. Single-chamber, rate modulated pacing may be most useful in the child with congenital heart block in whom AV block is not associated with retrograde conduction, although a single case of retrograde conduction with congenital complete heart block has now been described. While implantation of a dual-chamber pacemaker can be successful, growth may cause difficulty with the lead system and only a few DDD pacemakers can readily accommodate the rapid atrial rates of which a young person is capable without developing AV block at the upper rate interval (URI). While a relatively prolonged Wenckebach interval can be programmed to ameliorate sudden onset of AV block, (see Chapter 4, Comprehension of Pacemaker Timing Cycles) a single-chamber ventricular rate modulated device should be considered. A ventricular lead alone may give less long-term difficulty than both atrial and ventricular leads, and when full growth has been reached, an atrial lead can be added during a pacemaker upgrade. A rate modulated upper rate of 150 bpm will allow vigorous physical activity.

Exercise testing and proper programming can set sensitivity, responsiveness, and upper and lower rates to be adequate to reproduce effective ventricular rate modulation. When such exercise programming is undertaken, an approximation of the normal atrial response to exercise should be reproduced (Figure 10). The normal atrial response to exercise is the standard that should be met by all rate modulated devices. If single-chamber, the modulation is based on the sensor alone, if dual-chamber, it is based on the sensor and its interaction with the atrium.

Test of sensor function can be by specific exercise test or formal stress test such as the Bruce, Naughton, or the CAEP (see Table III) (Figure 11). The Holter monitor is probably a more reliable means of assessing rate response than any specific test. Nevertheless, if the patient is inactive on the day of ambulatory monitoring little response may be seen. A low level of response may also not allow distinction between an inactive day and an underresponsive unit. In any event, it cannot be assumed that programming to specific settings without exercise testing will be satisfactory for the individual patient (Figure 12). Several devices provide a sensor passive mode in which the sensor will not drive the stimulation rate but in which a histogram can be printed to indicate what rates have been determined by the sensor to be appropriate for the patient's activity level. These can assist during evaluation of sensor programming in providing a rapid, numerical indication of the pacemaker sensor response.

The single-chamber rate modulated pacemaker should not be programmed

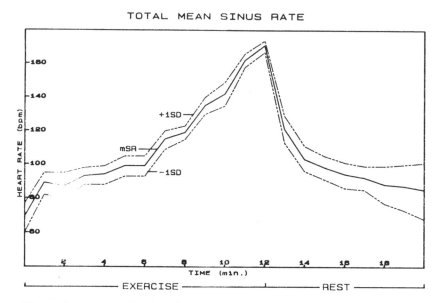

Figure 10. *This graphic display is of the overall mean sinus rate (mSR) ± one standard deviation of a group of normal volunteers of age 20 through age 70 during exercise testing.*

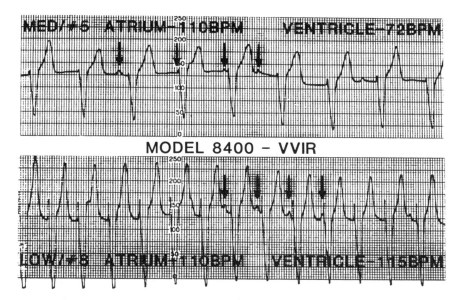

Figure 11. *Programming sensor sensitivity and responsiveness are essential to an appropriate response. In this analysis the atrial rate of approximately 110 per minute represents need, but the SENSITIVITY of MEDIUM and RESPONSIVENESS of level 5 do not produce a commensurate response. Programming to LOW (greater sensitivity to activity and 8 (greater responsiveness) yield a proportional response, i.e., equal to the atrial rate.*

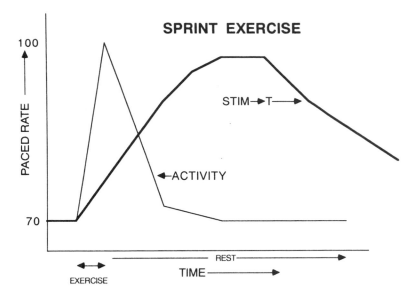

Figure 12. *The difference in onset of response of two different sensors, one rapid and the other relatively slower may be substantial. As a result of a short sprint exercise, the activity sensor increases its rate promptly and with rest returns to baseline. The stimulus to T sensor responds more slowly and, in this instance, the rate response occurs after the sprint has ended and persists during rest.*

to that rate modulated mode unless it is needed. In a person with episodic asystole, but who is largely in a normal spontaneous rhythm, it is unlikely that rate modulation programming will achieve exactly the correct rate modulation. Consequently, setting modulation to be excessively sensitive and/or responsive may cause ventricular stimulation when none is necessary. It is then probably wiser to provide a slower ventricular inhibited function merely to interrupt asystole, should it occur. Rate modulated atrial pacing should also be used when possible as it provides the equivalent of a dual-chamber rate modulated pacemaker. The status of AV conduction should be carefully assessed and the stimulation rate in the modulated mode should not be allowed to reach that rate at which onset of Wenckebach conduction occurs.

CARDIAC RHYTHMS SUBJECTED TO PACING

There are two broad rhythm categories that are subjected to cardiac pacing. One is that of disturbance of AV conduction (often referred to as AV node dysfunction). The second is sinus (SA) node dysfunction or sick sinus syndrome. Some patients have both AV and SA nodal (binodal) dysfunction. The characteristics of the two conditions are different. While ventricular bradycardia and asystole are indications for cardiac pacing common to both conditions, several modifying circumstances exist. Those with sinus node dysfunction usually are characterized by the presence of antegrade conduction and two thirds of them have retrograde conduction at some rate. Those with AV block, whether intermittent or fixed, have retrograde conduction less frequently, about one third of the time, at some paced rate (Chapter 2). Sinus node dysfunction is not progressive. Implant may be performed when arrhythmias and symptoms are most severe and both may recur, remain at the same level of severity, or be ameliorated over the long term. In AV block, the severity of the conduction disturbance is likely to be progressive. Both antegrade and retrograde conduction will deteriorate over time. The effect of ventricular stimulation, especially at different rates is quite different. Pacemaker syndrome, which results in part from the effects of retrograde conduction, occurs more frequently in sinus node dysfunction than AV node dysfunction. Ventricular pacing in sinus node dysfunction is more likely to be associated with echo beating and with pacemaker syndrome.

Retrograde conduction after ventricular stimulation occurs at some rate in about 45% of patients who require pacemaker implantation, but that incidence includes ventricular rates of 60–80 bpm. The effects of retrograde (VA) conduction producing decreases in peripheral arterial pressure and cardiac output occur either with single rate ventricular pacing or with small increases in paced ventricular rate when that rate does not exceed the lower physiological range. At a rate of 100 bpm only 25% of patients have 1:1 retrograde conduction and at 120 bpm and above fewer than 10% of patients will have retrograde conduction. As the main cause of pacemaker syndrome is retrograde conduction, it is possible that absence of VA conduction will allow decoupling of the atrium and ventricle at more rapid ventricular rates without deleterious effects. If so, some of the potential timing problems caused by dual-chamber pacemaker atrial and ventricular channel refractoriness and blanking, which occur at rapid paced atrial rates, may be avoided by a strategy of retaining atrial synchrony at slower rates and abandoning it at more rapid paced rates i.e., allowing sensor-driven ventricular rates at the upper end of the physiological range. However the issue of single- and dual-chamber pacing is eventually resolved, rate modulation is a standard and programmable mode of operation of a cardiac pacemaker.

SENSORS FOR CLINICAL PACING

The Atrium

The atrium has been the traditional sensor of body need. In patients with congenital heart block the ventricles may be moderately responsive in rate, and the overall result may be relatively normal cardiac output without AV synchrony or atrial drive of ventricular rate. Such ventricular responsiveness does not occur with postoperative heart block in the patient with congenital heart disease or with acquired heart block occurring later in life. In both instances ventricular rate is fixed (except that the idioventricular rate may slow or stop) and be unresponsive to body needs.

The atrium is a reliable sensor of body need for most people, but it may be dissociated from the ventricle via AV nodal disease and it may suffer its own disabilities caused by sinus node dysfunction, atrial fibrillation, flutter, and other supraventricular arrhythmias. In the presence of such dysfunction the atrium becomes an unreliable sensor of body needs. An even more significant technical impediment to the atrium as a sensor of body needs is the present requirement of a lead specifically to sense the atrium. The placement of two leads, one for the ventricle and the other for the atrium has never achieved popularity beyond about one -third of implants in the United States and even less in some other countries. This problem has persisted despite the widespread availability of leads deemed to be reliable and readily implanted.

Three ways of sensing atrial activity have been available:

a. The conventional lead that makes contact, either by active or passive fixation, with the atrial wall. This lead may sense or pace the atrium or do both.
b. A lead that senses atrial activity without direct contact with the atrium, i.e., is part of the ventricular lead, and therefore does not contact the atrial wall. This lead may sense atrial activity sufficiently discretely so that atrial synchrony can be provided for VDD pacing. Several such leads and pulse generators are available. One is named "dual atrial bipolar" (DAB) (See Chapter 3).
c. A similar lead as in (b) may sense atrial activity, but less reliably, so that the generator must have a slow response time and avoid falling back to the lower rate escape interval when a P wave is unsensed. The pacemaker rate then rises slowly to approximate the atrial rate and descends slowly. It never provides atrial synchrony, rather a ventricular rate that approximates the atrial rate. One such lead and pulse generator system had been in clinical evaluation but are no longer available.

All of these techniques are prey to the problems of atrial arrhythmia, and in the event of its persistence the only effective resolution may be return to single rate ventricular pacing. The first system (above) involves a second lead (clearly a less popular route), while the latter two involve a single lead only in which atrial sensing occurs via an electrode that is part of the ventricular lead.

Activity

During the early 1980s atrial synchronous (VDD) pacemakers were introduced that sensed atrial activity using a specific atrial lead (above) without the capability of pacing the atrium. With the advent of DDD generators, which are also capable of VDD pacing, most VDD generators fell from use. In one design the atrial channel input was replaced by input from a piezoelectric crystal which was part of the pulse generator case. This device was programmable, as was the original VDD generator, to three levels of sensitivity, corresponding to the three programmable levels of atrial electrogram amplitude and to ten levels of responsiveness that corresponded to programmable AV interval. In a single-chamber version, the device and its successors have become the most successful of rate modulated pacing systems and have been used in the atrium and in the ventricle. For ventricular use, it is programmable to four levels of sensitivity, the least sensitive referred to as HIGH, MEDIUM, then MEDIUM-LOW and the most sensitive LOW. There are also ten levels of responsiveness, numbered from 1, the least responsive, to 10, the most responsive.

The voltage developed by the crystal on the pacemaker case may be 5–50 mV at rest and as much as 200 mV during running or other vigorous activity. The most sensitive responsiveness, i.e., number 10, corresponds to an AV interval of 25 ms and the least sensitive, number 1, to an AV interval of 250 ms.

The response of the piezoelectric crystal results from episodic or continuous pressure. Most sensed events result from body movement, although imposed movement as from vehicular movement, sleeping face down, applying pressure to the device in its pectoral subcutaneous position, and tapping of the device can increase its rate.

In practice the response of the piezoelectric crystal is the most rapid of any of the sensors and movement causes as prompt a response as the normal atrium. The device seems to be tuned to a lower frequency limit of 2 Hz and an upper frequency limit of 70 Hz. The maximum frequency of body motion seems to be in the range of 0.1 to 4 Hz, and filtration above 8 Hz may be effective in reducing interference.

Piezoelectric crystal signals are emitted singly and their frequency and amplitude are determined within the device. These individual "on-off" signals are then counted and the pacemaker rate response is determined. Another use of the piezoelectric crystal is tuned similarly but with a somewhat lower upper frequency limit. The pacemaker rate is determined by integrating the vibrational forces to which the pulse generator is subjected. The former design sets the rate by detecting suprathreshold voltage emissions from the crystal which, in turn, are set by programming sensitivity. The later version integrates the electrical results of all vibrational forces. Clinical experience has suggested a somewhat smoother and more proportional response to workload, although the significance of the difference may not be great. Both approaches to the use of the piezoelectric crystal sensor produce relatively similar responses. Both respond rapidly, one more rapidly during walking, another somewhat more proportionally. Both suffer from greater responsiveness to body vibration than to actual activity. Both respond to walking up and down stairs so that ventricular rate may not be proportional for the effort expended while walking up or down a staircase.

For activity sensitive units, other physical activities that have little vibrational effect produce little pacemaker response. Handgrip, Valsalva maneuver, and standing produce minimal response. Jogging in place produces a prompt maximum response. Whether disproportionate response will occur with the other versions of piezoelectric crystal sensing remains to be determined. It must be emphasized that the idiosyncratic responses described remain relatively modest and have not limited the usefulness of the rate modulated approach. Indeed, the present field of rate modulated pacing, for single- and dual-chamber devices is dominated by activity sensing. Respiration and especially minute ventilation are of growing importance as are other physiologically based sensors.

ACCELEROMETER

The piezoelectric crystal bonded to the inside of the pulse generator case has been widely used and is maximally sensitive to up and down motion, such as occurs with walking, ascending and descending stairs, etc. This is generally

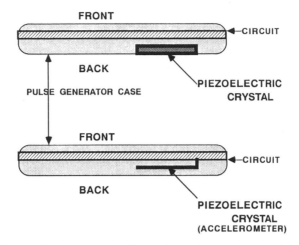

Figure 13. *Both the activity sensor and the accelerometer are based on the piezoelectric crystal. The orientation of the crystal is different in both, and that difference allows sensing of different kinds of motion. The activity sensor piezoelectric crystal is bonded to the back of the pulse generator can. The accelerometer is attached to the circuit board and lies free within the can. Both can be used with conventional leads.*

associated with the "heel strike rate." An alternative to this approach is to mount the crystal within the pulse generator case so that it is more sensitive to forward motion. The device is then called an accelerometer (Figure 13). Single- and dual-chamber accelerometer devices have been released for general use. It remains to be determined whether the activity sensing device or the accelerometer will be preferable or, as seems likely, that they will be similar (Figure 14).

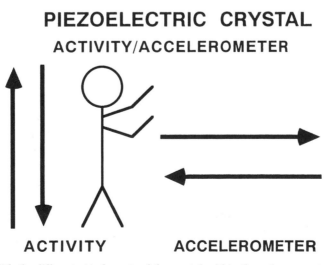

Figure 14. *With the different attachments of the crystal within the pulse generator the intent has been to change the responsiveness of the sensor from up and down, i.e., "heel strike," movement in the activity sensor to to-and-fro movement in the accelerometer.*

ENDOCARDIAL EVOKED POTENTIAL

QT Interval

It has been recognized since 1920 that the interval between the onset of the QRS complex and the end of repolarization i.e., the T wave, varies as a function of cardiac rate. The QT interval duration and the variation of rate result, at least in part, from the effect of circulating catecholamines, exercise, and the administration of some medications such as beta blockers. In 1979 Rickards was able to demonstrate in the presence of complete AV block that the interval between the stimulus beginning the ventricular depolarization and the end of repolarization i.e., the T wave, was abbreviated during activity even without change in the ventricular rate. Conversely the duration of the stimulus-T (or QT) interval was prolonged at rest. The duration of the interval could then be considered an indicator of activity and of the need for an increased ventricular paced rate, could participate in an algorithm, and in turn, drive a pulse generator. Because of the absence of an easily discernible repolarization wave the technique cannot be used for atrial pacing (Figure 15).

A single unipolar ventricular lead can sense the stimulus-T interval. The principle operates by pacemaker emission of a stimulus to drive the ventricle and sensing of the end of the resultant T wave. In the absence of a paced ventricular event the stimulus-T interval cannot be determined. Therefore, should the patient, during rest or activity, assume a ventricular rate more rapid than the pacemaker lower rate limit, no rate modulation sensing mechanism exists (Figure 16).

In the presence of ventricular pacing the emission of a stimulus causes the beginning of a 200 ms pacemaker absolute refractory period. No event can be sensed, particularly the depolarization of the ventricle. At the conclusion of 200 ms a new window for sensing begins. This window is specifically designed to

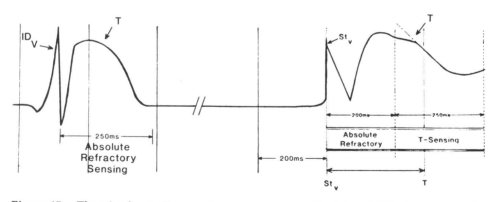

Figure 15. The stimulus to T pacemaker sensor measures the interval following a pacemaker stimulus to the end of the repolarization (T) wave of the ventricular response. To the left is a spontaneous event, sensing of which is followed by a conventional 250 ms interval of ventricular refractoriness. The event to the right is a pacemaker-induced contraction (St$_v$) followed by 200 ms of absolute refractoriness then by another 250 ms during which the T wave is sensed to set the Stimulus to T interval.

DETERMINATION OF STIMULUS TO T INTERVAL
AND PACING RATE DURING EVOKED POTENTIAL
→   PACING

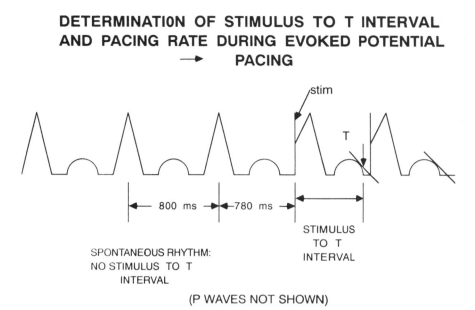

Figure 16. *During use of any evoked response as the sensor of pacer rate, the determination can only be made following a pacemaker stimulus. As long as the spontaneous ventricular rate is above (i.e., at a shorter coupling interval) the lower rate limit (i.e., the escape rate) no rate modulation occurs. Periodically the pacemaker "tests" the rate by emitting a stimulus at a shorter coupling interval than the existing cardiac rate so that a ventricular capture beat occurs and the stimulus to T interval can be determined.*

sense the T wave. During this interval the pulse generator can be programmed for sensitivity to the T wave and for the duration of sensing. The interval between the stimulus and the sensed T wave can then be determined and the rate accordingly modified. Following the T wave sensing interval the pacemaker becomes conventionally sensitive to ventricular activity until the end of the lower rate limit.

Should the coupling interval of the spontaneous ventricular rate be shorter (i.e., a more rapid rate) than the pacemaker lower rate limit, a QRS complex will fall during the conventional sensing interval that follows the absolute refractory period and the T sensing window. This will start another variety of cycle. In this instance the absolute refractory period is 250 ms in duration and is followed by normal ventricular sensitivity. Each such cycle will be abbreviated by 6.4 ms in duration so that eventually the abbreviated cycle will be shorter than the patient's spontaneous ventricular cycle length and a stimulus will be emitted. Once that stimulus is emitted the stimulus to T interval can be retested and the appropriate rate determined once again.

Because the T wave is of low amplitude and frequency content, maximum sensitivity must be available. High impedance leads generally attenuate the ventricular depolarization and repolarization electrograms and are therefore unsuitable for use with the stimulus-T pacemaker. Electrodes of generally low impedance such as large surface area, platinum-iridium, and porous and carbon tip electrodes seem better suited. Earlier 8 mm^2 electrodes such as the continuous (or ball-tip) lead, which had very low and satisfactory stimulation thresholds, seem unsuited for sensing the T wave.

The operation of the device as described may be problematic during alternation between paced and spontaneous ventricular activity. Therefore, two operating modes are available. The first is an operating mode in which it is assumed that there will be continuous pacing as exists during complete antegrade atrioventricular block. If this is not the case then another mode referred to as "tracking" is useful. The tracking mode operates by the abbreviation of the interval by 6.4 ms as described above. A difficulty with this approach is the assumption that the change in duration of the stimulus-T interval is linear between the lower and the upper rate limit. The interval is not linear and the algorithm which determines the change in rate as a function of the change in stimulus-T interval has been reworked to avoid the presumption of linearity and to provide a dynamic change in slope so that the response as a change in rate is different at different ventricular rates. Other difficulties with this device have been the absence of response in some patients who, for reasons as yet unclear, do not develop the same degree of abbreviation of the QT interval either during exercise or during emotion as is anticipated. Some investigations have suggested that the duration of the stimulus-T interval is independently influenced by changes in sympathetic tone as well as heart rate and that in some patients these influences may be in opposing directions. The stimulus-T interval is also affected by drugs such as beta blockers which will then modify the exercise response. The stimulus-T sensor has been combined with a piezoelectric sensor. This combination is now in clinical evaluation.

Paced Depolarization Integral

Another approach is based on the concept of the "ventricular gradient." If the endocardial electrogram voltages are integrated over a cardiac cycle, electrophysiological dispersion may be determined. Such dispersion may be measured via a right ventricular pacing electrode. This measurement, as the measurement of stimulus-T duration, depends on instantaneous recovery from post-stimulus polarization. The area of the post-stimulus ventricular depolarization gradient depends on the activity status of the myocardium. At implant the desirable gradient is set at a specific level of rest or activity and the pacemaker attempts to adjust the cardiac rate to retain the "normal" depolarization gradient area. The cardiac rate is thus adjusted with need. Both this technique and the stimulus-T measure the cardiac evoked potential and as such can determine whether a depolarization occurs after a stimulus. It is possible to increase stimulus energy if no depolarization follows a stimulus and consequently a technique of automatic threshold determination to provide safety by automatic increase in output as necessary (Figure 17). This sensor has been combined with the minute ventilation sensor in a single-chamber device now in clinical evaluation.

These two sensors (stimulus-T and paced depolarization integral) are especially able to evaluate the state of the myocardium. As such they are being investigated for use in distinguishing between a variety of ventricular arrhyth-

EVOKED POTENTIAL

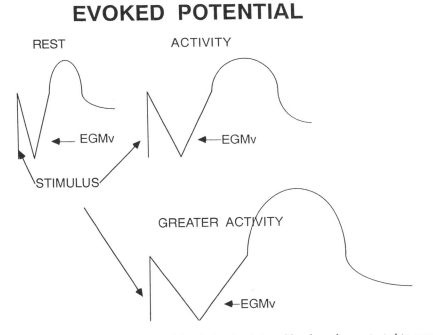

Figure 17. *Evoked Potential. The paced depolarization integral has been demonstrated to correlate with the activity status of the heart. A cardiac stimulus is required to begin sensing the result of the ventricular response. The width of the measured ventricular electrogram broadens with greater activity. It is then possible to correlate duration of depolarization with pacemaker rate.*

mias, especially in attempting to determine whether a tachycardia is ventricular or supraventricular in origin.

BODY TEMPERATURE

In 1951 Bazett, who in 1920 described variation in duration of ventricular systole (QT interval) as a function of activity, described a change in central body temperature as a result of the metabolism resulting from increased muscular activity. Skeletal muscular contraction is about 20% efficient; that energy not expended in actual movement is converted into heat which increases the local blood temperature. With maximum activity it is possible to increase central venous temperature from 37° C (98.6° F) to 38.5° C (101.3° F). A thermister in the central venous system, i.e., the right ventricle, can detect the change and increase the ventricular rate in response. The measurement of central venous pressure is thus a sensitive and reliable indicator of the metabolic state. Nevertheless deficiencies exist. The increase in temperature is not linear with activity and interrupted activity must be carefully assessed. In the absence of a linear relationship between temperature and cardiac rate each algorithm defines activity as a deviation in temperature from the immediately preceding level. Brief activity will result in a temperature and cardiac rate change. If the subject rests briefly and then resumes activity, the calculation of the temperature change begins at the new, and higher, temperature level which resulted from the first activity. The repeat activity may then raise the temperature proportionately less. Careful preparation of the algorithm to which this data is provided is therefore required (Figure 18).

The algorithm must account for multiple factors. These include a slow temperature rise because of two characteristics. The first is that an increase in central venous temperature is a relatively slow response to activity. Brief activity, such as a sprint (e.g., to catch a bus) may not produce a sufficient temperature change to increase the cardiac rate or, if it does, may have ended before the central temperature has risen, so that the physiological tachycardia will occur after the end of the activity. Another difficulty is the response to fever. While tachycardia normally is associated with hyperthermia, the device is unable to distinguish between a physiological increase in body temperature and an imposed hyperthermia. As a result, after a variable interval following the increase in temperature, rate will return to the lower setting, in effect disregarding the fever. Some modest changes in core temperature result from the ingestion of very warm or very cold foods. These too can inappropriately affect the pacemaker perception of body temperature and the cardiac rate. The biggest problem may be the difficulty in setting the device perception of the resting body temperature so that the baseline from which rate increases are calculated is properly leveled.

Still another problem is the site of the development of heat. The major site is the muscular mass of the lower extremities. With the onset of activity, local

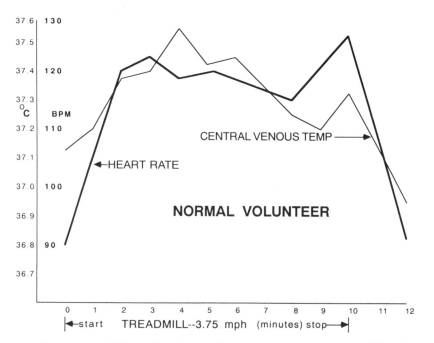

Figure 18. During treadmill exercise the central venous temperature, measured by a thermistor in the right ventricle, correlates well with the cardiac rate in a normal volunteer. This correlation allows the change in temperature to be used as an indicator of physiological need.

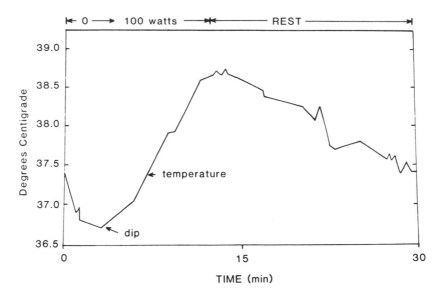

Figure 19.   *During measurement of central venous temperature the first flush of returning blood after the beginning of lower extremity activity is relatively cool, producing the centrally measured temperature dip. Warm blood follows, in this instance, producing a temperature increase of over 1.5° C. This response is sufficient to drive a rate modulated pacemaker. Rest allows core temperature to decline.*

blood is warmed and muscular movement propels the blood toward the central system. The initial blood arriving in the heart is at a lower temperature than the blood already there as blood from the extremities is normally cooler than central blood. The initial flush of blood therefore reduces the temperature and may falsely slow the cardiac rate when an increase is required. The algorithm must be sensitive to this change and must be able to correct the rate should the flush of cool blood not be followed by warmer blood. A common resolution for the problem is an increase in pacemaker rate to result from the temperature reduction, with a continued increase from the subsequent warm blood or a return to the lower rate if warm blood does not follow (Figure 19).

One implantable temperature regulated single-chamber pacemaker is commercially available that can respond to the temperature changes. Other devices, which had been in clinical evaluation, have not been commercially released. These manufacturers are now evaluating other sensors.

RESPIRATION

The linkage of respiration and heart rate is conceptually relatively recent. An almost linear relationship exists between minute ventilation and cardiac rate during exercise. While there is individual variation the correlation is close. Two factors that require measurement are respiratory rate and the tidal volume. Both systems use thoracic impedance measurement to estimate respiratory rate or respiratory rate and tidal volume, which constitute minute ventilation. The basis for this measurement is that oxygen consumption may be the single most physiological determinant of metabolic need. One technique of determining the respiratory rate is by impedance variations between the pacemaker case and a second lead implanted subcutaneously in the chest wall (Figure 20). This technique has been supplanted by a second electrode on the ventricular lead, eliminating the need for a second, i.e., chest wall lead. The interelectrode impedance can be measured by placing current impulses between the electrode tip and the pulse generator. By maintaining a pulse repetition rate (125 ms per cycle) and a brief pulse duration and low intensity, no adjacent muscle stimulation occurs and the current consumption from the pulse generator battery is sufficiently small so that there is little effect on device longevity (Figure 21).

The alternative approach calculates minute ventilation by impedance measurements made between a bipolar pacemaker lead and the pulse generator case. As above, short duration, low-amplitude constant current pulses one tenth to one hundredth of the level required either to stimulate the heart or to produce ventricular arrhythmias are delivered through the ring electrode and detected by the tip. The impedance of the system increases during inhalation and decreases during exhalation. The amplitude of these impedance changes is proportional to the tidal volume. Calculation of minute ventilation can readily be made as they are the product of frequency of respiration (breaths per minute) and tidal volume. Repetitive minute ventilation calculations continually update a timing mechanism that establishes the cardiac pacing rate. This respiratory pacemaker changes the cardiac stimulation rate in response to the rate of respiration and to the tidal volume, both of which make up minute ventilation—

RESPIRATORY SENSING PACEMAKER

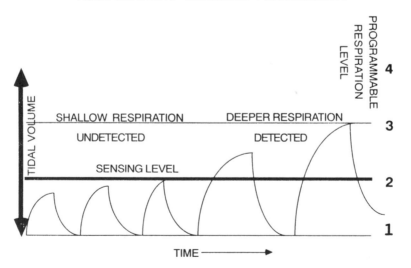

Figure 20. *In the respiratory sensing pacemaker that measures the depth and rate of respiration with a lead in the subcutaneous tissue, a sensing level and a resting cardiac rate are programmed. Should depth of respiration exceed the sensing level, stimulation rate increases. If the depth of respiration is adequate to be sensed and the rate increases, the cardiac rate increases further.*

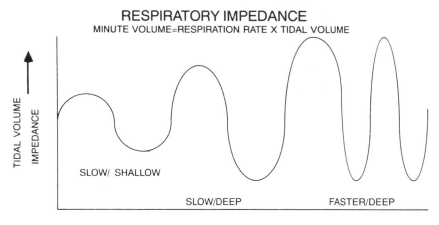

Figure 21. *The sensor of intrathoracic impedance to determine minute ventilation senses the depth and rapidity of respiration by changes in impedance. Increase in respiratory rate and/or depth produce increases in the cardiac paced rate.*

a value that has been demonstrated to correlate well with exercise. Upper and lower rate limits for the cardiac rate are established and are independent of the respiratory rate. Respirations greater than 60 breaths per minute will not increase the cardiac pacemaker rate but will trigger a return toward the lower rate limit. A lower rate limit is established as well. The constant current pulses can be detected by the conventional sensing circuit of the pulse generator and reduction of sensitivity may be required to allow unimpeded pacing. The measurement of minute ventilation, out of clinical evaluation in the United States, has achieved a significant role in rate modulated technology and is available in single-chamber and dual-chamber systems.

PRE-EJECTION INTERVAL

The interval between the beginning of electrical and mechanical systole in either the right or left ventricle has been referred to as the pre-ejection period or interval. This interval is mediated by autonomic influences that normally increase cardiac rate and the force and speed of contraction with metabolic need. The pre-ejection interval should then shorten with each of these stresses. This is, of course, a wholly physiological combination of events and varies with change in metabolic state. Active exercise involving movement or isometric exercise such as handgrip, emotion, and increase in circulating catecholamines and sympathetic tone all abbreviate the pre-ejection interval to a degree well correlated with atrial rate. In practice the potentially measured preejection interval during cardiac pacing will be between the ventricular pacemaker stimulus and the beginning of ventricular systole. The interval will be very different measured from the intrinsic deflection of a spontaneous beat to the beginning of mechanical systole (Figure 22).

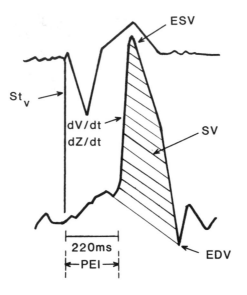

Figure 22.   *The measurement of myocardial mechanics following a pacemaker stimulus (ST$_v$) allows determination of the interval between the stimulus and beginning of the ventricular response. The pre-ejection interval (PEI), and the rate of development of the myocardial contraction, i.e., , the dV/dt of the upstroke velocity and the impedance of the system, dZ/dt, all change with contractility, which in turn changes with exercise. This system allows calculation of end systolic volume (ESV), end diastolic volume (EDV) and stroke volume (SV), all of which also change with physiological need.*

It remains important to correlate the pre-ejection interval of the right ventricle (which is measured by a pacemaker lead) with that of the left ventricle and to determine whether responsiveness, degree of response and its variation in duration are similar to that of the left ventricle. Presumably, measurement of electrical (depolarization) and mechanical events can be accomplished by a specialized right ventricular electrode. This parameter is better recorded during complete heart block, without spontaneous ventricular activity, as are other evoked potential measurements. To determine the appropriate cardiac rate when the spontaneous rate is more rapid than the lower rate limit episodic cardiac stimulation is required. Atrial pacing alone will probably not be possible. With a dual-chamber mode, the atrial rate can be driven by the response to episodic ventricular stimulation.

pH

In 1977 Cammilli made the first attempt to use a sensor other than the atrium. In so doing, he demonstrated that the pH of the mixed venous blood decreased by as much as 0.06 (became more acidotic) during activity. This effect is mediated by the production of lactic acid during anaerobic metabolism. The pacemaker rate was correlated with pH to increase with reduction in pH and return to normal as pH rose. The measurement of pH was by an iridium/iridium

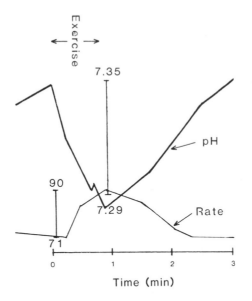

Figure 23. *Measurement of blood pH beginning with rest, continuing for 1 minute, then returning to rest is demonstrated graphically. The resting pH is 7.35. With the onset of activity it descends to 7.29, and the pacemaker rate increases from 72 bpm to 90 bpm. With rest pH rises and rate decreases. Redrawn from Cammilli et al: PACE 1978; 1:448–457.*

oxide electrode positioned in the right atrium, upon the pacemaker lead and a reference electrode of silver/silver chloride on the pacemaker case. The system was not investigated sufficiently so that despite a satisfactory initial response it is not now in clinical use (Figure 23).

OXYGEN SATURATION

During rest some 27% of oxyhemoglobin is reduced to hemoglobin with loss of oxygen to cells. During maximum activity some 80% of oxygen may be lost. Normal arterial oxygen saturation approximates 95%–98%, and normal mixed venous oxygen approximates 75% while breathing ordinary air. A drop of one third in mixed venous oxygen saturation to about 50% at maximum activity can occur. This can be measured with an optical oximeter and correlated with pacemaker rate (Figure 24).

STROKE VOLUME

The autonomic and humoral effects of exercise (as noted above) increase the cardiac rate and the force and speed of ventricular contraction. Because of increased contractile force and increased ventricular filling resulting from increases in venous return, the Frank-Starling law mandates an increase in stroke volume. Variation in intracardiac impedance results from changes in stroke vol-

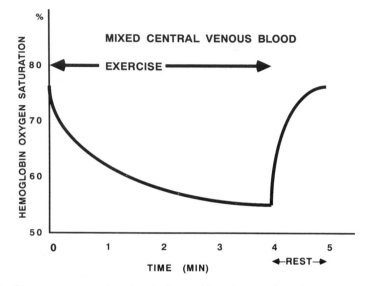

Figure 24. *Venous oxygen saturation declines with activity and can be measured by an intra-vascular oximeter on a pacemaker lead. During vigorous exercise central oxygen saturation may decline to 40%–60%, a level which can be detected and used to set the stimulation rate.*

ume. Impedance can be measured through high frequency impulses well below stimulation threshold between two electrodes in the right ventricle and placed on the pacing electrode. Right ventricular impedance is higher during contraction as the blood being ejected has a higher resistivity than the blood arriving in the ventricle.

RIGHT VENTRICULAR dP/dt

The sensor is a piezoelectric crystal bonded to a titanium diaphragm, part of a unipolar ventricular lead, and is set 3 cm proximal to the electrode. Deflection of the diaphragm produces pressure on the crystal which, in turn, yields a proportional voltage, monitored by the pulse generator during a 200-ms interval after each paced or sensed ventricular event to determine the escape interval. The appropriate pacing rate is determined by a rolling average of the previous ten measurements producing a smoothing effect on the actual rate. The sensor determines the first derivative (the rate of change [dP/dt]) of right ventricular pressure and the change in pulse generator rate is determined by the dP/dt_{max}. The dP/dt is increased by preload, i.e., myocardial fiber length and venous pressure and by afterload, the pulmonary artery pressure. Drugs, cardiac rate and autonomic tone each have a variable effect. The range of dP/dt may be between 200 and 700 mm Hg/sec. Higher cardiac rates are produced by greater rates of change.

The lead is unique to the system and is not usable with other pulse generators. The electrode is steroid eluting. The device has been successfully implanted outside of the United States and clinical evaluation has begun in the United States.

MAGNETIC BALL INDUCTANCE

Another version of the motion sensor is a magnetic ball 1.5 mm in diameter that rolls within an elliptical plastic housing with two coils, each wound in an opposite direction. The length of the housing is 3.6 mm and the outside diameter is 3.8 mm. As the ball moves within the metallic coil it generates an electromotive force proportional to the rate of its movement. This voltage can be measured and the pacemaker rate increase made proportional. The device is presently in clinical evaluation. Potential benefits include the ability to mount the entire sensor on the circuit board so that it will not be affected by pressure on the pulse generator can and it will be more responsive to three-dimensional movement and therefore possibly respond more proportionally to ascending and descending stairs. It may also be less sensitive to the site of implantation in the body, and during programming only a slope for responsiveness need be set. Neither programming of gain nor threshold will be necessary (Figure 25) (Table II).

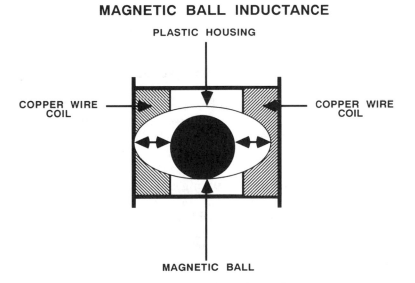

MAGNETIC BALL INDUCTANCE

PLASTIC HOUSING

COPPER WIRE
COIL

COPPER WIRE
COIL

MAGNETIC BALL

Figure 25.   *The magnetic ball inductance sensor operates by a magnetic ball rolling to and fro, depending on movement, within a plastic housing which is, itself, within two coils wound in opposite directions. Movement of the ball induces currents that can be measured and used to drive the pulse generator.*

Table II

	Activity	Temperature	Stim-T Interval	Paced Depolarization Integral	Minute Ventilation	Respiratory Rate	Stroke Volume	dP/dt	SO₂	pH	PEI
PERFORMANCE											
Physiological variable	NO	2	2	3	3	2	3	3	3	3	3
Response to emotion	NO	1	2	3	2	2	3	3	3	3	2
Closed loop	NO	2	2	3	2	1	2	2	2	2	2
Rapid response to onset of exercise	3	1	2	?	2	1	?	?	?	?	1
Decay after exercise	1	1	2	3	3	1	?	?	?	?	?
Drug sensitivity	NO	2	2	2	1	1	1	1	?	2	1
Effective in most conditions	2	2	2	2	2	1	?	?	2	2	2
SSI in atrium	3	NO	NO	NO	NO	NO	NO	NO	?	?	NO
Requires *stimulus* to function	NO	NO	YES	YES	NO	NO	YES	YES	NO	NO	YES
Noise immunity	1	2	1	1	1	2	1	?	?	?	?
Power consumption	1	1	2	2	2	2	2–3	?	?	?	?
Ease of combination with other variables	3	2	3	3	2	2	2	2	0	?	2
IMPLANTATION & MANAGEMENT											
Ease of implant	3	2	2	3	2	1	2	2	?	?	?
Post implant stability	3	2	2	2	3	2	?	?	?	?	
Standard lead	YES	NO	YES	YES	YES	YES	YES	NO	NO	NO	YES
Programming ease	2	1	1	3	1	2	?	?	?	?	1
Diagnostic ability	0	0	3	3	2	1	2	2	2	1	2
Routinely available	YES	YES	YES	NO	YES	YES	NO	NO	NO	NO	NO
Dual chamber	YES	NO	YES	NO	YES	NO	YES	NO	NO	NO	NO

1–least; 2–moderate; 3–most; ?–presently unclear.

RATE MODULATED PACEMAKER LONGEVITY

Sensors for rate modulation can be defined in many ways, one of which is the current drain required to operate the sensor. This must be considered in the context of the operation of the sensor device. In actual practice some of the sensors will draw less (or more) current than might be considered the theoretic drain.

In the nonrate modulated mode pacing is at a single rate and pulse generator operation is entirely conventional with programmability in rate, output, sensitivity, and possibly other functions. Only the drain for sensing cardiac function and the logic and output circuits exist. Each sensor requires some current drain. Some drain little, others much more. If the pulse generator is kept out of the rate modulation mode much of the time its longevity may be the same as that of other similar models. If the sensor is active, longevity will decrease because of: (1) the increase in average rate of stimulation; (2) the operation of the sensor.

The various piezoelectric sensors, as used in activity sensing pacemakers, drain little. The drain for sensing electrocardiographic changes such as that for the stimulus to T sensor is also relatively small. A change in stimulation rate drains relatively little. The circuit for sensing the output of the special sensor should be equivalent in drain to the atrial sensing circuit in a modern dual-chamber pacemaker, i.e., usually efficient, but not always so. The drain for a special sensor for impedance measurements as used in measurement of respiratory rate by impedance or the measurement of cardiac mechanics consumes more energy. The longevity of a single-chamber pacemaker with a piezoelectric sensor is likely to be similar to the longevity of a dual-chamber pacemaker operating in the VDD mode from the same manufacturer. The longevity of an impedance sensor single-chamber device is likely to be substantially reduced compared to that in the nonrate modulated mode. Other sensors are likely to fall between the two limits (Figure 26).

In some models programming the sensor "OFF" eliminates the battery drain for its operation with corresponding increases in pulse generator longevity. In others, sensor drain continues even when rate modulation is not operative. Pulse generator longevity is, therefore, not increased. Contemporary pulse generator design tends toward cessation of sensor drain when rate modulation is "OFF." In still others the sensor may be operative even when rate modulation is inoperative so that an assessment of the sensor-determined appropriate rate can be telemetered for programming purposes. In these models three sensor positions exist with corresponding battery drain: (1) active with rate modulation; (2) active without rate modulation; (3) inactive.

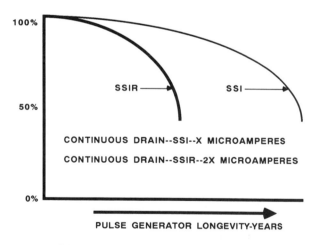

**RATE MODULATED PULSE GENERATOR
LONGEVITY**

Figure 26. *Some sensors require no battery drain for their operation. The only drain is for the logic system to handle the data received, much as in a dual-chamber pacemaker. This graph demonstrates the relative longevities of the same pulse generator in the rate modulated mode (SSIR) with a sensor that requires relatively large amounts of current drain for its operation and with the sensor OFF (SSI). Differential longevities are based on the continuous battery drain for sensor operation.*

LEAD SYSTEMS FOR RATE MODULATED PACING

Leads used with rate modulated pacemakers are either specialized or generally suitable for any pacing system. The difference is based on whether the sensor for rate modulation is within the pulse generator and whether the sensor is based on electrocardiographic data.

Conventional Unipolar and Bipolar Leads

Piezoelectric sensors (activity) are within the pulse generator, which may be either unipolar or bipolar and may be used with any lead that can be physically connected. The electrocardiographic sensor of stimulus to T requires a relatively normal to low-impedance (by modern standards) unipolar lead. Some older unipolar leads were of very high impedance and attenuated the electrogram sufficiently so that satisfactory stimulus to T interval measurement could not be achieved. In one model of respiration sensitive device, a conventional unipolar lead is used in association with a second subcutaneous lead, both required for delivering the current required to measure thoracic impedance. In newer models the second lead has been replaced by an electrode on the lead entering the heart and making it a specialized lead.

Bipolar Leads

Impedance measurements must be made between two intracardiac electrodes. Consequently, most thoracic impedance sensors require a bipolar lead as does the sensor of the evoked ventricular response. The lead may be a wholly conventional bipolar lead, but a unipolar lead is not suitable (see above).

Specialized Leads

All of the sensors that require an intravascular measurement also require a specialized lead. Measurement of intracardiac mechanics, temperature sensing with a thermistor, oxygen tension, and pH sensing all use an intravascular transducer and, therefore, need a specialized lead.

A major issue involved in the different leads to be used with different sensors is the possibility of pulse generator interchangeability at the time of pulse generator replacement. In the recent past virtually all lead and pulse generator systems had been interchangeable. New connectors (e.g., IS-1, VS-1) have caused some difficulty with adapters but aside from that virtually any pulse generator could be connected to any lead. This will no longer be the case should special leads come into widespread use, although none are commercially available in early 1993. Many patients now require pulse generator replacement after years of device service. Those sensors that are compatible with older leads can be used to upgrade to a rate modulated system. Pulse generators with sensors requiring a special lead will therefore be unsuitable or, alternatively, will require abandonment of an otherwise functional lead and placement of a new lead system.

SENSOR-DRIVEN IDIOSYNCRASIES

Problems can exist with the operation of the various sensors and their delivery of reliable signals to the pulse generator. The idiosyncrasy may be physiological or relate to the oversensing of some kinds of activity, the undersensing of others, and the lack of linearity in still others. For example, the stimulus to T sensor is quite nonlinear with the reduction of interval duration relatively large at the beginning of effort and much less so later as effort continues. The algorithm must be adjusted to accommodate differing intervals at different times of effort. Further, the stimulus to T interval seems to lose its flexibility with increasing patient age so that just when normal body mechanisms have lost their responsiveness so also may the stimulus to T interval.

The respiratory sensor using an accessory lead is sensitive to arm motion on the side of the pulse generator, and such movement, in the absence of an increase in respiratory rate, will increase the stimulation rate. The respiratory sensor based on intracardiac impedance measurement is readily affected by speaking and respiratory rate. Therefore, a more appropriate rate response occurs with an increase in respiratory rate while the patient is silent than when the patient is speaking. During speech the pacemaker rate will be slower and irregular. The temperature sensing pacemakers begin with a fall in central venous temperature and are slow to respond. Brief activity may be over before the cardiac rate increases. The activity, i.e., piezoelectric sensor, responds to what has been called the "heel strike" rate. In a simple way the "heel strike" rate and consequently the pacemaker rate is higher walking down steps than walking up steps even though the effort expended is substantially greater. Bicycle riding (moving and stationary) and swimming, both vigorous activities, produce a lesser sensor response. Direct pressure on the case of the piezoelectric sensor pulse generator increases its rate as does gently tapping the case. Such tapping will drive the rate rapidly and promptly.

Electromyographic interference (EMI) also can affect rate modulated pacemaker function. Despite the operation of the rate modulation sensor, output inhibition of unipolar systems can occur so that the sensor rate may increase but actual output may cease or the device may revert to the noise mode. Some devices are more sensitive to such effects than others and relate to the effectiveness of conventional interference rejection rather than the operation of the sensor.

RATE MODULATED PACEMAKER-MEDIATED TACHYCARDIA

Previous pacemaker-mediated tachycardias have resulted from a number of causes relative to sensing of some cardiac or noncardiac function. Indeed, the first description of a pacemaker-mediated tachycardia was the result of the sensing of retrograde atrial activation and produced the **endless loop tachycardia.** Other dual-chamber pacemaker-mediated tachycardias result from the sensing of pathological atrial activity and can follow sensing atrial fibrillation, flutter, and supraventricular tachycardias. While these are "pacemaker-mediated," they are not **endless loop.** Additional causes are oversensing pectoral muscle electromyographic interference with triggering of the ventricle and external electromagnetic interference with ventricular triggering.

Just as sensing normal or pathological atrial activity or signals that mimic atrial activity can produce a pacemaker-mediated tachycardia an additional source of input is the sensor present in many single- and dual-chamber implanted pacemakers. The activity, i.e., piezoelectric sensor, is sensitive to tapping with a finger. While at rest, tapping the device in the subcutaneous tissue will increase its rate, so that the rate of the device can be under patient or other control. A left-sided pulse generator may be sufficiently close to the cardiac apex thrust so that a variety of endless loop sensor-driven tachycardias occur, in which the apex thrust activates the pulse generator sensor which, in turn increases the rate of the apex thrust.

The respiratory impedance pulse generator is subject to increased rate resulting from hyperventilation, ipsilateral arm movement, and even speech. Some of these tachycardias can be controlled by programming and for other tachycardias it may be more difficult. Such a **sensor-mediated tachycardia** can result from the following causes:

1. Excessive sensor sensitivity: as the activity (piezoelectric) sensor does not respond to a physiological event its responsiveness is wholly under programming control and it may respond excessively so that slight motion may result in an excessive rate increase. Alternatively, it may be programmed to be underresponsive. In that instance some patients have tapped the pulse generator when in need of a rate response.
2. Lack of discrimination between noise and metabolic need: imposed motion such as from a vehicle may be interpreted as body motion requiring an increase in rate. Sleeping on the abdomen and therefore the pulse generator may provide pressure on the activity generator and cause an increase in rate.
3. Increased rate causing increased response, i.e., a kind of sensor-mediated endless loop: should a piezoelectric activity pulse generator be implanted on the left over the cardiac apex, the apical thrust may drive the pulse generator to increase its rate which will, in turn, drive the pulse generator to a higher rate until the upper rate limit is reached. Conversely, piezoelectric sensor responsiveness may be reduced if the generator is turned over in the subcutaneous tissue. The sensor is bonded to the back of the pulse generator where it is adjacent to muscle. If the sensor faces the subcutaneous tissue, responsiveness may be distinctly reduced. If a unipolar device is reversed in the subcutaneous tissue it may stimulate the local pectoral musculature and produce an increase in local motion which in turn may stimulate the pulse generator. The net effect on responsiveness may be variable.
4. Temperature deviation: For the central venous temperature sensing pacemaker, swallowing cold liquid or taking a hot bath will affect the pacemaker rate. Such a result may, indeed, partially mimic the physiological as the normal cardiac rate response to temperature is an increase in rate.

Amelioration of sensor- or atrial-driven pacemaker-mediated tachycardias can occur in several new pulse generators in which the operating mode can be automatically switched from DDDR with atrial responsiveness to VVIR in which the atrium is disregarded. (see below) Another alternative is automatic mode change to the VDIR mode (ventricular pacing, atrial and ventricular sensing in the rate modulated, inhibited mode). In both circumstance, the atrial rate can be monitored and the mode returned to DDD should the atrial rate and rhythm return to normal.

ASSESSMENT OF PACEMAKER PROGRAMMING AND EXERCISE RESPONSE

All dual- and single-chamber rate modulated pacemakers can be operated in the rate modulation insensitive mode. The single-chamber units can be programmed to SSI, and the dual-chamber units can be programmed to DDD and even lesser modes. The single-chamber inhibited (SSI) mode of operation is especially useful when a patient is deemed to have, for example, early AV block and requires a pacemaker to guard against episodic asystole but does not yet require continual pacing. Later, if fixed block should occur and continuous pacing be required, the rate modulated mode can be activated.

Programming the implanted rate modulated device, when it is in the modulation insensitive mode is identical to a conventional multiprogrammable pulse generator of single- or dual-chamber mode. In the rate modulated mode, output and conventional sensitivity to cardiac function is set as in the insensitive mode. However, in addition rate modulation settings are now required. Each device has settings specific to its own technology, but in general there are four categories of setting.

1. The sensitivity of the sensor to the physiological (or nonphysiological) event which is to set the rate;
2. The responsiveness of the sensor to physiological change;
3. The rate at which the cardiac rate will be increased by the sensor response;
4. The maximum and minimum rates that are to be achieved, one at rest and the other with maximum activity.

Each device is delivered with a default setting for the rate modulated mode, i.e., one which is deemed to be safe and effective in producing rate modulation during exercise. It is frequently unclear how programming should be accomplished and what settings should be sought. In setting a single-chamber pacemaker, an escape rate is set, usually a conventional rate of 60–70 bpm and no upper rate is required. In the patient capable of atrial synchronous pacing the atrium sets the rate. The lower rate may be set to allow atrial sensing at all times, i.e., at a rate of 40–50 bpm. Atrial sensitivity and refractoriness are then set so that the pacemaker will respond to each P wave in a 1:1 fashion until a specific upper rate is achieved, commonly between 100 and 175 bpm. Then a mechanism of upper rate limitation is established. The fact of atrial synchrony sets the responsiveness of the pulse generator in stimulating the ventricle (and sometimes the atrium). It is immediately apparent whether atrial synchrony is occurring and how the pacemaker is responding, even at rest during a programming sequence. For the rate modulated device the setting of the lower rate limit is about the same as for a single- or dual-chamber unit. Responsiveness and upper rate are different matters. A careful determination must be made so that the device is neither excessively responsive nor underresponsive. Proper response mimics that of the normal SA node. While it may be that it will be found that a different level of response is superior to that of the normal SA node, no such evidence now exists. The device may surely be underresponsive. At the usual default settings the increase in cardiac rate with modest and even severe exercise may be blunted and unrelated to the atrial response (Figure 27). That determination can only be made by some controlled challenge or formal exercise test protocol. Often the patient with the rate modulated pacemaker will not be able to use the programmable upper rate and a lesser maximum rate will be required. All of this can be ascertained by stress evaluation and the pacemaker response. The stress should be carefully selected to mimic reasonably normal activity. Those stress tests that evaluate the presence and severity of coronary artery disease may be excessively strenuous for the setting of sensor sensitivity and responsiveness and may not even give a result compatible with patient needs. As the activity sensor is by far the most widely used at present and that situation is likely to be so for a very prolonged period, the quirks of that sensor should be considered. A formal stress test is labor intensive and is likely not to be used

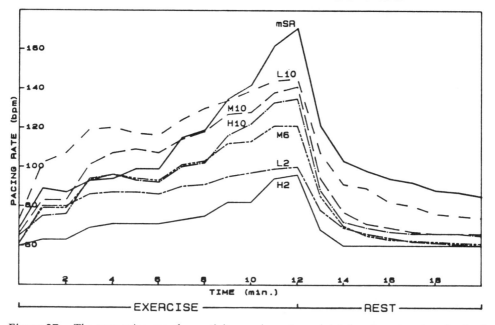

Figure 27. *The responsiveness of an activity sensing rate modulated system at various levels of SENSITIVITY AND RESPONSIVENESS is compared to the mean sinus rate (mSR) under similar test conditions. The pacemaker lower rate limit was set to 60 per minute, the upper rate limit to 150 per minute. The least RESPONSIVE AND SENSITIVE setting (H2) produces barely a response. The most (L10) produces an earlier and greater response than the atrium. Return to the lower rate limit with rest approximates the atrium. Even at maximum RESPONSIVENESS the pacemaker rate does not reach the atrial rate or the upper rate limit.*

at all while an evaluation that can be easily accomplished may, as a practical matter, provide significantly greater information.

EXERCISE TESTING AFTER PACEMAKER IMPLANT

During evaluation of the settings of a rate modulated pacemaker the lower limit of the modulation response is determined. In general an attempt to mimic the sinus rate should be made. If the atrium is in a persistent arrhythmia such as atrial fibrillation, flutter supraventricular tachycardia, or if AV block has been accomplished by interruption of the AV conduction system, the atrial rate cannot be a satisfactory guide to the ventricular rate and an assessment will be required of the lower rate, upper rate, and rate of increase.

1. The pacemaker is programmed to the settings to be tested;
2. The pacemaker rate is determined with the patient at rest. Fifteen minutes of supine, sitting, or standing rest are adequate to establish the lower sensor rate.
3. An exercise protocol is followed and the pacemaker response is recorded on the ECG. In some pacemakers a histogram of rates achieved can be read directly from the device (Figure 28). In a patient with a temporary pacemaker in place, especially if in sinus rhythm at the time of test, an activity sensitive pacemaker can be strapped to the chest and its response determined prior to implant. Sensors that depend on measurement of some body function, i.e., temperature, stroke volume, etc. cannot be tested in this way.
4. Care must be taken with activity sensing pacemakers to remember that cardiac demand and activity are independent and that the activity sensing pacemaker responds to activity rather than to workload. Consequently responsiveness may be greater to lesser activity and tempered with greater workload requirements. The protocol selected may influence apparent pacemaker responsiveness.
5. Different exercise protocols exist. Most are based on the traditional Bruce and Naughton protocols but as these are based on testing for coronary artery disease and not for setting of pacemaker responsiveness they may be less useful (Table III).

As in all protocols, the patient is continuously monitored by ECG and a knowledgeable technician must be in attendance. The goal is the establishment

Table III

Stage	Speed (mph)	Grade (%)	Duration (minutes)	Approx. Workload (METS)
Rest	Lying	Supine	1	0
I	1	0	2	1.9
II	2	0	2	2.6
III	2	3.5	2	3.4
IV	3	5.5	2	5.0
V	4	5.5	2	8.0
VI	5	5.5	2	12.0
Rest	sitting		8	0

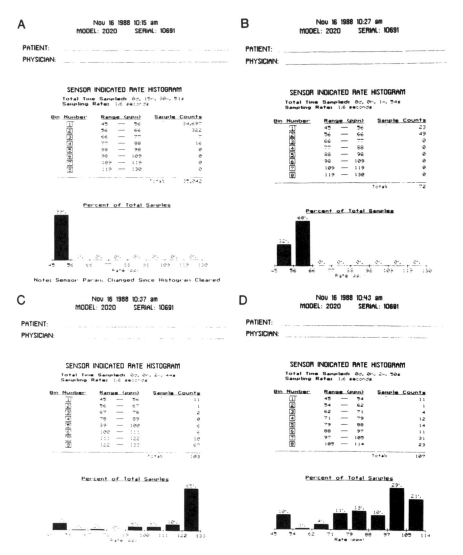

Figure 28. A rate histogram is available in several pulse generators and is useful in programming the best level of sensitivity and responsiveness. A. In a patient with chronotropic incompetence, a 15-hour recording shows that the pacemaker rate has not varied from a range of 45–56 when the lower rate setting had been at 50 bpm. B. During walking evaluation, with programming to modest sensitivity and responsiveness and with recordings made for several minutes, only a slight increase in responsiveness occurs, this time largely to 56–66bpm. C. With the pacemaker programmed to be much more sensitive and responsive, similar activity produces an excessive response near the programmed maximum. D. A more moderate programmed setting produces a response across the range of possible rates.

of a pacemaker rate similar to the spontaneous atrial rate or of a known rate response.

This protocol can be compared to a widely used CAEP protocol developed by Wilkoff, Harvey, and Blackburn and to the Bruce Protocol (Table IV).

Still, alternative approaches can be used without a treadmill but still requiring an ECG, Holter monitor, or telemetry ECG. A satisfactory setting can be created using a level walking protocol and a stairwell protocol. (Ferroconcrete building stairwells are reasonably standardized worldwide). Effort is controlled by time restraint using an electronic metronome which the patient wears. Level walk testing can be done at two levels:

> *Slow walk—2 minutes.* Each metronome beat is one step. Rates of 55–72 steps per minute are comfortable for most patients on a straight level course such as a hospital corridor. Walk is in one direction for one minute and then the reverse for another.
>
> *Rapid walk—2 minutes.* As above but the metronome is set for 100–120 steps per minute.

Table IV
Comparison of Treadmill Exercise Protocols

TIME	MMC McAlister Soberman Furman (modified Naughton) Speed/Grade/Mets (mph)/(%)	CAEP Wilkoff Harvey Blackburn Speed/Grade/Mets (mph)/(%)	Bruce Speed/Grade/Mets (mph)/(%)
1	STAGE 1 1.0/0/1.9	STAGE 1 1.0/2/2.0	STAGE 1 1.7/10/5
2			
3	STAGE 2 2.0/0/2.6	STAGE 2 1.5/3/2.8	STAGE 2
4			2.5/12/7
5	STAGE 3 2.0/3.5/3.4	STAGE 3 2.0/4/3.6	
6			
7	STAGE 4 3.0/5.5/5.0	STAGE 4 2.5/5/4.6	STAGE 3 3.4/14/9.5
8			
9	STAGE 5 4.0/5.5/8.0	STAGE 5 3.0/6/5.8	STAGE 4
10			4.2/16/13
11	STAGE 6 5.0/5.5/12.0	STAGE 6 3.5/8/7.5	
12			
13		STAGE 7 4.0/10/9.6	STAGE 5 5.0/18/16
14			
15		STAGE 8 5.0/10/12.1	
16			
17		STAGE 9 6.0/10/14.3	
18			
19		STAGE 10 7.0/10/16.5	
20			
21		STAGE 11 7.0/15/19.0	

CALCULATION OF WORKLOAD
STAIRWELL PROTOCOL

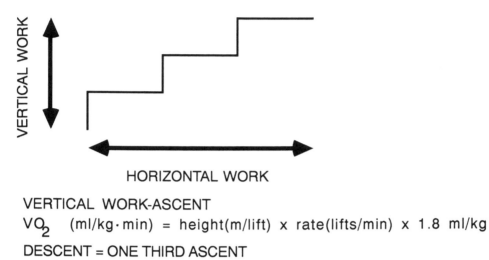

VERTICAL WORK-ASCENT

VO_2 (ml/kg·min) = height(m/lift) x rate(lifts/min) x 1.8 ml/kg

DESCENT = ONE THIRD ASCENT

SOBERMAN ET AL-1988

Figure 29. *A staircase is a good place to test rate modulation. The two means of stress, ascending and descending, are identical except that the work of ascending is three times that of descending. Regulation of the degree and variety of stress can further be modified by changing the rate of ascent and descent and whether that rate is equal, ascending, or descending.*

Stairway response: Once again the metronome sets the rate for the "standardized" stairwell. Three rates can be used, approximating 30 steps per minute as the slow rate, 60 steps per minute as the moderate rate and 90 steps per minute as the rapid rate. Record the ascending rates and the descending rates (Figure 29).

Total Work = Vertical Work ÷ Horizontal Work

The workload descending is about one third of that ascending the staircase (Figure 30) (Table V).

Table V
Maximum Workloads Achieved (Approximate)

Ascent		Descent	
Rate	Workload	Rate	(Workload)
(Steps/min)	(METS*)	(Steps/min)	(METS*)
30	3.5	30	2.0
60	6.5	60	3.0
90	9.0	90	4.0

* MET = 3.5 mL/kg min.

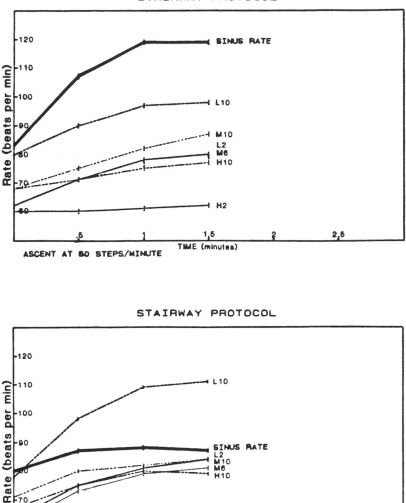

Figure 30. *These graphs represent a comparison of activity response to staircase ascent and descent. A paradoxical response is produced because of variation in "heel strike" vigor even when the rate of ascent and descent is controlled, in this instance at 60 steps/minute. The activity sensing rate modulated unit was strapped to the chest of a person with a normal cardiovascular system and programmed through six settings. The pacemaker lower rate limit was set at 60 bpm, the upper rate limit at 150 bpm. The sinus rate and the pacemaker stimulus rate were read from the ECG. ASCENT: The sinus rate reaches 120 bpm 1 minute after onset. Even maximum pacemaker sensitivity and responsiveness (L1O) only produces a rate of 95 bpm. Three conventional settings are well below the sinus node in rate response. DESCENT: The sinus rate reaches 85 bpm at about 1 minute after onset of exercise and then declines slightly. Three conventionally programmed settings follow the sinus rate as well.*

ELECTROCARDIOGRAPHY OF RATE MODULATED PACEMAKERS

Single Chamber

Electrocardiography is relatively simple. As in any electrocardiographic interpretation it must be remembered that the interval between one stimulus and the next varies and that the stimulation rate is a result of these individual variations. A smooth rate of acceleration or deceleration with continuous pacing provides a small variation from one stimulus to the next (Figure 31). If the sensor modifies its rate, but spontaneous events occur simultaneously and inhibit and recycle pacemaker output, then the interval between a sensed spontaneous event and the next pacemaker stimulus will vary depending on the sensor imposed escape interval. Interpretation of the ECG should consider the absence of a fixed pacemaker stimulus escape interval during sensor operation (Figures 32–34).

While the action of some sensors is electrocardiographically invisible except for changes in the escape interval, others produce an ECG mark. The two respiratory impedance sensor pacemaker models continually emit rapid small amplitude stimuli which can be seen readily on the ECG. These should be recognized as representing normal pacemaker function. In the absence of these

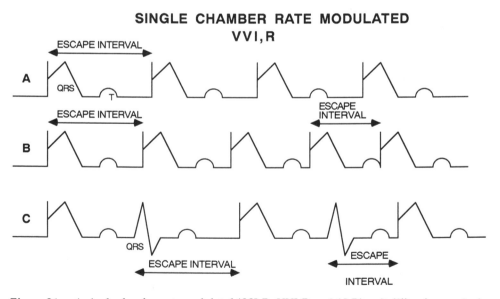

Figure 31. *A single-chamber rate modulated (SSI,R, VVI,R or AAI,R) unit differs from a single rate (SSI) unit as the escape (lower rate) interval can change because of the operation of the rate modulating sensor. In this diagram, a VVI,R unit is illustrated. In (A) operation is at or near the lower rate interval with a prolonged escape interval. In (B) the sensor progressively abbreviates the escape interval between stimuli. In (C) the escape interval between spontaneous beats and the succeeding stimulus is also abbreviated.*

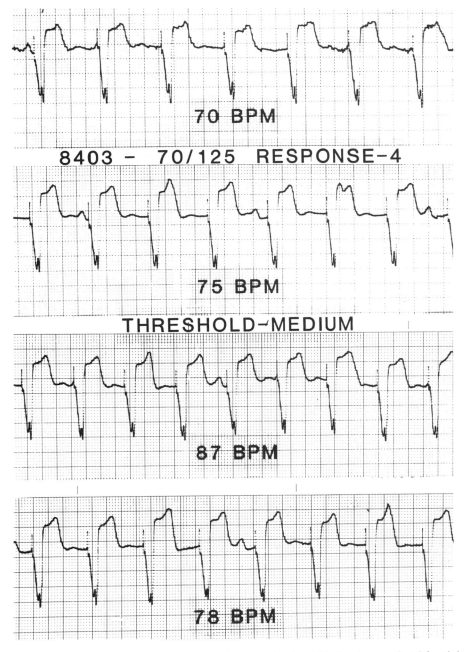

70 BPM

8403 - 70/125 RESPONSE-4

75 BPM

THRESHOLD-MEDIUM

87 BPM

78 BPM

Figure 32. *This elderly patient, with longstanding complete heart block and normal atrial activity, underwent replacement of a single rate single-chamber pacemaker by a single-chamber rate modulated unit. Despite relatively unresponsive settings the rate increase of only 17 beats per minute with activity produced a dramatic improvement in exercise tolerance.*

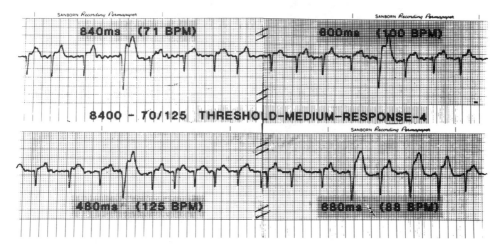

Figure 33. In addition to changing the interval between pacemaker stimuli, the rate modulating sensor changes the escape interval between a spontaneous event and the next paced event. In this instance, during atrial fibrillation with episodically slow ventricular response, the change in escape interval results from sensor operation. The escape varies between 840 ms (71 bpm) and 480 ms (125 bpm) depending on the sensor's state of activity response.

stimuli the pulse generator is in the "sensor off" mode and no modulation of rate or escape interval can be anticipated. In the presence of these stimuli, rate and escape interval modulation can be anticipated.

The stimulus to T wave sensor and the evoked potential sensor can only make a rate determination following a paced event. During pacemaker inhibition, i.e., with the sensor determining a rate which is less than the spontaneous rate, the sensor "tests" the cardiac status, i.e., the stimulus to T wave interval or the area under the curve of the evoked potential, by determining the actual rate (i.e., spontaneous QRS coupling interval) and emitting stimuli at a briefer coupling interval, stimulating the ventricle and determining what the pacemaker rate should be. Two possibilities then exist. The appropriate rate will be determined to be less than the spontaneous rate, and the pacemaker will return to its inhibited state and soon emit three test stimuli again; or the appropriate rate will be determined to be more rapid than the spontaneous rate and pacing will continue. During continuous pacing each QRS interval will be evaluated to determine an increase or decrease in rate.

Stimulation threshold can be determined by those pacemakers that test the response evoked by the ventricular stimulus. The two such devices are the stimulus-T device and the evoked ventricular response device. Possibly other devices will have similar capabilities. In each instance the measurement of a ventricular response to the pacemaker stimulus is part of sensor operation. In both instances the absence of a response, the T wave (Figure 35) in one and ventricular depolarization in the other (Figure 36) is interpreted as an ineffective stimulus and the pacemaker response can be an increase in stimulus amplitude.

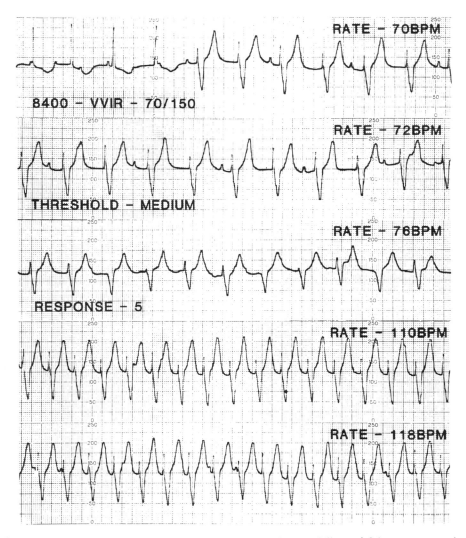

Figure 34. *A single-chamber rate modulated unit may be especially useful in a young patient with congenital heart block, allowing avoidance of an atrial lead. This five year old who had a syncopal episode had also been fixed in ventricular rate at about 70 bpm and had been markedly restricted in exercise tolerance. Following implantation of an activity responsive unit, even at modestly sensitive and responsive settings, she readily developed exercise rates as high as 118 bpm with marked improvement in exercise capacity.*

Single-Chamber Atrial Pacing

Single-chamber rate modulated ventricular pacing may restore rate variation with activity, but not the normal AV sequence. In the presence of sinus node dysfunction with intact AV conduction, atrial pacing will stabilize the atrial and ventricular rates. Rate modulated atrial pacing maintains the AV sequence and

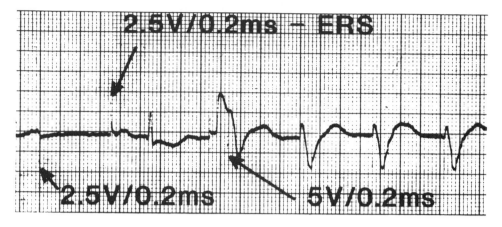

Figure 35. *Pacemakers that sense the ventricular response evoked by a pacemaker stimulus can determine whether one has, indeed, occurred. The first stimulus (left) is without ERS (evoked response sensing) and is below capture threshold. When ERS function is activated, the second stimulus, also without a ventricular response, is followed 170 ms later by a stimulus of double amplitude, i.e., from 2.5 V to 5.0 V and consequent ventricular capture.*

restores rate response to activity. Prolongation of the AV interval may, however, increase with higher paced rates. Should the AV interval prolong sufficiently, atrial contraction may occur early after the preceding ventricular contraction, so that, from a timing perspective, it may be hemodynamically a retrograde event rather than an antegrade event. The result of such prolongation may be "pacemaker syndrome" with the maintenance of the normal AV sequence, but not of a normal AV interval (Figure 37).

During dual-chamber pacing, whether rate modulated or not, the AV interval is programmably controlled. Although prolongation of the AV interval at upper rate operation with a sufficiently prolonged pseudo-Wenckebach interval

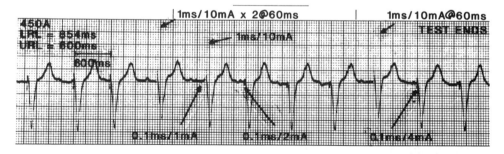

Figure 36. *A pacemaker that senses the ventricular evoked response can determine whether capture has occurred. This threshold tracking sequence begins with two pulses of 1 ms duration and 10 mA output separated by 60 ms, followed by a pulse of 0.1 ms duration and 1 mA amplitude, which does not capture, and is followed 60 ms later by a rescue pulse of 1 ms/10 mA. Next 0.1 ms/0.2 mA is tested and does capture. The pacemaker output is then stabilized at 0.1 ms/4 mA. Capture is determined at each stimulus and threshold is actively determined twice daily. The margin of output above threshold is kept small to conserve energy.*

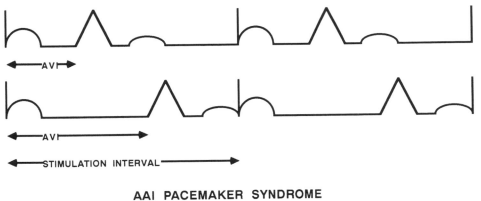

AAI PACEMAKER SYNDROME
(PROLONGATION OF AV INTERVAL)

Figure 37. *Atrial pacing in the presence of a normal interval between atrial contraction and ventricular response produces an increase in atrial and ventricular rate and maintains the normal AV sequence and depolarization pattern for the ventricle. If the AV interval prolongs, cardiac output may become inefficient, and if sufficiently prolonged, the pacemaker produced P wave and atrial contraction may fall after the preceding QRS, producing an effect akin to retrograde conduction and "pacemaker syndrome" during AAI pacing.*

may produce the same AV interval prolongation and the consequent "pacemaker syndrome," this effect can be avoided by proper programming. To avoid this effect during AAIR pacing, careful evaluation of the state of AV conduction, the Wenckebach point during atrial pacing, i.e., the atrial pacing rate at which Wenckebach periodicity occurs, should be evaluated at the time of implantation. Even if the paced AV interval is nonproblematic during implant, it may be affected later by the passage of time, progression of conduction system disease, or the administration of medication. The implantation of a dual-chamber pacemaker may resolve the problem. Virtually all can be programmed to the single-chamber atrial pacing mode. Should prolonged AV conduction occur or AV block develop, the ventricular channel can be programmably activated.

A potentially significant problem with atrial pacing is the effect of sensing the ventricular depolarization via the atrial lead. This effect in recycling the pacemaker and effectively slowing the atrial rate has long been recognized. It should be kept in mind during atrial rate modulated pacing and can often be clearly demonstrated via telemetry in which slowing of the atrial pacing rate may be associated with sensed events seen on the ECG interpretation channel. Use of bipolar rather than unipolar leads will almost always reject the far-field ventricular event.

Dual-Chamber

As a single timing interval exists in a single-chamber pacemaker, several exist in a dual-chamber device. The lower rate limit is set by the atrial and then the ventricular pacing rate at rest. The AV delay is also set and can be of fixed or modulated duration (Figure 38). The fixed AV delay will be of the same

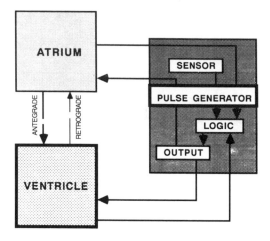

DUAL CHAMBER-RATE MODULATED
(DDDR)

Figure 38. *A diagrammatic representation of a dual-chamber rate modulated pacemaker shows inputs and outputs from atrium and ventricle. There are three signals that affect function of the logic system, that from the atrium, from the ventricle (both as in a conventional DDD pacemaker), and from the sensor. Each plays a role in setting the stimulation rate and, in some units, the rate modulated AV interval.*

duration at the lower rate limit, i.e., when both atrium and ventricle are being paced, and the upper rate limit or the maximum atrial tracking limit. A modulated AV delay will be set to be abbreviated at higher rates whether sensor-driven or spontaneous.

The upper rate limit, as determined by atrial tracking, is determined as in other DDD modes of operation (see Chapter 4) by the duration of atrial refractoriness. But, in the rate modulated (i.e., DDDR unit) a second and independent, i.e., sensor-driven upper rate limit, can exist. There can therefore be three different upper rate limits:

1. That determined by atrial refractoriness alone;
2. That set independently of atrial refractoriness, as in the conventional DDD pacemaker. It is always lower (i.e., at a longer RR interval) than that set by the duration of atrial refractoriness;
   Both of these exist in most conventional DDD models.
3. An upper rate limit based on the maximum sensor rate.

As in the conventional DDD mode the atrial refractory determined upper rate limit and that independently programmed may or may not be similar. Different upper rate mechanisms will result. In the DDDR mode all three upper rate limits may be the same, or all three may be different, resulting in markedly different pacemaker operation and ECG manifestation (Figure 39).

If all three are the same then, as the atrial rate rises, the atrium will be driven or sensed to drive the ventricle depending on which is at a shorter coupling interval. If the independently set upper rate limit is lower than that based on atrial refractoriness and the maximum sensor rate is equally low, then the

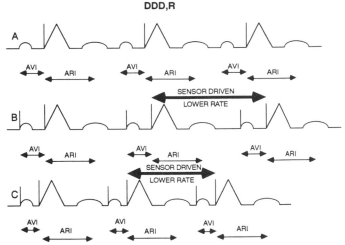

**DUAL CHAMBER RATE MODULATED
DDD,R**

Figure 39. *This is a diagrammatic representation of some of the operation of a DDDR pacemaker with AV interval modulation. For diagrammatic purposes the P wave is sensed at its beginning. The total atrial refractory interval is, as usual, the sum of the AVI and ARI. The upper rate for atrial tracking is determined by atrial refractoriness. With the decrease in AV interval, total atrial refractoriness decreases and the upper tracking rate increases. AVI = atrioventricular interval; ARI = atrial refractory interval, after the ventricular event (PVARP).*

upper rate will be manifested by conventional pseudoWenckebach operation. If the upper rate limit based on atrial refractoriness is lower than the maximum sensor-driven rate, then P waves may fall into the atrial refractory period after the ventricular event and be unsensed. Each will be followed thereafter by an atrial channel stimulus that:

1. may be competitive with the earlier unsensed P wave;
2. may produce a second P wave or a competitive atrial arrhythmia;
3. may fall into atrial refractoriness and be ineffective.

The electrocardiography of dual-chamber rate modulated pacemakers (see Chapter 9) can be extremely complex as the sensor setting, providing a third source of pacing interval setting (atrium, ventricle, and sensor) within the device, changes the conventional rules of pacemaker ECG interpretation (Figure 40). A device may be set so that AV block or pseudo-Wenckebach operation occurs or does not occur at the upper rate limit. AV intervals which are set to be reduced in duration at increasing atrial and sensor rates may be both reduced and simultaneously prolonged as the upper rate limit is approached and as Wenckebach operation is progressively invoked. Careful evaluation of each ECG and knowledge of operation of the device and its specific settings is mandatory (Figure 41).

The availability of a rate drive independent of the atrium has increased the utility of a previously infrequently used dual-chamber mode, DDI. In this mode the atrium is sensed and paced at the lower rate limit, but sensing of an atrial event does not cause emission of a ventricular stimulus after the programmed

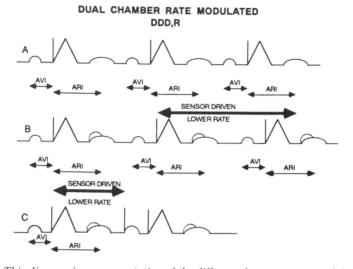

DUAL CHAMBER RATE MODULATED
DDD,R

Figure 40.   *This diagram is a representation of the difference between a sensor-driven upper rate and that based on response to atrial activity. As in the conventional DDD pacemaker the duration of total atrial refractoriness determines the upper rate of atrial tracking. But as there is another determinant of upper rate in operation, the two may result in different upper rates. For example, in diagram B the atrial rate and atrial refractoriness are such that the pacemaker is operating in the 2:1 AV block mode. As the sensor does not require a pacemaker rate more rapid, i.e., a ventricular coupling interval shorter than half the atrial rate, the pacemaker will stimulate the ventricle at half the atrial rate. In diagram C the pacemaker is still operating in the 2:1 AV block mode based on atrial refractoriness. However, sensor operation now indicates a rate higher than, i.e., a coupling interval briefer than, half the atrial rate. In this instance, despite the alternate blocked P waves, the atrium will be driven at a more rapid rate. AVI = atrioventricular interval; ARI = atrial refractory interval, after the ventricular event (PVARP).*

AV delay. In the presence of sinus bradycardia (i.e., spontaneous rate below the pacemaker escape rate) DDI, DVI (the atrium is never sensed), and DDD pacing are indistinguishable. During an atrial arrhythmia (atrial flutter or fibrillation) the DDD mode is commonly driven to the upper rate limit. The DVI mode produces atrial and ventricular stimuli at the programmed escape interval.

These drive the ventricle and are competitive with the atrium and may tend to fix the arrhythmia. The DDI mode produces only ventricular stimuli at the escape interval with the atrial channel inhibited by atrial activity. The DDI mode is particularly useful in a patient in whom sinus bradycardia (possibly medication induced) alternates with supraventricular arrhythmia. In the past, with the DDI mode a ventricular stimulation rate more rapid than the pacemaker escape rate (lower rate limit) could not exist. With dual-chamber rate modulation (DDIR), the ventricular stimulation rate is established independently of the atrial rate during sinus bradycardia (with maintenance of the normal AV sequence) with disregard of an atrial arrhythmia and without atrial competition, although with loss of the normal AV sequence. This mode is especially useful in pacing after AV node ablation for intractable, but episodic atrial arrhythmia. It provides rate modulation and the normal AV sequence during pacing of sinus bradycardia and rate modulation during ventricular pacing of atrial arrhythmia (Figure 42).

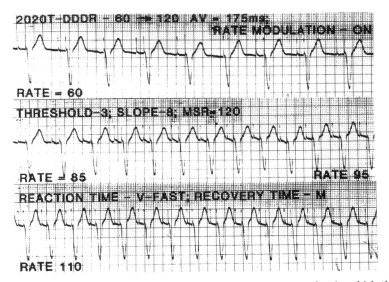

Figure 41. *An ECG of a dual-chamber rate modulated (DDDR) pacemaker in which the atrium is less responsive than the sensor to activity shows that at rest (upper line) atrium and ventricle are paced at a rate of 60 bpm (1000 ms). The AV interval has been programmed to 175 ms. Other rate and sensor functions (i.e., sensitivity and responsiveness) are shown. The rate increases progressively (middle line) and the AV interval is modulated and abbreviated with the increase in rate.*

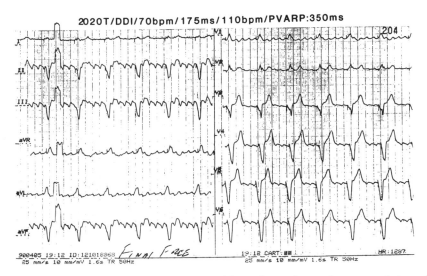

Figure 42. *This ECG shows the DDIR mode used for patients who may have normal sinus rhythm alternating with atrial arrhythmia such as atrial flutter. The DDIR mode was used in this patient following AV node ablation and production of complete AV block. The lower rate was set at 70 bpm, the sensor-driven upper rate 110 bpm, and the atrial refractory interval after the ventricular event at 350 ms. When atrial flutter occurred, the atrial flutter waves were sensed by the atrial channel and inhibited atrial channel output but did not start an AV interval (this is a usual function of the DDI mode). While this ECG was done at rest and the ventricular rate was 70 bpm, with activity the rate would have risen to that indicated by the sensor.*

Acknowledgments: Thanks should be given to the efforts of Drs. Hugh McAlister and Judith Soberman whose work forms a partial basis for this text.

BIBLIOGRAPHY

Alicandria C. Fouad FM, Tarazi RC, et al: Three cases of hypotension and syncope with ventricular pacing: Possible role of atrial reflexes. Am J Cardiol 1978; 42:137–142.

Alt E, Heinz M, Hirgstetter C, et al: Control of pacemaker rate by impedance-based respiratory minute ventilation. Chest 1987; 92:247–252.

Alt E, Hirgstetter C, Heinz M, et al: Rate control of physiologic pacemakers by central venous blood temperature. Circulation 1986; 73:1206–1212.

Alt E, Hirgstetter C, Heinz M, et al: Measurement of right ventricular blood temperature during exercise as a means of rate control in physiological pacemakers. PACE 1986; 9:970–977.

Alt E, Matula M, Theres H, et al: The basis for activity controlled rate variable cardiac pacemakers: An analysis of mechanical forces on the human body induced by exercise and environment. PACE 1989; 12:1667–1680.

Alt E, Matula M, Thilo R, et al: A new mechanical sensor for detecting body activity and posture, suitable for rate responsive pacing. PACE 1988; 11:1875–1881.

Alt E, Theres H, Heinz M, et al: A new rate-modulated pacemaker system optimized by combination of two sensors. PACE 1988; 11:1119–1129.

Anderson KM, Moore AA: Sensors in pacing. PACE 1986; 9:954–959.

Auerbach AA, Furman S: The autodiagnostic pacemaker. PACE 1979; 2:58–68.

Ausubel K, Furman S: The pacemaker syndrome. Ann Int Med 1985; 103:420–429.

Baig MW, Green A, Wade G, et al: A randomized double-blind, cross-over study of the linear and nonlinear algorithms for the QT sensing rate adaptive pacemaker. PACE 1990; 13:1802–1808.

Balke B, Ware R: An experimental study of physical fitness of Air Force personnel. US Armed Forces Med J 1959; 10:675–688.

Batey RL, Sweesy MW, Scala G, et al: Comparison of low rate dual chamber pacing to activity responsive rate variable ventricular pacing. PACE 1990; 13:646–652.

Bazett HC: An analysis of the time relationship of electrocardiograms. Heart 1920; 7:353–370.

Bazett HC: Theory of reflex controls to explain regulation of body temperature at rest and during exercise. J Appl Phys 1951; 4:245–262.

Bellamy C, Roberts D, Hughes S, et al: Comparative evaluation of rate modulation in new generation evoked QT and activity sensing pacemakers. PACE 1992; 15:993–999.

Benditt DG, Mianulli M, Fetter J, et al: Single chamber cardiac pacing with activity-initiated chronotropic response: Evaluation by cardiopulmonary exercise testing. Circulation 1987; 75:184–189.

Benditt DG, Milstein S, Buetikofer J, et al: Sensor-triggered, rate-variable cardiac pacing. Current technologies and clinical implications. Ann Int Med 1987; 107:714–724.

Bennett T, Sharma A, Sutton R: Development or a rate adaptive pacemaker based on the maximum rate-of-rise of right ventricular pressure (RV dP/dt max). PACE 1992; 15:219–234.

Bevegard S, Jonsson B, Karlof I, et al: Effect of changes in ventricular rate on cardiac output and central pressures at rest and during exercise in patients with artificial pacemakers. Cardiovasc Res 1967; 1:21–33.

Blanc J, Mansourati J, Ritter P: Atrial natriuretic factor release during exercise in patients successively paced in DDD and rate matched ventricular pacing. PACE 1992; 15:397–402.

Bloomfield P, Macareavey D, Kerr F, et al: Long-term follow-up of patients with the QT rate adaptive pacemaker. PACE 1989; 12:111–114.

Bruce RA, Kusumi F, Hosmer D: Maximal oxygen intake and nomographic assessment of functional aerobic impairment in cardiovascular disease. Am Heart J 1973; 85:546–562.

Brundin T: Temperature of mixed venous blood during exercise. Scand J Clin Lab Invest 1975; 35:539–543.

Callaghan F, Vollman W, Livingston A, et al: The ventricular depolarization gradient: Effects of exercise, pacing rate, epinephrine, and intrinsic heart rate control on the right ventricular evoked response. PACE 1989; 12:1115–1130.

Camm AJ, Garratt C, Paul V: Single-chamber rate adaptive pacing. J Electrophysiol 1989; 3:181–189.

Cammilli L, Alcidi L, Papeschi G: A new pacemaker autoregulating the rate of pacing in relation to metabolic needs. In Y Watanabe (ed): Cardiac Pacing. Proc Vth Internatl Symposium, Amsterdam, Excerpta Medica, 1977; 414.

Cammilli L, Alcidi L, Papeschi G, et al: Preliminary experience with the pH-triggered pacemaker. PACE 1978; 1:448–457.

Candinas RA, Gloor HO, Amann FW, et al: Activity-sensing rate responsive vs conventional fixed-rate pacing: A comparison of rate behavior and pt well-being during routine daily exercise. PACE 1991; 14:204–213.

Chin C-F, Messenger JC, Greenberg PS, et al: Chronotropic incompetence in exercise testing. Clin Cardiol 1979; 2:12–18.

Chirife R: Physiological principles of a new method for rate responsive pacing using the pre-ejection interval. PACE 1988; 11:1545–1554.

Chirife R, Spiodick DH: Densitography: A new method for evaluation of cardiac performance at rest and during exercise. Am Heart J 1972; 83:493–503.

Cohen TJ: A theoretical right atrial pressure feedback heart rate control system to restore physiologic control to the rate-limited heart. PACE 1984; 7:671–677.

Curtis AB, Vance F, Miller K: Automatic reduction of stimulus polarization artifact for accurate evaluation of ventricular evoked responses. PACE 1991; 14:529–537.

den Dulk K, Bouwels L, Lindemans F, et al: The Activitrax rate responsive pacemaker system. Am J Cardiol 1988; 61:107–112.

den Dulk K, Brugada P, Wellens HJJ: Tachycardia termination with a rate responsive pacemaker. Am J Cardiol 1987; 59:1424–1426.

Den Heijer P, Nagelkerke D, Perrins EJ, et al: Improved rate responsive algorithm in QT driven pacemakers—Evaluation of initial response to exercise. PACE 1989; 12:805–811.

Dickhuth HH, Bluemner E, Auchschwelk W, et al: The relationship between heart rate and QT interval during atrial stimulation. PACE 1991; 14:793–799.

Djordjevic M, Kocovic D, Pavlovic S, et al: Circadian variations of heart rate and STIM-T interval: Adaptation for nighttime pacing. PACE 1989; 12:1757–1762.

Donaldson RM, Fox K, Richards AF: Initial experience with a physiological rate responsive pacemaker. Br Med J 1983; 286:667–671.

Donaldson RM, Rickards AF: Rate responsive pacing using the evoked QT principle. A physiological alternative to atrial synchronous pacemakers. PACE 1983; 6:1344–1349.

Donaldson RM, Rickards AF: The ventricular endocardial paced evoked response. PACE 1983; 6:253–259.

Economides AP, Walton C, Gergely S: The ventricular intracardiac unipolar paced-evoked potential in an isolated animal heart. PACE 1988; 11:203–213.

Edelstam C, Hedman A, Nordlander R, et al: QT sensing rate responsive pacing and myocardial infarction: A case report. PACE 1989; 12:502–504.

Ellestad MH, Allen W, Wan MCK, et al: Maximal treadmill stress testing for cardiovascular evaluation. Circulation 1969; 39:517–522.

Epstein SE, Beiser GD, Stampfer M, et al: Characterization of the circulatory response to maximal upright exercise in normal subjects and patients with heart disease. Circulation 1967; 35:1049–1062.

Faerestrand S, Breivik K, Ohm O-J: Assessment of the work capacity and relationship between rate response and exercise tolerance associated with activity-sensing rate-responsive ventricular pacing. PACE 1987; 10:1277–1290.

Faerestrand S, Ohm OJ: A time-related study by Doppler and M-mode echocardiography of hemodynamics, heart size, and AV valvular function during activity-sensing rate-responsive ventricular pacing. PACE 1987; 10:507–518.

Fananapazir L, Bennett DH, Monks P: Atrial synchronized ventricular pacing: Contribution of the chronotropic response to improved exercise performance. PACE 1983; 6:601–608.

Fearnot NE, Evans ML: Heart rate correlation, response time and effect of previous exercise using an advanced pacing rate algorithm for temperature-based rate modulation. PACE 1988; 11:1846–1852.

Fearnot NE, Jolgren DL, Nelson JP, et al: Increasing cardiac rate by measurement of right ventricular temperature. PACE 1984; 7:1240–1245.

Fearnot NE, Smith HJ, Geddes LA: A review of pacemakers that physiologically increase rate: The DDD and rate-responsive pacemakers. Prog Cardiovasc Dis 1986; 29(2): 145–164.

Fearnot NE, Smith HJ, Sellers D, et al: Evaluation of the temperature response to exercise testing in patients with single chamber, rate adaptive pacemakers: A multicenter study. PACE 1989; 12:1806–1815.

Fetter J, Benditt DG, Mianulli M: Usefulness of transcutaneous triggering of conventional implanted pulse generators by an activity-sensing pacemaker for predicting effectiveness of rate response pacing. Am J Cardiol 1988; 62:901–905.

Fredman C, Bjerregaard P, Janosik D, et al: Unusual Wenckebach upper rate response of an atrial-based DD pacemaker. PACE 1992; 15:975–978.

French WJ, Haskell RJ, Wesley GW, et al: Physiological benefits of a pacemaker with dual chamber pacing at low heart rates and single chamber rate responsive pacing during exercise. PACE 1988; 11:1840–1845.

Furman S: Current advances in rate modulated pacing. Circulation 1990; 82:1081–1094.

Gammage M, Schofield S, Rankin I, et al: Benefit of single setting rate responsive ventricular pacing compared with fixed rate demand pacing in elderly patients. PACE 1991; 14:174–180.

Gesell RA: Auricular systole and its relation to ventricular output. Am J Phys 1911; 29: 32–63.

Gillette P: Critical analysis of sensors for physiological responsive pacing. PACE 1984; 7:1263–1266.

Goicolea de Oro A, Ayza MW, de la Llana R, et al: Rate-responsive pacing: Clinical experience. PACE 1985; 8:322–328.

Grace A, Newell S, Cary N, et al: Diagnosis of early cardiac transplant rejection by fall in evoked T wave amplitude measured using an externalized QT driven rate responsive pacemaker. PACE 1991; 14:1024–1031.

Griffin JC, Jutzy KR, Claude JP, et al: Central body temperature as a guide to optimal heart rate. PACE 1983; 6:498–501.

Hanich RF, Midei MG, McElroy BP, et al: Circumvention of maximum tracking limitations with a rate modulated dual chamber pacemaker. PACE 1989; 12:392–397.

Hatano K, Kato R, Hayashi H, et al: Usefulness of rate responsive atrial pacing in patients with sick sinus syndrome. PACE 1989; 12:16–24.

Hayes DL, Christiansen JR, Vlietstra RE, Osborn MJ: Follow-up of an activity-sensing, rate-modulated pacing device, including transtelephonic exercise. Mayo Clin Proc 1989; 64:503–508.

Hayes DL, Higano ST, Eisinger G: Electrocardiographic manifestations of a dual chamber, rate-modulated (DDDR) pacemaker. PACE 1989; 12:555–562.

Hedman A, Nordlander R: Changes in QT and Qa-T intervals induced by mental and physical stress with fixed rate and atrial triggered ventricular inhibited cardiac pacing. PACE 1988; 11:1426–1431.

Hedman A, Nordlander R: QT sensing rate responsive pacing compared to fixed rate ventricular inhibited pacing: A controlled clinical study. PACE 1989; 12:374–385.

Heiman DF, Helwig J: Suppression of ventricular arrhythmias by transvenous intracardiac pacing. JAMA 1966; 195:1150–1153.

Hermansen L, Ekblom B, Saltin B: Cardiac output during submaximal and maximal tread-mill and bicycle exercise. J Appl Physiol 1973; 29:82.

Higano ST, Hayes DL, Eisinger G: Sensor-driven rate smoothing in a DDDR pacemaker. PACE 1989; 12:922–929.

Higano ST, Hayes DL: P wave tracking above the maximum tracking rate in a DDDR pacemaker. PACE 1989; 12:1044–1048.

Hull RW, Snow F, Herre J, et al: The plasma catecholamine responses to ventricular pacing: Implications for rate responsive pacing. PACE 1990; 13:1408–1415.

Humen DP, Anderson K, Brumwell D, et al: A pacemaker which automatically increases its rate with physical activity. In: K Steinbach, et al. (eds): Cardiac Pacing. Darmstadt, Steinkopff Verlag, 1983, p 259–264.

Janicki JS, Weber KT: Equipment and protocols to evaluate the exercise response. In: KT Weber, JS Janicki (eds): Cardiopulmonary Exercise Testing: Physiologic Principles and Clinical Applications. Phila, WB Saunders, 1986, p 138–150.

Jolgren D, Fearnot N, Geddes L: A rate-responsive pacemaker controlled by right ventricular blood temperature. PACE 1984; 7:794–801.

Johnston SL, Bradding P, Watkins J: A simultaneous, noninvasive comparison with sinus rhythm, of two activity sensing, rate adaptive pacemakers, in an elderly population. PACE 1991; 14:20–27.

Judge RD, Wilson WS, Siegel JH: Hemodynamic studies in patients with implanted cardiac pacemakers. N Engl J Med 1964; 270:1391–1395.

Kappenberger LJ, Herpers L: Rate responsive dual chamber pacing. PACE 1986; 9:987–991.

Karlof I: Haemodynamic effect of atrial triggered versus fixed pacing at rest and during exercise in complete heart block. Acta Med Scand 1975; 197:195–206.

Karlof I: Haemodynamic studies at rest and during exercises in patients treated with artificial pacemaker. Acta Med Scand 1975; 3:195–206.

Kaye GC, Baig W, Mackintosh AF: QT sensing rate responsive pacing during subacute bacterial endocarditis: A case report. PACE 1990; 13:1089–1091.

Kristensson BE, Arnman K, Ryden L: The hemodynamic importance of atrioventricular synchrony and rate increase at rest and during exercise. Eur Heart J 1985; 6:773–778.

Kristensson BE, Arnman K, Smedgard P, et al: Physiological versus single-rate ventricular pacing: A double-blind cross-over study. PACE 1985; 8:73–84.

Kruse I, Ryden L: Comparison of physical work capacity and systolic time intervals with ventricular inhibited and atrial synchronous ventricular inhibited pacing. Br Heart J 1981; 46:129–136.

Kruse I, Ryden L, Duffin E: Clinical evaluation of atrial synchronous ventricular inhibited pacemakers. PACE 1980; 3:641–650.

Laczkovics A: The central venous blood temperature as a guide for rate control in pacemaker therapy. PACE 1984; 7:822–830.

Landman MAJ, Senden PJ, Van Rooijen V, et al: Initial clinical experience with rate adaptive cardiac pacing using two sensors simultaneously. PACE 1990; 13:1615–1622.

Langenfeld H, Schneider B, Grimm W, et al: The six-minute walk: An adequate exercise test for pacemaker patients? PACE 1990; 13:1761–1765.

Lau C-P: The range of sensors and algorithms used in rate adaptive cardiac pacing. PACE 1992; 15:1177–1211.

Lau C-P, Antoniou A, Drysdale M: Clinical experience with a minute ventilation sensing rate responsive pacemaker. Br Heart J 1988; 59:613–614.

Lau CP, Antoniou A, Ward DE, et al: Initial clinical experience with a minute ventilation sensing rate modulated pacemaker: Improvements in exercise capacity and symptomatology. PACE 1988; 11:1815–1822.

Lau CP, Antoniou A, Ward DE, et al: Reliability of minute ventilation as a parameter for rate responsive pacing. PACE 1989; 12:321–330.

Lau CP, Lee CP, Wong CK, et al: Rate responsive pacing with a minute ventilation sensing pacemaker during pregnancy and delivery. PACE 1990; 13:158–163.

Lau C-P, Leung W-H, Wong C-K, et al: Adaptive rate pacing at submaximal exercise: The importance of the programmed upper rate. J Electrophysiol 1989; 3:283–288.

Lau CP, Mehta D, Toff WD, et al: Limitations of rate response of an activity-sensing rate-responsive pacemaker to different forms of activity. PACE 1988; 11:141–150.

Lau CP, Ritche D, Butrous GS, et al: Rate modulation by arm movements of the respiratory dependent rate responsive pacemaker. PACE 1988; 11:744–752.

Lau CP, Stott JRR, Toff WD, et al: Selective vibration sensing: A new concept for activity-sensing rate-responsive pacing. PACE 1988; 11:1299–1309.

Lau C, Tai Y, Fong P: Clinical experience with an activity sensing DDDR pacemaker using an accelerometer sensor. PACE 1992; 15:334–343.

Lau CP, Tai YT, Fong PC, et al: Pacemaker mediated tachycardias in single chamber rate responsive pacing. PACE 1990; 13:1575–1579.

Lau CP, Tse WS, Camm AJ: Clinical experience with Sensolog 703: A new activity sensing rate responsive pacemaker. PACE 1988; 11:1444–1455.

Lau C-P, Wong C-K, Cheng C-H, et al: Importance of heart rate modulation on the cardiac hemodynamics during post exercise recovery. PACE 1990; 1277–1285.

Lau CP, Wong CK, Leung WH, Liu WX: Superior cardiac hemodynamics of AV synchrony over rate responsive pacing at submaximal exercise: Observations in activity sensing DDDR pacemakers. PACE 1990; 13:1832–1837.

Lee MT, Baker R: Circadian rate variation in rate-adaptive pacing systems. PACE 1990; 13:1797–1801.

Leitch J, Arnold J, Klein G: Should a VVIR pacemaker increase the heart rate with standing: PACE 1992; 15:288–294.

Lillehei CW, Varco RL, Ferlic RM, et al: Results of the first 2,500 patients undergoing open-heart surgery at the University of Minnesota Medical Center. Surgery 1967; 62:819–832.

Linde-Edelstam C, Nordlander R, Pehrsson K, et al: A double blind study of submaximal exercise tolerance and variation in paced rate in atrial synchronous compared to activity sensor modulated ventricular pacing. PACE 1992; 15:905–915.

Lindemans FW, Rankin IR, Murtaugh R, et al: Clinical experience with an activity sensing pacemaker. PACE 1986; 9:978–986.

Lipkin DP, Buller N, Frenneaux M, et al: Randomised crossover trial of rate responsive Activitrax and conventional fixed rate ventricular pacing. Br Heart J 1987; 58:613.

Maisch B, Langenfeld H: Rate adaptive pacing—Clinical experience with three different pacing systems. PACE 1986; 9:997–1004.

Maksud MG, Coutts KD, Hamilton LH: Time course of heart rate, ventilation and VO2 during laboratory and field exercise. J Appl Physiol 1971; 30:536–539.

McAlister HF, Soberman J, Klementowicz P, et al: Treadmill assessment of activity modulated pacemaker. PACE; 1989; 12:486–501.

McElroy PA, Janicki JS, Weber KT: Physiologic correlates of the heart rate response to upright isotonic exercise: Relevance to rate-responsive pacemakers. JACC 1988; 11:94–99.

McMeekin JD, Lautner D, Hanson S, et al: Importance of heart rate response during exercise in patients using atrioventricular synchronous and ventricular pacemakers. PACE 1990; 13:59–68.

Mond H, Strathmore N, Kertes P, et al: Rate responsive pacing using a minute ventilation sensor. PACE 1988; 11:1866–1874.

Moura PJ, Gessman LJ, Lai T, et al: Chronotropic response of an activity detecting pacemaker compared with the normal sinus node. PACE 1987; 10:78–86.

Muller OF, Bellet S: Treatment of intractable heart failure in the presence of complete atrio-ventricular heart block by the use of internal cardiac pacemaker: Report of 2 cases. N Engl J Med 1961; 265:768–772.

Murtaugh RA, Rueter JC, Watson WS: Activitrax clinical study report. Minneapolis, Medtronic Inc, October 1986.

Nappholtz T, Valenta H, Maloney J, et al: Electrode configurations for a respiratory impedance measurement suitable for rate responsive pacing. PACE 1986; 9:960–964.

Noll B, Krappe J, Goke B, et al: Influence of pacing mode and rate on peripheral levels of atrial natriuretic peptide (ANP). PACE 1989; 12:1763–1768.

Nordlander R, Hedman A, Pehrsson SK: Rate responsive pacing and exercise capacity. PACE; 1989; 12:749–751.

Oetgen WJ, Tibbits PA, Abt MEO, et al: Clinical and electrophysiologic assessment of oral flecainide acetate for recurrent ventricular tachycardia: Evidence for exacerbation of electrical Instability. Am J Cardiol 1983; 52:746–750.

Oldoyel KG, Rae AP: Double blind crossover comparison of the effects of dual chamber pacing (DDD), ventricular rate adaptive (VVIR) pacing on neuroendocrine variables, exercise performance, symptoms of heart block. Br Heart J 1991; 65:188–193.

Oto MA, Muderrisoglu H, Ozin MB, et al: Quality of life in patients with rate responsive pacemakers: A randomized, cross-over study. PACE 1991; 14:800–806.

Ovsyshcher L, Guetta V, Bondy C: First derivative of right ventricular pressure, dP/dt, as a sensor for a rate adaptive VVI pacemaker: Initial experience. PACE 1992; 15: 211–218.

Patterson JA, Naughton J, Pietras RJ, et al: Treadmill exercise in assessment of the functional capacity of patients with cardiac disease. Am J Cardiol 1972; 30:757–762.

Paul V, Garratt C, Ward DE, et al: Closed loop control of rate adaptive pacing: Clinical assessment of a system analyzing the ventricular depolarization gradient. PACE 1989; 12:1896–1902.

Pehrsson SK: Influence of heart rate and atrioventricular synchronization on maximal work tolerance in patients treated with artificial pacemakers. Acta Med Scand 1983; 214:311–315.

Penton GB, Miller H, Levine SA: Some clinical features of complete heart block. Circulation 1956; 13:801–824.

Pinsky WW, Gillette PC, Garson A Jr, et al: Diagnosis, management, and long-term results of patients with congenital complete atrioventricular block. Pediatrics 1982; 69:728–733.

Rickards AF, Donaldson RM: Rate responsive pacing. CPPE 1983; 1:12–19.

Rickards AF, Norman J: Relation between QT interval and heart rate. New design of physiologically adaptive cardiac pacemaker. Br Heart J 1981; 45:56–61.

Ritter PH, VAI F, Bonnet JL: Rate adaptive atrioventricular delay improves cardio-pulmonary performance in patients implanted with a dual chamber pacemaker for complete heart block. Eur JCPE 1991; 1:31–38.

Ross J Jr, Linhart JW, Braunwald E: Effects of changing heart rate in man by electrical stimulation of the right atrium. Studies at rest, during exercise, and with isoproterenol. Circulation 1965; 32:549–558.

Rossi P: Rate-responsive pacing: Biosensor reliability and physiological sensitivity. PACE 1987; 10:454–466.

Rossi P, Aina F, Rognoni G, et al: Increasing cardiac rate by tracking the respiratory rate. PACE 1984; 7:1246–1256.

Rossi P, Plicchi G, Canducci G, Rognoni G, Aina F: Respiration as a reliable physiological sensor for controlling cardiac pacing rate. Br Heart J 1984; 51:7–14.

Rossi P, Rognoni G, Occhetta E, et al: Respiration-dependent ventricular pacing compared with fixed ventricular and atrial-ventricular synchronous pacing: Aerobic and hemodynamic variables. JACC 1985; 6:646–652.

Ruiter J, Heemels J, Kee D, et al: Adaptive rate pacing controlled by the right ventricular prejection interval: Clinical experience with a physiological pacing system. PACE 1992; 15:886–894.

Ruiter JH, De Boer H, Begemann MJS, et al: The A-R interval as exercise indicator: A new option for rate adaptation in single and dual chamber pacing. PACE 1990; 13: 1656–1655.

Ryden L: Atrial inhibited pacing—An underused mode of cardiac stimulation. PACE 1988; 11:1375–1379.

Salo RW, Pederson BD, Olive AL, et al: Continuous ventricular volume assessment for diagnosis and pacemaker control. PACE 1984; 7:1267–1272.

Samet P, Bernstein WH, Medow A, et al: Effect of alterations in ventricular rate upon cardiac output in complete heart block. Am J Cardiol 1964; 14:477–482.

Samet P, Castillo C, Bernstein WH: Hemodynamic consequences of sequential atrioventricular pacing. Am J Cardiol 1968; 21:207–212.

Santomauro M, Fazio S, Ferraro S: Follow-up of a respiratory rate modulated pacemaker. PACE 1992; 15:17–21.

Sellers TD, Fearnot NE, Smith HJ, et al: Right ventricular blood temperature profiles for rate responsive pacing. PACE 1987; 10:467–479.

Sermasi S, Marconi M, Marzaloni M: Usefulness of 1-hour and 24-hour heart rate Holter inbuilt in new TX* rate adaptive pacemakers. PACE 1990; 13:1751–1754.

Shandling AH, Castellanet MJ, Thomas L, et al: Impaired activity rate responsiveness of an atrial activity-triggered pacemaker: The role of differential atrial sensing in its prevention. PACE 1989; 12:1927–1937.

Singer E, Gooch AS, Morse DP: Exercise induced arrhythmias in patients with pacemakers. JAMA 1973; 224:1515–1518.

Singer I, Brennan AF, Steinhaus B, et al: Effects of stress and beta blockade on the ventricular depolarization gradient of the rate modulating pacemaker. PACE 1991; 14:460–469.

Singer I, Olash J, Brennan AF, et al: Initial clinical experience with a rate responsive pacemaker. PACE 1989; 12:1458–1464.

Smedgard P, Kristensson B-E, Kruse I, et al: Rate-responsive pacing by means of activity sensing vs single rate ventricular pacing: A double-blind cross-over study. PACE 1987; 10:902–915.

Solti F, Renyi-Vamos F, Gyongy T: Atrial standstill: An indication for rate responsive pacing. PACE 1990; 13:830–832.

Stangl K, Wirtzfeld A, Heinze R, et al: First clinical experience with an oxygen saturation controlled pacemaker in man. PACE 1988; 11:1882–1887.

Stephenson SE Jr, Brockman SK: P wave synchrony. Ann NY Acad Sci 1964; 111:907–914.

Sugiura T, Kimura M, Mizushina S, et al: Cardiac pacemaker regulated by respiratory rate and blood temperature. PACE 1988; 11:1077–1085.

Sulke AN, Dritsas A, Chambers J, et al: Is accurate rate response programming necessary? PACE 1990; 13:1031–1044.

Sulke N, Pipilis A, Bucknall C, et al: Quantitative analysis of contribution of rate response in three different ventricular rate responsive pacemakers during out of hospital activity. PACE 1990; 13:37–44.

Sulke AN, Pipilis A, Henderson RA: Comparison of the normal sinus node with seven types of rate responsive pacemakers during everyday activity. Br Heart J 1990; 64:25–31.

Tyers GFO: Current status of sensor-modulated rate-adaptive cardiac pacing. J Am Coll Cardiol 1990; 15:412–418.

Vai F, Bonnet JL, Ritter Ph, et al: Relationship between heart rate and minute ventilation, tidal volume and respiratory rate during brief and low level exercise. PACE 1988; 11:1860–1865.

Van Hemel NM, Hamerlijnck RPHM, Pronk KJ, et al: Upper limit ventricular stimulation in respiratory rate responsive pacing due to electrocautery. PACE 1989; 12:1720–1723.

Vogt P, Goy JJ, Kuhn M, Leuenberger P, et al: Single versus double chamber rate responsive cardiac pacing: Comparison by cardiopulmonary noninvasive exercise testing. PACE 1988; 11:1896–1901.

Volosin KJ, Rudderow R, Waxman HL: VOOR–Nondemand rate modulated pacing necessitated by myopotential inhibition. PACE 1989; 12:421–425.

Webb SC, Lewis LM, Morris-Thurgood JA, et al: Respiratory-dependent pacing: A dual response from a single sensor. PACE 1988; 111:730–735.

Weber KT, Kinasewitz GT, West JS, et al: Long-term vasodilatory therapy with trimazosin in chronic cardiac failure. N Engl J Med 1980; 303:242–250.

Wiens RD, Lafia P, Marder CM, et al: Chronotropic incompetence in clinical exercise testing. Am J Cardiol 1984; 54:74–78.

Wilson FN, Macleod AG, Barker PS, et al: The determination and the significance of the areas of the ventricular deflections of the electrocardiogram. Am Heart J 1934; 10: 46–61.

Wilson JH, Lattner S: Apparent undersensing due to oversensing of low amplitude pulses in a thoracic impedance-sensing, rate-responsive pacemaker. PACE 1988; 11:1479–1481.

Wirtzfeld A, Heinze R, Stanzl K, et al: Regulation of pacing rate by variations of mixed venous oxygen saturation. PACE 1984; 7:1257–1262.

Zegelman M, Beyersdorf F, Kreuzer J, et al: Rate responsive pacemakers: Assessment after two years. PACE 1986; 9:1005–1009.

Zegelman M, Cieslinski G, Kreuzer J: Rate response during submaximal exercise comparison of three different sensors. PACE 1988; 11:1888–1895.

Chapter 12

THE IMPLANTABLE
CARDIOVERTER DEFIBRILLATOR

David R. Holmes, Jr.

Electrical stimulation as a treatment for cardiac arrhythmias dates back more than 200 years. Specifically, by the end of the nineteenth century, electrical stimulation had been used to not only induce but also to terminate ventricular arrhythmias. From 1899 to 1900, J.F. Prevost and F. Batelli published their observations in open and closed chest experiments with cardiac fibrillation and defibrillation. In this century, the volume of data increased rapidly with observations on defibrillation induction and the vulnerable phase of the cardiac cycle stimulation threshold, intraoperative defibrillation, and then extension from the open to closed chest setting. The pioneering efforts and continued intense investigation by Michel Mirowski and his colleagues, and Schuder et al. have culminated in the development of the current implantable cardioverter defibrillators (ICDs), which now occupy a central place in the treatment of patients with ventricular arrhythmias. From its initial conception by these investigators in the late 1960s and the first description in 1970, the device has overcome many hurdles including initial skepticism by the medical community, biological and technical questions, as well as practical considerations. Early debate was intense. It centered around questions as to whether the arrhythmia could be sensed appropriately and by what specific sensor, for example, pressure versus electrical activity, whether patients at risk for the arrhythmia could be identified, and whether societal costs were warranted. An early editorial (Lown) concluded that the rationale for some current bioelectronic development is best exemplified by "It was developed because it was possible." Despite such controversy, Michel Mirowski continued vigorous investigation on an implanted defibrillator system that some authorities thought "represented an imperfect solution in search of a plausible and practical application."

Major early issues involved (1) electrode design, (2) development of batteries capable of generating multiple high energy (≥ 30 J) shocks with a fast charge time, (3) circuitry efficient enough to allow the device to have a reasonable longevity, and (4) high gain sensing circuits and algorithms to detect arrhythmias.

From these beginnings, there has been an evolution of technology that has resulted in rapid growth in the field. From the first human implant performed February 4, 1980, the number of implants has increased so that with one manufacturer's device, the automatic implantable cardioverter defibrillator (AICD™, Cardiac Pacemakers Inc. [CPI], St. Paul, MN), there is a worldwide experience through October 1991 of 25,000 implants. After a 5-year period of clinical trials, device modification, and review by federal agencies, Food and Drug Administration approval was granted in 1985. Currently, one other device is now available (Pacer-Cardioverter-Defibrillator [PCD℠], Medtronic, Minneapolis, MN). A third device, Cadence℠, Ventritex, Sunnyvale, CA) is awaiting final approval. Other devices can be expected to be approved in the near future.

During this last decade, there have been four factors that have played a major role in increasing utilization of the ICD: (1) improved device design and performance, (2) improved manufacturing processes that increased the number of devices available for implantation, (3) expanded patient and physician comfort and experience with the device, and (4) concern about the safety and efficacy of long-term antiarrhythmic drug therapy. The findings of the Cardiac Arrhythmia Suppression Trial (CAST), which documented increased mortality in patients with coronary artery disease undergoing antiarrhythmic drug treatment of ventricular arrhythmias, must not be underestimated in this regard. With its great emphasis on the potential proarrhythmic effects of drugs, this study has further stimulated interest in ICDs.

There is increasing data on the reliability and utility of ICDs in a variety of clinical settings. This data comes from many sources including industry registries, which have the largest number of patients but also the potential for biased reporting, single center institutional experiences, and multicenter data. Devices have been increasingly reliable, although defining performance and reliability is difficult. Early devices were able to deliver a nominal 25- to 30-J shock after detection using rate or rate and morphology criteria. Using discrete component designs, these units had a device reliability of 87.6% at 1 year, decreasing to 49.7% at 2 years, and satisfactory performance of 82.2% and 31.3% at these time intervals (CPI Registry data). This data documents more recent devices with hybrid circuits have 1- and 2-year reliability of 98.7% and 95.4%, respectively and satisfactory performance of 98.4% and 91.8% at these same time intervals.

The most recent Bilitch Report summarized a 13-center experience with 3102 ICDs from March 1982 through December 1992 (Figure 1). There is now experience with multiple devices from multiple manufacturers. Earlier models, for example, CPI 1510 and 1520, had a substantial decline after 18 months). Most recent models are substantially more reliable with ≥ 90% of the units surviving out to 30–36 months. Battery depletion is the typical failure mode after that time as can be seen in the Bilitch Report on device failures from October to December 1991 (Table I).

There is no question that these devices can be used to successfully treat ventricular tachycardia or ventricular fibrillation and return the patient to normal sinus rhythm (Figure 2). Longer term follow-up of patients receiving these devices has documented a low incidence of arrhythmic sudden cardiac death compared to what might have been expected in a "similar" cohort of patients treated without the device. Both single and multicenter data are available. Within each patient group treated, there is substantial variation in baseline demographics and need for concomitant antiarrhythmic drug therapy. These may have important implications for assessment of comparative outcome.

The largest survival follow-up experience is the CPI industry data base which includes 15,862 patients. In this data base, survival was excellent with > 95% of patients free of sudden death at 4 years. An increasing amount of

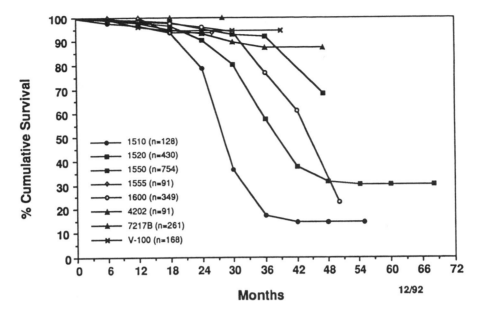

Figure 1. *Performance of implantable cardioverter defibrillator pulse generators by model number. Those models with some generators still in service are listed if 90 or more units have been implanted (CPI models 1510, 1520, 1550, 1555, 1600; Telectronics model 4202; Medtronic model 7217B; Ventritex model V-100). Courtesy of the Bilitch Report, April, 1993.*

potentially less biased data is becoming available. In the most recent Bilitch ICD registry of 1737 patients, the total all-cause mortality was 19.8% at 3 years, while at 6 years, mortality was 33.1% (Figure 3). More data is available on a smaller subset of 1281 patients from this registry. In this group, the mean ejection fraction was 34.3%. During follow-up, 231 patients (18%) died. As would be ex-

Table I
Incidence and Mode of Failure of ICDs Bilitch Report October 1, 1991– December 31, 1991

ICD	Number in Series	Number Failed	Implant Duration (Months)	Failure Mode
CPI				
1500	128	1	35	Battery depletion
1510	128	1	33	Battery depletion
1520	428	20	29, 30, 32, 33, 33, 33, 35, 36, 36, 37, 37, 37, 38, 38, 39, 39, 40, 40 43, 53	Battery depletion
1550	719	3	21, 27, 30	Battery depletion
1600	194	1	36	Battery depletion
Ventritex				
V-100	83	1	6	Battery depletion

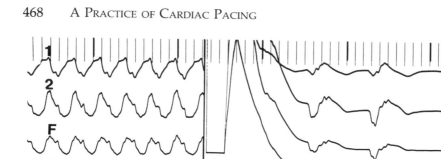

Figure 2. *Successful termination of ventricular tachycardia with 34 J in a patient with a Medtronic PCD®. Note backup bradycardia VVI pacing.*

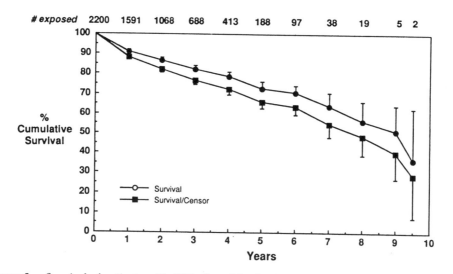

Figure 3. *Survival of patients with ICDs from March 1982 to December 1992. The upper line is overall patient survival whether or not any ICD device remains implanted. The lower line is censored for those devices that have been removed and not replaced (n = 109) and for those lost to follow-up (n = 127). In each instance patient survival is credited to the date of removal or lost to follow-up and then data thereafter censored. Courtesy of the Bilitch Report, April 1993.*

pected, the most common cause of death was a cardiac arrhythmia, seen in 41%, although 37% of patients died a nonarrhythmic cardiac death. The cumulative survival from an arrhythmic death at 1, 3, and 5 years was 96%, 92%, and 87%, respectively, while the survival from all-cause cardiac death was 93%, 90%, and 76%. Given the mean ejection fraction of 34%, these survival rates look encouraging. In another recent large experience (Winkle), even better results have been reported in 555 ICD treated patients in whom the 1- and 4-year sudden death free survival rates were 98.5% and 96.0%, respectively. Recently, data has become available dealing with the cost-effectiveness of the ICD (Larsen). In this small study, the actual variable costs of hospitalization and follow-up care were used for 21 patients receiving an ICD and 43 patients treated with amiodarone. In this small study, life expectancy with an ICD was 50% greater than that associated with amiodarone treatment. Lifetime costs of a device that required replacement at 24 months were substantially greater than if a device could reliably last >36 months.

Although sudden death rates are markedly reduced in most reported patient series, the incidence of total cardiac death and noncardiac death remains high. Given the underlying severity of the cardiac disease, this is not unexpected. As previously mentioned, in the Bilitch Registry, cumulative survival at 5 years was 64% and survival from all-cause cardiac death was 76% in 1281 patients receiving an ICD. In another series of 270 patients, at 3 years there was a sudden death rate of 4.4% but an additional 13.4% of patients died of nonsudden cardiac death (Winkle).

There is concern regarding the documentation of the efficacy of ICDs. These concerns have included (1) the possibility that patients who receive the ICD did not truly need the device and were not at increased risk of sudden death, (2) patients receiving ICDs have more advanced heart disease and thus may be prone to nonsudden cardiac death even if the ICD functioned appropriately, and (3) methodologic problems in assessment of follow-up of patients following ICD implantation. In this latter regard, the question has been raised as to whether survival should be calculated from the time of the first shock instead of from the time of implantation? This has important implications for the definition of a successful procedure; for example, if many patients have the device but it never discharges, should that be defined as a success?

Intense efforts are focused on identifying patients most apt to benefit from ICD implantation. Algorithms are being developed that include clinical and angiographic factors as well as concomitant therapy such as revascularization to predict patient subgroups most likely to benefit. If widely applicable and reliable, these algorithms may help to optimize patient selection. Given the cost of this technology and the concerns about resource allocation, such attempts to optimize patient selection will become increasingly important.

Available studies on the outcome of patients with an ICD have significant limitations. Patient selection factors can influence results. In addition, proarrhythmic medication effects, as seen in the CAST trial, and coronary revascularization could have a profound impact upon results. The optimal means to assess the relative merits of different treatment strategies are randomized controlled studies. Several studies are either planned or currently underway (Table II). A German (Hamburg) trial randomizes patients with cardiac arrest and inducible ventricular tachycardia or ventricular fibrillation to drug treatment (either propafenone, metoprolol, or amiodarone) versus ICD, while a Canadian trial randomizes patients with ventricular fibrillation, cardiac arrest, or sustained ventricular tachycardia and syncope to either amiodarone or an ICD. These trials involve patients with established lethal ventricular arrhythmias. The Multicenter Automatic Defibrillator Implantation Trial (MADIT) compares a prophylactic ICD with conventional treatment for patients with low ejection fraction and nonsustained ventricular tachycardia. The CABG Patch trial is comparing ICD or conventional therapy in patients with depressed ejection fraction and positive signal-averaged electrocardiography who are undergoing coronary bypass graft surgery. Other randomized trials, the Sudden Death Prevention Study (SDPS)

Table II
Randomized Trials of ICD

Hamburg Cardiac Arrest Study:
Patient population—cardiac arrest and inducible ventricular tachycardia or ventricular fibrillation
Randomization—ICD vs drug therapy (propafenone, metoprolol or amiodarone)
Primary endpoint—cardiac arrest or sudden death

Canadian Implantable Defibrillator Study:
Patient population—ventrciular fibrillation, cardiac arrest or syncope, and sustained ventricular tachycardia
Randomization—ICD vs amiodarone
Primary endpoint—arrhythmic death

MADIT (Multicenter Automatic Defibrillator Implantation Trial):
Patient population—coronary artery disease, ejection fraction ≤0.35, nonsyncopal, nonsustained ventricular tachycardia, inducible ventricular tachycardia at study
Randomization—ICD vs conventional pharmacological therapy
Primary endpoint—arrhythmic death

CABG (Coronary Artery Bypass Graft) Patch Trial:
Patient population—undergoing CABG, ejection fraction ≤36%, positive

SA-ECG
Randomization—ICD vs conventional pharmacologic therapy
Primary endpoint—all-cause mortality, nonfatal ventricular arrhythmia

Dutch Prospective Study of the AICD as First-Choice Therapy
Patient population—prior myocardial infarction, cardiac arrest within 3 months, inducible ventricular tachycardia, or ventricular fibrillation
Randomization—ICD vs conventional drug therapy
Primary endpoint—cost effectiveness, costs per year of life saved

---

and Defibrillator Implantation as a Bridge to Later Transplantation (DEFIBRLAT) are also in the planning stage. These trials will identify the optimal role for these devices in specific patient subsets.

A Dutch trial is also studying the cost-effectiveness of ICD implantation as a first-choice therapy in patients with coronary artery disease, prior infarction, and resuscitated cardiac arrest. Patients will be randomized to either initial ICD or conventional therapy that initially attempts drug therapy.

The AICD™ (Cardiac Pacemakers Inc., St. Paul, MN) and the PCD™ (Medtronic Inc., Minneapolis, MN) have been approved for use by the Food and Drug Administration. Final approval is expected for Cadence™ (Ventritex, Sunnyvale, CA). The number of models is expected to expand significantly. The Health Care Financing Administration (HCFA) has approved Medicare coverage for the device. Initially, approval required an inducible ventricular arrhythmia at the time of electrophysiological study prior to implantation and reserved implantation as a treatment of last resort. As of July 1991, this has been revised so that HCFA does not require the ICD to be reserved as a last resort.

In addition, preoperative electrophysiological inducibility is no longer required. This issue of "noninducibility" is particularly important in patients with cardiomyopathy. Patients with cardiomyopathy and sustained ventricular tachycardia or ventricular fibrillation are at increased risk of recurrent arrhythmias or sudden death. Despite this, only 50%–70% are found to have an inducible arrhythmia at the time of electrophysiological study; in the remainder, serial drug testing is not possible to optimize therapy. In patients with hypertrophic cardiomyopathy and known sustained arrhythmias, electrophysiological testing is also less helpful in predicting risk of subsequent events and selecting effective therapy. The change in preoperative electrophysiological inducibility requirements will help optimize the care of many of these patients. Other groups that may benefit from the change in guidelines include those with prolonged QT syndromes and those who have arrhythmias following repair of congenital heart disease.

CURRENT ICD SYSTEMS

There has been rapid evolution in the technology of ICDs. Early devices were designed to recognize and treat only ventricular fibrillation. While effective, these early devices were large, nonprogrammable, and had short battery lives. In addition, they did not have backup bradycardia pacing and could not effectively treat some patients with ventricular tachycardia. New groups of ICDs are now available. Devices currently under development or in clinical trials are even more sophisticated (Table III) and include antibradycardia and antitachycardia pacing, low- and high-amplitude shock, programmability, and telemetry.

Table III
Devices Available or Under Evaluation, 1993

	CPI Ventak P	CPI PRx	Intermedics RES Q	Medtronic PCD	Siemens Siecure	Telectronics AIP	Telectronics Guardian	Ventritex Cadence
Weight (grams)	240	220	220	N/A	220	269	270	237
Programmable rate/energy	Yes	Yes	Yes	Yes	Yes	Yes	Yes	Yes
Bradycardia pacing	No	Yes	Yes	Yes	Yes	Yes	Yes	Yes
Antitachycardia pacing	No	Yes	Yes	Yes	Yes	Yes	No	Yes
Waveforms	M	M	B	M, S	N/A	M	M	M, B
Minimum energy (joules)	0.1	0.1	0.1	0.2	2.5	0.5	3	0.1
Maximum energy (joules)	30	32	40	34	40	30	30	38
Tiered therapy	No	Yes	Yes	Yes	Yes	Yes	No	Yes
Committed	Yes	No	Yes	No (VT) Yes (VF)	Yes	No	No	No
Stored electrograms	No	No	No	No	N/A	"snapshot"	No	Yes
Noninvasive EPS	No	Yes	Yes	Yes	Yes	Yes	No	Yes

M = monophasic; B = biphasic; S = sequential; N/A = not available.

ICD EVOLUTION

Devices are now broadly grouped into generations based upon their functions.

1. First generation ICDs were either not programmable or only programmable to the extent that the device could be noninvasively altered with a magnet to a "standby mode."
2. Second generation ICDs are more complex but include antibradycardia pacing capability, limited programmability, and may have telemetry.
3. Third generation ICDs are the most complex. In addition to antibradycardia pacing, they have antitachycardia pacing capability, extensive programmability, and telemetry. These devices (for example, CPI-PRx™, PCD™, and Cadence™) will allow performance of noninvasive electrophysiological testing and the ability to store and read electrograms after a shock has occurred.

Another important third generation feature is waveform programmability. This will be particularly true as nonthoracotomy systems become more widely used; in general, these nonthoracotomy systems appear to require higher energy levels than epicardial defibrillation. Both monophasic and biphasic waveform pulses have been studied (Figure 4). The latter may be associated with a decrease in voltage and energy requirements for defibrillation. Although, in general, biphasic waveforms are more efficient than monophasic waveforms, differences are variable between patients and dependent upon which configuration electrode system is used. For patients with marginal defibrillation thresholds, or particularly patients with a nonthoracotomy system, these differences in defibrillation efficacy may be important. Other factors may also be important such as the shape or tilt of the waveforms, although these are less well studied. New devices will be programmable to allow for either monophasic or biphasic waveforms.

As devices have evolved, the concept of *tiered therapy* has also become im-

CAPACITOR DISCHARGE PATTERNS

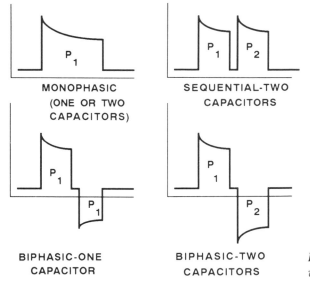

MONOPHASIC
(ONE OR TWO
CAPACITORS)

SEQUENTIAL-TWO
CAPACITORS

BIPHASIC-ONE
CAPACITOR

BIPHASIC-TWO
CAPACITORS

Figure 4. *Monophasic and biphasic waveform pulses.*

portant. Tiered therapy involves programmable differential responses to a specific arrhythmia. As such, it requires accurate sensing of a variety of different arrhythmias. New detection algorithms are becoming available that include rapidity of onset of the ventricular arrhythmia to distinguish the arrhythmia from sinus tachycardia, and rate stability to help in the differentiation from atrial fibrillation (Table IV). The ICDs with these features will be extensively pro-

Table IV
Ventricular Arrhythmia Detective Criteria with a Third Generation ICD
(PCD™)

Ventricular Tachycardia Detection		
Parameter	Range	Nominal
Enable	On/off	Off
NOI*	4–52	16
TDI**	280–600 msec	400 msec
Stability	Off/30–130 msec	Off
Onset criteria enable	On/off	Off
RR%	56–97	81
Onset counter enable	On/off	Off
Ventricular Fibrillation Detection		
Parameter	Range	Nominal
Enable	On/off	Off
FDI†	240–400	320
NOI**	6–30	18

* Number of intervals to select; ** tachycardia detection interval; † Fibrillation detection interval.

grammable and will allow improved specificity of detection of both ventricular tachycardia and ventricular fibrillation.

Other improvements in sensing will also be required. In early and current units, once the tachycardia detection criteria were met, the capacitors were charged and the shock was delivered (committed discharge). With nonsustained ventricular tachycardia, the arrhythmia could, therefore, initiate the discharge and then have spontaneously terminated prior to device discharge so that the patient received the subsequent shock after return to normal sinus rhythm. This

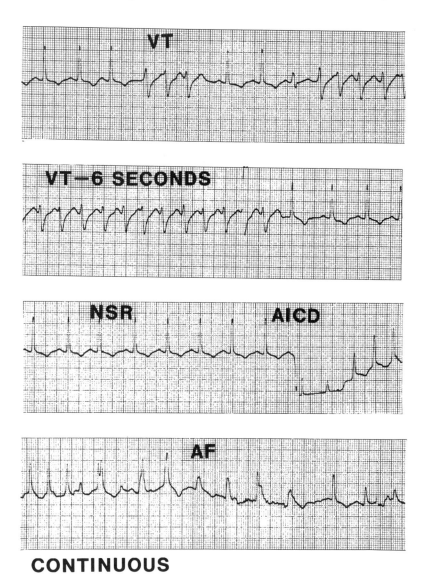

CONTINUOUS

Figure 5.   Induction of atrial fibrillation. In this patient, the ICD senses nonsustained ventricular tachycardia. The committed device then discharges after the nonsustained ventricular tachycardia has terminated spontaneously. This results in atrial fibrillation.

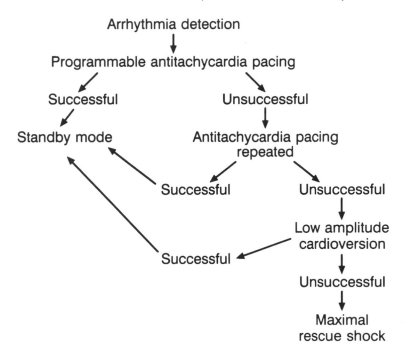

Figure 6. *Arrhythmia detection and treatment.*

shock was uncomfortable and also carried with it the potential to reinitiate the ventricular arrhythmia or another arrhythmia (Figure 5). Some new third generation ICDs will be programmably noncommitted and permit sensing throughout the time it takes for capacitor charging. This feature requires that the arrhythmia continue until charging is complete; if the arrhythmia spontaneously terminates during this time, the shock is aborted.

With these improvements in sensing capabilities, tiered therapy with a variety of antitachycardia pacing modes is possible and expands the number of patients who can be treated although it adds substantial complexity.

Overdrive pacing has been widely used for terminating tachycardia (see Chapter 13). It will potentially terminate all types of reentrant arrhythmias. Although it has been commonly used during electrophysiological testing, it has only been used infrequently for the treatment of ventricular tachycardia with implantable units because of concerns that stable ventricular tachycardia could be accelerated to a hemodynamically unstable arrhythmia or converted to ventricular fibrillation. Third generation ICDs have the capability of antitachycardia pacing and then low output shock before delivery of the maximum output defibrillation energy (Figure 6). After arrhythmia detection, the selected antitachycardia pacing therapy is administered (Figures 7 and 8). The device then analyzes the effect of pacing on the arrhythmia. If successful, it will revert to its standby mode; if bradycardia is present, it will pace. However, if tachycardia persists or has accelerated, additional antitachycardia pacing therapies will be administered. If these are not successful, a low-amplitude cardioversion may

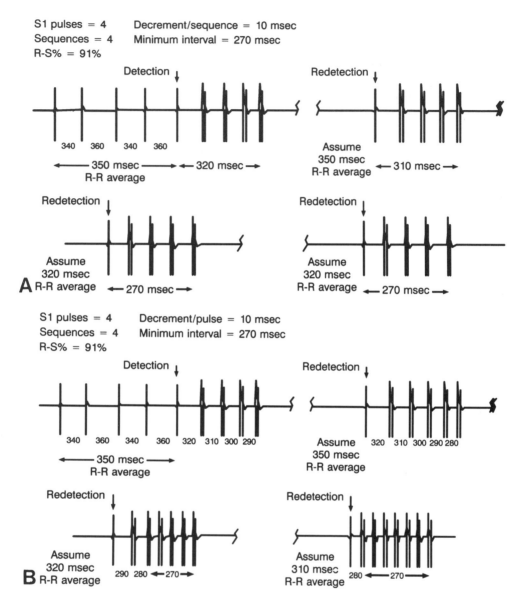

Figure 7. Both ramp (A) and burst (B) therapy are possible. With ramp therapy, after arrhythmia detection, a train of impulses is delivered with a programmable decrement. If the arrhythmia continues or accelerates, the cycle of the delivered impulses decreases. With burst therapy, a train of impulses with the same repetitive cycle length is delivered after detection of any specific arrhythmia. If the arrhythmia accelerates, the burst cycle length decreases.

be attempted or failing this, a maximal rescue shock of approximately 30 J is administered (Figure 9). Two or three levels or zones of detection will be available so that multiple discrete arrhythmias can potentially be treated in a single patient. Each zone will have preset programmed detection criteria, then pacing, then low energy cardioversion or, finally, rescue shock defibrillation.

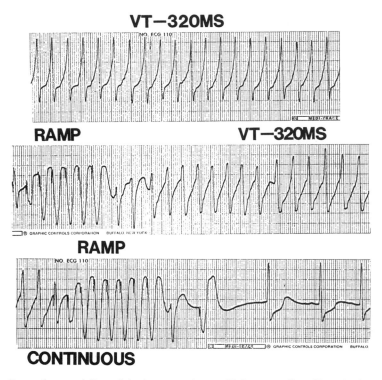

Figure 8. *Ramp therapy delivered during a continuous Holter recording. Ventricular tachycardia (cycle length 320 msec) is treated initially with ramp therapy but fails. The device recycles and delivers a second therapy which restores normal rhythm.*

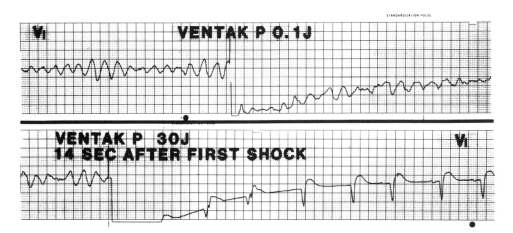

Figure 9. *During ventricular fibrillation, a 0.1-J shock with the Ventak P™ is ineffective. Fourteen seconds after the first shock, a maximal output shock of 30 J converts the patient to normal rhythm.*

DESCRIPTION OF CURRENT ICDs

At the present time, two devices are available, the CPI Ventak P™ model 1600 and the Medtronic PCD™. The Ventritex Cadence™ should be available shortly.

The Ventak P™ 1600 is smaller and lighter than prior CPI devices, but is still rather large (10.1 × 7.6 × 2.0 cm and weighs 235 g). The projected device life of the two lithium-silver vanadium pentoxide batteries is approximately 4–5 years.

This device, which can treat either ventricular tachycardia or fibrillation, has two independently programmable arrhythmia detection algorithms: (1) a rate sensing channel, and (2) a morphology sensing channel (Probability Density Function). The programmable rate sensing channel monitors intrinsic R waves. The nominal rate criterion is 155 bpm although it can be programmed from 125–200 bpm. If the ventricular arrhythmia is slower than the rate cutoff, detection will not occur. It has been recommended that the rate cutoff be 10 bpm less than the rate of spontaneous monomorphic ventricular tachycardia. If polymorphic ventricular tachycardia is present, the rate cutoff should be lower because not all ventricular depolarization may reach the voltage threshold required for sensing.

The second detection algorithm involves Probability Density Function (PDF). The PDF was developed as a morphology criterion (Figure 10). The concept was that rhythms have specific and characteristic waveform profiles. During sinus rhythm or supraventricular tachycardia, a large portion of the transcardiac electrogram is isoelectric. This is different than ventricular tachycardia or fibrillation in which there is a relative absence of isoelectric potentials on the electrocardiogram. Narrow complex well-organized ventricular tachycardia, such as fascicular tachycardia, may not meet PDF criteria. Conversely, supraventricular tachycardia with a marked interventricular conduction delay may satisfy the PDF criteria. If PDF is on, both rate and morphology criteria must be met. Alternatively, rate criteria alone can be used. A minimum of eight tachycardia complexes (usually 2–5 seconds) are required. Once the detection criteria are met, the pulse generator delivers the shock. Some data suggest that PDF causes significantly decreased battery life due to current drain. Depending upon the specific situation, the increased specificity of arrhythmia detection supplied by adding PDF may be worth the tradeoff of decreased battery life.

After arrhythmia detection, there is a first shock delay programmable from 2.5 to 10 seconds. This is necessary to ensure that the arrhythmia is sustained, and is extremely important in patients with nonsustained ventricular tachycardia to prevent delivery of a shock after the patient's rhythm has spontaneously reverted to normal sinus rhythm. If the arrhythmia continues throughout the delay, the pulse generator charges its capacitors to deliver the programmable first shock. The shock energy level is selected based upon the results of programmed ventricular stimulation, tachycardia induction, and cardioversion/defibrillation determined at the time of postoperative testing and can vary from 0.1 to 30 J. Following this initial shock, if the rhythm persists, a second shock is delivered after charging the capacitor. This sequence can be repeated up to

PROBABILITY DENSITY FUNCTION

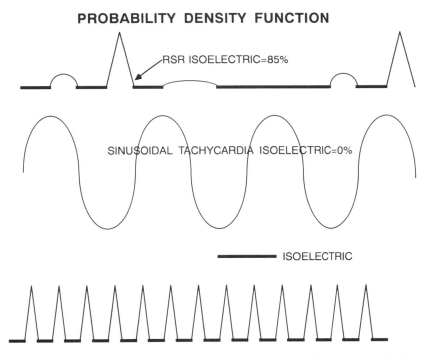

Figure 10. *Schematic diagram of the probability density function. During sinus rhythm (top), the majority of the transcardiac electrogram is isoelectric. During wide complex ventricular tachy-cardia or ventricular fibrillation, there is marked absence in isoelectric potentials (middle). During narrow complex tachycardia (bottom), the amount of isoelectric intracardiac electrogram is in be-tween. As can be imagined, narrow complex ventricular tachycardia, i.e., fascicular tachycardia, may not meet PDF criteria.*

a total of 5 shocks. In current FDA approved devices, only the first shock has programmable energy levels; all subsequent shocks are delivered at 30 J. After the 5-shock sequence, the pulse generator does not deliver additional shocks if the arrhythmia persists. Backup bradycardia pacing is not available in this model, although in subsequent generations it will be available.

PCD™

The current PCD™ (7217B) is 10.1 × 7.0 × 2.0 cm and has a mass of 197 g. The projected life of the lithium-silver vanadium oxide batteries depends upon the programmed bradycardia pacing parameters, the ratio of paced-to-sensed events, the pacing load, and the frequency of high-voltage capacitor charging and ranges from approximately 3.6 to 5.4 years.

This device can also be used to treat ventricular tachycardia or ventricular fibrillation. There are two independently programmable detection and treatment procedures.

Ventricular Fibrillation

For ventricular fibrillation, there are two programmable parameters for detection, a programmable ventricular fibrillation interval criteria with a programmable fibrillation detection interval (FDI) and a fibrillation event counter (Table IV). The ventricular fibrillation detection criteria are designed to detect a very rapid rate and requires that ≥75% of the previous intervals are shorter than the programmable FDI. The second programmable parameter is the number of intervals (NOI) to detect. Ventricular fibrillation detection occurs when the number of intervals shorter than the FDI is equal to the number of intervals required for detection.

The PCD℠ can deliver up to four defibrillation therapies for each ventricular fibrillation episode detected. Each therapy is a high energy defibrillation shock programmable for stored energy (leading edge voltage) as well as pulse width. In addition, each therapy is programmable to consist of either a single shock or two high voltage pulses. Defibrillation therapy is committed and once the charging cycle begins, a shock will be delivered. After a ventricular fibrillation therapy, the device returns to the programmed settings and scans for either recurrent ventricular fibrillation or bradycardia. Ventricular tachycardia detection is automatically halted for 64 events (either paced events, sensed events, or therapy), after each ventricular fibrillation detection that initiates a ventricular fibrillation therapy. This is designed to avoid detection of nonsustained ventricular tachycardia that may follow ventricular fibrillation therapy.

Ventricular Tachycardia

For ventricular tachycardia detection, there are up to four separately programmable parameters (Table IV). Any programmed ventricular tachycardia criteria must be met for any episode. These include Tachycardia Detection Interval, Interval Stability Criteria, Onset Criteria, and the Number of Intervals (NOI) required to Detect. The Onset Criteria are used to prevent false detection of ventricular tachycardia during an episode of sinus tachycardia, while the Interval Stability Criteria are used to prevent detection of atrial fibrillation as ventricular tachycardia.

After detection of ventricular tachycardia, there are three programmable ventricular tachycardia therapy categories: Burst, Ramp, and Cardioversion. Burst therapy is rate adaptive; as such, the PCD℠ delivers a burst of impulses at a calculated percentage of the tachycardia rate. Ramp therapy is also rate adaptive and delivers a programmable train of progressively shortening cycle length impulses to treat tachycardia (Figures 7 and 8). Cardioversion therapy can be programmed as either a single pulse, two simultaneous pulses, or two sequential pulses separated by a short period of time. Delivery of the cardioversion pulse is synchronized to the second nonrefractory sensed event after the charging cycle is completed. Following cardioversion, after a 300 msec blanking period, a 520 msec refractory period, and a bradycardia escape interval of 1000 msec, the device resumes surveillance.

Other features of the PCD™ include backup programmable VVI pacing, the ability to perform noninvasive programmed ventricular stimulation for electrophysiological testing, and telemetry capacity.

CADENCE™

The Ventritex Cadence™ weighs 240 g and is 9.72 × 8.21 × 2.36 cm. This device is a multiprogrammable antitachyarrhythmia device with backup bradycardia pacing. On the current model, up to three different tachyarrhythmias can be detected. Detection of tachycardia involves both a programmed rate criterion and a programmable number of intervals. The tachycardia algorithm also incorporates features that detect a sudden onset in rapid rate and a parameter that detects sustained tachycardia in the event that the therapy delivered is not successful (Extended High Rate [EHR]).

Ventricular fibrillation is detected using a rate criterion. An important aspect is an automatic gain control circuit as compared to a fixed sensitivity circuit. By changing the sensitivity based upon the detected signal amplitude, the automatic gain control allows sensing of a large range of input signals and decreases the chance of either undersensing or oversensing.

Following detection of fibrillation, the high voltage capacitors charge; after charging, the continued presence of the arrhythmia is confirmed before delivery of the shock. This minimizes the chance of delivering a shock after nonsustained ventricular tachycardia has spontaneously terminated.

The device is extensively programmable in four major configurations: (1) defibrillation alone with a maximum of six synchronous shocks with variable programmable output and either monophasic or biphasic waveform; (2) defibrillation as well as antitachycardia treatment for single tachycardia detection criteria. With this configuration, tachycardia therapy includes antitachycardia pacing and synchronous cardioversion shocks; (3) defibrillation as well as antitachycardia treatment for two different tachycardia discriminations. For each of the last two configurations, the EHR parameter can be selected to facilitate treatment of sustained arrhythmias that do not respond to initial therapy; (4) bradycardia pacing alone. This device has the capability for extensive data storage including electrograms, real-time electrogram transmission, rate, sequence, andnumber of arrhythmias, type of therapy delivered, and the number of aborted shocks. In addition, battery voltage, residual high voltage capacitor voltage and pacing lead impedance can also be assessed.

LEAD CONFIGURATION

The lead systems used have changed considerably. Currently there are three types of leads: ventricular patch leads, conventional epimyocardial screw-in electrodes, and endocardial leads. Each of the manufacturers has their own unique systems. Adapters are available, however, for conversion of some of the leads.

TRANSCARDIAC PATCH ELECTRODES

CPI

The titanium mesh ventricular patch electrodes monitor the electrical waveforms for the PDF circuit in addition to delivering the cardioverting/defibrillating energy. The standard patch has a 14-cm^2 surface area while the larger patch is 28 cm^2. Defibrillation thresholds typically are lowest with the largest electrode surface area. The decision to use a specific patch configuration, for example, a large and a small patch or a patch and a superior vena cava transvenous lead, depends upon the cardiac anatomy and left ventricular size, need to perform other procedures such as bypass grafting, and the defibrillation thresholds. The patches are fixed to the parietal pericardium with synthetic, nonabsorbable suture material at opposite ends to prevent migration. Typically, a 28-cm^2 patch is placed on the posterolateral left ventricle and the other patch (another 28-cm^2 size) placed over the septum anteriorly.

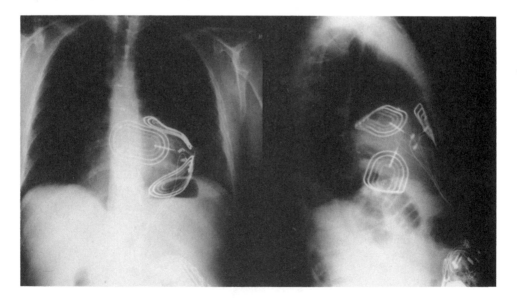

Figure 11. PA and lateral chest x-rays in a patient who has undergone PCD™ implantation using a three-patch system. With a three-patch system either sequential or simultaneous pulses can be delivered. A two-patch system may also be used.

Cadence™

The Cadence™ patch electrodes are also titanium mesh. Two patch sizes (19 cm^2 and 38 cm^2) are available. As is true with CPI systems, DFTs are typically lowest with the largest electrode surface area.

ENDOCARDIAL ELECTRODES

PCD™

The PCD™ patch electrodes are a plantinum alloy. There are three patch sizes with surface areas of 370 mm^2, 660 mm^2, and 840 mm^2, respectively. The latter usually have the lowest DFT (Figure 11).

CPI

A superior vena cava spring lead may be used instead of one of the patches for monitoring PDF function and serves as the anode or cathode. This lead is 100 cm long and has a 10-cm^2 surface area (Figures 12 and 13). It is placed in the venous system near the junction of the right atrium and the superior vena cava. When the spring lead and a left ventricular patch are utilized, the threshold may be higher than when two patches are used. Another potential disadvantage is that there may be dislodgment of the spring lead.

A transvenous right ventricular endocardial lead is also currently in clinical trials. This tripolar 14 Fr lead has a distal spring electrode with a surface area of 3 cm^2 and a proximal spring electrode of 5 cm^2. These are separated by 10–16 mm. This lead can be used alone or in combination with a subcutaneous patch.

Transvene™

The largest nonthoracotomy implantation experience is with the PCD™. The transvenous system consists of a 10.5 Fr multipolar active fixation lead for placement in the right ventricular apex. The active fixation electrode is the cathode. There have been two versions. In one there is a second distal ring electrode 5 mm proximal to the tip; this was used for bipolar pacing and sensing. The other model did not have this additional distal ring electrode; instead, the defibrillating coil electrode was used. The defibrillation electrode is 50 mm long and provides a conduction surface area of 205 mm^2; it is located 22 mm from the tip.

The second lead is a 7.0 Fr monopolar defibrillation lead with a 50-mm coil electrode and a surface area of 90 mm^2 which is placed either in the coronary sinus or in the superior vena cava. Using these leads, a variety of configurations are available (Table V).

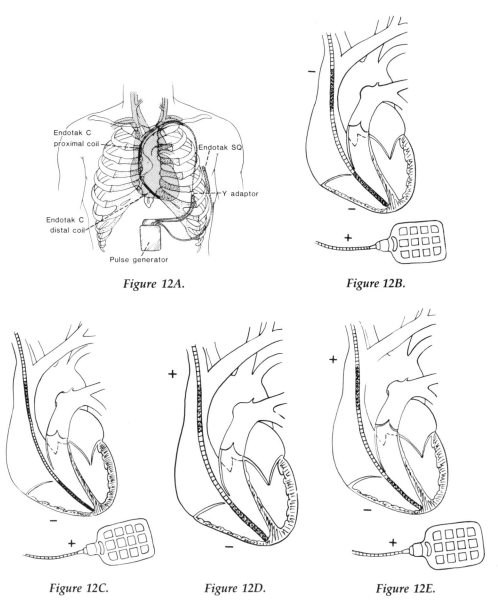

Figure 12A.

Figure 12B.

Figure 12C.

Figure 12D.

Figure 12E.

Figure 12A. *An Endotak system involves pulse generator, tripolar tined transvenous catheter with a proximal and distal coil, and a subcutaneous patch (Endotak SQ). The Y adaptor is used for various lead connections. **B.** One option involves use of both the proximal and distal coils of the transvenous lead system as the common cathode (−) with the subcutaneous patch as the anode (+). **C.** A second option uses the distal coil as cathode (−) and the subcutaneous patch as the anode (+). **D.** A third option uses the proximal coil as the anode (+) and the distal coil as the cathode (−) without a patch. **E.** A fourth option uses the distal coil as the cathode (−) and both the proximal coil and subcutaneous patch as the anode (+).*

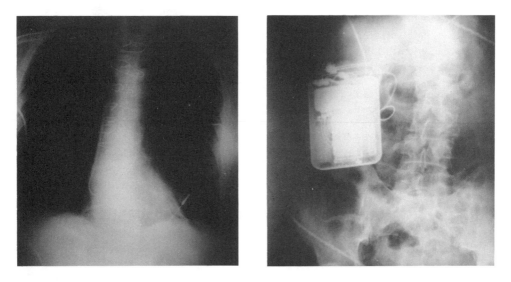

Figure 13A. *PA chest x-ray of a nonthoracotomy lead system with an Endotak C and SQ lead (Cardiac Pacemakers, Inc., St. Paul, MN). Arrows indicate the patch electrode in the subcutaneous tissue.* **B.** *The pulse generator is placed in an upper abdominal pocket on the right side.*

Table V
Defibrillation Complications

Transvene™

- Right ventricle to superior vena cava and subcutaneous patch used for sequential or simultaneous pathway;
- Right ventricle to coronary sinus and subcutaneous patch used for sequential or simultaneous pathway;
- Right ventricle to coronary sinus and superior vena cava used for sequential or simultaneous pathway;
- Right ventricle to coronary sinus used for single pathway;
- Right ventricle to subcutaneous patch used for single pathway;
- Right ventricle to superior vena cava used for single pathway.

EPIMYOCARDIAL ELECTRODES

CPI

Conventional epimyocardial electrodes can also be used in place of the endocardial lead for rate sensing and maintaining R wave synchrony. These should be placed within 1 to 2 cm of each other on either the right or left ventricle. Medtronic 4915 or 6917A leads are very satisfactory as are CPI 4313 or 4320 leads.

Cadence℠

No epimyocardial system is required other than the transcardiac patches. Usually for pacing and sensing, a bipolar endocardial lead is used.

IMPLANTATION COMBINATIONS

Given the number of electrodes available, several implant combinations are possible.

Epimyocardial System

If only epimyocardial systems are used, two patch electrodes are placed for PDF analysis (only for CPI systems) and defibrillation, and two epimyocardial electrodes are used for rate sensing and R wave synchronizing. Selection of the patch size will depend upon what other procedures are planned and the details of the cardiac anatomy and size. As has been mentioned, larger patch sizes usually are associated with improved defibrillation thresholds.

Combined Epimyocardial and Endocardial Systems

A variety of options are available. Nonthoracotomy systems employing sequential shocks from a SVC coil to right ventricular apex (RVA) or a coronary sinus lead to RVA may not require patch electrodes. Usually, however, at least one patch electrode is used with either a second patch electrode or in combination with the superior vena cava spring lead as the anode. In combined systems, the transvenous bipolar endocardial lead can be used for rate sensing and R wave synchronization. In one of our institutions, a single left ventricular patch lead is placed during thoracotomy and then combined with the spring lead and a transvenous rate sensing lead.

Transvenous Systems

Development of a complete transvenous system can be expected to become the dominant approach for ICD implantation. At Montefiore Hospital approximately 90% of the past 50 new ICD implants, have been transvenous. At the present time, both Endotak™ and Transvene™ implants require a subcutaneous patch so that they are not completely transvenous but are nonthoracotomy.

PATIENT SELECTION

NASPE has developed a consensus statement based upon currently available data for patient selection of ICD (Table VI). Patients are grouped into three classes: Class I: consensus exists that an ICD is indicated; Class II: consensus does not exist but an ICD is a therapeutic option to be considered; Class III: an ICD is not generally justified. Such classifications are only to be interpreted as guidelines requiring clinical interpretation. For Class I indications, the ICD should at least be strongly considered as a treatment option or may be considered the treatment of choice. Expansion of these classification schemes will be dy-

---

Table VI
Patient Selection Criteria for ICD

Class I

1. One or more episodes of spontaneous sustained ventricular tachycardia or ventricular fibrillation in a patient in whom electrophysiological testing and/or spontaneous ventricular arrhythmias cannot be used accurately to predict efficacy of other therapies.
2. Recurrent episodes of spontaneous sustained ventricular tachycardia or ventricular fibrillation in a patient despite antiarrhythmic drug therapy (guided by electrophysiological testing or noninvasive methods).
3. Spontaneous sustained ventricular tachycardia or ventricular fibrillation in a patient in whom antiarrhythmic drug therapy is limited by intolerance on noncompliance.
4. Persistent inducibility of clinically relevant sustained ventricular tachycardia or ventricular fibrillation at electrophysiological study, on best available drug therapy or despite surgical/catheter ablation, in a patient with spontaneous sustained ventricular tachycardia or ventricular fibrillation.

Class II

1. Syncope of undetermined etiology in a patient with clinically relevant sustained ventricular tachycardia or ventrciular fibrillation induced at electrophysiological study in whom antiarrhythmic drug therapy is limited by inefficacy, intolerance, or noncompliance.

Class III

1. Sustained ventricular tachycardia or ventricular fibrillation mediated by acute ischemia/infarction or toxic/metabolic etiologies, amenable to correction or reversibility.
2. Recurrent syncope of undetermined etiology in a patient without inducible sustained ventricular tachyarrhythmias.
3. Incessant ventricular tachycardia or ventricular fibrillation.
4. Ventricular fibrillation secondary to atrial fibrillation in the Wolff-Parkinson-White syndrome in a patient whose bypass tract is amenable to surgical or catheter ablation.
5. Surgical, medical, or psychiatric contraindications.

---

namic and highly dependent upon the results of further controlled and randomized studies. Such expansion will also depend upon continued evolution of the technology.

In addition to indications for ICDs, the following contraindications must also be kept in mind:

1. slow, well-tolerated ventricular tachycardia. In these patients, the arrhythmia may either not be detected by the device (Figure 14) or the patient may receive a discharge while awake. This is less of a problem with current new devices that allow low energy cardioversion, but a discharge may still cause significant patient distress and, in selected circumstances, may limit use.
2. Recurrent nonsustained ventricular tachycardia that cannot be controlled pharmacologically but which is of sufficient duration to initiate a device discharge. In these patients, the nonsustained ventricular tachycardia may initiate discharges (Figure 5).
3. Recurrent supraventricular tachycardia including atrial flutter or fibrillation, particularly in patients with bundle branch block that cannot be controlled

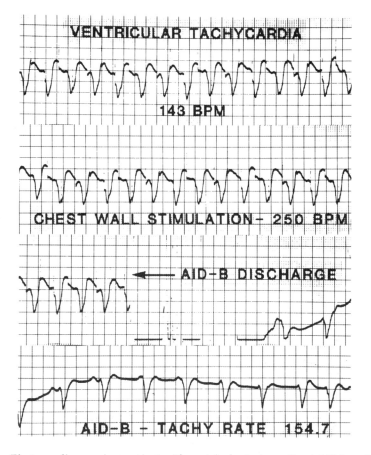

Figure 14. *Electrocardiogram in a patient with ventricular tachycardia at 143 bpm that was too slow to meet detection criteria. The patient was then subjected to chest wall stimulation that was sensed by the device and a shock was delivered with return to normal rhythm.*

pharmacologically but which may be sufficient to meet device criteria and trigger a discharge.
4. Patients with such severe underlying cardiac disease or extracardiac disease that will limit survival to <6–12 months.
5. ICD implantation is contraindicated in centers without experienced personnel including electrophysiologists, cardiovascular surgeons, and nursing personnel needed for initial implantation, screening, and follow-up of these patients.
6. Patients who are unwilling or unable to accept the limitations of the device.

Evolving technology may impact greatly on some of these relative contraindications. Some of the new devices will or already have satisfactorily resolved the first three relative contraindications. ICDs with antitachycardia pacing can be used to treat slow ventricular tachycardia; third generation devices can program the number of intervals of ventricular tachycardia necessary for detection to resolve the problem of nonsustained ventricular tachycardia; finally, in patients with recurrent atrial fibrillation, stability detection algorithms may be useful.

PATIENT EVALUATION

Preoperative

In all patients in whom an ICD is contemplated, a baseline electrophysiological study is required to document the underlying ventricular arrhythmia. Drug testing is performed in all patients to determine if a successful drug regimen can be identified thus avoiding an ICD. The effect of drugs on the rate and duration of tachycardia should also be assessed. If drug therapy slows the tachycardia and makes it nonsustained or very well tolerated, the device may also discharge while the patient is awake. (These issues are particularly important if drug therapy is changed after device implantation.) The use of amiodarone is important in that it may increase defibrillation thresholds while at the same time alter the ease of ventricular tachycardia induction. If amiodarone is to be used chronically, a steady state should be reached, if possible, before testing with the drug and continued through the time of surgery. It is also important to remember that amiodarone has been associated with an increased incidence of noncardiogenic pulmonary edema following thoracotomy.

Because some current devices deliver multiple tiers of therapy with antitachycardia pacing as well as low- or high-energy cardioversion and finally defibrillation (Figures 7, 8), preimplantation electrophysiological testing will be even more important to document one or several arrhythmias and their response to variable treatments. Prior to electrophysiological evaluation or implantation, a thorough evaluation should be undertaken to exclude remediable cause for the ventricular arrhythmia, for example, electrolyte disturbances or uncontrolled congestive heart failure. These should be corrected before baseline evaluation.

It is also important to thoroughly evaluate the underlying heart disease with assessment of left ventricular function and the presence of myocardial ischemia and coronary angiography. This is required for planning such additional operative interventions as coronary artery bypass graft surgery, aneurysmectomy, or electrophysiologically guided surgical resection of the tachycardia focus. The presence of ongoing ischemia should be treated before device implantation.

Preoperative assessment also includes evaluation of the need for permanent pacing. Unipolar pacemakers are contraindicated because ICD sensing of the pacemaker stimulus artifact may trigger spurious discharges by double or triple counting, or sensing the stimulus artifact during ventricular fibrillation may cause failure of the ICD to deliver appropriate therapy. Patients with unipolar pacemakers already implanted should have these pulse generators replaced with bipolar systems. Alternatively, in some of these patients, if only VVI pacing is required, an ICD with bradycardia pacing may be all that is required. Polarity has important implications for specific pulse generators. Some current units are polarity programmable and automatically reset to unipolar pacing as a default or backup mode in the presence of a defibrillating shock that may require pulse generator replacement. A unit that will remain bipolar is optimal.

A final preoperative evaluation is psychosocial. The patients and their families must be able to understand and accept potential complications with the device and the follow-up requirements. One of the most important limitations is the restriction of driving. In the initial experience with ICDs at many centers, patients were completely restricted from driving. This restriction was based upon the underlying arrhythmia, for example, ventricular tachycardia or fibrillation. Some centers have relaxed this recommendation although there may also be specific state guidelines. Similar driving guidelines exist for many patients with recurrent syncope and cardiac arrhythmias. These limitations must be carefully discussed and understood by the patient and the family.

Operative Techniques

ICD implantation approaches are evolving rapidly. At present, there are two alternative approaches, either thoracotomy or transvenous. Although thoracotomy implants currently account for the majority of procedures, in a manner analogous to cardiac pacing, with the development of transvenous leads, the transvenous approach will eventually dominate. With current systems, in carefully selected patients at selected centers, success rates of 75%–85% can be achieved with a transvenous route.

Transthoracic Approach

Several transthoracic approaches are used. If other cardiac surgery, for example, aneurysmectomy or coronary artery bypass graft surgery is planned, a median sternotomy is used. With this approach, the primary cardiac surgical procedure is carried out using standard techniques. After the primary operation is completed, the patient is rewarmed and left only on partial cardiopulmonary bypass. A large patch electrode is sutured on the left ventricle, usually the apex. It is placed as far as possible from the bypass graft distal arterial anastomoses (if they have been performed as part of the primary surgery). The epicardial screw-in electrodes used for sensing are also fixed to the left ventricle. If the ventricles are large enough, a second large patch electrode is placed on the right ventricle; otherwise, a smaller patch electrode is used. The leads are then tunneled to the location of the pulse generator in the left upper quadrant of the abdomen. While the median sternotomy approach affords the greatest access to and visualization of the heart, it carries with it a higher risk of infection; in addition, it may make subsequent cardiac surgical procedures more difficult.

In patients undergoing primary implantation without other cardiac surgery, other approaches are more frequently used. Each has advantages and disadvantages. A left lateral thoracotomy is often used because it provides the best exposure for placement of left ventricular patches and can minimize the chance of inadvertent injury to previously placed bypass grafts. A subxiphoid approach is also used although, depending upon details of patient anatomy, the left ventricular apex may be harder to reach and exposure may be limited. With this approach, infection rates have been decreased. Finally, a subcostal approach is also possible (Figure 15). With any of these approaches, intrapericardial placement is most common although in some centers, extrapericardial placement is used unless defibrillation energy requirements are too high. With extrapericardial placement, subsequent development of a pericardial effusion could *theoretically* affect thresholds, although in actual practice this has not been documented. The advantage of extrapericardial placement may be most apparent in patients who have previously undergone cardiac surgery in whom a difficult dissection may be required for intrapericardial placement. Initial data from one manufacturer (Medtronic, Inc.) shows no difference in DFTs between intra- and extrapericardial patch placement.

Tunneling of the leads to the pocket should be done with great care to avoid mechanical trauma to the lead body, electrode, electrode plate, or pin. The use of a Penrose drain or a chest tube over the lead during tunneling can help protect the integrity of the lead; traction is placed on the Penrose drain or chest tube around the lead rather than on the lead itself.

After the leads have been implanted, the generator pocket is fashioned usually in the left upper quadrant of the abdomen either in a subcutaneous position or behind the belly of the rectus muscle. Due to the size of the device, migration or erosion can occur. Several approaches have been described to prevent this. One option includes placement between the anterior and posterior rectus sheaths. Another option is placement in either a conventional nonabsorbable Dacron pouch (Parsonnet pouch) or an absorbable collagenous pouch to stimulate formation of a solid fibrous capsule.

Recently, thoracoscopy has been used for implantation (Figure 16). Using this approach, implantation of the patch and epicardial pacing/sensing leads provides more conventional ICD placement but with only a minimal thoracotomy. As the majority of implantations become completely transvenous, thoracoscopy may never be widely used.

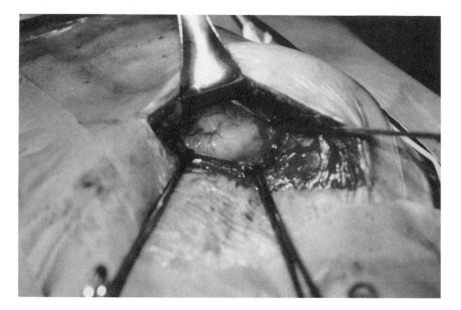

Figure 15A. *ICD implantation may be accomplished via a left subcostal incision. The chest is rotated approximately 30° with the left side up, and the lower portion of the left chest is further elevated with a sand bag. The pericardium is approached extrapleurally. The pericardium is opened to expose the cardiac apex.*

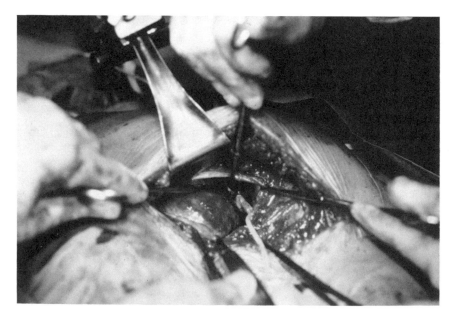

Figure 15B. *With the pericardium retracted, the left ventricular patch is positioned and sutured at its corners to the epicardium.*

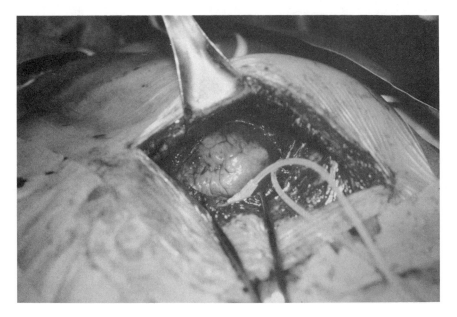

Figure 15C.   *The right ventricular patch is then placed and also sutured to the epicardium.*

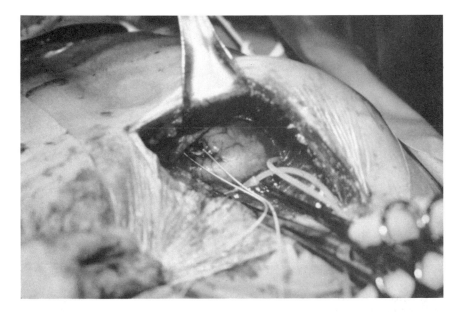

Figure 15D.   *The two 4951 epimyocardial leads for sensing a tachyarrhythmia are placed between the two patches. The four leads are tunneled to the subcutaneous tissue of the left upper quadrant and are attached to the ICD pulse generator. The entire procedure is accomplished via a single incision with general, endotracheal anesthesia.*

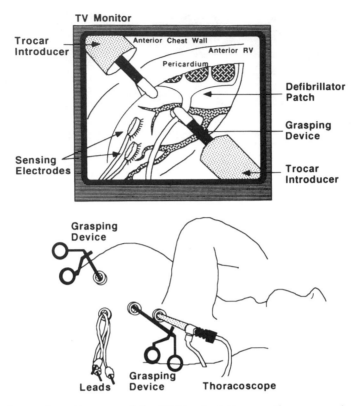

Figure 16.   *A new alternative approach for ICD implantation uses thoracoscopy for placement of patches and sensing electrodes. This is less invasive than traditional thoracotomy. Courtesy of Howard Frumin, M.D., Sinai Hospital, Detroit, MI.*

Nonthoracotomy Lead Implantation

The worldwide experience with the Medtronic 7216A/7217 ICD has recently been documented. Of 660 patients, 226 had endocardial leads while 434 had epicardial leads. Perioperative mortality was substantially decreased with the former (0.4% vs 5.5%, P < 0.001). Nonthoracotomy lead systems may be of particular importance in patients who have undergone prior cardiac surgery. At the present time, three manufacturers provide endocardial ICD leads, each with two defibrillating electrodes and a pacing/sensing electrode. With these, defibrillation may require just the two intracardiac electrodes or may require a patch lead placed in the subcutaneous tissue of the left chest wall.

With one of the devices (CPI), a nonepicardial 12 Fr tripolar endocardial catheter was tested that allowed rate and PDF sensing as well as shock delivery. The distal end of the endocardial lead had tines for passive fixation. A screw-in endocardial lead is also available. A proximal spring electrode had a surface area of 617 mm^2, while the distal spring electrode had a surface area of 295 mm^2.

This lead was used in combination with a subcutaneous patch electrode with a surface area of 2800 mm^2 placed in the left chest wall, usually over the left ventricular apex. With this device, four configurations were available: (1) both endocardial springs as cathode with the patch as anode, (2) the distal spring as cathode while the proximal spring and patch were anodal, (3) the distal spring as cathode and proximal spring as anode, and (4) the distal spring as cathode and the patch as anode. The second configuration with the distal spring as cathode and the proximal spring and patch as anode was most successful. During follow-up of this system, a high incidence of patch lead fracture and oversensing with subsequent inappropriate shocks was documented. A new endocardial system is being evaluated that does not require a patch and seems to avoid fracture.

Other systems are being tested for complete transvenous use. A three transvenous lead system (Transvene™) can be used—coronary sinus, right ventricular, and superior vena cava with several possible configurations. The leads are positioned using the cephalic, subclavian, or jugular systems for venous entry. If a subclavian approach is chosen, the venous entry site should be kept as lateral as possible to avoid damage to the lead from compression forces related to the costoclavicular ligament. The coronary sinus lead is positioned in the distal coronary sinus with the tip just under the left atrial appendage. If the coronary sinus lead cannot be advanced far enough so that the proximal end of the defibrillation coil is within the ostium of the coronary sinus, it should not be used. The tip of the superior vena cava lead is positioned at the right atrial/superior vena cava junction and the right ventricular lead is positioned in the apex of the right ventricle (Figure 17).

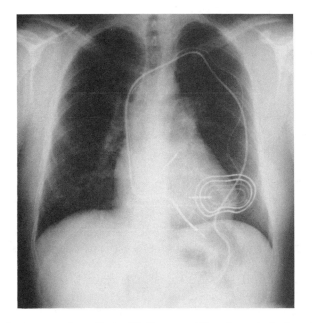

Figure 17.   *PA chest x-ray of a patient with Transvene™ system. A single patch was required.*

With these three lead systems, a number of combinations can be tested (Table V). They may be tested in conjunction with a temporary cutaneous patch over the left ventricular apex at the fifth intercostal space. If an effective configuration is found that terminates ventricular fibrillation and has an adequate defibrillation threshold (usually ≤18 J), a subcutaneous patch can then be implanted. In some patients, this system can be implanted without the subcutaneous patch. Implantation of transvenous systems may require multiple inductions of the ventricular arrhythmia and subsequent defibrillations to test the different electrode configurations because defibrillation thresholds may be marginal. This need for multiple inductions must be kept in mind if the patient's clinical condition is very unstable. If the DFTs are unacceptably high with a transvenous approach, a thoracotomy procedure may then be performed.

If thresholds and performance are satisfactory, a subcutaneous patch lead is then implanted. While typical placement is subcutaneous, it may be submuscular or even directly on the rib periosteum. It should be placed along the left anterior or mid-axillary line over the fourth or fifth intercostal space. The patch may need to be repositioned to fulfill defibrillation criteria (<18 J). The leads are then tunneled to the location of the pulse generator pocket and connected. Following implantation, the system should be checked again for efficacy.

IMPLANTATION AND ANESTHESIA REQUIREMENTS

General anesthesia is required for ICD implantation. Initially when all systems were placed via a thoracotomy route, implantation was performed in the operating room. With the shift toward transvenous systems (either solely or in combination with a subcutaneous patch), in some institutions the entire implantation is now performed in the catheterization laboratory.

OPERATIVE TESTING

After lead implantation, pacing and sensing thresholds are evaluated. It is important to note the position of the leads for follow-up or in case thresholds are found to be high. Specific testing protocols vary. Testing can be performed with a conventional pacing system analyzer. R waves on the patch electrodes should be >1–2 mV while R waves on the screw-in epicardial or endocardial leads should be >5 mV. Pacing thresholds are checked on the screw-in epicardial leads and should be <1.5 V at 0.5 ms pulse duration connected in a bipolar configuration. If thresholds are high, epicardial contact should be checked. The leads may need to be repositioned. Implant lead impedances should be recorded as well as electrograms that should be obtained during sinus rhythm and ventricular tachycardia.

After the pacing and sensing thresholds have been checked, the DFT is measured, which is critical to the success of ICD implantation. It is best described as a dose-response curve where the greater the shock amplitude delivered, the more likely that successful defibrillation will be accomplished. The number of measurements made is finite because of the need for induction of ventricular fibrillation, so that DFT is said to exist when from 60%–90% of induced arrhythmias are terminated successfully. If only 60% of shocks defibrillate, however, the lead/electrode system should be revised.

For measurement of DFT, ventricular tachycardia or fibrillation is induced using either AC current or ramp pacing. Bipolar stimulation is used so that maximum energy is directed to the heart. Typically, following induction of ventricular fibrillation, an initial shock is programmed at 18 J. Following successful conversion, two additional defibrillations are performed with progressively lower energy. The DFT should be reproducibly <15–20 J. If the arrhythmia induced is ventricular tachycardia, the DFT is likely to be lower. If DFTs are acceptable, then the ICD is connected and successful defibrillation documented after repeat arrhythmia induction. A 10-J safety margin is recommended.

Occasionally, defibrillation thresholds are excessively high. The frequency of this is variable, but it may occur in up to 15%–20% of implants. Such high thresholds may be associated with prior cardiac surgery or extensive myocardial damage with depressed left ventricular function. Elevated thresholds may also be the result of poor epicardial contact or insufficient patch electrode surface area. Patch size varies among manufacturers. If thresholds are high, larger patches may be tried. Alternatively, the lead polarity may be reversed or the configuration changed, for example, from a patch and spring superior vena cava electrode to two patches. Care should be taken to separate the patches, cover the largest amount of ventricular myocardium, and approximate the largest angle (ideally 180°). Other reasons for elevated DFTs are amiodarone therapy, hyperkalemia, cold cardioplegia, or hypothermia used for associated procedures, i.e., valve replacement or coronary bypass surgery. After the patient's device has been checked and found to adequately defibrillate ventricular fibrillation, it is implanted. During surgical closure, the ICD usually is deactivated because electrocautery may trigger device discharge. Following surgery, the device is reactivated for sensing ventricular fibrillation. Care should be taken during this time to document false-positive discharges, for example, from sinus tachycardia.

Three to four days postoperatively, the patient is brought back to the electrophysiology laboratory for final evaluation and testing of the unit. The specific protocol used varies depending upon the clinical setting, the specific arrhythmia, and the device used. For energy programmable units, energy response curves can be generated and the device then programmed to optimize longevity but maintain safety. Some centers only perform follow-up tests if antiarrhythmic drugs have been added that may affect DFTs or if there was concern at the time of implantation as to the safety margin and efficacy of the unit.

With newer generation programmable devices, the importance of postoperative testing will increase—particularly when tiered therapy devices are used to treat ventricular tachycardia by pacing techniques or with low-energy cardioversion (Figures 7–9). Some of these new generation devices can be used to perform programmed ventricular stimulation without the need for placing a venous catheter in the ventricle, making postoperative testing easier and safer.

Postoperative electrophysiological testing is required in those patients with antitachycardia pacing devices. In these patients, the ventricular arrhythmia/ arrhythmias to be treated must be induced using programmed ventricular stimulation and the response to rapid overdrive pacing assessed. Stimulation strategies that terminate the tachycardia are identified and the device programmed accordingly. Although such strategies may allow for treatment of a larger number of patients using device strategies, they have dramatically increased the complexity of the evaluation and continued follow-up care.

FOLLOW-UP

Close follow-up of patients with ICDs is essential. Patients are given identification cards identifying their specific device. In addition, they are instructed to wear a medical alert identification bracelet. Patients are also followed by a phone system. At the present time, some devices that incorporate pacing modalities are investigational. For these investigational devices, protocols may be predetermined. Otherwise patients should be seen every 2 to 3 months at which time pacing thresholds, R wave amplitude, and oversensing of R wave with induction of myopotentials by isometric exercise are checked. In addition, the charge times are measured. The charge time represents the time it takes for the batteries to charge the storage capacitor to a nominal 25–35 J. Depending upon the specific device, measurement of charge time varies. For example, for some older CPI devices, the second magnet test charge time is the reliable indicator based upon the fact that capacitor deformation/reformation changes after the capacitor has been inactive. For other devices, charge time can be measured without the need for an initial test.

Each device has an elective replacement indicator (ERI) dictated by the manufacturer. In most current devices, ERI is based on voltage measurement and not charge time. When end of life is reached, elective replacement is indicated.

During follow-up, patients are instructed to contact the implanting center for any device discharge. If symptoms of arrhythmia, for example, syncope or sustained palpitations occur, followed by a discharge, the patient usually is instructed to go to the nearest emergency room. If a single discharge occurs in the absence of any symptoms, the patient is instructed to call the implanting center. If no other untoward event occurs, nothing further is required in the latter situation. If multiple shocks have occurred in the absence of symptoms, however, the patient is instructed to return for reevaluation to determine the cause. In such a setting, hospitalization with continuous electrocardiographic monitoring is often required. Sinus tachycardia or atrial fibrillation with rates greater than that set for tachycardia detection are among the most frequent causes of inappropriate discharge (Figure 18). In addition, nonsustained or self-terminating ventricular tachycardia may also be the cause (Figure 5). Evaluation includes electrocardiography, ambulatory monitoring, exercise testing (particularly if the discharges are related to exertion), and a phonogram from the device. Evaluation of the cycle lengths stored prior to the shock can assist in troubleshooting. In addition, some of the new devices have electrogram storage

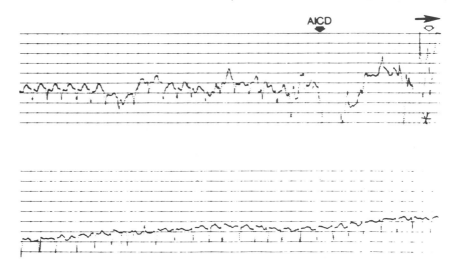

Figure 18. *Supraventricular tachycardia is sensed by the ICD as a ventricular arrhythmia and is shocked. Courtesy of Marshall S. Stanton, M.D., Mayo Clinic, Rochester, MN.*

capability that may be of particular help in assessing asymptomatic device discharges.

COMPLICATIONS

Operative Complications

These complications are affected by the patient population undergoing implantation. In patients with very poor left ventricular function or severe extracardiac diseases, there may be substantial morbidity and even mortality.

MORTALITY AND MORBIDITY

Hospital mortality rates of approximately 4%–5% have been documented. In some patients, mortality has been related to congestive heart failure while in other patients, refractory ventricular arrhythmias have developed. As previously discussed, perioperative mortality with transvenous endocardial systems is substantially lower.

Nonfatal complications occur in up to 15% of patients. They may result in substantial morbidity and prolong the hospital stay. Some are related to underlying diseases and comorbid conditions. Others relate to the surgical procedure itself.

Pulmonary complications are perhaps the most frequent early postoperative complications and include atelectasis, infiltrates, pleural effusions, and pneumothorax. Adult respiratory distress has been reported following implantation;

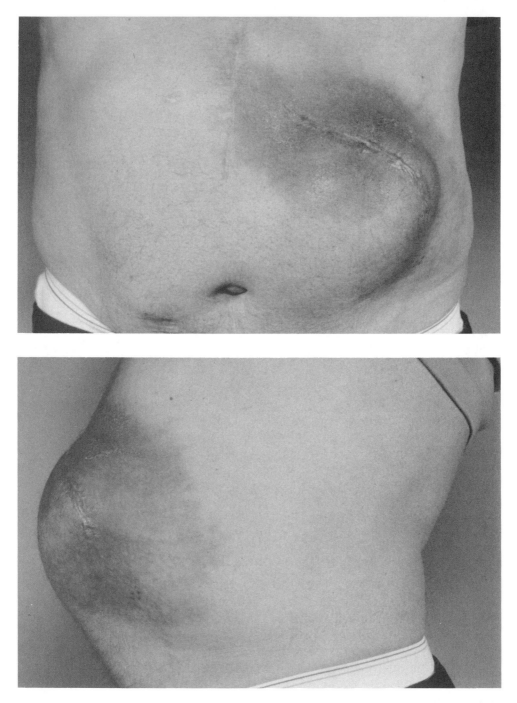

Figure 19. *Abdominal wall swelling and tenderness after ICD implantation in a patient with an infected device.*

although anecdotal data suggests a potential relationship between this condition and chronic amiodarone toxicity, further investigation is needed. Other complications include bleeding, congestive heart failure, and cerebrovascular accidents. Unusual types of bleeding have been reported including erosion of epicardial vessels by the patches. This has been reported early postoperatively but is extremely uncommon.

ICD INFECTIONS

Infections following ICD implantation occur with a frequency of 5%–6%. Although immediate postoperative infections can occur, there is usually a delay of weeks to months following implantation with local erythema, tenderness, or a draining sinus (Figure 19). Systemic signs with fever and leukocytosis are relatively common although sepsis is rare. *Staphylococcus aureus* and *epidermidis* have been cultured most commonly, the former usually from earlier infections and the latter from patients who present later. In such patients, CAT scans may be helpful in localizing an abscess. As is true with other pulse generators, complete removal of the ICD and lead system usually is required. The question of sterilization and reuse in the same patient has been explored. In a preliminary experience, the safety and efficacy of ethylene oxide sterilization and reuse has been demonstrated, which could result in substantial cost savings. As is true with permanent pacemakers, infective endocarditis prophylaxis is not recommended for a patient with an ICD.

Generator pack erosion may also occur, particularly in thin patients. Threatened erosion with thinning of the skin, pain, and erythema may be treated by pocket revision. Once actual erosion has occurred, replacement of the pulse generator may be necessary to prevent infection. If an endocardial lead has been used, it may migrate or cause superior vena cava thrombosis.

Device Malfunction

Early devices had complications related to pulse generator fabrication including early battery depletion secondary to corrosion of the glass insulator and loss of the hermetic seal. Random component failure continues to occur as does premature battery depletion. The batteries, however, have a finite longevity. Lead fractures may also occur and cause either device failure or inappropriate shocks (Figures 20, 21).

Spurious Discharges

Spurious discharges are defined as a device discharge in the absence of sustained ventricular tachycardia or ventricular fibrillation (Figure 22). Most patients with prolonged ventricular tachycardia or ventricular fibrillation will have associated symptoms. Unless the patient is being monitored, it is impossible to identify the exact cause of the discharge, which may range from device mal-

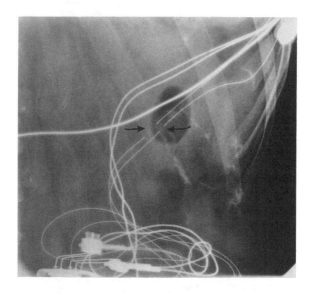

Figure 20. *Flat x-ray of abdomen following blunt trauma in a patient with an ICD. Two lead fractures are apparent.*

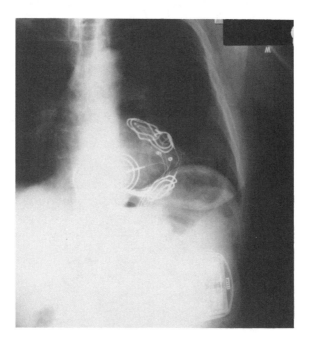

Figure 21. *X-ray documenting wrinkling of the superior patch in a patient with a three patch system. This may cause malfunction.*

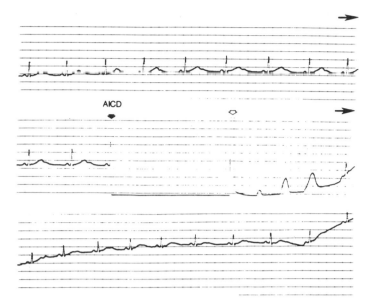

Figure 22.   *Electrocardiogram in a patient with a spurious discharge during normal sinus rhythm. Acknowledgment: Marshall S. Stanton, M.D., Mayo Clinic, Rochester, MN.*

function to sensing supraventricular tachycardia, or atrial fibrillation with rapid ventricular response, sinus tachycardia, nonsustained ventricular tachycardia, myopotentials, extraneous environmental artifacts, or signals from electrocautery devices. Spurious discharges may be difficult to evaluate and prevent. They are also very bothersome for the patient and may result in psychological disability. Careful patient selection and treatment of other types of tachycardia are important to limit the frequency of spurious discharges. Spurious discharges may be frequent, however, and have been documented in up to 40% of some series. As has been mentioned, patients are instructed to report any asymptomatic device discharges. This is important for monitoring device performance and efficacy as well as for ensuring optimal patient care.

ICD INTERACTIONS AND PACEMAKERS

Interactions with pacemakers and ICDs are of substantial clinical concern (Table VII). One of the first groups of interactions was inappropriate ICD discharge as a result of defibrillator device sensing of pacing artifacts (Figure 23). Unipolar pacemakers can result in device discharge from double sensing of the unipolar stimulus artifact and the QRS electrogram. Although these problems are most common with unipolar pacemakers, they have also been documented with bipolar devices. Dual-chamber devices are even more of a problem, particularly unipolar dual-chamber devices which should not be used.

In addition to inappropriate ICD discharge, there may also be inappropriate inhibition. During ventricular fibrillation, the permanent pacemaker may not

Table VII
Potential Pacemaker/Defibrillator Interactions

- Inappropriate defibrillator discharge due to "over-counting" of pacemaker stimuli;
- Defibrillator inhibition due to pacemaker failure to sense ventricular fibrillation;
- Transient pacemaker failure to sense and/or capture after defibrillator discharge;
- Defibrillator deactivation by magnet;
- Inappropriate defibrillator discharge due to magnet application to permanent pacemaker and resultant asynchronous pacing;
- Defibrillator-discharge reprogramming of polarity-programmable pacemaker from bipolar to unipolar.

sense the ventricular arrhythmia and thus continue to deliver a pacing artifact that may then be sensed by the ICD as regular cardiac activity, preventing detection (Figure 24). Again, this is more of a problem with unipolar pacemakers. Attempts should be made to optimally place the sensing electrodes of the ICD at the time of implantation to avoid far-field sensing of pacemaker stimuli. This potential interaction must be closely evaluated at the time of implantation.

Other interactions involve magnet application that can result in defibrillation deactivation, inappropriate discharge, or reprogramming. Some devices (CPI 1500, 1510, 1520, 1550, and 1660) can be inactivated with magnet application for 30 seconds; therefore, it is important to assess the status of the device after pacemaker programming. Programming the pacemaker can result in ICD discharge. This interaction is complex and depends upon whether the programmer uses an electromagnetic or radiofrequency signal, as well as the specific ICD used. For this reason, it has been recommended that the ICD be transiently inactivated during pacemaker programming for some ICDs. Finally, the pacemaker may revert to Elective Replacement Indication (ERI) or Power On Reset (POR) as a result of a shock artifact. In either case (ERI or POR), the pacemaker may revert to VVI at 65 bpm.

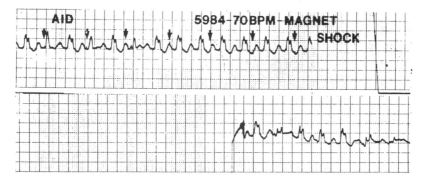

Figure 23. The interaction of a pacemaker and an implanted defibrillator must be carefully monitored. It is possible that pacemaker stimuli will be sensed and treated as ventricular contractions. In this electrocardiogram, each stimulus was treated as a ventricular event and each paced QRS and each spontaneous QRS added to the count. As the total exceeded the tachycardia criterion, the ICD was discharged.

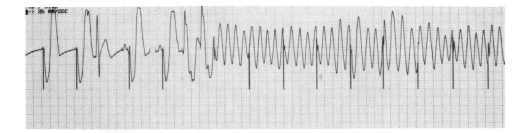

Figure 24. *During ventricular fibrillation, the VVI pacemaker continues to fire resulting in nondetection of the arrhythmia by the ICD. Courtesy of Mr. Joe Fetter, Medtronic, Inc., Minneapolis, MN.*

Inactivation of ICDs by pacemaker programming can also rarely occur as a result of electromagnetic interference even by household appliances. The magnetic field strength necessary to close the reed switch, thus disabling sensing and discharge, is approximately 10 gauss at the surface of the device. Such electromagnetic interference needs to exceed the deactivation time of 30 seconds. Unexplained failure of an ICD secondary to deactivation of the unit should raise the question of electromagnetic interference.

Another group of interactions includes the aftereffects of defibrillator discharge on pacing. Temporary increases in pacing thresholds have been documented following defibrillation. While failure to capture in this setting can occur, it usually lasts for <10 seconds. New devices have incorporated a postshock high-output pacing option that should effectively solve this. In addition, sensing thresholds may also be temporarily affected following defibrillation. Although the potential for long-term increases in pacing thresholds as a function of recurrent defibrillation is possible, it has not been well documented.

In addition to interactions with conventional pacemakers are those interactions of ICDs and pacemakers used to treat tachyarrhythmias. Third generation devices with antitachycardia and bradycardia pacing as well as programmable output shocks will make these interactions obsolete. In patients with recurrent ventricular tachycardia, pacing may be used to convert the arrhythmia to normal sinus rhythm. Some of these patients may experience only lightheadedness with their arrhythmia and not loss of consciousness. In these patients, the use of antitachycardia pacing has been evaluated and may be very effective. A concern, however, has been the potential for antitachycardia pacing to accelerate a relatively stable ventricular arrhythmia or convert it to ventricular fibrillation that could not be treated with pacing techniques. For this reason, combined procedures involving both antitachycardia pacemakers and implantable ICDs have been used in small selected series. In these very selected series, the majority of episodes of ventricular tachycardia could be terminated with antitachycardia pacing. ICD discharge was only rarely required. This approach requires extensive preimplantation testing to document the reliability of the pacing as well as the efficacy of the ICD should acceleration of the arrhythmia occur.

DRUG INTERVENTION AND ICD

Antiarrhythmic drugs are used in the majority of patients in whom ICDs are considered. In addition, these drugs are often used following implantation. There are a number of potential interactions between drugs and these devices. Some of these interactions are theoretical, some are anecdotal, and some are a cause of significant and potentially frequent concern (Table VIII).

One of the most important concerns is the potential to change (either increase or decrease) DFT. This is of particular importance at the time of ICD implantation but also may continue to affect outcome. Amiodarone, because of its common use for lethal ventricular arrhythmias, has been studied. There is controversy about its effect. Some anecdotal cases have documented high DFT while on amiodarone with a lowering of DFT after cessation of the drug. In other series of patients, there has either been an increase in DFT with amiodarone or no difference compared to patients not receiving amiodarone. Whether these differences relate to drug dose, duration of therapy, or even route of administration is not clear. Class IC drugs such as flecainide and encainide also have been shown in experimental animal preparations to be associated with an increase in DFT, whereas Class IA agents have usually not had an effect. These interactions must be kept in mind if unexpected problems with DFT are encountered. In general, if possible, ICD implantation should be performed without drugs known to alter DFT. If the patient subsequently needs such a drug, the ICD should be retested. Lidocaine increases DFT experimentally; if lidocaine is given during implantation to treat frequent ventricular ectopy, this must be kept in mind.

An equally important interaction between drugs and the ICD are those which affect the underlying arrhythmia. Changes in cycle length may affect sensing of the arrhythmia or may affect the hemodynamic response to the arrhythmia. This is of particular importance in current defibrillate-only systems; if the initial arrhythmia was unstable fast ventricular tachycardia associated with collapse and then successful device discharge with high energy, the outcome

---

Table VIII
Antiarrhythmic Drugs and ICDs Potential Interactions

- Interactions which change DFT;
- Changes in cycle length of sustained ventricular arrhythmias;
- Alterations in the specific arrhythmia, for example, a change from sustained ventricular tachycardia to nonsustained ventricular tachycardia;
- Changes in conduction that may affect QRS morphology thus potentially affecting PDF morphology of either ventricular tachycardia or supraventricular tachycardia.

may be optimal; if, however, antiarrhythmic therapy slows the rate of the arrhythmia so that the patient does not lose consciousness but the device still discharges, it may result in an unacceptable clinical outcome, for example, the patient feels the shock. Drugs may also convert sustained arrhythmias to nonsustained arrhythmias that may trigger discharge in committed devices after the arrhythmia has terminated spontaneously. New generation devices that reassess the rhythm after completing the charge cycle should greatly improve this problem. Alternatively, drugs may have a proarrhythmic effect leading to more frequent discharge. These considerations may be magnified with the new generations of ICDs that allow for pacing for treatment, low energy cardioversion, or defibrillation. If, after implantation of an ICD, antiarrhythmic therapy is changed substantially, consideration must be given to reevaluation of the unit and its effect on the arrhythmia to be treated. This will become easier with devices that allow noninvasive electrophysiological testing.

Other interactions of drugs and ICDs are possible. Drugs may affect QRS morphology, which in turn may affect morphology recognition of tachycardia. Also, drugs may alter escape rhythms following defibrillation making pacing backup support more important.

CONCLUSIONS

ICDs have moved to occupy a central place in the management of potentially lethal ventricular arrhythmias. The number of new devices able to treat these arrhythmias is increasing. Such devices will allow treatment of a wider number of patients because of the development of improved sensing algorithms, antitachycardia pacing, bradycardia pacing, and tiered therapy. As the new devices become more complex, pre- and postoperative testing and follow-up become more rigorous.

At the present time, ICDs appear to have dramatically decreased sudden death mortality. All-cause mortality remains significant reflecting surgical mortality as well as the underlying pathophysiological substrate of patients receiving these devices with extensive coronary arterial disease and depressed ventricular function or severe cardiomyopathy.

With further advances, ICD technology should become safer and easier to implant. The eventual role of these new devices will depend upon their documented safety and efficacy, the results of the randomized trials of devices versus drugs or surgery, and the issue of the cost of health care, which is assuming increasing importance.

BIBLIOGRAPHY

Bardy GH, Troutman C, Poole JE, et al: Clinical experience with a tiered-therapy, multiprogrammable antiarrhythmic device. Circulation 1992; 85:1689–1698.
Epstein AE, Kay GN, Plumb VJ, et al: Combined automatic implantable cardioverter-defibrillator and pacemaker systems: Implantation techniques and follow-up. J Am Coll Cardiol 1989; 13:121–131.

Kim SG, Fisher JD, Furman S, et al: Exacerbation of ventricular arrhythmias during the postoperative period after implantation of an automatic defibrillator. J Am Coll Cardiol 1991; 18:1200–1206.

Larsen GC, Manolis AS, Sonnenberg FA, et al: Cost effectiveness of the implantable cardioverter defibrillator: Effect of improved battery life and comparison with amiodarone therapy. J Am Coll Cardiol 1992; 19:1323–1334.

Lawrie GM, Griffin JC, Wyndham CRC: Epicardial implantation of the automatic implantable defibrillator by left subcostal thoracotomy. PACE 1984; 7:1370–1374.

Lehmann MH, Saksena S: NASPE Policy Statement-Implantable Cardioverter Defibrillators in Cardiovascular Practice: Report of the Policy Conference of the North American Society of Pacing and Electrophysiology. PACE 1991; 14:969–979.

Lown B, Axelrod P: Implanted standby defibrillators (Editorial). Circulation 1972; 46:637–639.

Mirowski M, Mower M, Gott VL, et al: Transvenous automatic defibrillator: Preliminary clinical tests of the defibrillating subsystem. Trans Am Artif Organs 1972; 18:520.

Mirowski M, Mower MM, Staewn WS, et al: Standby automatic defibrillator: An approach to prevention of sudden death. Arch Intern Med 1970; 126:158–161.

Mirowski M, Reid PR, Mower MM, et al: Termination of malignant ventricular arrhythmias with an implanted automatic defibrillator in human beings. N Engl J Med 1980; 303:322.

Moore SL, Maloney JD, Edel TB, et al: Implantable cardioverter defibrillator implanted by non-thoracotomy approach: Initial clinical experience with the redesigned transvenous lead system. PACE 1991; 14:1865–1869.

Prevost JL, Batelli F: Sur quelque effets des decharges electriques sur le coeur mamifres. Comptes Rendus Seances Acad Sci 1899; 129:1267.

Saksena S, Parsonnet V, Pantopoulos D, et al: Implantation of a cardioverter/defibrillator without thoracotomy using a triple electrode system. J Am Med Assoc 1988; 259:69–72.

Schuder JC, Stoeckle H, Gold JH, et al: Experimental ventricular defibrillation with an automatic and completely implanted system. Trans Am Soc Artif Organs 1970; 16:207–212.

Schuder JC, Stoeckle H, West JA, et al: Ventricular defibrillation in the dog with a bielectrode intravascular catheter. Arch Intern Med 1973; 132:286–290.

Song SL: The Bilitch Report. Performance of implantable cardiac rhythm management devices. PACE 1992; 15:475–486.

The Cardiac Arrhythmia Suppression Trial (CAST) Investigators. Preliminary report: Effect of encainide and flecainide on mortality in a randomized trial of arrhythmia suppression after myocardial infarction. N Engl J Med 1989; 321:406–412.

The Cardiac Arrhythmia Suppression Trial (CAST) II Investigators. Effect of the antiarrhythmic agent moricizine on survival after myocardial infarction. N Engl J Med 1992; 327:227–233.

Troup PJ, Chapman PD, Olinger GN, et al: The implanted defibrillator: Relation of defibrillating lead configuration and clinical variables to defibrillation threshold. J Am Coll Cardiol 1985; 6:1315–1321.

Wiggers CJ: The physiologic basis for cardiac resuscitation from ventricular fibrillation: Method for serial defibrillation. Am Heart J 1940; 20:413–422.

Winkle RA, Mead RH, Ruder MA, et al: Long-term outcome with theautomatic implantable cardioverter-defibrillator. J Am Coll Cardiol 1989; 16:1353–1361.

Winkle RA, Mead RH, Ruder MA, et al: Ten year experience with implantable defibrillators. (abstract) Circulation 1991; 84:II-416.

Zoll PM: Resuscitation of the heart in ventricular standstill by external electrical stimulation. N Engl J Med 1952; 247:768.

Zoll PM, Linethal AJ, Gibson W, et al: Termination of ventricular fibrillation in man by externally applied electric shock. N Engl J Med 1956; 254:727.

Chapter 13

PACING FOR TACHYCARDIA

David R. Holmes Jr.

Rapid developments in the fields of pacing and electrophysiology have significantly altered the approach to the patient with both supraventricular and ventricular tachycardia. New approaches such as the widespread use of radio-frequency catheter ablation to treat supraventricular tachycardia due to either atrioventricular nodal reentry or pre-excitation syndromes, as well as the on-going development of third generation implantable cardioverter defibrillators (ICDs) with combined antitachycardia pacing, backup bradycardia support, and cardioversion or defibrillation, have greatly impacted upon patient selection criteria for antitachycardia pacing. In addition, concern about the long-term safety and efficacy of antiarrhythmic drug regimens has been heightened as a result of the proarrhythmic effects seen with multiple antiarrhythmic medications in the CAST trial. These events will continue to impact on pacing for tachycardia.

There are two broad groups of approaches for antitachycardia pacing: (1) pacing for prevention of tachycardia, and (2) pacing for termination. With the latter, combined devices with cardioversion or defibrillation capability have become increasingly important. Before either of these approaches are used, it is necessary to identify the specific arrhythmia and the setting in which it occurs. In some patients, detailed electrophysiological assessment is required while in others, rhythm strips supply all of the information needed.

PACING FOR PREVENTION OF TACHYCARDIA (Table I)

Elimination of Bradycardia

The most common reason for pacing to prevent tachycardia is to eliminate bradycardia. The typical sequence is bradycardia followed by escape supraventricular or ventricular arrhythmias, some of which may be sustained (Figures 1 and 2). In this setting, the tachycardia is usually the result of bradycardia, and the bradycardia is often symptomatic and would require pacing in any event. Pacing prevents arrhythmias by one of several mechanisms including: (a) shortening diastole and providing less opportunity for ectopic escape beats, (b) suppressing junctional escape rhythms or retrograde P waves that may collide with sinus P waves or conduct to the atrium at a time when it is vulnerable to develop reentry, (c) decreasing the variability in the rate of recovery of excitability, and (d) decreasing the dispersion of refractoriness that is aggravated by bradycardia (this reduces the likelihood of reentrant arrhythmias). In addition to providing

Table I
Rhythms Amenable to Pacing

Prevention of Tachycardia	Termination of Tachycardia

● Bradycardia-dependent
   atrial flutter
   atrial fibrillation
   supraventricular tachycardia
   junctional escape beats
   ventricular ectopy
   ventricular tachycardia
	● Paroxysmal supraventricular tachycardia
	   atrioventricular nodal reentry
	   atrioventricular reentry
	   intra-atrial reentry
	   atrial flutter
	● Ventricular tachycardia (ICD backup)

a physiological support of the cardiac rate, permanent pacing may improve hemodynamics in patients with organic heart disease, and may decrease ischemia or reduce myocardial stretch. These effects may lessen atrial and ventricular ectopy, thus decreasing the precipitating or triggering events for tachycardia.

Bradycardia followed by an escape arrhythmia is relatively common in patients with sinus node dysfunction and may result in recurrent tachycardia.

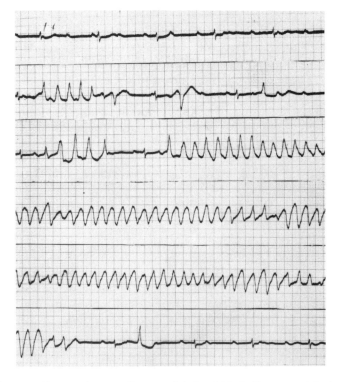

Figure 1. *Electrocardiogram documenting complete heart block. Escape ventricular ectopy results in nonsustained ventricular tachycardia and torsades de pointes. Permanent pacing may suppress ventricular ectopy and prevent ventricular tachycardia.*

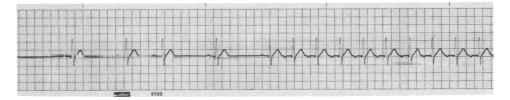

Figure 2. *Underlying sinus bradycardia with atrial premature contractions that result in supraventricular tachycardia.*

Support of the base rate and avoidance of atrial bradycardia may prevent tachycardia without the need for antiarrhythmic agents. Bradycardia-dependent ventricular arrhythmias, either in the setting of sinus node dysfunction or atrioventricular (AV) block, may also be improved or even eliminated by providing a physiological base rate support. It must be emphasized that identification of bradycardia followed by tachycardia is essential to improve the likelihood that pacing may prevent tachycardia in these patients. Ambulatory or in-hospital monitoring is necessary to document the typical sequence of bradycardia then tachycardia. Detailed invasive electrophysiological assessment may not be required in this setting.

Overdrive Suppression

Arrhythmias may also be prevented by overdrive suppression, particularly in patients with ventricular ectopy. Suppression by atrial overdrive may be more effective than ventricular overdrive, particularly if there is hemodynamic benefit achieved by maintaining AV synchrony. Increasing the paced rate results in suppression of ectopy and thereby decreases the precipitating event for tachycardia. This technique has its widest application in temporary pacing. While treatment of either the underlying cardiac disease or the cause of the arrhythmias is being undertaken, temporary overdrive pacing may be useful. In those with symptomatic, drug resistant arrhythmias, permanent overdrive pacing also may be helpful.

Ventricular arrhythmias associated with QT prolongation syndromes are particularly well suited for overdrive pacing. The QT prolongation may be drug related, in which case the accompanying ventricular arrhythmias can be managed by temporary atrial pacing until the offending drug has been withdrawn, or may be idiopathic or congenital. In the latter, if temporary pacing is effective, a permanent overdrive unit may be implanted.

The pacing rates chosen for overdrive suppression vary. The rate used may be significantly slower than the rate of tachycardia to be suppressed. If the patient is in tachycardia at the onset of pacing, tachycardia is terminated by overdrive suppression. The pacing rate needed for the initial overdrive termination is then gradually decreased until the lowest rate that will prevent tachycardia from recurring is reached. This rate then is continued. Alternatively, the pacing rate is initially set at 5 to 10 beats above the intrinsic normal rate and gradually increased until prevention of recurrent arrhythmias is achieved. The final rate should be the lowest rate that suppresses tachycardia. This concept is particularly important in the patient with arteriosclerotic heart disease or valvular heart disease in whom increasing the rate may aggravate hemodynamics or ischemia, and actually worsen the arrhythmia.

Other forms of preventive pacing have been evaluated. Subthreshold stimulation has been used to prevent a subsequent threshold stimulus from fully depolarizing cardiac cells. This subthreshold stimulus acts by prolonging local refractoriness. It requires that the inhibitory subthreshold stimulus be applied in close proximity to the site of origin of tachycardia that has limited its development. High current strength has also been used to prevent tachycardia. This approach also requires delivery of high current close to the site of origin. Finally, delivery of single or multiple extrastimuli at another or multiple other sites after an initiating impulse can prevent macro-reentrant tachycardia. These approaches remain investigational. They are all limited by the fact that inhibition is site-dependent and requires careful, precise localization of the reentrant circuit or initiating impulse location; time-dependent requiring very specific but potentially variable intervals to be effective; and voltage-dependent. These considerations may limit their practical utility.

PACING FOR TERMINATION OF TACHYCARDIA (Table I)

Pacing is more commonly used for terminating paroxysmal tachycardia. This is widely used during electrophysiological testing and has achieved increasing clinical utility as a therapeutic approach. Evaluation of the role of pacing in the termination of tachycardia is complex and involves consideration of the two major mechanisms of tachycardia—reentry and automaticity. Differentiation of these two mechanisms is based in part upon findings at the time of electrophysiological study. Supraventricular or ventricular arrhythmias that can be induced and terminated by single or multiple critically timed premature extrastimuli or rapid stimulation are felt to be reentrant. Automatic arrhythmias are those that cannot be reliably induced and terminated by stimulation techniques. This differentiation is arbitrary and overlap exists, particularly in triggered automatic arrhythmias. Even though this is arbitrary, it is very useful particularly as it relates to pacing for tachycardia. It follows that pacing is more useful in arrhythmias that can be reliably induced and then terminated by stimulation techniques, for example, reentrant arrhythmias.

REENTRY

Reentry is the most common mechanism of tachycardia. It may occur at any level within the conduction system and requires three conditions (Figure 3).

RE-ENTRY CONDITIONS

1. Two pathways connected proximally and distally, forming the limbs of the reentrant circuit.

   The two limbs need not be anatomically distinct but only functionally different in terms of terms of electrophysiological properties of impulse conduction and refractoriness.

2. Differential conduction of the impulse down the two limbs.

   This differential conduction may be the result of autonomic tone, electrolyte changes, or anatomical abnormalities such as fibrosis, infarction, dilatation, or hypertrophy.

3. Unidirectional block in one pathway which allows antegrade conduction in one limb and retrograde conduction via the other limb.

   It is dependent on the refractory periods of each limb and can be affected by drugs, metabolic changes, autonomic tone, and structural abnormalities.

In patients with reentry arrhythmias, tachycardia can be initiated in the electrophysiological laboratory by single or multiple extrastimuli or a train of premature impulses (Figures 4A and B). These impulses, if appropriately timed,

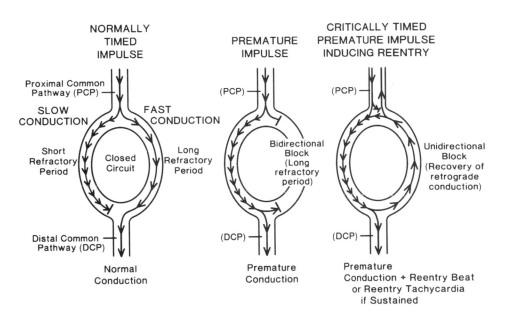

Figure 3. Schematic diagram of dual AV nodal pathways and AV nodal reentry. Proximal and distal common pathways are shown. The two limbs of the reentrant circuit are characterized by different conduction and refractory properties. The slow-conducting pathway (alpha) has a short refractory period. During sinus rhythm, impulses are conducted down the fast pathway (beta). A premature conduction (middle panel) is blocked in the fast pathway because of its long refractory period, and is conducted down the slow pathway. A critically timed premature conduction (right panel) can induce an atrial echo or reentrant paroxysmal supraventricular tachycardia. (From Brandenburg RO, Fuster V, Giuliani ER, et al: Cardiology: Fundamentals and Practice. Yearbook Medical Publishers, Chicago, 1987. By permission of the Mayo Foundation.)

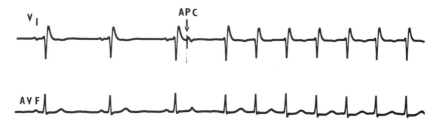

Figure 4A.   *Induction of supraventricular tachycardia by atrial premature complexes (APC). The prolonged PR interval following the APC is the result of block in the fast pathway and conduction down the slow pathway (see Figure 3).*

change conduction or refractoriness (or both) in the reentrant circuit and can either start or terminate an existing tachycardia. During the tachycardia, premature impulses or a train of impulses (burst pacing) can invade one or both limbs of the reentrant circuit and, by capturing the circuit or interrupting it, terminate the tachycardia (Figure 5).

Atrioventricular nodal tachycardia is the most common and prototypical

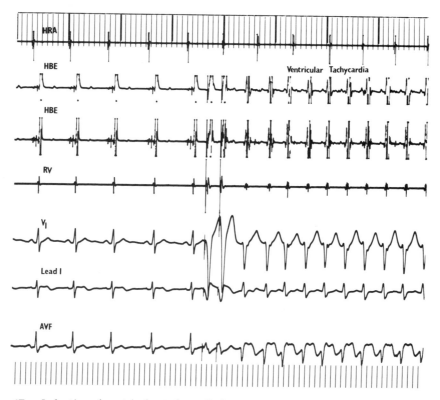

Figure 4B.   *Induction of ventricular tachycardia by premature ventricular beats. After five sinus beats, two ventricular premature contractions (VPCs) are delivered, resulting in sustained ventricular tachycardia. HRA = high right atrium; HBE = His bundle electrogram; RV = right ventricular electrogram.*

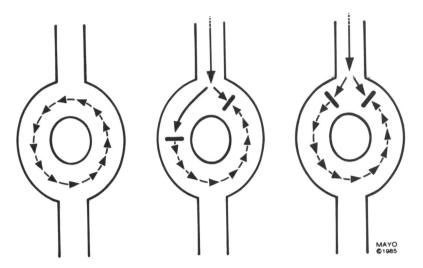

Figure 5. *Schematic of the effect of atrial stimulation on AV nodal reentry tachycardia. Reentrant arrhythmia circuit is shown on the left. An impulse may invade one limb of the circuit and block in the other limb (middle panel), or may block in each limb, interrupting the reentrant circuit and terminating tachycardia. (By permission of the Mayo Foundation.)*

reentrant arrhythmia. In patients with this electrophysiological substrate, there are two functional limbs within the AV node: the alpha limb, characterized by slow conduction but rapid recovery (shorter refractoriness) and the beta limb, characterized by faster conduction but slow recovery (longer refractoriness). There is increasing information on the physiological substrate in these patients. Detailed electrophysiological mapping has documented that the junction of the slow pathway and the atrium is located near the coronary sinus and posterior to the atrioventricular node. In some patients, the slow pathway has multiple atrial insertions, while in others there may be multiple slow pathways. A premature impulse (Figure 3) arriving at the AV node is conducted down the alpha pathway but is blocked in the beta pathway because of its slower recovery. When the impulse reaches the distal common pathway, the beta pathway has recovered so that the impulse can travel in a retrograde direction and set the stage for AV nodal reentry. All reentrant arrhythmias share these common features, for example, two functional pathways, connected proximally and distally with differential conduction, and refractoriness in each limb that allows for unidirectional block in one pathway. Electrophysiological assessment of the mechanism is essential prior to consideration of pacing for termination of tachycardia.

To terminate reentrant arrhythmias, the stimuli must penetrate and capture the reentrant circuit and adequately depolarize it so that reset does not occur. Several factors affect termination. These include the following: (1) the site of stimulation. If the site of stimulation is remote from the reentrant circuit, particularly if conduction to the reentry circuit is delayed by associated conduction system disease, the ability to terminate tachycardia is decreased. Conversely, delivering single or multiple extrastimuli in close proximity to the reentrant circuit increases the chance of termination. (2) Characteristics of the reentrant circuit include cycle length and entrance and exit of cardiac impulses to and from the remainder of the heart. In general if the tachycardia is fast and the circuit small and remote, termination will be more difficult. Conversely with a slow tachycardia and large reentrant circuit, for example, slow atrioventricular reentrant tachycardia, a single stimulus close to the site of reentry may be very effective. The importance of these parameters can be assessed in the electrophysiological laboratory by determining how difficult it is to terminate tachycardia and what stimulation protocol is needed, for example, single extrastimuli versus rapid cardiac pacing. Analysis of these factors is of utmost importance in evaluating a patient for pacing for tachycardia.

Automatic Arrhythmias

Automatic arrhythmias may occur at any level within the heart. These arrhythmias arise from disorders in impulse formation, compared to reentry, which is related to impulse propagation. Automatic arrhythmias may arise in areas capable of spontaneous impulse formation, for example, the AV node or the atria, or may arise as the result of abnormalities, such as ischemia, which allows spontaneous depolarization of tissues that do not normally depolarize spontaneously, for example, ventricular muscle. Automatic arrhythmias usually cannot be terminated in the laboratory by electrical stimulation, therefore pacing techniques for termination are not usually successful. However, if these automatic arrhythmias are bradycardia-dependent, then pacing to prevent tachycardia may be very successful.

CRITERIA FOR SELECTION OF PATIENTS

Pacing is only one of an expanding number of treatment options for patients with tachycardia (Table II). These treatment methods are sometimes complimentary and used in combination, and at other times are used alone. In the past, drug therapy was the standard treatment of choice. Recent advances have changed this. Drug therapy now remains *one* of the treatments available but not *the* treatment of choice. This is the result of new advances in catheter therapy as well as the fact that in some patients drugs either do not work or are associated

---

Table II
Therapy for Recurrent Paroxysmal Tachycardia 1992

Pharmacological:	conventional, investigational drugs
Catheter Based:	RF ablation, DC ablation, alcohol/sclerosing agent, arterial injection
Pacing:	antitachycardia pacing, antitachycardia pacing + defibrillation backup
Surgical:	ablation of accessory pathway, cryosurgical modification AV node, endocardial resection, aneurysmectomy

with significant cardiac toxicity, for example, proarrhythmia, AV block, or worsening of left ventricular function. In addition, noncardiac toxicity remains a problem. These issues are particularly important in young patients who face a long duration of therapy for intermittent tachycardia. Current options to standard drugs include investigational agents, radiofrequency or surgical ablation, endocardial resection, left ventricular aneurysmectomy, electrophysiologically guided endocardial resection, pacemakers, and implantable cardioverter defibrillators. Selection of the most appropriate method of treatment depends on clinical factors, the specific arrhythmia, the availability of investigational drugs and devices, and the experience of the physician treating each patient.

Identification of patients who may be candidates for pacemaker termination of tachycardia follows electrophysiological assessment during which the tachycardia is induced by extrastimuli or rapid pacing. The mechanism of tachycardia and the pathophysiological substrate are identified, for example, intra-atrial reentry, AV nodal reentry, or atrial flutter; the stability and hemodynamic consequences of the arrhythmia are assessed. Once tachycardia is induced, a careful search for specific termination sequences is made. To consider permanent pacing for the treatment of paroxysmal tachycardia, one must repeatedly demonstrate its efficacy and safety. Efficacy and safety usually are documented repetitively with temporary pacing, during which time the arrhythmia must be repeatedly induced and safely and reliably terminated. It is important to remember that changes in position, autonomic tone, and medications may affect initiation and termination of tachycardia.

Patient selection criteria are evolving. The most important are documented efficacy and safety and patient symptoms. If the patient's symptoms are very minimal and attacks can be easily self-terminated, or if the arrhythmia can be completely prevented by relatively easily eliminating the substrate, for example, radiofrequency ablation of an accessory pathway, even though pacing is very effective and safe, it may not be used. The most suitable patients are those with infrequent but significantly symptomatic episodes that cannot be self-terminated. Many of these patients have required repeated, urgent medical evaluations. Pacing may be an excellent alternative to long-term daily administration of medications to prevent infrequent attacks. In other patients, medications may be ineffective in preventing tachycardia, or may be associated with significant side effects, and pacing may be the treatment of choice. Many antiarrhythmic medications are especially unsuitable in young women who may become pregnant.

In patients with very frequent episodes of tachycardia, each of which could be terminated by pacing, the potential for rapid battery depletion exists. Concomitant antiarrhythmic therapy may be required to decrease the frequency of tachycardia in this situation.

Supraventricular Arrhythmias

Radiofrequency ablation has significantly changed the management of arrhythmias that may be suitable for pacing for tachycardia. Ablation has now become the treatment of choice for patients with symptomatic isolated pre-excitation syndromes (Figure 6). In these patients, electrophysiological mapping and then delivery of radiofrequency energy at either the site of atrial or ventricular insertion is curative for atrioventricular reentrant tachycardia eliminating the need for either medications or antitachycardia pacing. If catheterization ablation is not possible, then other options become more important. Radiofrequency ablation has also been applied in patients with paroxysmal supraventricular tachycardia secondary to atrioventricular nodal reentry (Figures 7A and B). In these patients, the slow conducting pathway that usually inserts into the posteroseptal region near the coronary sinus is identified and ablated leaving conduction via the fast pathway intact. This also is curative in the large majority of patients with a low incidence of significant side effects, although atrioventricular block has been reported. When successful, it results in no further tachycardia and obviates the need to take any cardiac medications. This technique may also be able to be applied in other patients with reentrant arrhythmias, for example, intra-atrial reentrant tachycardia if mapping techniques improve. Such developments will decrease the use of antitachycardia pacing for supraventricular arrhythmias. Prior to widespread use of radiofrequency ablation, some of these patients would have been ideal for current antitachycardia pacing modalities.

Other supraventricular arrhythmias may also be treated with pacing. As previously mentioned, in patients with sinus node dysfunction and bradycardia-

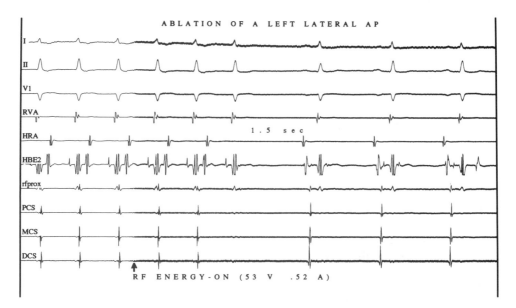

Figure 6. Radiofrequency ablation in a patient with a left lateral accessory pathway. During macro-reentrant tachycardia, radiofrequency energy is applied (arrow), resulting in ablation of the pathway and termination of tachycardia. RVA = right ventricular apex; HRA = high right atrium; HBE = His bundle electrogram; rfprox = radiofrequency probe; PCS, MCS, and DCS = proximal, mid, and distal coronary sinus, respectively. (Courtesy of Douglas L. Packer, M.D., Mayo Clinic, Rochester, MN.)

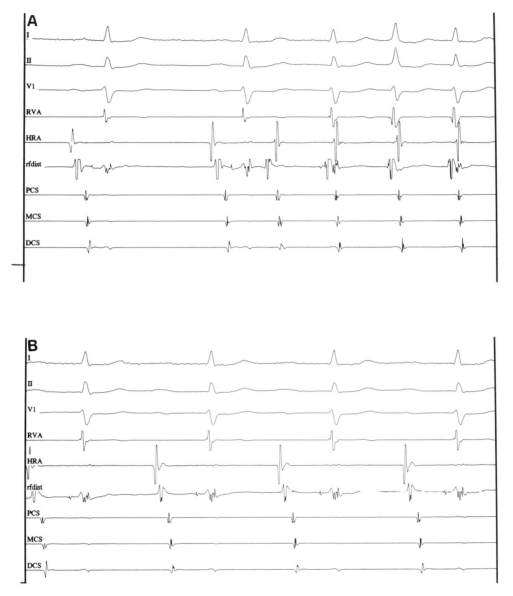

Figure 7. *Electrograms from a patient with AV nodal reentry tachycardia. (A) At baseline, first and second beats, conduction is via the fast pathway. Tachycardia is initiated (third beat) by an impulse that blocks in the fast pathway and then conducts antegradely down the slow pathway. (B) Following radiofrequency ablation, fast pathway conduction is eliminated; AV conduction is via the slow pathway. Reentry cannot take place. RVA = right ventricular apex; HRA = high right atrium; PCS = proximal coronary sinus; MCS = mid coronary sinus; DCS = distal coronary sinus; rfdist = radiofrequency catheter distal recording.*

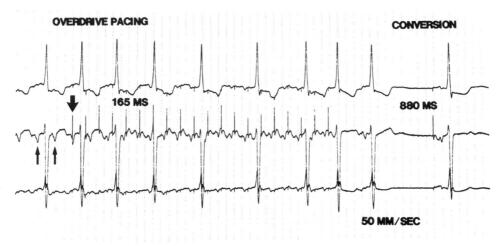

Figure 8. *Electrocardiogram from a 14 year old with a Mustard procedure for complete transposition of the great arteries. The patient had recurrent atrial flutter with 2:1 atrioventricular conduction (small arrows left). An Intertach 262–12™ pacemaker was implanted. After sensing the arrhythmia, the device delivers an overdrive burst (large arrow) at a cycle length of 165 msec for 20 pulses. This converts the patient to sinus rhythm. The device then paces AAI because of sinus slowing. (From Fukushige J, Porter CJ, Hayes DL, et al: Antitachycardia pacemaker treatment of postoperative arrhythmias in pediatric patients. PACE 1991, Part I; 14:546–556.)*

dependent escape rhythms, for example, atrial fibrillation or other atrial tachycardia, pacing may be very effective and has been found to be associated with an increased chance of remaining in sinus rhythm during follow-up. A small but expanding group of patients include those with recurrent atrial flutter (Figure 8). Some of these patients have congenital heart disease and are status post corrective surgical operations such as Fontan or Mustard procedures. In these patients, burst overdrive pacing may be very effective.

The long-term results of pacing for supraventricular tachycardia are variable and depend upon the specific arrhythmia, the clinical setting in which it occurs, for example, postoperative congenital heart disease patients versus patients with no underlying structural disease, the specific device used, and the definition of success used. With initial devices, during longer term follow-up, success rates declined. This resulted from the fact that over time the electrophysiological properties of the tachycardia changed, for example, cycle length and limited flexibility of termination modes. With newer software-based multiprogrammable antitachycardia units, e.g., Intertach 262–12 and 262–16™, successful longer outcome has been maintained in carefully selected patients, and the need for adjunctive antiarrhythmia medications has decreased. In these patients, antitachycardia pacing results not only in decreased need for medications but also a decreased number of hospital admissions and therefore improved quality-of-life.

Ventricular Arrhythmias

There has been substantial concern about antitachycardia pacing for the treatment of recurrent sustained ventricular tachycardia. It has been effective in very selected patients, most commonly using overdrive burst pacing. The major issue in these patients has been the potential for the pacing strategy to result in acceleration of the tachycardia, conversion to another arrhythmia, for example, ventricular tachycardia to ventricular fibrillation, or to result in adverse hemodynamic consequences for the patient. These concerns greatly limited stand-alone antitachycardia pacing for ventricular tachycardia. With the initial development of ICDs, there was an increase in interest and several small series of patients were treated with two devices simultaneously—an antitachycardia pacemaker and a backup ICD for ventricular fibrillation or tachycardia not responsive to pacing. These device combinations were very costly and had the problem of device interactions, for example, the ICD sensing the pacing treatment as ventricular tachycardia. New third generation ICDs with multiple tiers of antitachycardia pacing and backup cardioversion and defibrillation as well as bradycardia pacing should greatly expand the use of this approach (Figure 9). These multiprogrammable antiarrhythmic devices have been found to reduce the need for antiarrhythmic drugs, minimize the use of delivery of painful or inappropriate spurious shocks, and prevent the need for two devices (see Chapter 12). Other therapies are also becoming available for these patients. Radiofrequency catheter ablation has been found to be safe and effective in patients with ventricular tachycardia but without structural heart disease. However, these patients with ventricular tachycardia but without structural heart disease represent only a small minority of all patients with ventricular tachycardia. If these ablation techniques can be applied in more patient subsets in the future, this may impact upon antitachycardia pacing. The majority of these patients, however, will need defibrillator backup.

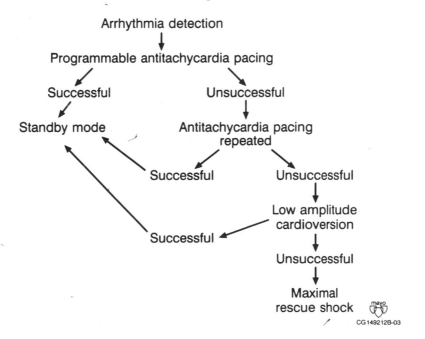

Figure 9. *Arrhythmia detection and treatment.*

PATIENT EVALUATION

Patient evaluation includes both invasive and noninvasive testing (Table III). The presence or absence of associated diseases that may impact on the arrhythmia or its treatment should be evaluated. The spontaneous characteristics of the arrhythmia should be studied, if possible, to determine precipitating events. Careful invasive assessment is a cornerstone. This defines the mechanism of tachycardia and the underlying pathophysiological substrate. During this, tachycardia is induced, and its stability and hemodynamic consequences are assessed. If the patient is a good candidate from a clinical treatment standpoint, then the baseline electrophysiological study is modified for extensive testing of tachycardia initiation or termination. In some patients this may be performed at the time of a second electrophysiological study. The effectiveness of different pacing sites and modes, the stability of the atrium or ventricle to the stimulation protocol during tachycardia, and the presence of associated electrophysiological abnormalities are assessed. Repeated testing is necessary to be certain that the stimulation protocol used does not cause adverse results, for example, acceleration of the tachycardia or conversion to another arrhythmia. In patients with supraventricular tachycardia, more aggressive pacing algorithms, for example, more rapid pacing, may result in an increased potential for atrial fibrillation. This must be kept in mind during follow-up. In some patients, multiple arrhythmias are present with different cycle lengths. The response of each specific arrhythmia to pacing must be evaluated. Ideally, a pulse generator similar to the one to be implanted should be used for termination testing. In addition to multiple attempts at termination in the laboratory, the patient may be sent to the intensive care unit with a temporary pacemaker in place to allow for repeated testing over the next several days. If antiarrhythmic drugs are to be used in conjunction with the pacemaker, the patient should be evaluated while on the specific drug regimen prior to receiving the permanent pacemaker. This is important because antiarrhythmic drugs may affect tachy-

---

Table III
Patient Evaluation

- Characterize Spontaneous Tachycardia (Monitoring and/or Electrophysiological Testing)
    Electrophysiological mechanism, rate, precipitating factors, frequency, response to medications, hemodynamic stability.
- Electrophysiological Assessment
    Characterize anatomical pathophysiological substrate, associated abnormalities, stability of tachycardia, identify optimal termination sequences, ascertain adverse effects of stimulation, evaluate effects of medication on rate and stimulation, assess requirement for backup pacing, defibrillation.
- Subsequent Testing
    Repeated induction and termination of tachycardia to document continued safety and efficacy of stimulation strategy using devices similar or identical to those to be implanted. Evaluate effects of time, changes in autonomic tone, and any antiarrhythmic medications to be used on initiation and termination.

---

cardia cycle length and termination parameters that may require a change in the stimulation protocol. In patients receiving a third generation ICD, postoperative testing is essential to select the specific tiered therapy. Increasing the number of attempts at tachycardia termination prior to implantation can help ensure continued efficacy of the device after permanent implantation.

SAFETY CONCERNS AND PACING

Selection of antitachycardia pacing must take into account safety issues.

1. The potential for converting one arrhythmia, such as stable ventricular tachycardia, to ventricular fibrillation.
2. The conversion of a stable ventricular tachycardia to one that is more severe, cannot be terminated by the implanted device, or will convert to fibrillation either spontaneously or when termination is attempted automatically.
3. Rapid 1:1 AV conduction during high rate atrial pacing.
4. Accurate detection of the tachycardia, either automatically by the pulse generator or manually during well-tolerated tachycardia by patients who have patient-activated units.
5. Prompt termination of the arrhythmia.
6. Maintenance of stimulation sequences that are stable over time and that will reliably terminate the tachycardia under a variety of clinical conditions.

Even with reliance on stringent criteria prior to implantation, during follow-up, in a sizable number of patients (up to 20%–50%), the ease and ability of terminating tachycardia will change. The ability to use these implanted devices to initiate tachycardia and evaluate its termination noninvasively following implantation may also be helpful.

DEVICE DESIGN

There are two major device types: those that require patient interaction and those with automatic tachycardia detection and treatment.

Patient Interactive Devices

As detection algorithms have improved, patient interaction devices have become uncommon. Such devices are for the most part of historical interest. To use an interactive device, the patient must be able to detect tachycardia accurately, tolerate it until it is terminated, operate the pacemaker unit, and then recognize return to normal sinus rhythm.

There are two basic types of devices, one with an implanted power source, and the other with a power source supplied by an external electromagnetically coupled unit.

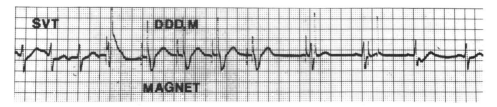

Figure 10. *Underdrive dual-chamber pacing in patient with supraventricular tachycardia (SVT). Application of magnet terminates tachycardia.*

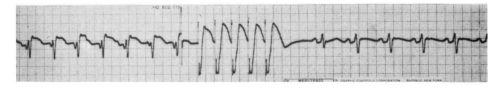

Figure 11. *Stable recurrent ventricular tachycardia at 110 bpm. The patient recognizes the arrhythmia and terminates it by a short burst of pacing at 150 bpm from the radiofrequency pacemaker.*

Implanted Power Source

Devices with an implanted power source range from a conventional pacemaker to sophisticated antitachycardia pacing devices. For some patients in whom underdrive pacing is effective for termination, application of a conventional magnet that converts the pulse generator to an asynchronous mode is all that is needed (Figure 10). More sophisticated units are now available that can be programmed to deliver a variety of stimulation sequences and which can also be used for noninvasive initiation of tachycardia.

External Power Source

Hand-held radiofrequency units also have been used in the past (Figure 11). The pulse frequency was adjustable in a wide range up to 400 pulses per minute. This device had the advantage of small size because it was a receiver only and did not need sophisticated tachycardia detection systems. Although effective in carefully selected patients, it had the disadvantage of limited flexibility in stimulation protocol. It also had the disadvantage that the patient had to be able to identify the pathological versus a physiological arrhythmia such as sinus tachycardia.

AUTOMATIC DEVICES

For automatic devices, accurate sensing is essential (Tables IV and V). Because stimulation techniques can induce as well as terminate tachycardia, if abnormal sensing occurs, for example, from electromyographic interference, and

Table IV
Tachycardia Detection

- High rate:
  - Number of intervals required: 5–99 (increments of 1)
  - Interval: 614 msec (98 bpm) to 266 msec (226 bpm) in 10.24 msec increments
- Sudden onset delta: 20–502 msec in 10.24 msec increments
- Rate stability:
  - Number of intervals required: 8–250 (increments of 1)
  - Delta: 15–149 (± 5) msec in 10.24 msec intervals
- Sustained high rate:
  - Number of intervals required: 6–10,000 (increments of 1)

Tachycardia detection criteria used by one of the current software based multiprogrammable pacemakers (Intertach II™).

if the device paces during normal sinus rhythm, it may actually initiate tachycardia. Detection algorithms have become progressively more sophisticated (Table VI). Early units had rate-only sensing. This led to spurious detection of sinus tachycardia as an arrhythmia. More recent devices have several programmable criteria including rate, sudden onset, rate stability, and sustained high rate. These help to decrease the chance of spurious detection and treatment of a nonpathological arrhythmia. Other systems under development rely on biological and physiological sensors such as mixed venous oxygen saturation. In patients with more than one arrhythmia, for example, intermittent atrial flutter or atrial fibrillation with a rapid ventricular response and also paroxysmal AV nodal reentry, detection of both arrhythmias may be problematic. A variety of medications may be required, including beta blockers, to reduce the maximum sinus rate, or other antiarrhythmic drugs to eliminate one tachycardia, leaving only one to be electrically terminated. It is essential that the patient's spontaneous tachycardia rate be faster than the programmed detection rate criteria. For example, if the tachycardia rate is usually 175–180 bpm, the detection criteria

Table V
Detection Algorithm Combination

1. High rate alone
2. High rate and sudden onset
3. High rate and sudden onset *or* sustained high rate
4. High rate and rate stability
5. High rate and rate stability *or* sustained high rate
6. High rate and sudden onset and rate stability
7. High rate and sudden onset and rate stability *or* sustained high rate
8. High rate and sudden onset *or* high rate and rate stability
9. High rate and sudden onset *or* high rate and rate stability *or* sustained high rate

Tachycardia detection algorithm combinations using criteria seen in Table IV with one current antitachycardia pacemaker (Intertach II™).

Table VI
Antitachycardia Pacing Functions

Burst, Single Extrastimulus, Double Extrastimulus
- Number of pulses: 1–250 (increments of 1)
- Delay: Fixed; fixed and scanning; adaptive; adaptive and scanning
  Interval to treatment:
  Fixed: 3–653 msec in 2.56 msec increments
  Adaptive: 50%–100% of tachycardia interval in 5% increments
  Scanning: incremental, decremental
             Step size: 2.6–38.4 msec in 2.56 msec increments
             Number sequences: 1–8
             Number steps: 2–31 (increments of 1)
- Burst cycle   Fixed, fixed and scanning, or autodecremental; adaptive;
  length: adaptive and scanning or autodecremental
  Interval to treatment:
  Fixed: 151–614 msec in 2.56 msec increments
  Adaptive: 50–100% of tachycardia interval in 5%
                                        increments
  Autodecremental: 2.6–38.4 msec in 2.56 msec increments
  Scanning: incremental, decremental
  Minimum burst cycle length: 148–614 msec in 2.56 msec increments
  Number of attempts: 1–31

Antitachycardia pacing functions are extensively programmable. The number of options available allow more patients to be treated but also greatly increase the complexity of treatment (Parameters-Intertach II™).

must be <170 bpm or the pacemaker will not recognize the tachycardia. Difficulties may occur if the tachycardia rate detection criteria is less than the maximum sinus rhythm. This is of concern in several clinical circumstances including:

1. slow tachycardia, for example, rates of 130–140 bpm;
2. a sinus rate faster than the tachycardia criterion, for example, sinus tachycardia during exercise;
3. more than one arrhythmia, for example, intermittent atrial flutter or fibrillation with rapid ventricular response and also paroxysmal AV nodal reentry. In this circumstance, depending on the rate of the two tachycardias, the pacemaker may only detect one.

As has been mentioned, new sensing algorithms should improve detection and facilitate correct treatment.

After recognition of tachycardia by the pulse generator, preset stimulation sequences (identified at the time of electrophysiological testing to be safe and effective) are automatically delivered to terminate a tachycardia (Figure 12). After each stimulation sequence, the pulse generator senses either return to sinus rhythm and is inhibited or senses tachycardia and repeats the stimulation sequence. For third generation ICDs, low energy cardioversion or backup defibrillation are also available (see Chapter).

The management of tachyarrhythmias by implantable devices is a highly

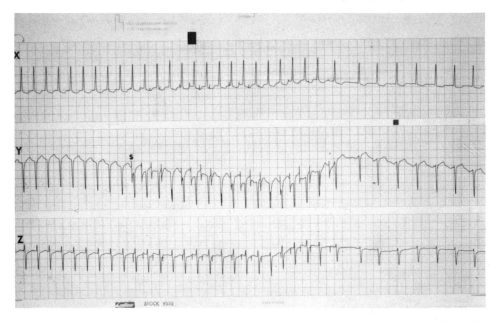

Figure 12.   *Three-lead electrocardiogram from a patient with recurrent supraventricular tachycardia. An implantable automatic overdrive pacemaker detects supraventricular tachycardia, and delivers a train of impulses (S) that terminates the arrhythmia, restoring sinus rhythm.*

complex and evolving clinical effort, requiring the maximum of comprehension of the tachycardia and the means of its termination (Table VI). In addition to terminating tachycardia, current devices allow for performance of a limited electrophysiological study noninvasively by stimulation through the pulse generator. This may be of help in follow-up if the tachycardia changes or the device is not effective. Current devices also have counters that can document the frequency of tachycardia and the frequency of conversion sequences used for termination. Finally, adaptive devices are available that compile the most successful termination sequences. When tachycardia occurs, these successful sequences are initially tried before others are used.

STIMULATION STRATEGIES FOR TERMINATION OF TACHYCARDIA (TABLE VII)

Underdrive Pacing

Underdrive pacing may be used for either supraventricular or ventricular tachycardia (Figure 10). The ability to terminate tachycardia by one or more than one extrastimulus depends on the characteristics of the reentrant circuit. During tachycardia, extrastimuli may be able to invade and capture a portion of the reentrant circuit, thus disrupting the circling wave front. Underdrive pacing may be performed manually by magnet application, changing an implanted

Table VII
Stimulation Strategies

- Underdrive (Single or Dual Chamber)
    Asynchronous
    Scanning
        sequential, incremental, decremental, adaptive table
- Overdrive (Single Chamber)
    Fixed rate burst
    Adaptive burst
    Tachycardia cycle length-dependent
    Autodecremental burst
    Scanning/shifting burst
    Ultra-rapid stimulation

inhibited pacemaker to an asynchronous unit (Figure 6). The pacemaker then stimulates asynchronously with stimuli falling at different times of the cardiac cycle. There is often a range of critical coupling intervals between the QRS complex and the extrastimulus during which one, two, or more stimuli delivered during this "time window" can terminate the tachycardia by capturing and changing the reentry circuit. Both single- and dual-chamber units have been used.

Single-Chamber Devices

Single-chamber devices can be used for both atrial and ventricular arrhythmias. These are most effective in patients with slow tachycardia, a large reentrant circuit, a wide termination time window, and in patients in whom the single stimulus can be delivered in close proximity to the reentrant circuit. This mode is not frequently used either because these criteria are not often met, it is not effective, or the time to termination is long. When found to be effective, however, underdrive pacing is a reasonable and safe option. Although tachycardia acceleration is uncommon, it may occur (Figure 13).

Dual-Chamber Devices

Dual-chamber pacemakers may be particularly useful in patients with atrioventricular reentry due to accessory pathways (Figure 14). The rationale is that nearly simultaneous capture of both atrium and ventricle may prevent continuation of the reentry circuit. Underdrive dual-chamber pacing is again more effective in patients with a wide range of coupling intervals that can terminate tachycardia and in patients with slower tachycardia rates. Because there is random stimulation during the cardiac cycle, termination of tachycardia may be delayed. Stimulation during the atrial vulnerable period may occur with the potential for inducing atrial fibrillation; this may promptly return to normal sinus rhythm or may be sustained. The potential for ventricular stimulation with induction of ventricular tachycardia or ventricular fibrillation must also be studied in the electrophysiological laboratory prior to implantation.

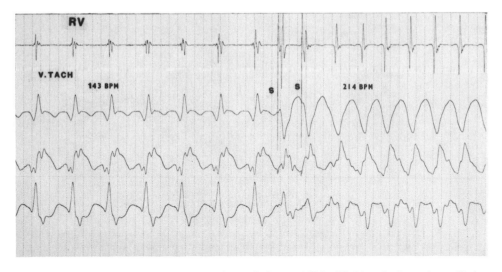

Figure 13. *Acceleration of ventricular tachycardia by two VPCs (S). Ventricular tachycardia (rate 143 bpm) induced during electrophysiological study. Two underdrive extrastimuli (S) are delivered, resulting in acceleration of VT to 214 bpm.*

Scanning Pacemakers

Scanning is a variety of underdrive pacing (Figure 15). Patient activated and automatic scanning devices are available. After detection of tachycardia and activation, these units introduce an extrastimulus or multiple extrastimuli at progressively shorter coupling intervals during diastole. Scanning during diastole maximizes the chance of prompt stimulation during the range of coupling intervals in which the tachycardia can be terminated. In addition, it is adaptive and thus can deal with the problem of a variable termination zone. Finally, because the stimuli are triggered off of sensed beats, the chance of stimulation during the vulnerable period may be decreased. Several pacing modalities have been used including sequential, incremental, or decremental scanning. Other

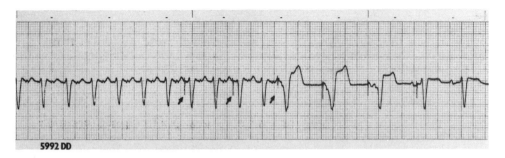

Figure 14. *Dual-demand pacemaker in patient with recurrent atrioventricular reentry secondary to bypass tract. After detection of tachycardia, the pacemaker stimulates both atrium and ventricle (arrows) and terminates tachycardia.*

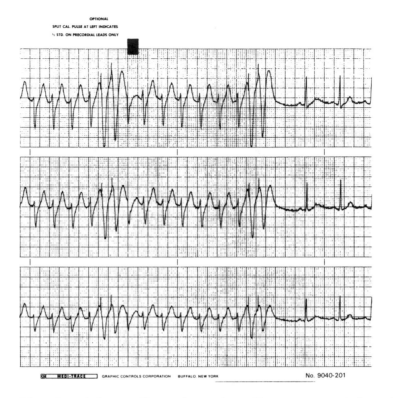

OPTIONAL
SPLIT CAL. PULSE AT LEFT INDICATES
½ STD. ON PRECORDIAL LEADS ONLY

MEDI-TRACE   GRAPHIC CONTROLS CORPORATION   BUFFALO, NEW YORK   No. 9040-201

Figure 15. *Three-channel electrocardiogram in a patient with recurrent ventricular tachycardia. An implantable patient-activated scanning pacemaker has been implanted. The first pair of coupled extrastimuli fail to terminate tachycardia, the second pair successfully return the patient to normal sinus rhythm.*

forms incorporate a self-searching mode and adaptive table scanning (Figure 16). With decremental scanning, the initial extrastimulus is delivered at a slightly shorter interval than the tachycardia cycle length and then progressively shorter coupling intervals are used until termination. If a single stimulus is ineffective, then two can be programmed. For incremental scanning, a similar sequence is performed in reverse beginning just beyond the refractory period determined at the time of electrophysiological study. Such units are extensively programmable. This is important because the tachycardia may vary under different circumstances. Changes in autonomic tone, posture, activity, or drug concentration level can all influence the rate of the tachycardia and affect its response to pacing. Even though scanning is effective, the mean duration of pacing prior to termination may be up to 1 to 1½ minutes. It is therefore important to select patients with well-tolerated tachycardia.

Some new pacing systems include an adaptable table scanning or adaptive scanning with memory. For this, the most successful stimulation protocols previously used are stored in the pacemaker and are used first at the time of subsequent tachycardia. Self-searching modes are also available in which the stimulation protocol is adjusted automatically depending upon the effect of

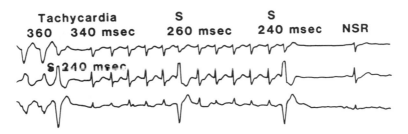

Figure 16. *Adaptive scanning. During a wide QRS complex tachycardia at CL 360 msec, the last beat of a scanning sequence (S) at 240 msec converts the wide QRS complex tachycardia to a narrow complex tachycardia at a faster rate of 340 msec. The pacing system senses the arrhythmia and adapts the next extrastimulus to be delivered at 260 msec. The second extrastimulus is then delivered at 240 msec and terminates tachycardia. (From Holmes DR Jr., Vlietstra RE: Interventional Cardiology. Philadelphia, F.A. Davis Publishers, 1989, with permission of the Mayo Foundation.)*

stimulation on tachycardia. These may help to decrease the time required for successful termination of tachycardia.

Overdrive Pacing

Overdrive pacing has been a widely used method of terminating tachycardia. It has the advantage that it is often more effective than underdrive pacing and results in more prompt return to normal sinus rhythm. It will potentially terminate all types of reentrant arrhythmias. It also has the potential for accelerating arrhythmias or converting tachycardia to fibrillation (Figure 17). For this reason it has been more commonly used in patients with supraventricular tachycardia although in the past in some patients with slow stable ventricular tachy-

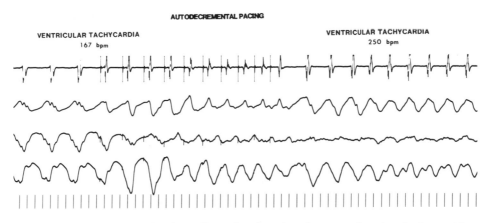

Figure 17. *Autodecremental tachycardia acceleration. Autodecremental pacing during rapid ventricular tachycardia, resulting in tachycardia acceleration associated with hemodynamic compromise. (From Holmes DR Jr., Vlietstra RE: Interventional Cardiology. Philadelphia, FA Davis Publishers, Philadelphia, PA, 1989, with permission of the Mayo Foundation.)*

cardia, it has been used after extensive testing (Figure 8). Currently, in patients with ventricular tachycardia, if pacing for tachycardia is selected, a combined antitachycardia pacing and defibrillation third generation ICD should be used.

The rate required for termination varies. In general, a rate approximately 25% faster than the tachycardia rate is required for termination. Pacing at slower rates that are just slightly faster than the rate of tachycardia may entrain the arrhythmia without terminating it. Alternatively, with very fast stimulation rates, the arrhythmia may be changed from an organized tachycardia to fibrillation. With supraventricular tachycardia and rapid pacing, atrial fibrillation may result; this is sometimes transient and then returns to normal sinus rhythm. In patients with enhanced AV nodal conduction or a rapidly conducting accessory pathway, the potential for rapid 1:1 conduction also exists. Stimulation sequences should be as short as possible, and limited to that required for termination. In general, 5–10 capture beats are sufficient, although in patients with atrial flutter postoperatively, 20–30 capture beats may be required. If that sequence is not effective, a slightly more rapid rate should be tested.

For ventricular arrhythmias, overdrive pacing is commonly used during electrophysiological testing. Similar concerns exist as for supraventricular tachycardia, namely that the more rapid the stimulation, the greater the chance of acceleration of the arrhythmia or conversion to ventricular fibrillation, and the less well tolerated.

Combined burst pacing/scanning devices have been developed that combine scanning and burst techniques. These include autodecremental burst pacing, scanning burst (concertina/accordion), and shifting burst modes (Figures 18, 19). With autodecremental pacing, after tachycardia detection, the first stimulus cycle length is delivered at a slightly shorter (programmable) cycle length. Each subsequent stimulus cycle length is decreased by similar degree. Shifting or scanning burst modes offer a different approach with the introduction of premature impulses at a specific delay following a tachycardia complex. A burst or multiple extrastimuli is then administered. A final method of overdrive pacing uses ultra-rapid stimulation at 3000–6000 per minute. Pacing is initiated in the refractory period and timed to give one or two captures after the refractory

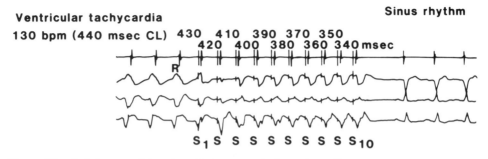

Figure 18.   *Autodecremental pacing. During ventricular tachycardia, 10 ventricular extrastimuli (S) are delivered in an autodecremental fashion. The decremental value (D) is 10 msec. CL = cycle length; R = last spontaneous tachycardia beat. (From Holmes DR Jr., Vlietstra RE: Interventional Cardiology. Philadelphia, F.A. Davis Publishers, 1989, with permission of the Mayo Foundation.)*

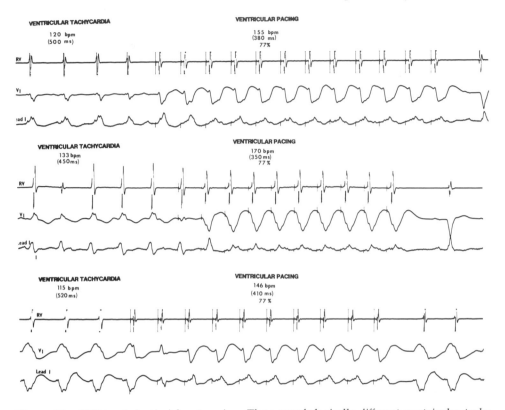

Figure 19. *Shifting (adaptive) burst pacing. Three morphologically different ventricular tachycardias in the same patient. Burst is synchronized to R wave during tachycardia, and burst rate is programmed to be 77% of the tachycardia cycle length. RV = right ventricular electrogram. Electrocardiographical leads: V_1, I. (From Holmes DR Jr., Vlietstra RE: Interventional Cardiology. Philadelphia, F.A. Davis Publishers, 1989, with permission of the Mayo Foundation.)*

period. The role that these combination devices will have for the treatment of ventricular arrhythmias remains unclear although with backup defibrillation, they may be very important.

SUMMARY

The number of options available for patients with paroxysmal tachycardia is increasing. For patients with AV nodal reentry tachycardia or atrioventricular reentry tachycardia from pre-excitation syndromes, radiofrequency ablation will play an increasingly primary role. Antitachycardia pacing for patients with these and other supraventricular arrhythmias is often very effective in addition but will be used relatively infrequently. For patients with recurrent ventricular tachycardia, however, device use will increase. The widespread availability of third generation devices with antitachycardia pacing, backup cardioversion, and defibrillation will greatly expand the patient population that will benefit.

At the present time, the technique has gone beyond the ability of casual users to understand and manage the systems. This has important implications for the follow-up care and evaluation of these patients. At present, the decision to use any of these technology approaches must be made after the most careful analysis of the clinical setting and the specific arrhythmia. Electrophysiological testing, an essential part of this decision making, is required to document the mechanism of arrhythmia and the safety and efficacy of the tachycardia termination technique. Careful follow-up is required to make sure the devices perform in the manner for which they are intended. Repeated electrophysiological testing, either using the pacemaker itself or tachycardia induction with temporary transvenous pacemakers, may be required.

BIBLIOGRAPHY

Akhtar M, Gilbert CJ, Al-Nouri M, et al: Electrophysiological mechanisms for modification and abolition of atrioventricular junctional tachycardia with simultaneous and sequential atrial and ventricular pacing. Circulation 1979; 60:1443–1454.

Bardy GH, Troutman C, Poole JE, et al: Clinical experience with a tiered therapy, multiprogrammable antiarrhythmia device. Circulation 1992; 85:1689–1698.

Bennett MA, Pentecost BL: Suppression of ventricular tachyarrhythmias by transvenous intracardiac pacing after acute myocardial infarction. Br Med J (Clin Res) 1970; 4: 468–470.

Calvo RA, Saksena S, Pantopoulous D, et al: Sequential transvenous pacing and shock therapy for termination of sustained ventricular tachycardia. Am Heart J 1988; 115: 569–575.

Camm HJ: Design of Pacing Algorithms for Tachycardia Termination or Prevention. In B Luderitz B, S Saksena (eds.) Interventional Electrophysiology. Mount Kisco, NY, Futura Publishing Company, 1991, pp. 141–153.

Case CL, Gillette PC, Ziegler VL, et al: Successful treatment of congenital atrial flutter with antitachycardia pacing. PACE 1990; 13:571–573.

Cheng TO: Transvenous ventricular pacing in the treatment of paroxysmal atrial tachyarrhythmias alternating with sinus bradycardia and standstill. Am J Cardiol 1968; 22:874–879.

Critelli G, Grassi G, Chiarello M, et al: Automatic "scanning" by radiofrequency in the long-term electrical treatment of arrhythmias. PACE 1979; 2:289–296.

DiSegni E, Klein HO, David D, et al: Overdrive pacing in quinidine syncope and other long QT-interval syndromes. Arch Intern Med 1980; 140:1036–1040.

Fisher JD, Johnston DR, Furman S, et al: Long-term efficacy of antitachycardia pacing for supraventricular and ventricular tachycardias. Am J Cardiol 1987; 60:1311–1316.

Fromer M, Gloor H, Kus T, et al: Clinical experience with the Intertach 262–12 pulse generator in patients with recurrent supraventricular and ventricular tachycardia. PACE 1990; 13:1955–1959.

Fromer M, Gloor H, Kus T, Shenasa M: Clinical experience with a new software-based antitachycardia pacemaker for recurrent supraventricular and ventricular tachycardias. PACE 1990; 13:890–899.

Fukushige J, Porter CJ, Hayes DL, et al: Antitachycardia pacemaker treatment of postoperative arrhythmias in pediatric patients. PACE 1991; 14:546–556.

Gillette PC, Zeigler VL, Case CL, et al: Atrial antitachycardia pacing in children and young adults. Am Heart J 1991; 122:844–849.

Holt P, Crick JCP, Sowton E: Antitachycardia pacing: A comparison of burst overdrive, self searching and adaptive table scanning programs. PACE 1986; 9:490–497.

Jackman WM, Beckman KJ, McClelland JH, et al: Treatment of supraventricular tachycardia due to atrioventricular nodal reentry by radiofrequency catheter ablation of slow pathway conduction. N Engl J Med 1992; 327:313–318.

Jackman WM, Wang X, Friday KJ, et al: Catheter ablation of accessory atrioventricular pathways (Wolff-Parkinson-White syndrome) by radiofrequency current. N Engl J Med 1991; 324:1605–1611.

Jung W, Mletzko R, Manz M, et al: Comparison of two antitachycardia pacing modes in supraventricular tachycardia. PACE 1991; 14:1762–1766.

Jung W, Mletzko R, Manz M, et al: Long-term therapy of antitachycardia pacing for supraventricular tachycardia. PACE 1992; 15:179–187.

Li CK, Shandling AH, Nolasco M, et al: Atrial automatic tachycardia—reversion pacemakers: Their economic viability and impact on quality of life. PACE 1990; 13:639–645.

McComb JM, Jameson S, Bexton RS: Atrial antitachycardia pacing in patients with supraventricular tachycardia: Clinical experience with the Intertach pacemaker. PACE 1990, Part II; 13:1948–1954.

Medina-Ravell V, Maduro C, Mejias J, et al: Use of dual-demand AV sequential (DVI, MN) pacemakers in the management of supraventricular tachycardias. Cardiovasc Clin 1983; 14:227–238.

Nathan AW, Creamer JE, Davies DW, et al: Clinical experience with a software based tachycardia reversion pacemaker. PACE 1986, Part II; 9:1312–1315.

Nazari J, Fujimura O, Kuo CS, et al: Treatment of atrioventricular nodal reentry with antitachycardia pacing. Intermedics, Inc. 1990.

Osborn MJ, Holmes DR: Antitachycardia pacing. Clin Prog Electrophysiol Pacing 1985; 3:239–269.

Pless BD, Sweeney MB: Discrimination of supraventricular tachycardia from sinus tachycardia of overlapping cycle length. PACE 1984, Part II; 7:1318–1324.

Porter CJ, Fukushige J, Hayes DL, et al: Permanent antitachycardia pacing for chronic atrial tachyarrhythmias in postoperative pediatric patients. PACE 1991; 14:2056–2057.

Preston TA, Haynes RE, Gavin WA, et al: Permanent rapid atrial pacing to control supraventricular tachycardia. PACE 1979; 2:331–334.

Ruskin JN, Garan H, Poulin F, et al: Permanent radiofrequency ventricular pacing for management of drug-resistant ventricular tachycardia. Am J Cardiol 1980; 46:317–321.

Schneller SJ: Intertach II: New antitachycardia pacemaker. Cardiol Trends 1990; p 37.

Shandling AH, Li CK, Thomas L: Sustained effectiveness of an atrial antitachycardia pacemaker during follow-up. PACE 1990; 13:833–838.

The Cardiac Arrhythmia Suppression Trial (CAST) Investigators. Preliminary report: Effect of encainide and flecainide on mortality in a randomized trial of arrhythmia suppression after myocardial infarction. N Engl J Med 1989; 321:406–412.

The Cardiac Arrhythmia Suppression Trial II Investigators: Effect of the antiarrhythmic agent moricizine on survival after myocardial infarction. N Engl J Med 1992; 327: 227–233.

Wettstein EH, Rotenberg WB, Adler SC: Trends in supraventricular antiarrhythmic drug therapy after implantation of an antitachycardia pacemaker. Intermedics, Inc. 1991.

Wilkoff BL: Treatment of concealed Wolff-Parkinson-White syndrome with antitachycardia pacing. Intermedics, Inc. 1990.

Chapter 14

PACEMAKER COMPLICATIONS

David L. Hayes

Pacemaker complications are relatively infrequent. They can occur intraoperatively, soon after implantation, or at a time distant from implantation (Table I). Environmental or device-related pacemaker complications and the effect of drugs on the pacing system are discussed in Chapter 18, "Practical Considerations."

EARLY COMPLICATIONS

Pain/Ecchymoses

Most patients undergoing pacemaker implantation have some discomfort at the site of the incision in the early postoperative period. Although the incision is usually small, the operation is not different from any other surgical procedure, and mild analgesics may be required. (Although aspirin may be an effective analgesic it could potentially aggravate bleeding/ecchymoses at the incision site.) Mild ecchymoses around the incision are not uncommon.

Pneumothorax

Access to the subclavian vein, commonly used for implantation of an endocardial pacemaker lead, usually is accomplished by subclavian vein puncture with a modified Seldinger technique. The vein usually is approached blindly. Because of the relationship of the subclavian vein to the apex of the lung, the possibility of lung injury and traumatic pneumothorax (Figure 1) or hemopneumothorax (Figure 2) are always present. Hemothorax can be caused by laceration of the subclavian artery and hemopneumothorax by laceration of the lung and the subclavian artery. In a patient with unusual anatomy of the chest wall or clavicle, the subclavian vein can be displaced and the usual landmarks used for subclavian puncture can be altered. Anatomy must be taken into account before subclavian puncture is undertaken. In the patient with unusual anatomy, when there is concern that the subclavian vein may be displaced, peripheral injection of contrast media and fluoroscopic guidance of the subclavian puncture may help to minimize complications. (See Chapter 8, "Permanent Pacemaker Implantation.")

If pneumothorax occurs, it may manifest during the pacemaker procedure or as late as 48 hours after implantation. Prompt chest x-ray after subclavian venipuncture is very useful. Indications that pneumothorax has occurred are as

Table I
Pacemaker Complications

Early Complications	Late Complications	Early or Late Complications
Pain/ecchymoses	Skin erosion	Lead dislodgment
Pneumothorax	Skin adherence	Pacemaker-related
Hematoma formation	Thrombosis	arrhythmias
Lead perforation	Radiation damage	Twiddler's syndrome
Intraoperative lead	Pacemaker failure	Abnormalities induced by
damage	High thresholds	medical equipment*
Subcutaneous	Lead fracture or	Infection
emphysema	insulation defect	Pacemaker syndrome
Thoracic duct injury		Pacemaker allergy
Air embolism		Pulse generator
Brachial plexus injury		malfunction
Subclavian artery		Loose lead/connector
puncture		block interface

* See Chapter 18, Electromagnetic Interference

follows: (1) aspiration of air during the subclavian puncture when the exploring needle is either introduced or removed; (2) unexplained hypotension; (3) chest pain; (4) respiratory distress.

Following subclavian puncture, the lung fields should be visualized intra-operatively with fluoroscopy and postoperatively with a chest radiograph. A pneumothorax that collapses the apex of the lung only to the second or third interspace or involves less than 10% of the pleural space probably can be ob-

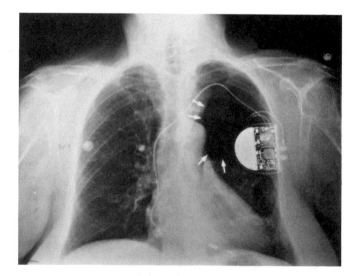

Figure 1. *Left pneumothorax after pacemaker implantation, a complication of subclavian puncture.*

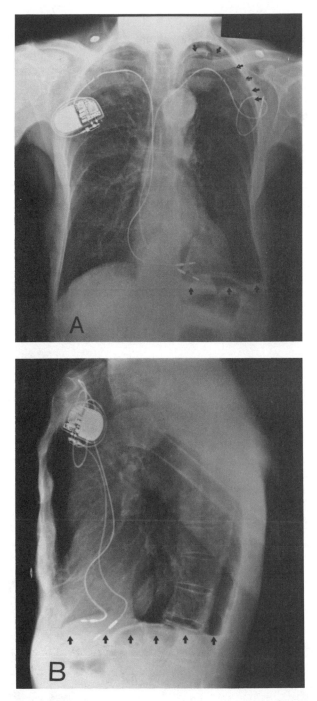

Figure 2. *PA* ***(A)*** *and lateral***(B)*** *chest x-rays demonstrating a left apical pneumothorax after an unsuccessful attempt to place a second lead via the left subclavian vein. (The ventricular lead on the left had been abandoned because of an insulation defect.) In addition to the apical pneumothorax there is also a fluid level due to a hemothorax. The new lead was subsequently placed via the right subclavian without further complication.*

served without chest tube placement. A chest tube should be considered if any of the following exist: (1) a pneumothorax of greater than 10%; (2) respiratory distress; (3) hemopneumothorax.

There are other potential complications of subclavian venous entry including inadvertent arterial puncture, air embolism, arteriovenous fistula, thoracic duct injury, and brachial plexus injury. Meticulous attention is required to minimize these risks.

Hematoma Formation

Because local ecchymoses are common after pacemaker implantation, a small or large ecchymosis that is not expanding is treated by observation only.

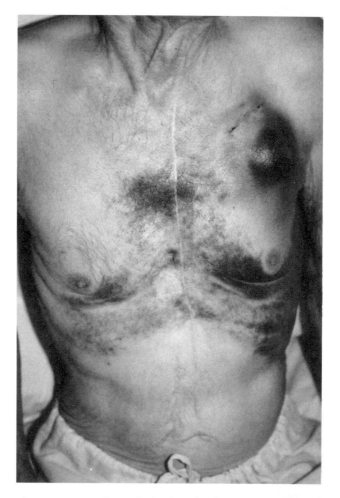

Figure 3.   *Large hematoma over the newly implanted pulse generator. Extensive ecchymoses can be seen inferior to the pacemaker as well as midsternum and in the inframammary area. The patient had undergone aortic valve replacement during the same hospitalization, and the sternal and inframammary ecchymoses were in part due to the recent sternotomy.*

A discrete hematoma formation at the site must be dealt with on the basis of its secondary consequences (Figure 3). If there is continued bleeding or if pain from the hematoma cannot be managed with mild analgesics, consideration should be given to evacuating the hematoma. If it does not compromise the suture line or skin integrity, it should be observed without intervention. Because it is ineffective and increases the risk of infection, early hematoma aspiration should not be attempted. Late aspiration may be attempted carefully in a sterile procedure after the hematoma has liquefied. However, in most cases late aspiration is unnecessary.

To avoid hematoma formation, patients should have a normal prothrombin time before pacemaker implantation, and heparin administration should have been discontinued at least 6 hours before implantation. Ideally, the patient should not have recently taken aspirin or other platelet-inhibitory drugs. Antiplatelet drugs may be the most common cause of hematoma formation. In patients who have been receiving platelet-inhibitory drugs, hemostasis during implantation often is difficult. Whether pacemaker implantation should be delayed in elective patients on platelet-inhibitory drugs remains controversial. Careful attention to hemostasis prior to closure of the incision should prevent complications in most patients on platelet-inhibitory drugs.

In patients who require therapeutic anticoagulation, a 48-hour delay after implantation is wise before resuming full heparinization. Warfarin (Coumadin) administration usually can be started safely 24 hours after implantation, but 48 hours is preferable if this will not compromise the patient. It should be started at the patient's maintenance dose and not at higher doses that would be used to initiate therapy. The absolute timing for reinstitution of anticoagulants varies from patient to patient. Anticoagulation at greater than therapeutic levels can result in late hematoma formation.

Although not practiced by these authors, a technique has been described for pacemaker implantation in the fully anticoagulated patient. This involves use of topical thrombin and cryoprecipitate within the pacemaker pocket at the time of implantation.

Subcutaneous Emphysema

Subcutaneous emphysema may occur as a complication of subclavian puncture. In the presence of subcutaneous emphysema, the patient should be evaluated for associated pneumothorax.

If subcutaneous emphysema extends to the pacemaker pocket in a unipolar pacemaker or a polarity-programmable pacemaker programmed to the unipolar configuration, pacemaker malfunction occurs. If air accumulates in the pacemaker pocket it may result in insulation of the unipolar anodal plate with subsequent failure to pace. (In a polarity-programmable pulse generator where pacing and sensing can be independently programmed for polarity, it may be possible to see failure of either pacing or sensing rather than failure of both depending on how the polarity of each had been programmed.) Gentle pressure on the pacemaker site to express the air should restore normal pacemaker function.

Arterial Lead Puncture and Cannulation

Subclavian artery puncture is a well-recognized complication of subclavian vein puncture. It usually is easily recognized by the pulsating nature of the blood return and/or the aspirating syringe being filled under pressure. If this is recognized promptly and the needle removed, it is unlikely that a problem will result. A hemothorax may occur if the artery is lacerated, but this is an extremely rare complication.

One of the complications of the subclavian puncture technique is arterial entry and introduction of the lead(s) into the subclavian artery, the aorta, and the left ventricle (Figure 4). Frequently, arterial entry will be recognized readily because of the pulsatile flow of saturated (crimson) blood. Arterial entry may be entirely unrecognized because of desaturation of the arterial blood, making it appear venous, or loss of pulsatile arterial flow because of hypotension or diminution of the arterial pulse pressure. Once within the great arteries, passage

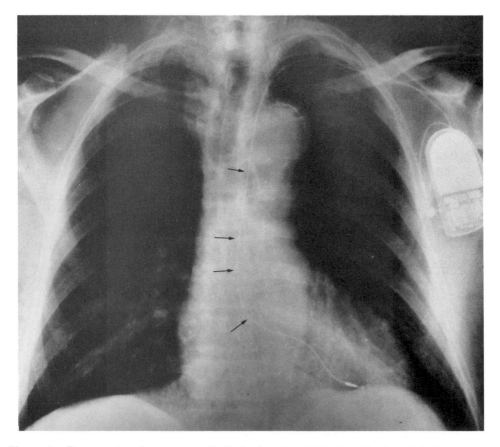

Figure 4. *Permanent pacing system with the lead inadvertently placed in the subclavian artery and the lead positioned in the left ventricle. From the anteroposterior view it is difficult to tell that the lead is in the left ventricle. The black arrows emphasize the course of the lead which is more leftward than expected for a vena cava/right ventricular course.*

of the lead into the left ventricle will be as easy as passage into the right ventricle via the venous system.

As pacemaker implantation is likely to be performed under fluoroscopy, arterial entry can be recognized by the passage of the lead well within the cardiac silhouette and medial to the usual course of lead entry. The passage into the left ventricle, as viewed in the AP projection, will be similar, but well medial to entry into the right ventricle. If a lateral view is used (this is not common), then a right ventricular lead will be anterior, i.e., posterior to the sternum, while a left ventricular lead will be in the posterior aspect of the heart.

Electrograms and stimulation thresholds are likely to be sufficiently similar between right and left ventricles so as not to offer a distinction. The ECG in right ventricular pacing is of a left bundle branch block pattern and during left ventricular pacing is of a right bundle branch block pattern. Association of posterior x-ray position and electrocardiographic right bundle branch block pattern is diagnostic of left ventricular placement.

While left ventricular pacing may be permanently secure, it has been associated with thrombus formation, embolization, and consequently stroke. Reports of long-term uncomplicated left ventricular endocardial pacing exist, but the risk of embolization continues. Removal of the left ventricular lead should be undertaken if it is recognized early after implant. If it is recognized years after uncomplicated pacing and antiplatelet anticoagulation can be performed, it may be safe to leave the endocardial lead in place. Sufficient data is not yet available.

A pacing lead may also be placed in the left ventricle by passing it across an unsuspected atrial or ventricular septal defect. In a patient with a ventricular septal defect, endocardial pacing should be avoided because the potential exists for small emboli to cross the ventricular septal defect that potentially could cause symptoms in the arterial circulation.

Lead Perforation

Lack of symptoms after ventricular perforation by a lead is not uncommon. The only sign may be a rising stimulation threshold. In other patients, the signs may include:

1. right bundle branch block paced rhythm when the lead has been placed in the right ventricle (depending on the lead position it is also possible to see an RBBB pattern when the lead is within the right ventricular cavity);
2. intercostal muscle or diaphragmatic contraction;
3. friction rub after implantation;
4. pericarditis, pericardial effusion, or cardiac tamponade.

The diagnostic techniques used to identify ventricular perforation are x-ray (Figure 5), electrocardiography, and two-dimensional echocardiography (Figure 6). Once a perforation has been identified, the lead must be withdrawn and repositioned. Lead withdrawal usually is uncomplicated. Pericardial bleeding or tamponade may result, but this complication is rare.

If the patient demonstrates mild symptoms or signs compatible with lead perforation, i.e., pericardial pain, friction rub, but a persistent perforation cannot be identified, it is reasonable to observe the patient. If the symptoms and/or

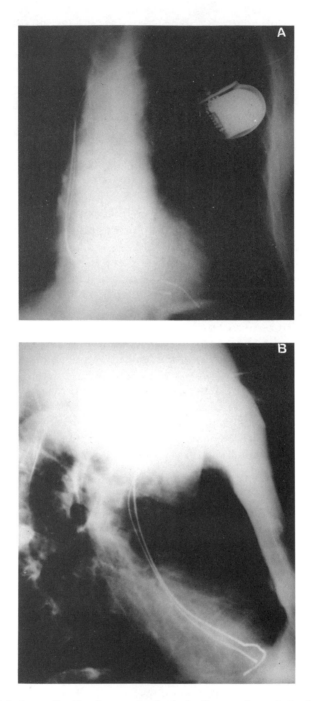

Figure 5. *Ventricular perforation by a pacing lead. **A.** On a posteroanterior film, although the lead can be seen to cross the border of the diaphragm, perforation is difficult to diagnose. **B.** On a lateral projection, however, the perforating lead extends past the end of the pacing lead within the ventricle, enters the pericardium, and forms a curve in the pericardial space.*

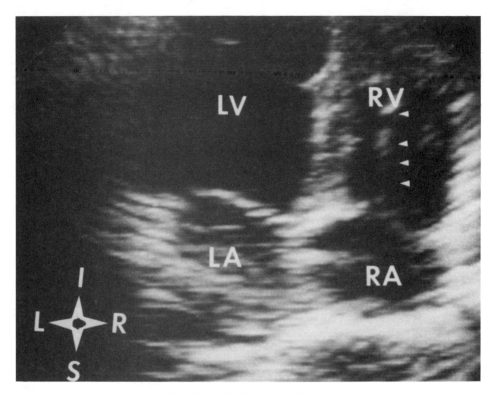

Figure 6. *An echocardiogram identifies a lead (arrowheads) in a correct right ventricular apical position. I = Inferior; L = left; LA = left atrium; LV = left ventricle; R = right; RA = right atrium; RV = right ventricle; S = superior.*

signs resolve during a 24- to 48-hour time period, lead repositioning will probably not be necessary. If an echocardiogram reveals a small pericardial effusion but no definite perforation, serial echocardiograms should be performed to insure that the effusion is not hemodynamically significant or enlarging.

Lead Damage

Lead damage during pacemaker implantation may be more common than is recognized. Damage of silicone rubber insulated leads seemed to occur less frequently in the past, but polyurethane insulated leads are more vulnerable to mishandling during the operative procedure. Both types of leads are easily cut by scissors or scalpel, and repair is difficult. Polyurethane leads can be easily damaged by placement of a ligature directly around the lead itself. To secure the lead, the protector sleeve provided on most polyurethane leads or a "butterfly" sleeve that can be secured around the lead and then to the underlying support structures should be used (Figure 7).

It is also possible to damage the lead during the implant procedure with the stylet, i.e., the stylet may be forced at an angle through the conductor and the surrounding insulating material. If this is recognized during the procedure the lead should be removed and repaired or discarded.

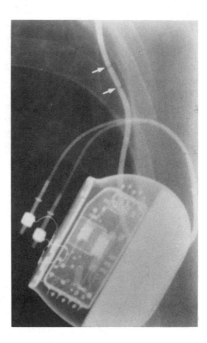

Figure 7. *Two indentations on the pacemaker lead are ligature compression of the insulating material. This anomaly has been referred to by some as "pseudofracture." Polyurethane leads can be damaged easily by tight ligatures.*

LATE COMPLICATIONS

For the purpose of this chapter the "late" post-implantation period is defined as being beyond 1 month post-implant, and the complications that are discussed subsequently usually are seen after 1 month. However, it is possible that any complication can be seen at an early date.

CAUSES OF EROSION

1. An indolent infection.
2. The pacemaker pocket formed at the time of surgery is too small for the implanted pulse generator.
3. The pulse generator is implanted too superficially, especially in children and small-framed adults

   in whom lack of adipose tissue results in the pacemaker being "tight" despite adequate pocket size.
4. The generator is implanted too far laterally in the anterior axillary fold.

Erosion

Although erosion of the pulse generator through the skin usually occurs long after implantation, it is most often related to the implantation technique (Figure 8). Erosion is a rare complication that may occur in four situations.

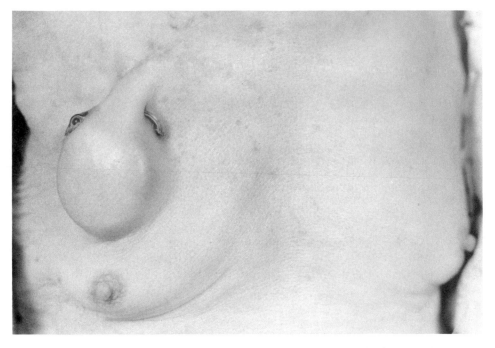

Figure 8. *Extrusion of an implanted pacemaker placed excessively lateral. The pacemaker is very adherent to the skin and the pocket is tight. Portions of the lead and pacemaker are exposed.*

Although there are several causes of erosion, infection is the most common. When pacemaker erosion occurs, the only choice is surgical revision of the pacemaker site. If associated with infection, the entire system (pulse generator and lead) must be removed and a completely new pacing system implanted at a clean site. In rare situations it may be possible to revise the pacer site, enlarge the "pocket," and fashion a satisfactory skin flap. Revision can only be undertaken in the absence of infection. It should be noted that infection may be present even in the absence of purulent material and therefore cultures should be obtained and proven negative prior to pocket revision.

Skin Adherence

Adherence of the pulse generator to the skin strongly suggests the presence of an infection, and salvage of the site may not be possible. Impending erosion (skin thinned to the point of transparency) should be dealt with as an emergency. Once the skin is broken, infection is virtually certain; while it is still closed, the pacemaker is protected. If revision is accomplished before the pacemaker has fully eroded and become contaminated, the original pacemaker can be reimplanted if infection is not present. In this setting, the original site can be successfully revised and reused. Cultures should be obtained in all such circumstances.

Thrombosis

Thromboembolic complications after permanent pacemaker implantation are rare. If thrombosis involves the superior vena cava, axillary vein, or area around the pacemaker lead in the right atrium or right ventricle, several problems can develop.

1. Occlusion of the superior vena cava and superior vena cava syndrome.
2. Thrombosis of the superior vena cava, right atrium, or right ventricle with hemodynamic compromise or pulmonary embolism.
3. Symptomatic thrombosis of the subclavian vein with an edematous painful upper extremity.

Partial or silent inconsequential thrombosis is common and usually is clinically insignificant (Figure 9). Such partial or silent thrombosis may be of significance at the time of pacing system revision. Thrombosis limits venous access, and it may be necessary to alleviate an obstruction either for symptomatic relief or to improve venous access enough to allow placement of a new pacing lead. Venous obstruction as a result of a chronic pacing lead can be relieved with balloon venoplasty (Figures 10 A and B).

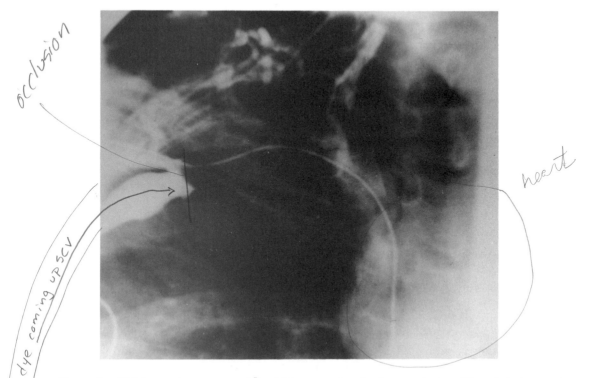

Figure 9. Still frame of a venogram of the right upper extremity shows occlusion of the subclavian vein. The patient had clinical venous insufficiency.

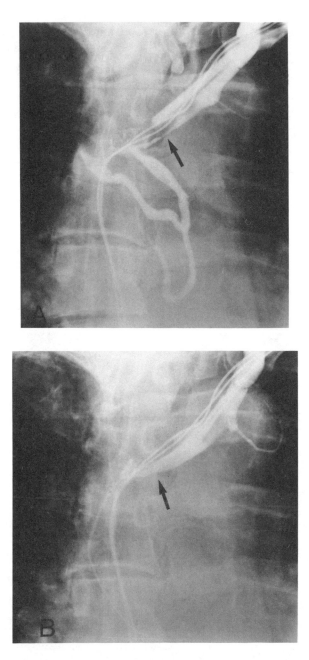

Figure 10. **A.** *Initial venogram, revealing high-grade stenosis of left innominate vein and large bridging collateral venous channels around area of stenosis (arrow).* **B.** *Postvenoplasty venogram, demonstrating large opening in area of previously noted stenosis (arrow). Dilation was sufficient to allow passage of pacemaker lead. (From Spittell PC, Vlietstra RE, Hayes DL, et al: Venous obstruction due to permanent transvenous pacemaker electrodes: Treatment with percutaneous transluminal balloon venoplasty. PACE 13:271–274, 1990, with permission.)*

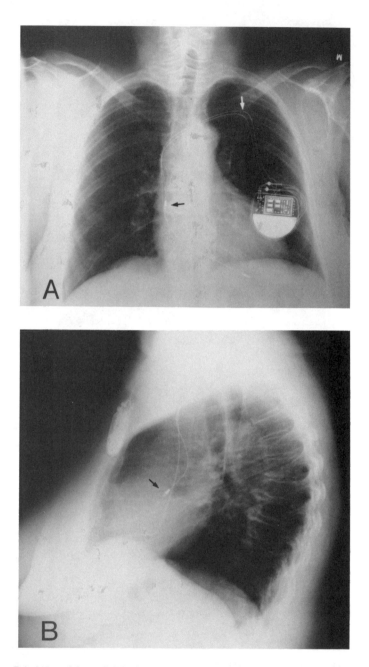

Figure 11. PA **(A)** and lateral **(B)** chest x-ray of a patient with a dual-chamber pacing system. The white arrow points to a fracture of the atrial lead. The fracture has occurred at the clavicular edge. The fracture is noted by the white arrow on the PA chest x-ray and close-up **(C)**. (Incidentally noted is unacceptably shallow atrial lead placement, black arrow that is better appreciated on the lateral view.)

Lead Fracture and Insulation Defect

Lead malfunction due to fracture or insulation defect is most commonly seen in the late post implant period. Lead fracture, common in the early years of cardiac pacing, has become less common as conductor technology has evolved (Figure 11). Additional examples of fracture may be found in Chapter 10, "Pacemaker Radiography." Lead fractures most often occur adjacent to the pulse generator or near the site of venous access, i.e., at a stress point. However, fracture has also been reported of more distal portions of the pacing lead. Although uncommon, direct trauma may result in damage to the pacing lead. When lead fracture does occur, it usually is necessary to replace the lead. A fracture of a unipolar lead near the connector can sometimes be managed by replacing the connector with the expectation of long-term stability. If a fracture of a bipolar lead occurs and the pacemaker is polarity programmable, it may be possible to restore pacing by reprogramming to the unipolar configuration. This is a short-term solution and should not be a substitute for replacing the lead.

Polyurethane and silicone are used as insulating materials for most permanent pacing leads. In the early 1980s, concern arose about the long-term performance of the polyurethane lead because of the early failure of several specific polyurethane leads. In these specific leads, difficulties in manufacturing were identified that appear to have been limited to those leads and were not indicative of overall polyurethane experience. However, because some concern remains about long-term performance of polyurethane leads, newer silicone-insulated leads have emerged. Newer technology has allowed a smaller diameter for silicone leads, so that handling differs little between the newer silicone leads and polyurethane leads, which were traditionally of smaller diameter.

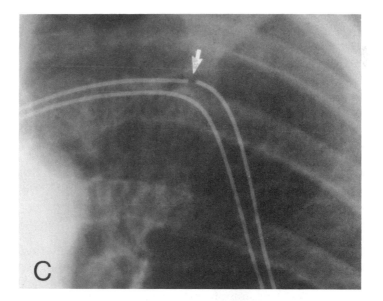

Figure 11C. Close-up view.

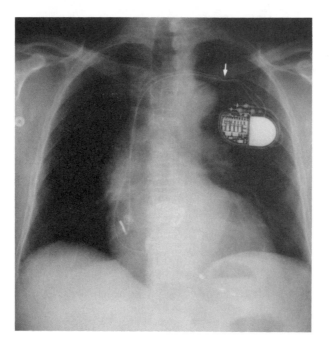

Figure 12. *Posteroanterior chest x-ray of a patient with a dual-chamber pacing system. The arrow points to a "crimp" in the pacing lead. The leads are being crimped between the clavicle and first rib. This patient subsequently developed an insulation failure of the ventricular lead. (The ventricular pacing lead is tripolar. The third pole is for impedance measurements as part of a rate adaptive pacing system.)*

Insulation defects of polyurethane leads have also been described at stress points, crush injury, specifically at the costoclavicular space when placed via the subclavian puncture technique (Figure 12), and at the site of ligatures, even when a suture sleeve is used. In bipolar coaxial leads, the insulation defect often occurs internally, i.e., the layer of insulation between coils, as opposed to an external, outer surface, insulation defect. (See Chapter 2, "Basic Concepts.")

Exit Block

Exit block has been defined in several ways. The most commonly accepted clinical definition is high pacing thresholds, often progressive, that cannot be explained on the basis of radiographic dislodgment or perforation. (If normal thresholds are achieved and maintained after repositioning the lead then the term "exit block" does not apply.) In true exit block, stimulation thresholds are often excellent at the time of implant, but instead of displaying the usual acute rise at 3 to 6 weeks with a subsequent decrease and plateau, the threshold remains high. Exit block is uncommon and appears to represent an abnormality at the myocardial tissue/electrode interface. The cause is controversial. It is felt by some to be a problem with the lead design and others believe it to be an intrinsic problem of the patient's myocardium that results in excessive reaction to the electrode. Higher pulse generator output, i.e., 10 V, may be satisfactory for the patient while other patients may exceed the high output capacity of the pacemaker. Steroid-eluting leads are often effective in preventing exit block.

Battery Depletion

Battery depletion is an expected occurrence as the power supply of a pulse generator is consumable and should not be considered a complication in most patients. If the pulse generator displays end-of-life characteristics at a point in time much earlier than expected, other potential problems should be explored. Early battery depletion may be due to inappropriate programming to unnecessarily high output or excess current drain caused by a loss of lead integrity. The manufacturer should also be consulted for data regarding the pulse generator performance, that is, predicted versus observed pulse generator longevity in other patients.

When battery depletion is very advanced it may not be possible to program the pacemaker. At other times attempting to program a pacemaker at an advanced stage of battery depletion may result in sudden complete loss of output (Figure 13).

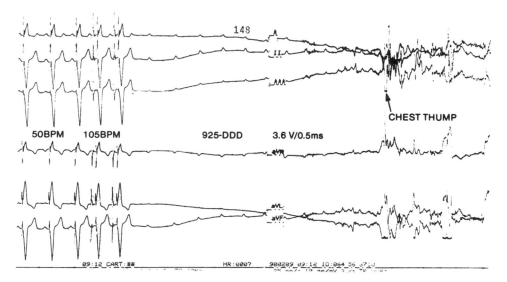

Figure 13. *Electrocardiogram taken during programming of a DDD pacemaker that had reached end-of-life (EOL) indicators. When programmed to a faster rate there was suddenly no output. Ventricular asystole occurs until a chest thump is delivered and a native rhythm occurs.*

EARLY OR LATE COMPLICATIONS

Lead Dislodgement

Active and passive fixation mechanisms common to current pacing leads have significantly reduced the incidence of lead dislodgment. Secondary intervention rates for dislodgment should be well below 2% for ventricular leads and below 5% for atrial leads. Dislodgement has been classified by some as "macrodislodgment" and "microdislodgment." Macrodislodgment is radiographically evident and microdislodgment is not. Adequate lead position is assessed by posteroanterior and lateral chest x-rays (Figures 14–16). It must be remembered that lead placement by chest x-ray may appear excellent in the patient with a "microdislodgment." (Also see Chapter 10, "Pacemaker Radiography.") There are other more unusual types of dislodgment (Figure 17). Although rare, ventricular lead dislodgment by atrial contraction has been reported. Other causes include lead migration. For this to occur the lead must be detached from the pulse generator, either intentionally when a lead is abandoned and allowed to migrate into an intravascular position or, rarely, when the lead is not adequately secured in the pacemaker connector block.

Loose Connector Block Connection

Intermittent or complete failure of output can occur due to a loose connection at the pacing lead/connector block interface. This usually occurs because the lead has been inadequately secured at the time of pacemaker implant. It may also occur because of a poor fit between the lead and pacemaker even though they are allegedly compatible. Specifically, a side-lock connector has been demonstrated to be insecure in connecting with one model of VS-1 connector. When there is a loose connection, manipulating the pacemaker may reproduce the problem. The poor connection may be evident radiographically (Figure 18).

Pacemaker Related Arrhythmias

Supraventricular and ventricular arrhythmias are often encountered during pacemaker implantation. They are discussed in Chapter 8, "Permanent Pacemaker Implantation."

In the early postoperative period, "tip extrasystoles" may be seen. These are ventricular complexes of similar morphology of the paced beats because they originate at the same site as the paced beats. They are not preceded by a pacemaker stimulus. Tip extrasystoles most often occur during the first 24 to 48 hours after implantation and usually resolve spontaneously. It is rarely necessary to pharmacologically suppress tip extrasystoles.

The "runaway pacemaker," a sudden increase in pacing rate caused by circuit malfunction, is rare with present-day pulse generators, but was more common with earlier pulse generators. Should runaway occur, the pulse gen-

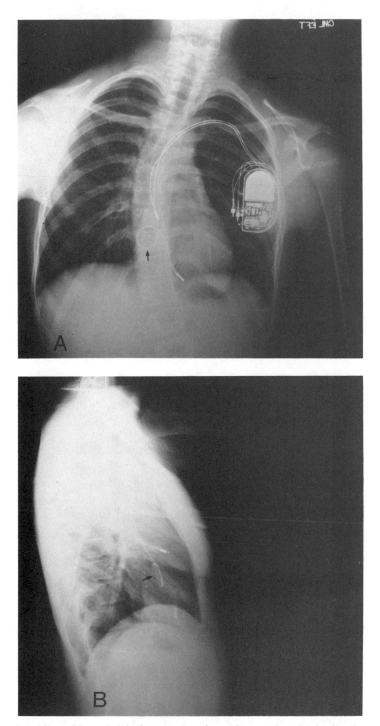

Figure 14. PA **(A)** and lateral **(B)** chest x-rays of a patient with a single-chamber ventricular pacing system. The ventricular lead has dislodged and there is a large loop in the ventricular lead (arrow).

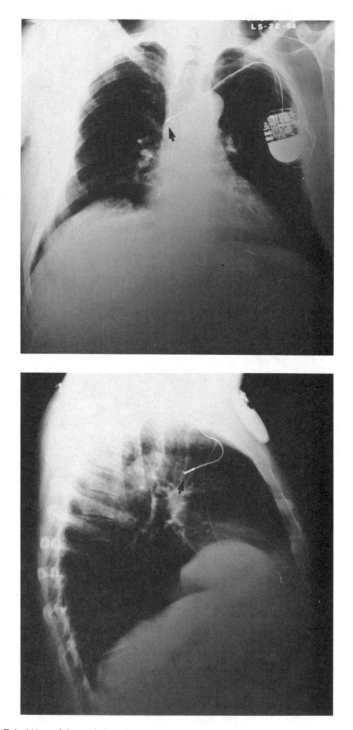

Figure 15.   PA **(A)** and lateral **(B)** chest x-ray of a patient with a dual-chamber pacing system. The atrial lead has been displaced into the superior vena cava. The arrow notes the tip of the atrial lead.

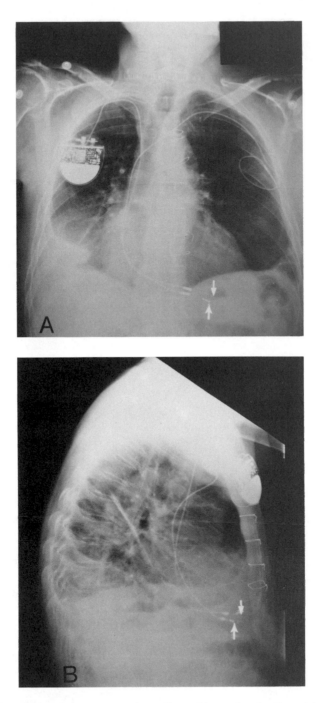

Figure 16. *PA and lateral chest x-rays of a patient with an abandoned ventricular pacing lead that had been placed via the left subclavian vein. The newly placed lead was placed via the right subclavian vein. The PA (A) and lateral (B) chest x-ray obtained shortly after placement of the new ventricular lead demonstrates the relationship of the ventricular lead tips. The patient subsequently developed intermittent failure to pace and sense.*

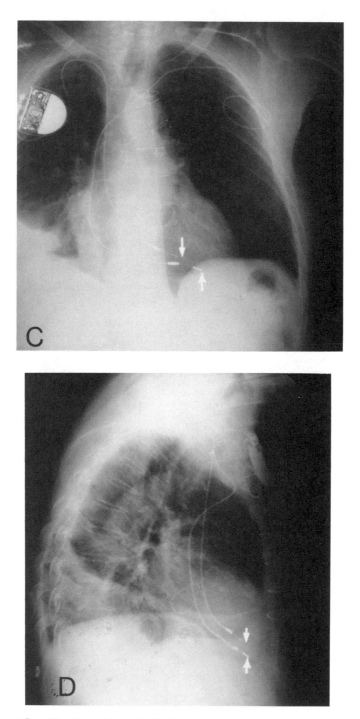

Figure 16 (contd).   *PA* **(C)** *and lateral* **(D)** *chest x-ray obtained after the pacing abnormalities occurred that demonstrates dislodgment of the newly placed ventricular lead. The dislodgment is easy to appreciate when compared to the stable position of the abandoned ventricular lead.*

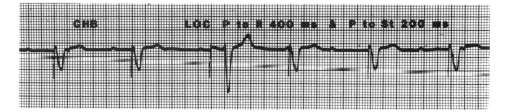

Figure 17. *Electrocardiogram from a patient with complete heart block (CHB) and a ventricular (VV) pacemaker. When the intrinsic P wave occurs within 200 ms of the ventricular pacing artifact there is failure to capture. At other times ventricular capture is normal. Atrial contraction results in enough ventricular lead movement in this patient to result in transient lack of contact with the endocardial surface and failure to capture.*

erator must be disconnected. In an emergency, the lead may be cut and the transected lead used with an external pulse generator. In other situations, prompt removal of the pulse generator is required and, if possible, should be accomplished under sterile conditions (Figure 19). If the "runaway" spontaneously stops, the pulse generator should still be removed because the circuitry is unreliable, and it is likely that runaway will recur. "Runaway pacemaker" can occur as a complication of therapeutic radiation (see above).

Although permanent pacing is used to suppress ventricular rhythm disturbances, it may also induce ventricular ectopy. Figure 20 demonstrates a paced patient in whom ectopy persisted until the pacemaker was programmed to a rate low enough that the patient's intrinsic rate dominated. Asynchronous pacing may also result in rhythm disturbances if the cardiac chamber is paced during a "vulnerable" period. Figure 21 shows a ventricular rhythm disturbance due to VOO pacing. Atrial rhythm disturbances can be a result of asynchronous atrial pacing.

Endless loop tachycardia is another well-recognized pacemaker related rhythm disturbance, which is discussed in Chapter 9, "Pacemaker Electrocardiography" and Chapter 4, "Comprehension of Pacemaker Timing Cycles."

Twiddler's Syndrome

Purposeful or absentminded "twiddling" or manipulation of the pulse generator by the patient has been named "twiddler's syndrome." Manipulation may cause axial rotation of the pacemaker, twisting of the lead, and eventual fracture or dislodgment of the lead. The pulse generator usually is not damaged. The syndrome commonly occurs when the pacemaker sits loosely in the pacemaker pocket (Figure 22) either because the pocket was too large or because the pacemaker migrated.

If the problem has occurred because of pacemaker migration or a poorly fashioned pacemaker pocket, the pocket should be revised. This problem may be prevented by placing the pacemaker in a Parsonnet pouch, which is a snugly fitting Dacron pouch that reduces migration and torsion of the pacing system

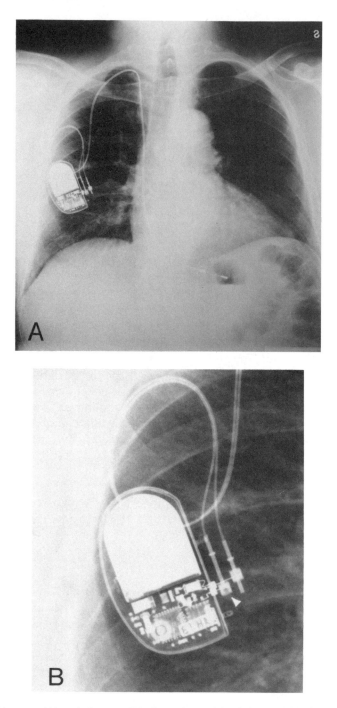

Figure 18.   *PA x-ray (A) and close-up (B) of a patient with a bifurcated bipolar ventricular lead and pacemaker. The patient presented with intermittent failure to output. Close inspection reveals that the inferior pin is not securely in the connector block. At the position of the white arrowhead the connector pin should be seen protruding through as it does in the upper pin.*

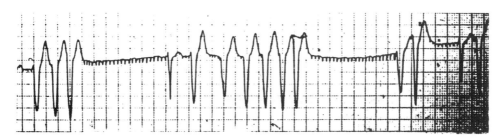

Figure 19.   An electrocardiogram of a runaway bipolar pacemaker. A pacemaker stimulus and the depolarization are followed by erratic pacing, which if sufficiently rapid and sustained may lead to ventricular fibrillation. During the pauses, close inspection of the electrocardiogram reveals pacemaker artifacts occurring at a very rapid rate.

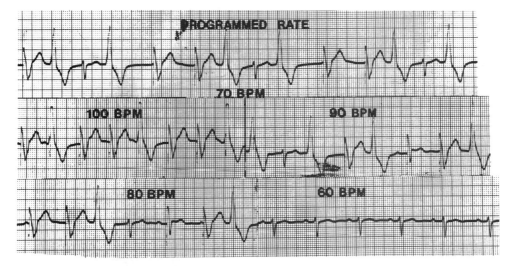

Figure 20.   Electrocardiogram from a patient with a ventricular pacing system in whom ventricular stimulation results in ventricular ectopy. Five different programmed rates are shown. In the uppermost panel at the programmed rate of 70 bpm there are frequent ventricular premature contractions (VPCs). These persist at all rates except 60 bpm, which is slow enough to allow the patient's intrinsic rhythm to predominate.

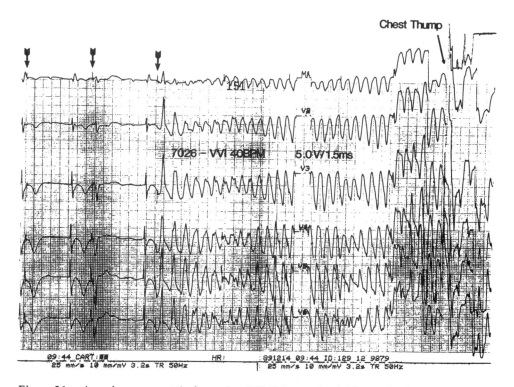

Figure 21.   *Asynchronous ventricular pacing (VOO) in a patient with complete heart block results in ventricular tachycardia. The black arrows note the first three pacing artifacts. The third stimulus occurs at a point when the ventricular myocardium is vulnerable and ventricular tachycardia is initiated.*

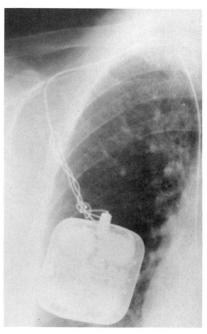

Figure 22.   *Twiddler's syndrome. The pacemaker was placed in a too large pocket and the patient was able to manipulate it. Manipulation caused lead twisting, which can cause fracture.*

by promoting tissue ingrowth and stabilization of the pacemaker, fixation of the pulse generator by an anchoring suture, and/or anchoring the lead to the pre-pectoral fascia by a sleeve.

Extracardiac Stimulation

Extracardiac stimulation usually involves the diaphragm or pectoral muscle. Diaphragmatic stimulation may be due to direct stimulation of the diaphragm (usually stimulation of the left hemidiaphragm) or stimulation of the phrenic nerve (usually stimulation of the right hemidiaphragm). The potential for diaphragmatic stimulation should be tested at the time of implantation. If any stimulation is noted with 10 V stimulation, the pacing lead should be repositioned. Because this testing is usually accomplished with the patient in a supine position, it does not eliminate the possibility of diaphragmatic stimulation when the patient is upright. Diaphragmatic stimulation occurring during the early post-implant period may be due to either micro- or macrodislodgment of the pacing lead. (Although perforation of the myocardium by the pacing lead may result in diaphragmatic pacing, perforation occurs uncommonly.) It may be diminished or alleviated by decreasing the voltage output and/or pulse width. (An adequate pacing margin of safety must be maintained after decreasing the output parameters.) Local muscle stimulation occurs much more commonly with unipolar than bipolar pacemakers and is usually noted in the early post-implant period.

Pectoral muscle stimulation may also be due to an insulation defect of the pacing lead, current leakage from the connector or sealing plugs, erosion of the pacemaker's protective coating, or from rapid high-amplitude atrial output in a unipolar dual- chamber pacemaker. If the problem is due to an insulation defect on either a unipolar pacemaker or the pacemaker lead, the stimulation may be minimized by decreasing the voltage output and/or pulse width, but it may be necessary to replace the defective portion of the system. (If an activity-sensing rate adaptive pacemaker is in place, muscle stimulation may result in sensor activation and inappropriately rapid pacing rates for a given level of activity.) Pectoral muscle stimulation is less common with bipolar than unipolar pacemakers. If pectoral muscle stimulation occurs in a polarity-programmable pacemaker that is programmed, unipolar reprogramming to the bipolar configuration may alleviate the problem.

When pectoral muscle stimulation occurs in the late post-implant period in a patient with a unipolar pacing system, erosion of the pacemaker's protective coating should be suspected (Figure 23). Unipolar pulse generators are insulated on one side, generally that opposite to the side engraved with the pulse generator identification. The insulated side should be placed toward muscle and the noninsulated side toward subcutaneous tissue. The integrity of the insulation material can be damaged during handling or, it seems, deteriorate with time. Should that occur, two circumstances may follow. The first is that electromyographic interference (EMI) may occur and inappropriately inhibit the pulse generator. Alternatively, a small area of defect may shunt a relatively high current density to the muscle causing a local twitch with each stimulus. This is especially true in the case of the atrial stimulus in a pulse generator with a

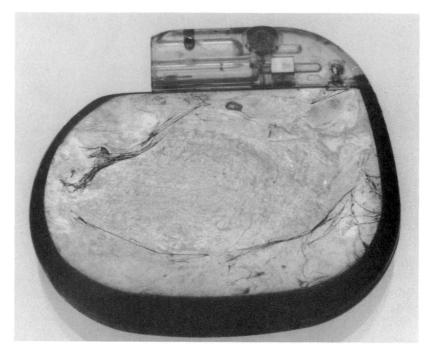

Figure 23. *Deterioration of the insulating cover of a unipolar pacing device. The patient developed pectoral muscle stimulation when the insulating material was no longer intact.*

superfast recharge circuit. If this has occurred, it may not be possible to program an atrial channel output sufficiently low to avoid local muscle stimulation. This may be particularly problematic in a patient with chronotropic incompetence who requires continued atrial stimulation. In this unusual situation, muscle stimulation will likely be present to some degree at even the lowest programmable pulse width and/or voltage.

If this problem occurs with a DDD pacemaker and the pacemaker can be programmed to the VDD mode in which there is no atrial stimulation but the patient can maintain AV synchrony via P-synchronous pacing, muscle stimulation may be avoided. If there is no possibility of ending atrial channel stimulation, operative intervention will be required. Once the insulation defect is found, an accessory silicone rubber boot may be placed on the generator. Alternatively, the pulse generator may be replaced. This condition is unusual but has been seen by the authors on several occasions.

Pacemaker Infection

The incidence of infection after pacemaker implantation should certainly be less than 2% and in most series has been less than 1%. Careful attention to surgical details and sterile procedures are of paramount importance in avoiding pacemaker site infection. The prophylactic use of antibiotics before implantation and in the immediate post-operative period remains controversial. Most studies do not show any significant difference in the rate of infection between patients who have had prophylactic administration of antibiotics and those who have not. Irrigation of the pacemaker pocket with an antibiotic solution at the time of pacemaker implantation may help to prevent infection.

Pacemaker infection must be recognized and be treated properly. It may appear as:

1. Local inflammation and abscess formation in the area of the pulse generator pocket.
2. Erosion of part of the pacing system through the skin with secondary infection.
3. Fever associated with positive blood cultures with or without a focus of infection elsewhere.

The most common clinical presentation is infection around the generator; septicemia is an uncommon mode of presentation. Early infections usually are caused by Staphylococcus aureus, are aggressive, and are often associated with fever and systemic symptoms. Late infections commonly are caused by *Staphylococcus epidermidis* and are more indolent—usually without fever or systemic manifestation. Treatment for both organisms requires removal of the entire infected pacing system, pulse generator, and leads. Other organisms may be involved in either early or late infections (Table II).

There is some controversy about how to proceed once the infected system has been removed. A one-stage surgical approach involves implantation of a new pacing system at a distant clean site after explantation of the infected pacing system. Others favor removal of the infected system, temporary pacing, if required, and antibiotic management in the interim, and implantation of a new system at a later date. (See Lead Removal-Chapter 19, "Troubleshooting").

Table II
Organisms Documented in Pacing System Infections

Frequently Identified	
Staphylococcus epidermidis	*S. aureus*

Less Frequently Identified	
Klebsiella pneumoniae	*Peptostreptococcus*
Enterobacter cloacae	*Micrococcus*
Pseudomonas aeruginosa	*a-Hemolytic streptococcus*
Escherichia coli	*b-Hemolytic streptococcus*
Proteus mirabilis	*Flavobacterium*
Alcaligenes faecalis	*Propionibacterium*
Serratia marcescens	

Isolated Reports	
Candida albicans	*Hemophilus parainfluenzae*
Petriellidium boydii	*Actinobacillus actinomycetemcomitans*
Mycobacterium avium	*Aspergillus flavus*

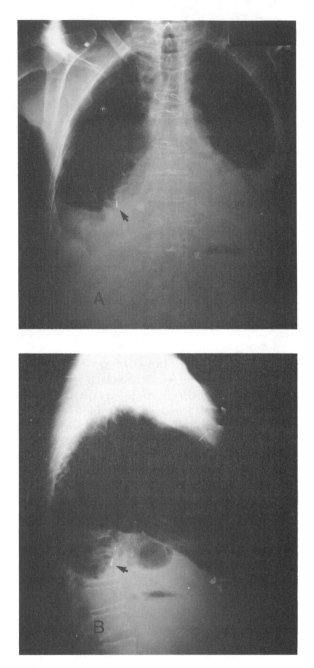

Figure 24.   *PA and lateral chest x-rays of a patient with a retained lead fragment. This patient had undergone surgery for mitral valve replacement, and at the time of surgery the previously implanted endocardial pacing system was removed. A portion of the transvenous ventricular lead was only partially removed because it could not be removed from the right ventricular wall despite considerable traction to the point of inversion of the free wall of the right ventricle. The lead was transected and a portion of the lead left in place. On the postoperative chest x-ray this retained fragment is noted by the arrow.*

Retained Lead Fragments

Multiple leads can be left in place as long as none of the leads have been part of an infected system (see Chapter 10). If the pacing system is infected, it is essential that the entire lead be removed. Chronically implanted tined leads can be difficult, if not impossible, to remove. Several techniques have been described to remove chronically implanted leads. (See Chapter 19, "Troubleshooting.") It is possible that a portion of the lead, specifically, portions of the "tines" may be left in an endocardial position. Complications as a result of a noninfected portion of a pacing lead being left embedded in the endocardium following attempted extraction are unusual. A mobile, or nonembedded, portion of the lead could potentially embolize into the pulmonary circulation. Figure 24 demonstrates a chest x-ray where a portion of the pacing lead has been retained.

Pacemaker Syndrome

Pacemaker syndrome, which results from loss of atrioventricular synchrony and ventriculoatrial conduction, is described in Chapter 5, "Hemodynamics of Cardiac Pacing."

Pacemaker Allergy

Allergy to the pacemaker itself is a very rare but reported complication. Usually, the allergy is to the pulse generator can but the patient may be allergic to any exposed portion of the pacing system. The most common materials used in a pacing system that may be responsible for an allergy include titanium, epoxy, silicone rubber, and/or polyurethane. Proof of such an allergy requires sophisticated allergy testing, and correction of the problem may require changing to another type of system. Some of the cases of "allergy" are, in reality, low-grade *S. epidermidis* infections, which should be treated as infections rather than allergies. No diagnosis of allergy should be made until infection has been carefully and thoroughly ruled out.

BIBLIOGRAPHY

Alt E, Volker R, Blomer H: Lead fracture in pacemaker patients. Thorac Cardiovasc Surg 1987; 35:101–104.

Antonelli D, Turgeman Y, Kaveh Z, et al: Short-term thrombosis after transvenous permanent pacemaker insertion. PACE 1989; 12:280–282.

Baumgartner G, Nesser HJ, Jurkovic K: Unusual cause of dysuria: Migration of a pacemaker generator into the urinary bladder. PACE 1990; 13:703–704.

Byrd CL, Schwartz SJ, Gonzales M, et al: Pacemaker clinic evaluations: Key to early identification of surgical problems. PACE 1986; 9(6 Pt 2):1259–1264.

Chauvin M, Brechenmacher C: Muscle stimulation caused by a pacemaker current leakage: The role of the insulation failure of a polyurethane coating. J Electrophysiol 1987; 1:326–329.

Choo MH, Holmes DR Jr, Gersh BJ, et al: Permanent pacemaker infections: Characterization and management. Am J Cardiol 1981; 48:559–564.

Cooper D, Wilkoff B, Masterson M, et al: Effects of extracorporeal shock wave lithotripsy on cardiac pacemakers and its safety in patients with implanted cardiac pacemakers. PACE 1988; 11:1607–1616.

Dalvi BV, Rajani RM, Lokhandwala, et al: Unusual case of pacemaker lead migration. Cathet Cardiovasc Diagn 1990; 21:95–96.

Den Dulk K, Lindemans FW, Bar FW, et al: Pacemaker relatedtachycardias. PACE 1985; 5:476–485.

Fetter J, Patterson D, Aram G, et al: Effects of extracorporeal shock wave lithotripsy on single chamber rate response and dual chamber pacemakers. PACE 1989; 12:1494–1501.

Flaker GC, Mueller KJ, Salazar JR, et al: Total venous obstruction following atrioventricular sequential pacemaker implantation. PACE 1983; 6:815–817.

Fyke FE 3d: Simultaneous insulation deterioration associated with side-by-side subclavian placement of two polyurethane leads. PACE 1988; 11:1571–1574.

Furman S: Pacemaker emergencies. Med Clin North Am 1979; 63:113–126.

Furman S, Behrens M, Andrews C, et al: Retained pacemaker leads. J Thorac Cardiovasc Surg 1987; 94:770–772.

Gabry MD, Behrens M, Andrews C, et al: Comparison of myopotential interference in unipolar-bipolar programmable DDD pacemakers. PACE 1987; 10:1322–1330.

Giroud D, Goy JJ: Pacemaker malfunction due to subcutaneous emphysema. Int J Cardiol 1990; 26:234–236.

Goudevenos JA, Reid PG, Adams PC, et al: Pacemaker-induced superior vena cava syndrome: Report of four cases and review of the literature. PACE 1989; 12:1890–1895.

Grace AA, Sutters M, Schofield PM: Balloon dilatation of pacemaker induced stenosis of the superior vena cava. Br Heart J 1991; 65:225–226.

Higano ST, Hayes DL, Spittell PC: Facilitation of the subclavian-introducer technique with contrast venography. PACE 1990; 13:681–684.

Iliceto S, Di Biase M, Antonelli G, et al: Two-dimensional echocardiographic recognition of a pacing catheter perforation of the interventricular septum. PACE 1982; 5:934–936.

Lau CP, Cheung KL, Mok CK: Biventricular perforation by a temporary pacing electrode: Recognition from the lateral chest radiograph. Int J Cardiol 1989; 24:368–371.

Lee ME, Chaux A: Unusual complications of endocardial pacing. J Thorac Cardiovasc Surg 1980; 80:934–940.

Marketwitz A, Hemmer W, Weinhold C: Complications in dual chamber pacing: A six-year experience. PACE 1986; 9(6 part 2):1014–1018.

Mazzetti H, Dussaut A, Tentori C, et al: Transarterial permanent pacing of the left ventricle. PACE 1990; 13:588–592.

Mickley H, Andersen C, Nielsen LH: Runaway pacemaker: A still existing complication and therapeutic guidelines. Clin Cardiol 1989; 12:412–414.

Mugge A, Gulba DC, Jost S, et al: Dissolution of a right atrial thrombus attached to pacemaker electrodes: Usefulness of recombinant tissue-type plasminogen activator. Am Heart J 1990; 119:1437–1439.

Nanda NC, Barold SS: Usefulness of echocardiography in cardiac pacing. PACE 1982; 5: 222–237.

Parry G, Goudevenos J, Jameson S, et al: Complications asssociated with retained pacemaker leads. PACE 1991; 14:1251–1257.

Parsonnet V, Bernstein AD, Lindsay B: Pacemaker-implantation complication rates: An analysis of some contributing factors. J Am Coll Cardiol 1989; 13:917–921.

Peters MS, Schroeter AL, van Hale HM, et al: Pacemaker contact sensitivity. Contact Dermatitis 1984; 11:214–218.

Spittell PC, Hayes DL: Venous complications after insertion of a trasvenous pacemaker. Mayo Clin Proc 1992; 67:258–265.

Spittell PC, Vlietstra RE, Hayes DL, et al: Venous obstruction due to permanent trans-venous pacemaker electrodes: Treatment with percutaneous transluminal balloon venoplasty. PACE 1990; 13:271–274.

Stroobandt R, Willems R, Depuydt P, et al: The superfast atrial recharge pulse: A cause of pectoral muscle stimulation in patients equipped with a unipolar DDD pacemaker. PACE 1989; 12:451–455.

Winner SJ, Boon NA: Transvenous pacemaker electrodes placed unintentionally in the left ventricle: Three cases. Post Grad Med J 1989; 65:98–102.

PART III.

PRACTICAL MANAGEMENT

Chapter 15

PACEMAKER FOLLOW-UP

Seymour Furman

The function of implanted pacemaker systems is variable. Lead or generator failure and intercurrent medical events affect the interaction of pacemaker system and patient. Pacemaker systems with long-lived power sources and hermetically sealed complementary metal oxide semiconductor (CMOS) circuitry provide stability and longevity, but the interaction between the pacemaker and the patient has become correspondingly more complex. Patient welfare requires continued observation to reduce the incidence of sudden and unpredicted pacemaker system failure, detect substandard performance of some models, and produce maximum longevity of those units capable of prolonged operation. It should be remembered that for the patient's safety all failures to pace are equivalent, whether caused by lead or electronic failure or power source depletion. Approximately 80% of lithium pulse generators remain capable of function 8 years after implantation. However, newer generators, especially those that are sensor driven and dual chamber, have briefer anticipated longevities so that the expectations of recent times may not be achieved. As half of patients with implanted pacemakers survive about 7 years, many patients do not have a second intervention. Nevertheless, lead fractures and displacements, infections, and sudden "no output" electronic failure remain important considerations. They can be avoided in a variety of ways. A substantial portion of pulse generator and lead failures result from a systematic hardware defect. Since these usually are eventually known to the industry, the physician responsible for a patient's follow-up will be notified in order to evaluate the individual patient risk for pacemaker system malfunction.

PACEMAKER FOLLOW-UP SYSTEMS

All pacemaker follow-up systems should have the capability to perform the following functions:

The pacemaker clinic analyzes the patient's pacemaker electrocardiogram, stimulus waveform, the range of programmability, sensing and pacing thresholds, the stability of patient-pacemaker interaction, and physiological response to yield maximum rhythmic stability without pacemaker syndrome. The wound is evaluated for comfort and freedom from infection.

Programming is important for single-chamber pacemakers. It is even more important for dual-chamber pacemakers where decisions concerning atrial pacing and sensing and ventricular pacing and sensing have significant impact on device longevity, whether the various chambers will be paced or sensed appropriately, and whether maximum hemodynamic and rhythmic benefit will occur.

PACEMAKER FOLLOW-UP SYSTEMS

All pacemaker follow-up systems should:

1. Predict impending pacemaker system failure before the patient is at risk;
2. Ascertain the nature of the malfunction when failure is about to occur or has occurred;
3. Record patient location should a pattern of systematic pulse generator or lead failure develop or recall occur;
4. Develop statistical data specific for one clinic or that is part of a much larger database;
5. National standards in the United States (and elsewhere) are now in the process of evolving to follow all patients with implantable pacemakers so that their location is known should notification concerning defective or suspect hardware be required.

ORGANIZATION OF A PACEMAKER CLINIC

PACEMAKER CLINIC ORGANIZATION

1. Patients should be seen on a consistent schedule, not solely when symptoms return. The early schedule should be based on electrode(s) stability so that patients are seen soon after implant of a new electrode and pulse generator. They need not be seen soon after pulse generator replacement.
2. Pacemaker records should be kept separate from the hospital record system, be immediately retrievable, and contain:
   a. patient data, i.e., name, age, identification number, address, and phone number;
   b. pacemaker data, i.e., model and serial number and updated records of rate, electrocardiogram, and other indicators of function.
3. Patients should be subjected to:
   a. x-ray annually or as necessary to note electrode and pacemaker position in a growing child;
   b. 12-lead ECG at each visit—both pacing and with the pacemaker inhibited;
   c. a rhythm strip in the free-running and magnet modes in a lead in which pacer artifacts and P and QRS complexes are readily discernible;
   d. recording of the pulse generator stimulus in the free-running and magnet modes and representative programmed functions;
   e. programming of programmable and dual-chamber pacemakers to a variety of functions with recording of representative waveforms, rates, and other significant programmable factors;
   f. evaluation of the stimulation and sensing thresholds of atrium and ventricle;
   g. measurement and recording of the pacemaker rate in the free-running and magnet modes;
   h. evaluation of the implant wound site;
   i. Evaluation of sensor function.

It is probably not wise to provide general medical or cardiologic follow-up in the pacer clinic.

DEMOGRAPHIC PATIENT DATA

A major part of follow-up is having records available of patient location and all pacemaker related data. Patients should be easily identifiable and their location known. A patient registry with this information will probably be developed independently of a physician's records in the near future. Knowledge of each patient's location is a herculean task and is very likely beyond the reasonable ability of any physician or clinic. Patients who have a pacemaker implanted sometimes improve, within a few minutes, from life-threatening illness to being asymptomatic. Symptoms can return equally rapidly if the pacer system fails. After pacemaker implantation, such patients may forget that they are well managed but not cured. As the device has a finite longevity that depends on how frequently it stimulates the heart, how it is programmed, and whether it is single- or dual-chamber, no specific number can be placed on the longevity of any single device. Leads also have a finite longevity although it is far less certain how long that is. Random fractures continually occur, but at an apparently accelerating rate after about 10 years of implant. Still, technology has improved to the point that lead systems introduced over the past 15 years (excluding those few that are intrinsically defective) are extremely durable with a very low failure rate, even after many years (see Chapter 2).

Patients with implanted pacemakers, whether pacer-dependent or not, require follow-up. In preparation for a possible recall, it may be wise to determine which patients are to be considered "pacer-dependent" and require early intervention should system unreliability occur.

Recall, generated by manufacturer, government regulators, or the physician responsible for follow-up, may be required. Physician generated recall, i.e., elective pulse generator removal because of a physician perceived problem, is more difficult than ever before. Warrantee replacement is based on manufacturer acceptance of the recall condition. Until that is acknowledged, physician generated recall may be difficult and expensive. It will be important to locate patients and to have additional information, such as the degree of pacer dependency and the consequent potential for injury, should the pacemaker system be subject to sudden "no-output" failure. Computerized databases are useful for this purpose. Most manufacturers maintain computer records of patients with pacemakers of their manufacture (see national registry, above). It is important that the physician cooperate by providing pacemaker registration at implant, reporting pulse generator removal, and reporting a patient's death. These computerized reports can be very useful at the time of recall, should one occur. Data provided to the manufacturer is also available to other physicians in the event of an emergency. Patients carry little information beyond a registration card, and often, even that is not available. It has been our observation that patients who have received several pacemaker identification cards over the years will keep them all. Sometimes a patient will keep an earlier card and discard the current card.

As the manufacturer of most pacemakers can be identified on x-ray (Figure 1), manufacturers' records can be the best source of information about a patient who has developed an emergency away from his customary medical attention. Even better than a manufacturer generated list (which is commonly incomplete or erroneous or both) is one generated and maintained by the individual physician. One issue may be the patient who moves to another physician's care. She/he may not be in any manufacturer's record provided to the "new" following physician. Adequate documentation may be beyond the capability of any physician (especially given the low level of present-day reimbursement) and has not yet been given over to an industry-government registry.

The twin bases of any pacemaker clinic are follow-up and the quality of record keeping. Follow-up should be organized, not haphazard. A schedule should be established with patient and clinic staff so that there is little uncertainty concerning the constancy and schedule of follow-up. Records of each visit should be available for comparison with earlier visits. Rate changes and alterations in other functions, such as shape or amplitude of the oscilloscopic artifact, assume importance largely in comparison with previous data. The oscilloscopic photograph of an implanted polyurethane lead that shows a modest change

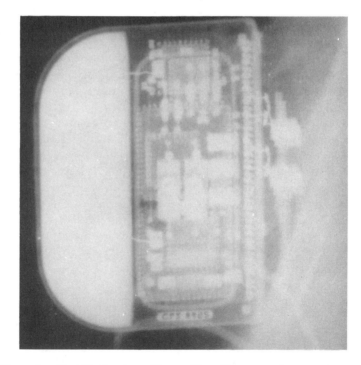

Figure 1. *Pacemaker identification is readily possible with newer pulse generators—most contain written identification of the pulse generator model and manufacturer on a radiopaque label. In this unit the manufacturer and model are readily visible.*

may herald deterioration of the polyurethane. Such a change may occur before clinical manifestation and may be detectable only in comparison with an earlier, presumably "normal" finding. This is especially important as at least one implanted lead is in Class I or "danger to life and/or health" status.

Those generators that allow telemetry of lead impedance may be especially useful if a sudden increase in impedance exists since this indicates that a lead fracture may have occurred. Alternatively, a decrease in lead impedance may herald insulation deterioration (see Chapter 16, Telemetry). Still, it is not known what degree of change may (or may not) be associated with beginning fracture or insulation deterioration before any clinical or electrocardiographic manifestations exist. Relatively few impedance telemetry pulse generators were in use during the major era of lead deterioration and inadequate information exists whether those that were available were valuable in detecting impending failure before clinical manifestation.

PULSE GENERATOR END OF LIFE

A pulse generator has reached its end of life when the power source has been depleted to the point at which it cannot drive the circuit reliably or if failure is impending. Electronic circuit-caused end of life occurs when the pulse generator is no longer operating within its design specifications and has become unreliable, erratic, or unsafe but the cause is not battery failure or depletion. End of life is not necessarily associated with clinical manifestations. Indeed it is better to determine that end of life has been reached before clinical manifestations occur. The magnet pacemaker rate may be at battery depletion level while otherwise normal function exists. Nevertheless, the unit will be at end of life.

Determination of end of life may be difficult. A pulse generator that has begun to show change, for example, a shift in some, or all, programmed rates, but in which overall operation seems stable may still have years of satisfactory operation. Consultation with the manufacturer may be desirable, but it is the physician's responsibility to decide whether a pulse generator or any other device should be left in place. If a device is operating out of specification (accurate documentation is mandatory), its removal is the physician's option and decision.

Barring intercurrent events, all pulse generators will go to battery depletion end of life if they remain in service for a sufficient (but highly variable) period. Many lithium silver chromate powered pulse generators went to battery depletion in 4 to 5 years while some of the earliest lithium iodine cell models remain functioning 10 to 15 years after implant with no clearly defined model longevity expectation. The lithium thionyl chloride cells with a high voltage and large energy capacity went from apparently normal function to depletion within days or weeks, too short a period to follow realistically. For them, end of life was a statistically determined period. The time when the first of these units failed was the time to remove them all, electively. Some lithium cupric sulfide cell single-chamber models (only used by the Cordis corporation) behaved in a similar manner, though less precipitously. Originally designed to indicate battery depletion by a 10% decline in rate, sudden failures appeared after a 3% rate change had occurred. Consequently a 3% decline in the magnet rate became the indication of battery depletion. Few of these units remain in service.

Rate change has been the primary indication of battery depletion since manufacture of the first pacemakers. At present, all pulse generators decrease rate with battery depletion, but different pulse generators may have different criteria. Early lithium iodine generators relied on the increasing battery impedance to slow the rate of the circuit, and 6%–7% rate decrease was an indication of depletion with both the magnet and free-running rates in parallel. With a gradual shift to digital circuits, increasing battery impedance with depletion was not allowed to produce a gradual rate change in the free-running mode. Two different approaches were widely, but not universally, adopted. In one, the free-running rate is stable almost to impending battery exhaustion, and the magnetic rate (usually 90 or 100 bpm) is different from the usual programmed rate (see Chapter 2). Battery depletion indicators (up until the end of battery life) appear in the magnet rate only. Changes in free-running rate appear only late after end of life (EOL). In one series, a gradual rate decline occurs in the magnet mode with rate stability in the free-running mode. Battery depletion is indicated at 7% for some models and 16% for others. Another approach is stability of the programmed free-running rate with a step function rate decline in the magnet rate with 15% decline indicating battery depletion. Other rates in other models are used to indicate end of life. The characteristics of the pacer used must be known. It is recommended that the physician's manual be packed with each pacemaker.

RECALL

Recall of defective devices is important in the management of pacemaker patients. Follow-up will detect routine battery depletion well. It may not detect earlier than anticipated battery depletion, sudden electronic failure, and the two most dangerous but uncommon failure modes, sudden "no-output" and "runaway," which are electronic in origin. A failure pattern, rather than random failure, in a pacemaker model population should be dealt with in a different fashion than continued routine follow-up. In the event the patient is believed to be at risk, the device should be electively replaced. The individual physician should not be dissuaded from action by a manufacturer or by the absence of a formal recall by a governmental agency. Industry may have inadequate data (or judgment) and government may be too slow in reaching a decision. For example, the physician may determine that battery depletion is occurring in an orderly fashion but at a time when it is unanticipated, and, therefore, follow-up should be at briefer intervals. Follow-up intervals should then be adjusted. The physician may decide that end of life characteristics are not smooth, i.e., that sudden no output failure may occur without detectable warning when the battery is fully depleted. Such pulse generators should be electively removed. Indeed a physician's insistence that the warranty be provided earlier than a manufacturer's intention may cause the manufacturer to issue a change in anticipated end of life behavior. Such an event has occurred in the author's experience.

The "recall" mechanism, whether it involves more intense observation or actual replacement of a defective device, is an integral part of follow-up. It should be used sparingly, but it should be used. If device replacement is elected, patients who are at greater risk should be operated on early, those at lesser risk, later. With the more formal recognition of pacemaker recall, physicians will receive a manufacturer generated list of patients who require careful observation. These manufacturer generated lists are required by regulatory agencies and should be reviewed carefully. While manufacturers approach these "advisory" notices with dread, the physician should consider them as a means of assistance in patient management. The physician should assess the accuracy of a manufacturer generated list.

The need for device elective replacement may also be based on the degree of follow-up required. While in some circumstances, a patient can be monitored telephonically weekly, or more frequently, the shortest realistic routine clinic follow-up interval is 1 month. Patients who require follow-up at lesser intervals probably should have elective replacement. Therefore, as a general rule, if a device can go from apparently normal function to gross malfunction or absence of function in less than a month, it should be electively replaced.

The problem of polyurethane lead deterioration is potentially of greater magnitude. The number of leads at risk is greater than any pacemaker model ever subjected to recall, and the incidence of failure for some models is 20% or more (Figure 2). It is likely that failure of these leads is time-dependent—with

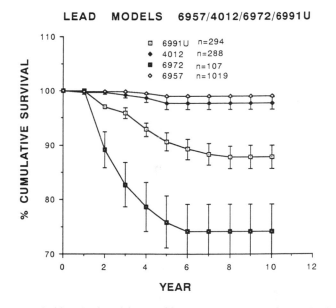

Figure 2. *The survival of four lead models, roughly contemporaneous, from a single manufacturer. Model 6957 had a prolonged satisfactory service in use. Model 4012 was not as good, although superior to the other two leads. Model 6991U had a failure rate of approximately 10% by the end of a decade, while for model 6972 almost 25% of the leads had failed. Recognition of the potential for such events and dealing with them before clinical failure occurs avoids the possibility of clinically manifested failure.*

the passage of more time, more leads will fail. While a pulse generator can be removed easily, a lead is far more difficult. A polyurethane lead subjected to extraction may fragment and embolize. A polyurethane lead undergoing deterioration in situ may deteriorate in a way so far undetermined and cause a far greater problem. Such potential fragmentation has not yet been demonstrated to be a clinical problem.

It is important when replacing a pulse generator implanted on a lead such as models 6972, 6990U, 6991, 4012, and 1016T (and to a lesser extent other leads known to behave relatively poorly) to recognize that the lead is very likely to be defective, no matter how long after it has been implanted and even if it tests well noninvasively. The best course is to remove the lead from function (either physical removal or to abandon it in place) and implant a new lead. Some areas of the lead such as that immediately adjacent to the connector will be visible during pulse generator replacement and deterioration can be seen. Other segments such as those adjacent to the ligature and sleeve holding the lead in place may not be approachable and are known to be vulnerable.

Physician management of a recall can be described as follows:

1. Knowledge that a recall is underway;
2. Assessment of the nature of the recall. One involving progressive lead deterioration or sudden no-output failure or runaway is far more dangerous than, for example, premature battery depletion;
3. Determination of all patients who are at risk (these include patients the physician/clinic is following who are registered with the manufacturer and those unknown to the manufacturer);
4. Determination of the degree of risk for each individual patient;
5. Triage of the patients into groups in which, for example, (a) no change in follow-up is required; (b) more intense follow-up is required; (c) early device removal and replacement is required.

Runaway pulse generator is not a significant problem among pacemakers, but it is the most potentially lethal complication. Should such an issue arise, these generators should be removed as soon as feasible after notification.

PACEMAKER DEPENDENCY

The term pacemaker dependency has been used to indicate those patients at substantial risk should a pacer fail. While widely used, the term is undefined, and different knowledgeable physicians use different criteria, often resulting in substantial confusion. The issue is especially important to regulators who will want to assess the overall risk to a patient population and to the physician who must assess intervention for his/her patients. While there is no general agreement concerning the method of definition of pacemaker dependency, the authors suddenly inhibit pacemaker output during a clinic visit and assess the state of the underlying rhythm. Asystole is permitted for a maximum of 4 seconds. This unpaced rhythm is a clue to the degree of risk. There is little doubt that patients may be at different levels of risk at different times. A patient with complete heart block will not have syncope each time sudden pacemaker failure occurs but, if restored to AV block from a paced rhythm, will certainly enter a category of increased risk. The estimates (all inaccurate to a lesser or greater degree) of patient pacer dependency range from 5% to 30%.

For practical purposes, a patient is pacer-dependent if the sudden (from one beat to the next) loss of pacing will result in a Stokes-Adams episode, serious injury, or death. Questions of definition and even more questions of how to make the clinical determination of potential sudden injury or death exist. During inhibition of the pacemaker, dependency is determined in the following way: if no escape rhythm (or ventricular tachycardia) occurs the patient is pacemaker-dependent (Class I). If the ventricular escape rhythm is complete AV block with atrial fibrillation or sinus rhythm, the patient is substantially pacemaker dependent (Class II). If escape is by a lesser degree of AV block or sinus bradycardia of 30 bpm or less, the patient is moderately dependent (Class III). If escape is by regular sinus rhythm of normal rate (50 or more bpm), the patient is not pacer-dependent (Class IV). As patients vary in pacer dependency from time to time, the worst assessment a patient ever has defines the status. In making these determinations, a patient who has had syncopal episodes because of infrequent but documented asystole before pacemaker implant clearly does require pacing, even if not for more than a few minutes each month. The patient will probably test as nondependent on each follow-up visit. The greatest caution and wisdom must be exercised during evaluation of pacer dependency (Figure 3).

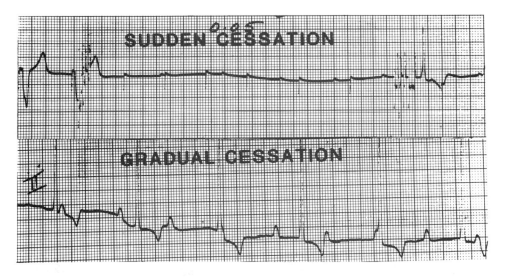

Figure 3. *Pacemaker dependency is a commonly used but not well understood term. Certainly the circumstance of failure to pace is a determinant of the cardiac response. In this patient, ECGs recorded several minutes apart show prolonged asystole following sudden cessation of pacing (above) and a satisfactory escape rhythm with complete AV block following gradual cessation of pacing (below).*

FOLLOW-UP SCHEDULES

The schedule for follow-up of implanted cardiac pacemakers in the United States is largely determined by Medicare regulations. A new schedule published during October 1984 revised the previously announced schedule.

The transtelephonic monitoring contact consists of a determination of the pacemaker rate in the free-running and magnet modes and ECGs in both the free-running and magnet modes. The free-running ECG and the magnet ECG should be of at least 30 seconds duration unless specifically contraindicated. Medicare requires that these ECGs and rates be part of a permanent record.

Different categories are now established for single- and dual-chamber pacemakers and for pacing systems of proven durability and for those of less well-known durability. The criteria for longevity are those that have been recommended by the Intersociety Commission for Heart Disease (ICHD) Resources. The data used to make the determinations are published periodically in *PACE*. Guideline I is for those pacemakers that have not yet developed sufficient exposure and have not met the criteria. Guideline II is for those pacemakers that have met the ICHD criteria. The two operative criteria for longevity and end of life decay are:

1. 90% or better cumulative survival at 5 years following implant;
2. an end of life decay or less than a 50% drop of output voltage and less than 20% deviation of magnet rate, or a drop of 5 bpm or less, over a period of 3 months or more.

Table I

GUIDELINE I. The majority of pacemakers.

SINGLE-CHAMBER PACEMAKERS		
1st Mo.	2nd Mo.–36th Mo.	37th Mo.–Failure
Every 2 weeks	Every 8 weeks	Every 4 weeks

DUAL-CHAMBER PACEMAKERS			
1st Mo.	2nd Mo.–6th Mo.	7th Mo.–36th Mo.	37th Mo.–Failure
Every 2 weeks	Every 4 weeks	Every 8 weeks	Every 4 weeks

GUIDELINE II. The minority of pacemaker systems (pacemaker and leads) for which sufficient long-term clinical information exists to assure that they meet the standards of the Inter-society Commission for Heart Disease Resources (ICHD) for longevity and end-of-life decay.

SINGLE-CHAMBER PACEMAKERS			
1st Mo.	2nd Mo.–30th Mo.	31st–48th Mo.	Thereafter
Every 2 weeks	Every 12 weeks	Every 8 weeks	Every 4 weeks

DUAL-CHAMBER PACEMAKERS			
1st Mo.	2nd Mo.–30th Mo.	31st–48th Mo.	Thereafter
Every 2 weeks	Every 12 weeks	Every 8 weeks	Every 4 weeks

As two criteria are involved, it is possible for a pacemaker to meet one and not the other. For example, a model may meet the 90% survival criterion and yet, once end of life is reached, failure may be sudden. Alternatively, failure may be orderly but sooner than 5 years. The Medicare guidelines also recognize the influence of lead longevity on the longevity of the entire pacing system but do not clearly define the schedule alterations that will be based on lead requirements. Because of the various complexities related to the criteria for pacemaker system longevity and single- and dual-chamber pacemakers, follow-up schedules are likely to be variable and perhaps even the source of uncertainty (Table I).

TRANSTELEPHONIC MONITORING

Telephonic monitoring is the most useful technique available for the long-term observation of patients with implanted cardiac pacemakers. As the total number of these patients increases, face-to-face observation becomes relatively more difficult and cumbersome. As face-to-face follow-up in the pacemaker center becomes more complex, it should be reserved for the extensive work-up necessary to analyze pacemaker malfunction and establish proper pacemaker settings. Clinic monitoring on a frequent basis for prolonged periods is burdensome for staff and patients and should be replaced by transtelephonic monitoring. Transtelephonic monitoring is very useful in overall follow-up of the paced patient.

Telephone monitoring with rate determination and an ECG can be used at frequent intervals following pacemaker implantation to ascertain electrode stability. Later, longer intervals between contacts will be appropriate and, as the unit ages, at shorter intervals.

PURPOSES OF TELEPHONIC MONITORING

1. Careful pacemaker follow-up to achieve maximum safety and longevity.
2. Careful and frequent observation of pulse generators and lead systems in models known to have a high incidence of electronic failure, lead fracture, or insulation deterioration, or observation of devices that are no longer operating normally but clear-cut malfunction hasn't been demonstrated.
3. Electrocardiographic monitoring for an intercurrent arrhythmia.
4. Follow-up as a laboratory resource for the physician in overall responsibility for a patient's welfare.
5. Provision of pacemaker follow-up to areas remote from a pacemaker clinic and for patients unable to travel.
6. Provision of technical expertise for facilities without that capability, such as a nursing home.
7. Follow-up of patient location.

The accuracy of telephone monitoring in detection of battery depletion is not matched by that of electronic monitoring because of the ease and frequency of the transmissions. The single area of failure has been the inability to detect impending lead fracture or insulation deterioration which, unfortunately, is usually not detectable by any means in advance of distinct ECG changes in pacemaker function.

Rate and ECG

Transmission of rate and ECG is now the standard of transtelephonic monitoring, providing rate for determination of battery and electronic status and ECG to confirm cardiac capture and sensing. The ECG is the universally recognized indicator of cardiac activity and is mandatory for any follow-up system since normal or abnormal function is readily recognized. The ECG clearly demonstrates pacemaker malfunction early or late after implant and is invaluable for the detection of intercurrent arrhythmias that occur with pacemaker malfunction or despite normal pacemaker function. Even stimulation threshold can be determined if the implanted unit has a magnet-activated automatic threshold determination such as the Vario system provided by several manufacturers (Figure 4).

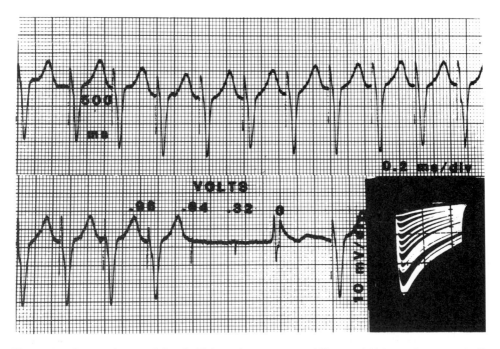

Figure 4. *Automatic test of threshold is an important capability, and if it can be magnetically activated as in the "Vario" system, threshold can be determined via the telephone. In this illustration each stimulus is $\frac{1}{15}$ the voltage below each preceding stimulus. The inverted stimulus at the right is a zero voltage mark. The threshold is 0.96 V. Whenever the magnet is removed from the pacer during the cycle, the output returns to its programmed setting.*

A wide variety of monitors for patient use exists. Some equipment has been carefully designed to be easy to use, with comfortable wrist or axillary electrodes, positive coupling between the telephone handset and monitor, and convenient hand application of the monitor. Other equipment is small and light but practically unusable. Some ECGs are easy to read, while others are virtually impossible to read. In selection of equipment, the capabilities of the usual patient (average age 70 years) and the ease or complexity of use should be the primary consideration.

Record Keeping

Records are of prime importance in knowledge of when failure will occur in an individual patient and for the collection of data concerning an entire model, to indicate when careful follow-up or elective replacement (see Recall) should be undertaken. As large groups of patients are followed by a single facility, routine secretarial effort becomes inadequate to maintain satisfactory observation of the patient population. Under these circumstances, computer generated record keeping facilities become mandatory. At Montefiore Medical Center the transtelephonic monitoring clinic is based on human interpretation and computerized record storage.

The computer provides the list of daily calls to be made and includes time, name, identification number (a 4-digit number unique to our facility), and telephone number. Once the operator selects a patient on that list, the patient's previous data, including pacemaker model, date of implant, date of the last telephone call, free-running and magnet rates at that time, and an abbreviated indication of overall pacemaker function are displayed on the screen. Additionally, the percent decline of magnetic rate since pacemaker implantation, the indicator of elective replacement, is displayed. All of the specific data, including the quality of electrocardiographic capture and sensing and overall function for the last eight contacts are also displayed. The nurse/technician then proceeds with telephone transmission of data and the interpretation of a telephonically transmitted ECG. With the transmission completed, the computer prompts the operator with requests for free-running and magnetic rate to three significant figures. It then prompts operator interpretation of the quality of capture and sensing, and the overall summary of the quality of pacing. When all of this has been entered, the computer will ask whether the next call is to be on a monthly or weekly schedule. Once one or the other is selected, it will recommend a date. Holidays (updated annually) and weekends are programmed into memory so that those dates are not selected. The operator can override the computer recommendation and assign another date. At the conclusion of the test procedure, a line printer provides a report with the free-running and magnet ECG as well as a full report of the transmission and appropriate interpretation. Each report is a history of the entire transtelephonic record and allows the physician who reads the report to acquaint himself with all of the data specific to that patient. The paper report can serve as a backup for computer failure. It also can be mailed to other facilities or physicians (Figure 5). A variety of commercial computer record keeping programs designed for pacemaker follow-up now exist.

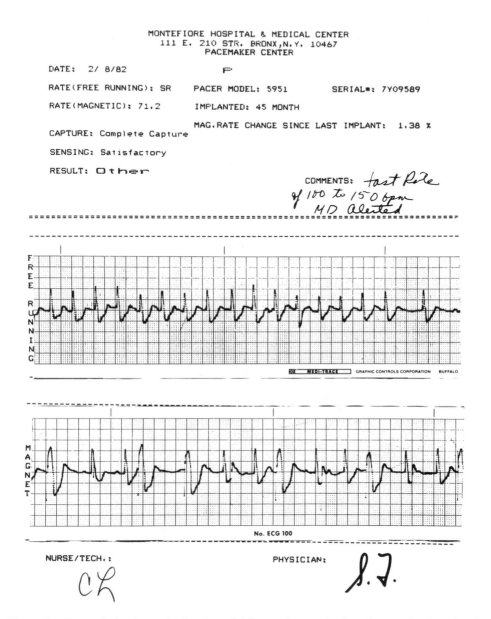

MONTEFIORE HOSPITAL & MEDICAL CENTER
111 E. 210 STR. BRONX,N.Y. 10467
PACEMAKER CENTER

DATE: 2/ 8/82   F

RATE(FREE RUNNING): SR   PACER MODEL: 5951   SERIAL#: 7Y09589

RATE(MAGNETIC): 71.2   IMPLANTED: 45 MONTH

                            MAG.RATE CHANGE SINCE LAST IMPLANT: 1.38 %
CAPTURE: Complete Capture

SENSING: Satisfactory

RESULT: Other

COMMENTS: fast Rate
of 100 to 150 bpm
MD alerted

NURSE/TECH.:

PHYSICIAN:

Figure 5. *Transtelephonic monitoring is useful for routine monitoring of pacemaker function. In addition, intercurrent arrhythmias can be detected. In this instance, an arrhythmia, possibly atrial fibrillation, was detected during normal pacemaker function. Only a 1.38% rate decline had occurred, and sensing and capture were documented. The free-running rhythm strip is shown above and the magnet strip below.*

ELECTROCARDIOGRAPHY IN TRANSTELEPHONE MONITORING

ECG transmission provides interpretive difficulties and artifacts that are similar to conventional electrocardiography and clearly indicate failure to capture, sense, or both. A few artifacts are unique to transtelephonic monitoring. The most serious is that caused by the use of a single-lead rhythm strip, usually lead I (right arm, left arm) in which the QRS or the pacemaker artifact may be isoelectric or, for some other reason, insufficiently diagnostic. Another lead should be selected and transmission repeated. The diagnostic lead can be used thereafter. Telephone noise frequently is picked up from continuous interference and electrical transients. Both usually are readily detected. Reversal of the limb leads is easily detected and is of little consequence. Motion artifacts occur frequently. Troublesome 60-Hz interference can exist with all systems, although the stimulus rate and the ECG usually can be discriminated. Because the determination of rate in the magnet mode requires a magnet to be held over the pacemaker, its movement (as in a patient with Parkinson's disease) can cause a variety of artifacts including brief inhibition of the pacer. Respiratory movement is recognized, as on a conventional ECG, by a slow rhythmic oscillation of the baseline (Figure 6).

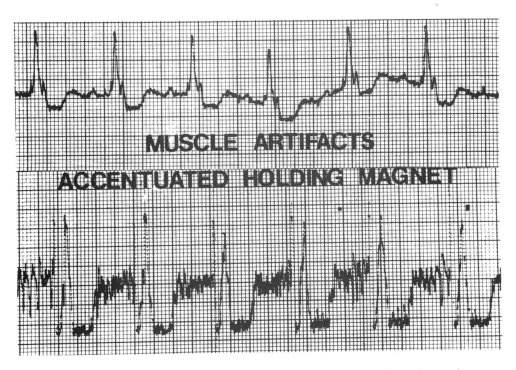

Figure 6. *The ECG is readily transmitted by telephone. A variety of artifacts also can be transmitted. In this instance, the muscle artifacts caused by magnet application are readily seen. The pacemaker is not inhibited or triggered.*

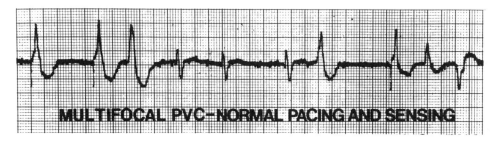

Figure 7.   *Multifocal premature contractions can be detected as they are here. Ventricular capture and sensing of all of the foci are demonstrated.*

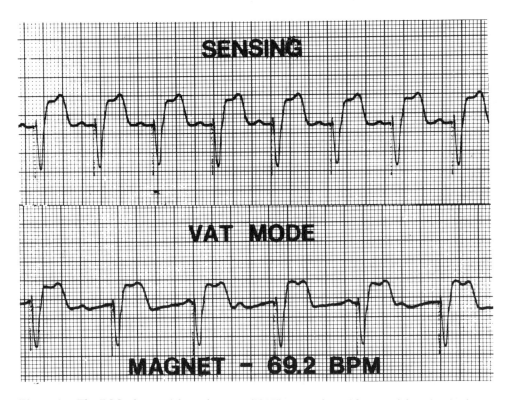

Figure 8.   *The ECG of an atrial synchronous (VAT) pacemaker with normal function is shown. Atrial sensing and ventricular capture are demonstrated as is a "normal" magnet rate indicative of satisfactory function of the power source.*

A wide variety of pathology may be detected with ECG monitoring. Included are the range of pacemaker malfunctions: rate change and loss of pacing or sensing, or both. Relatively common intercurrent findings are multifocal premature ventricular contractions, tachycardia, atrial fibrillation, and other arrhythmias.

The induction of a competitive, magnet-produced rhythm to detect pacemaker rate is almost always without meaningful effect. Pacemaker-produced premature ventricular contractions (PVC) occur but are not sustained and only rarely do multiple PVCs require cessation of use of the magnet. No episode of competitively induced ventricular fibrillation or sustained tachycardia has occurred in our patients followed by telephone (Figure 7).

Dual-chamber transtelephonic monitoring represents additional problems and complexities. Some dual-chamber telephonically monitored ECGs are extremely difficult to read. Equipment for interpretation of the ECG and rate is now as widely available as it is for single-chamber pacemakers. The increasing use of dual-chamber pacemakers makes monitoring of those devices important despite the associated difficulties (Figure 8).

RECURRENT SYMPTOMS AFTER PACEMAKER IMPLANT

It is often assumed that once a pacemaker is implanted all symptoms will, and should, vanish. Indeed, many patients make that assumption and refer all intercurrent illness or later symptoms to pacemaker malfunction. Some will even date remote symptoms such as those of the musculoskeletal system from the time of pacer implant. These are very dangerous miscalculations. Each patient who has an implanted pacemaker should have a general medical physician and/ or a cardiologist who will care for all nonpacemaker-related conditions.

Recurrent symptoms fall into the general categories of noncardiac symptoms, which are usually readily separated from the implanted pacemaker; nonpacemaker cardiac symptoms, such as those related to congestive heart failure, angina, or myocardial infarction; and those which approximate the symptoms that necessitated the pacemaker implant in the first instance. Some patients will have been implanted who had been relatively asymptomatic and may even be asymptomatic with lead or pacemaker failure. An increasing number of patients are being implanted for asymptomatic (or minimally symptomatic) electrocardiographically detected arrhythmias, for example, AV block, sick sinus syndrome with long pauses but with minimal symptoms. Although this approach is controversial, it seems to be widely practiced and is usually appropriate.

In our own evaluation and that of others, some 8% to 10% of patients will complain of return of symptoms, such as dizziness, syncope, palpitations, shortness of breath, angina, or edema only some of which may be pacemaker related. About one-third of symptoms result from some pacemaker malfunction, the remainder will be of cardiovascular origin unrelated to the pacemaker. One of the recognized causes of recurrent symptomatology is the pacemaker syndrome.

The pacemaker syndrome occurs in lesser or greater degree during single-chamber ventricular pacing and results from:

1. Cyclic atrial and ventricular synchronization, which causes cyclic variation of cardiac output and of peripheral blood pressure.
2. Retrograde conduction and entrainment of the P wave. Such an event can cause a marked drop in cardiac output, a feeling of pressure in the precordium (sometimes analogous to angina), and pounding in the neck and chest resulting from cannon waves in the jugular venous system and the pulmonary vasculature.

The pacemaker syndrome can be very severe in some patients, although almost one-quarter of patients paced only from the ventricle have been estimated to have some level of severity. It can be diagnosed by noting fluctuation in peripheral blood pressure, by physical examination, and the finding of cannon waves in the neck. The diagnosis can often be made by history alone. Management is by restoration of the normal AV sequence. If a patient with sinus bradycardia is paced at a more rapid rate from the ventricle, P waves may be entrained retrograde. Lowering the ventricular paced rate in order to prevent asystole but allow sinus bradycardia will restore the normal AV sequence. Atrial or dual-chamber pacing usually is preferred (Figure 9).

Symptoms may recur because of episodic pacemaker inhibition. Unfortunately, this is a common occurrence, existing in almost one-third of patients with unipolar inhibited pacemakers. About one-half of those affected will be symptomatic. Pacemaker inhibition by electromyographic inhibition (EMI) occurs almost exclusively in unipolar systems in which sensing is of the pectoral musculature adjacent to the pacemaker. If a pacemaker is inhibited, the patient will return briefly to the unprotected circumstance. If that is asystole, syncope

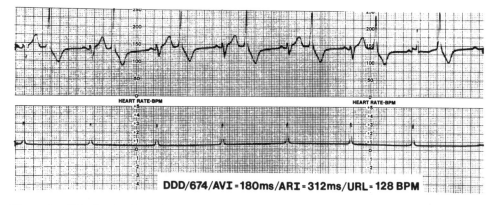

DDD/674/AVI=180ms/ARI=312ms/URL=128 BPM

Figure 9. Echo beating is readily determined on Holter monitoring. This recording, with a pacemaker channel (below), demonstrates echo beating following each ventricular stimulus. Atrial sensing, ventricular capture, coupled VPCs, and normal recycle are all demonstrated.

may occur. In dual-chamber pacemakers, the devices may be both inhibited and triggered. Unusual arrhythmias may occur, and an endless loop tachycardia can be started by EMI.

The test for EMI pacemaker effect is the provocation of pectoral muscle activity by raising a weight or vigorously pressing the hands together during electrocardiographic monitoring. A very large number of unipolar pacemakers will be affected, but the incidence will be falsely positive. Ambulatory monitoring is a much more realistic approach that will detect EMI very well in daily usage (Figure 10).

Evaluation of returned symptoms can be a difficult undertaking. Pacemaker function should be carefully evaluated. Chest x-ray should be read for intermittent lead fracture and lead displacement. Fluoroscopy may be useful. Physiological evaluation and ambulatory monitoring is useful in any unusual situation. In the end, the 90% of patients who have returned symptoms for reasons other than the pacemaker will be treated for tachyarrhythmias, hypertension, angina, or primary neurological conditions, as necessary.

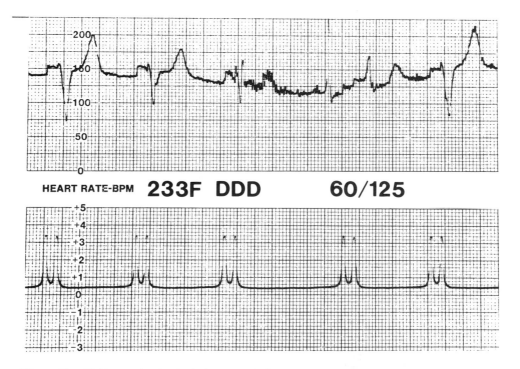

Figure 10.   *Holter monitoring is the best means of correlating symptoms with ECG findings. This is especially true for electromagnetic inhibition with pacemaker inhibition or false triggering. In this instance, the upper channel is a conventional ECG and the lower channel is that of the stimuli emitted by the pacemaker. Here, the EMI is seen clearly on the ECG, and inhibition of the pacemaker is clearly indicated.*

TELEMETRY

Pacemaker telemetry is noninvasive transmission of data from the implanted pulse generator to an external receiver. Both physiological and hardware data may be transmitted. Telemetry has been available in limited format for almost a decade. It has become more complex and will assume progressively greater importance as electronic computer based memory becomes more widely used and as electronic capability for data analysis and processing becomes more sophisticated.

Telemetry was initially devised for the transmission of hardware data such as the state of the pulse generator battery. Battery impedance, which rises progressively in a lithium iodine cell, corresponding to battery depletion is a good indication of the longevity remaining in a pulse generator (Figure 11). Lead impedance, also a measurable parameter, should lie within a narrow range, approximately that at implant. If impedance rises, lead fracture may have occurred. If it falls, insulation disruption or short circuit in a bipolar lead may have occurred. A low impedance will result in rapid depletion of a pulse generator, and reliable data of low impedance should be an indication for intervention or a resetting of the time of impending depletion and, therefore, the need for reschedule of follow-up.

More recently, additional hardware telemetry has become available includ-

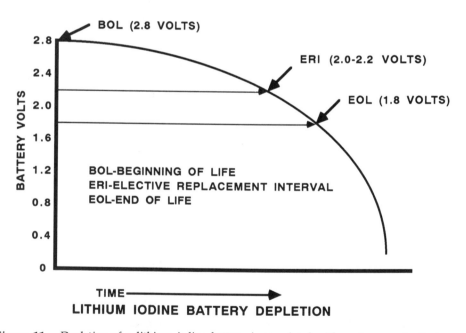

Figure 11. Depletion of a lithium iodine battery is associated with an increase in its internal impedance and progressive decline in output voltage. At beginning of life (BOL) output voltage is 2.8 V, elective replacement interval (ERI) is at 2.0–2.2 V, and at the end of life (EOL) is at 1.8 V. The actual output of the pulse generator measured at the terminals may be different depending on output programming.

ing pulse longevity, pulse amplitude in one or two channels, and the current drain from the battery and refractory intervals set for atrial and ventricular channels. Other telemetric capabilities include the display of upper and lower rates and the entire range of sensitive and refractory intervals after pacemaker programming.

Recently available telemetric capabilities are of memory data concerning pacer use and even sensor use, distinct from actual stimulation. Several pulse generators now have a memory for the number of stimuli emitted. If uncertainty exists concerning how frequently pacing is required, the counters can be reset to zero at each visit and read at a subsequent visit. If visits are sufficiently frequent and pacing sufficiently infrequent, the number of pacer stimuli can be counted. These memory banks are presently limited in capacity so that frequent pacing will overwhelm the data storage capability. With the progressive development of high density memory chips, it is likely that some variety of ambulatory ECG monitoring will be possible.

Despite all the hardware telemetry, this is of less present and potential utility than the availability of telemetry of physiological data. It is likely that some physiological functions will be telemetered in the near future. As physiological sensing pacemakers can set a stimulation rate based on pH, pCO_2/pO_2, or some other physiological parameter, that data can be telemetered out of the pulse generator for the physician's information.

Important present telemetry is that of the electrogram and of ECG interpretation channels. Electrogram telemetry can give an indication of the quality of the signal sensed by the pacemaker and which signal triggers its function. Telemetry can be of the atrial and/or the ventricular channels or both. Such telemetry indicates the quality of the EGM and can be invaluable in determining the nature of a malfunction caused by lead displacement, poor EGM amplitude, slew rate, or lead fracture. Atrial EGM telemetry can be useful in detecting a retrograde P wave and determining timing and existence of retrograde conduction. Not all EGM transmission is at an adequately high frequency to be valuable, some is not yet calibrated (Figures 12 and 13). A telemetry channel may not have similar frequency characteristics to a sensing channel so that direct comparison may not be possible.

ECG interpretation channels are at least equally important. The highly complex ECGs now being developed from dual-chamber pacemakers may not be capable of interpretation without assistance from pacemaker-generated markers. An EGM transmission is of a physiological signal, even when it may be of less than interpretable quality. A marker is an indication of how the pacemaker interprets a specific cardiac event. Simultaneous recording of marker information and an ECG can indicate what is being sensed and how the pacemaker deals with the sensed event. For example, a P wave that occurs too late in the lower rate interval cycle, which is always between ventricular events, may be sensed but unused by a VDD pacemaker to begin an AV interval. An anomalously short AV interval is thus explained. The absence of ventricular sensing and ventricular pacer stimuli on ECG and the presence of atrial sense markers and markers of ventricular stimuli clearly indicate ventricular lead fracture. ECG interpretation channels are invaluable (Figures 14 and 15).

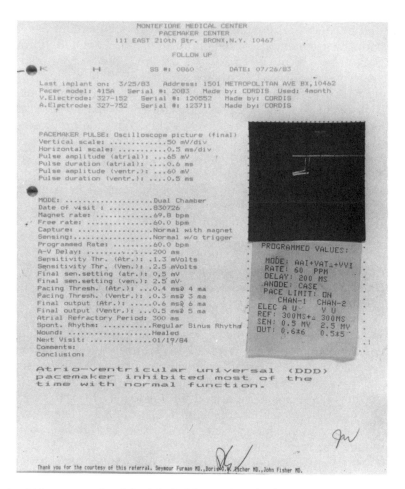

Figure 12. *Telemetry may be of physiological data such as the electrogram or it may be of hardware data only. In this instance, hardware data only is transmitted and is provided on a paper tape printout. This provides information concerning sensitivity, output, rate, and refractory settings. The tape is attached to a site made available on the clinic visit form. The oscilloscopic photograph is also attached to the form. The remainder of the format, uniquely designed for each pulse generator, is computer generated from patient data stored in the computer and information generated during the clinic visit.*

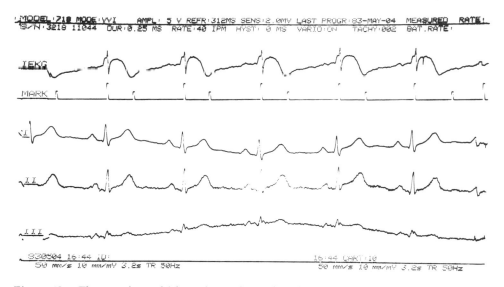

Figure 13.   *The use of a multichannel recorder with alphanumeric capabilities is invaluable. In the first channel telemetric text concerning model, mode, serial number, and date of last programming along with other data is recorded on paper from the programmer telemetry. Channel two is that of the telemetered intracardiac electrogram, and channel three is a marker indicating the instance of sensing and the duration of pacemaker refractoriness. Below are three ECG channels and then a "housekeeping" channel with date, time, paper speed, and patient identification.*

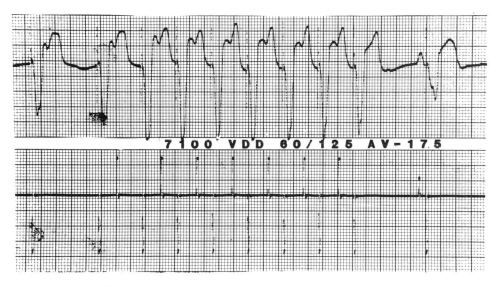

Figure 14.   *ECG interpretation channels are useful in indicating what a pacemaker senses and how it responds. Simultaneous ECG and ECG interpretation channels, with the ECG interpretation channel as the lower of the two, during endless loop tachycardia is shown. The upward markers are atrial events, the taller indicating a sensed event that starts a timing cycle, the lower, a sensed but unused event. The downward markers are ventricular pace markers. The ventricular escape interval is 1000 ms. The minimum interval between ventricular events is 480 ms. The retrograde P wave is sensed 260 ms after the ventricular event, and after a delay, readily measured as 220 ms, a ventricular stimulus is emitted. Bottom right, no retrograde P wave occurs. The next P wave appears too late to begin a full AV interval and is indicated by a lower mark.*

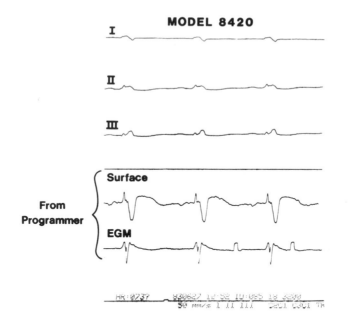

Figure 15. *Electrogram telemetry is especially valuable when compared to surface leads on a multichannel recorder. In this 5-channel recording, leads I, II, III are compared with both a telemetric transmission of the electrogram (surface) and a higher frequency direct telemetric recording (EGM). The timing and quality of the EGM can be determined readily via the telemetered EGM.*

HOLTER MONITORING

Ambulatory ECG monitoring is a most effective means of determining satisfactory pacemaker function. In the presence of a malfunction that has occurred or has been provoked by daily activity, there is no technique that provides greater accuracy for determination of the state of the function of the pacemaker device and patient interaction. Passive ECG, even with provocative testing, can frequently detect malfunction of an implanted pacemaker and is, of course, the basic technique. However, it is often impossible to duplicate specific daily events and, certainly, it is impossible to record for a prolonged period. Ambulatory monitoring frequently will distinguish between false-negative results in the pacer center and false-positive results. False-positive results can be troublesome when pacer inhibition is found in the pacer center and its finding cannot be correlated with clinical findings (Figure 16).

Provocative tests of pacemaker function can detect failure to a substantial degree, but many episodes can only be detected by continuous ambulatory monitoring. Episodic events such as brief runs of endless loop tachycardia, which occur only during a brief return of retrograde conduction, can be detected as a source of symptoms by ambulatory monitoring and frequently not during passive ECG. Events related to daily activity, EMI, loss of capture in a specific body position, or activity and the effect of sleep or activity on patient-pacemaker interaction can be readily demonstrated (Figure 17).

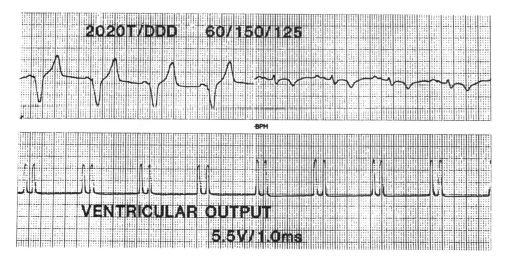

Figure 16. Subtle changes that may not be apparent on a passive ECG will appear on a Holter recording. In this recording the upper tracing is of the ECG, the lower the pacemaker stimuli. With the AV delay set at 150 ms, the lower rate limit is 60 bpm and the upper rate limit 125 bpm. The left tracing shows atrial and ventricular pacing with capture of both chambers. With an acceleration in the atrial rate the atrial channel did not stop emitting stimuli, demonstrating a loss of atrial sensing and with emission of ventricular channel stimuli loss of ventricular capture was also demonstrated. While the atrium was not captured, each atrial channel stimulus fell during atrial refractoriness so that loss of ability to capture cannot be diagnosed.

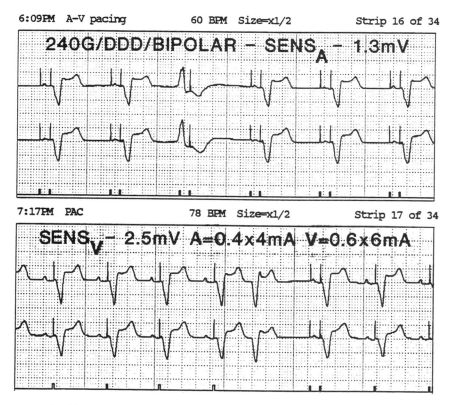

Figure 17. A Holter recording of a bipolar dual-chamber pacemaker demonstrates normal atrial and ventricular capture (above) with a single unsensed premature ventricular contraction with atrial and ventricular stimuli superimposed. The pacemaker stimuli are shown at the bottom of the trace as single or double marks. Below, the tracing demonstrates normal atrial sensing and tracking and ventricular stimuli that capture the ventricle. A single premature ventricular capture is ap-

PACEMAKER CLINIC

The pacemaker clinic represents an organized effort to detect abnormal pacemaker function. The overall management of the implanted patient or group of patients involves knowledge of the specific functional capabilities of the pacemaker system, i.e., the pulse generator and lead system and the anticipated variety of failure modes. If the lead system is known to have a proclivity for deterioration of the insulation material, such as has occurred in some models of polyurethane leads, then careful evaluation of sensing function, loss of capture, or high threshold and early battery depletion is to be anticipated as these can be the earliest manifestation of impending system failure. If a generator has a tendency to sudden no output failure then that generator must be handled differently than those generators that experience has indicated will deplete slowly and in an orderly fashion. Once these considerations are understood and noted, it should be further understood that transtelephonic monitoring is an integral part of follow-up as clinic visits are time consuming and labor intensive. Large numbers of patients are best managed by transtelephonic monitoring punctuated by annual visits to the pacemaker center during which time more extensive investigation of the pacemaker status, including x-ray, programming, and determination of the underlying cardiac function, can be determined.

During a pacemaker center visit the patient is logged in on a schedule. The schedule for follow-up is the single most important consideration because it determines that follow-up will indeed occur (Table II). The patient should be connected to a multichannel ECG recorder in which at least three (or better, six) channels simultaneously will be recorded. The pacer site is inspected. The wound should be clean and not tender. The pacemaker should be freely mov-

---

Table II

Clinic visits may be mixed with transtelephonic monitoring but the schedule guideline is

SINGLE-CHAMBER PACEMAKERS

Twice-1st 6 months (following implant)

THEN

Once-Every 12 months

DUAL-CHAMBER PACEMAKERS

Twice-1st 6 months (following implant)

THEN

Once-Every 6 months

able, and the overlying skin should be of normal color. If the skin is tight, tender, or erythematous, then infection may be present. If discomfort exists and infection is suspected, then the wound should be irrigated and cultures performed. For wound culture, the skin is carefully cleansed and painted with antiseptic solution (iodine is preferred) and a needle directed to the pulse generator. The passage of the needle will be stopped by the generator itself and clean or infected fluid will lie in a space around the generator. A syringe filled with isotonic saline from an intravenous infusion bottle rather than from solution used to dilute medication (such solutions contain bacteriostatic preservative and will defeat attempts at culture) should be used. The pacer site is irrigated and the fluid withdrawn and placed in infusions for aerobic and anaerobic culture. A confirmed culture of a pathogen requires removal of the pacemaker hardware.

If the initial ECG demonstrates normal pacing with appropriate sensing and pacing in each channel, then the pacemaker should be inhibited to determine the underlying cardiac rhythm —a determination which is useful in following the progression or improvement in the rhythmic basis for original implantation and to determine whether pacemaker dependency exists (Figure 18).

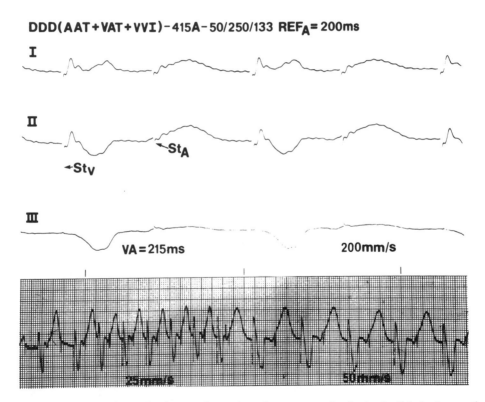

Figure 18. *Retrograde conduction can be evaluated on an ongoing basis. In this instance, the DDD pacemaker is programmed to the atrial triggered mode so that the instant of sensing the P wave is marked by an emitted stimulus. In a multichannel recording (100 mm/s) the ventricular stimulus interval to the atrial "mark" stimulus is 215 ms. The same recording is possible with slightly less accuracy on a conventional electrocardiograph at 50 mm/s (below).*

If the pacemaker is entirely inhibited by spontaneous cardiac rhythm, then a magnet should be placed over the pulse generator. The (almost) universal response to placement of a magnet over the pulse generator is the asynchronous mode of operation during which capture in the atrium and the ventricle can be determined. The threshold of capture should then be tested to ascertain whether it is stable or even lower in relation to a previous determination or whether it has deteriorated (increased). All programmable pacemakers will allow such determination, and several have mechanisms that allow rapid, automatic determination of threshold operated either via the pulse generator or the programmer. If threshold is stable, no further intervention is required. If a pulse generator has a specific threshold testing capability, that should be used. Programming output progressively down to loss of capture with rescue by an "Emergency" programming button is less satisfactory as the emergency output is often slow and may take 5–8 seconds before higher output stimulation begins (Figure 19).

Check of sensing threshold can be accomplished by setting the dual-chamber pacemaker in the single-chamber mode initially, ventricular then atrial. If the unit is then set below the spontaneous cardiac rate, appropriate inhibition indicates satisfactory sensing of spontaneous cardiac activity. The sensitivity settings of the pacemaker can then be altered to determine the actual threshold and the sensitivity set appropriately. A major portion of the issue of sensitivity

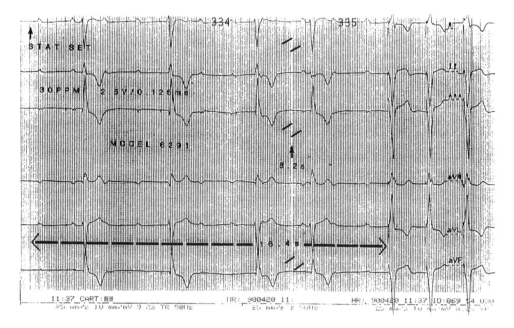

Figure 19. Use of the emergency output feature on a programmer may be very slow and allow a long period of asystole. In this patient with complete AV block threshold was taken below capture level and the "STAT SET" (emergency) button activated. More than 16 seconds elapsed, sufficiently long for the patient to be symptomatic, before the higher output occurred. This patient had a satisfactory underlying idioventricular rhythm and was asymptomatic at rest.

is the secondary effect of sensitivity to electromagnetic and electromyographic interference. If a higher output for cardiac stimulation is set than is necessary and if no adjacent structures (such as intercostal musculature or diaphragm) are stimulated, there are no secondary effects other than earlier battery depletion. The sensitivity setting, if higher than necessary, allows inappropriate sensing and, therefore, inappropriate response to noncardiac signals (Figure 20).

When all of the determinations and appropriate settings have been made, the maintenance of records is the most important consideration. Thresholds of sensing and stimulation, the presence or absence of retrograde conduction and the possibility of endless loop tachycardia, final sensitivity settings, and final outputs should be recorded in a format that allows retention of all data and its

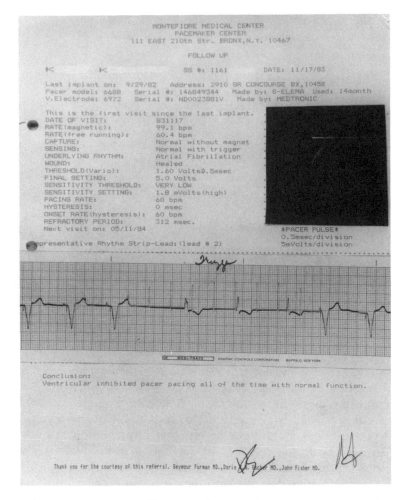

Figure 20. *The computer-generated clinic report designates historical data (top), the characteristics of the oscilloscopic artifact (center), and the data derived at the time of the visit. This includes mode of operation, rate, atrial and ventricular sensing thresholds, and final outputs. A summary of function is at the bottom. All data is retained in computer memory.*

AUTOMATED PACEMAKER FOLLOW-UP (CLINICAL)
1. COMPUTER ASSISTED

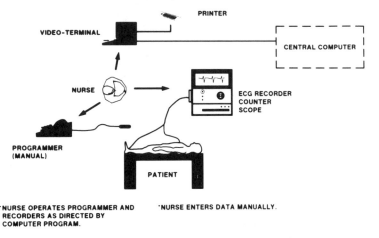

*NURSE OPERATES PROGRAMMER AND   *NURSE ENTERS DATA MANUALLY.
RECORDERS AS DIRECTED BY
COMPUTER PROGRAM.

Figure 21.   *Follow-up is computer assisted at Montefiore Medical Center. The computer contains data on all patients, records of their previous visits, and instructions and guidance on programming each of the pacemakers in use. The patient is attached to a counter, ECG, and oscilloscope. The nurse operates the program, derives data in cooperation with directions from the computer, and enters data into the computer. At the conclusion of the test procedure, all data have been entered into the computer, verified, and are in permanent memory. A printout, immediately available from a printer in the examination room, is provided for the chart and transmission to the referring physician.*

ready access. This is especially important in modern multiprogrammable dual-chamber pacemakers in which contents of memory may contain additional information concerning the number of spontaneous and paced events and given some indication of the need of pacing. With such large volumes of information, only computer maintained databases can process, retain, and generate a paper copy of the appropriate data (Figure 21).

SECONDARY INTERVENTION

The quality of the application of pacemaker therapy and effectiveness of follow-up is based on the stability of the lead system, quality of the electrodes, durability of the power source, and pulse generator programmability. Operator and follow-up capability is also intrinsic to the quality of the result. Unlike an operative procedure that does not involve the implantation of hardware, the use of a cardiac pacemaker requires improvements in hardware and personnel to improve the result. One measure of such improvement is the time to the first intervention after pacemaker implant. This has been calculated for the years 1965, 1970, 1975, 1977, 1980, and 1982. The earlier pacemaker eras were less technologically stable and secondary intervention occurred much earlier. The time by which 10% of patients and then 50% of patients had the first reintervention was calculated in months (Figure 22).

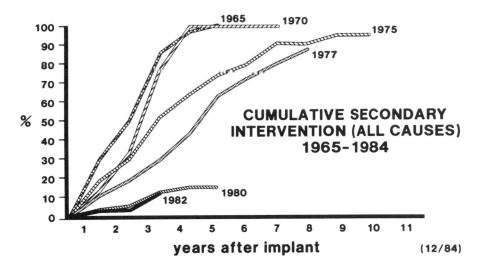

Figure 22. The interval from implant to the first reintervention has prolonged over the years. Ten percent of patients implanted during 1965 had a secondary procedure by the end of 3 months, 50% by the end of 24 months, and all had a secondary procedure by the end of 60 months. Those implanted during 1982 had 2.8% secondary interventions by the end of 2 years and fewer than 10% by the end of 3 years. The increased rate of reintervention was caused by exhaustion of short duration dual-chamber pulse generators and polyurethane lead failures. Interventions for more recent years are still fewer in number.

Despite the increasing complexity of cardiac pacing involving multiprogrammability, dual-chamber pacing, and rate responsiveness, the overall result has been a stability of therapy, which means that for pacemakers implanted during 1980 only 10% of devices will have undergone reintervention 4 years later. For those implanted during 1982 only 2.8% have undergone reintervention 2 years later. The dramatic improvement of stability and durability of implanted pacing is remarkable.

BIBLIOGRAPHY

Benedek M, Furman S: Semiautomatic computer follow up for transtelephone patients. PACE 1983; 6:316.

Bilitch M, Hauser R, Goldman B, et al: Performance of cardiac pacemaker pulse generators. PACE 1985; 8:276–282.

Brevik K, Ohm OJ: Myopotential inhibition of unipolar QRS-inhibited (VVI) pacemakers assessed by ambulatory holter monitoring of the electrocardiogram. PACE 1980; 3: 470–478.

Byrd CL, McArthur W, Stokes K, et al: Implant experience with unipolar polyurethane pacing leads. Pace 1983; 6:868–882.

Chardack WM, Gage AA, Federico AJ, et al: Five years' clinical experience with an implanted pacemaker: An appraisal. Surgery 1965; 58:915–922.

Choo MH, Holmes DR JR, Gersh BJ, et al: Permanent pacemaker infections: Characterization and management. Am J Cardiol 1981; 48:559–564.

Davies G, Siddons H: Prediction of battery depletion in implanted pacemakers. THORAX 1973; 28:180.

Dreifus LS, Pennock RS, Feldman M, et al: Experience with 3835 pacemakers utilizing transtelephonic surveillance. Am J Cardiol 1975; 35:133.

Edhag O, Elmqvist H, Vallin HO: An implantable pulse generator indicating asystole or extreme bradycardia. PACE 1983; 6:166–170.

Erbel R: Pacemaker syndrome. Am J Cardiol 1979; 44:771–772.

Escher DJW, Furman S: Oscilloscopic and recent other methods of implantable pacemaker follow-up. Ann Cardiol Angeiol 1971; 20:503.

Fisher JD, Escher DJW, Hurzeler P, et al: Recurrent syncope or dizziness after pacemaker implantation. Clin Res 1978; 26:231A.

Furman S: Cardiac pacing and pacemakers: V. Analysis of pacemaker malfunction. Am J Cardiol 1977; 94:378–379.

Furman S: Cardiac pacing and pacemakers: VIII. The pacemaker follow-up clinic. Am Heart J 1977; 94:795–804.

Furman S: Transtelephone pacemaker monitoring. In EK Chung (Ed): Artificial Cardiac Pacing: Practical Approach. 2nd ed. Williams & Wilkins, Baltimore 1984, pp 345–358.

Furman S, Escher DJW: Transtelephone pacemaker monitoring. Five years later. Ann Thorac Surg 1975; 20:326–338.

Furman S, Parker B, Escher DJW: Transtelephone pacemaker clinic. J Thorac Cardiovasc Surg 1971; 61:827–834.

Goldman B, MacGregor D: Management of infected pacemaker systems. CPPE 1984; 2:220–235.

Greatbatch W, Lee JH, Mathias W, et al: The solid-state lithium battery; A new improved chemical power source for implantable cardiac pacemakers. IEEE Trans Biomed Eng 1971; 18:317.

Gribbin B, Abson CP, Clarke LM: Inhibition of external demand pacemakers during muscular activity. Br Heart J 1974; 36:1210–1212.

Hanson J: Sixteen failures in a single model of bipolar polyurethane-insulated ventricular pacing lead. PACE 1984; 7:389–394.

Hellend J: Pacemaker lead complications: Clinical significance and patient management. Medtronic News 1983; 13:8–14.

Hoffmann A, Jost M, Pfisterer M, et al: Persisting symptoms despite permanent pacing. Incidence, causes and follow-up. Chest 1984; 85:207–210.

Jacobs LJ, Kerzner JS, Diamond MA, et al: Myopotential inhibition of demand pacemakers: Detection by ambulatory electrocardiography. Am Heart J 1981; 101:346–347.

Judson P, Holmes DR, Baker WP: Evaluation of outpatient arrhythmias utilizing transtelephonic monitoring. Am Heart J 1979; 97:759–761.

Katzenberg CA, Marcus F, Heusinkveld R, et al: Pacemaker failure due to radiation therapy. PACE 1982; 5:156–159.

Laurens P: Nuclear-powered pacemakers: An eight-year clinical experience. PACE 1979; 2:356–360.

Lewis KB, Criley JM, Nelson RJ, et al: Early clinical experience with the rechargeable cardiac pacemaker. Ann Thorac Surg 1974; 18:490–493.

Lillehei RC, Romero LH, Beckman CB, et al: A new solid-state, long-life, lithium-powered pulse generator. Ann Thorac Surg 1974; 18:479–489.

MacGregor DC, Covvey HD, Noble EJ, et al: Computer-assisted reporting system for the follow-up of patients with cardiac pacemakers. PACE 1980; 3:568–588.

MacGregor DC, Noble EJ, Morrow JD, et al: Management of a pacemaker recall. J Thorac Cardiovasc Surg 1977; 74:657.

Mantini EI, Majors RK, Kennedy Jr, et al: A recommended protocol for pacemaker follow-up: An analysis of 1,705 implanted pacemakers. Ann Thorac Surg 1977; 24:62–67.

Mitsui T, Mizuno A, Hrsegawa T, et al: Atrial rate as an indicator for optimal pacing rate and the pacemaking syndrome. Ann Cardiol Angeiol 1971; 20:371.

Morse D, Fernandez J, Lemole G: A four year study of 123 programmable pacemakers. Chest 1976; 70:436.

Morse DP, Tesler UF, Lemole GM: The actual lifespan of pacemakers. Chest 1973; 64: 454.

Mymln D, Cuddy TE, Sinha SN, et al: Inhibition of demand pacemakers by skeletal muscle potentials. JAMA 1973; 223:527.

Parsonnet V: Cardiac pacing and pacemakers VII. Power sources for implantable pacemakers Part 1. Am Heart J 1977; 94:517–528.

Parsonnet V, Myers GH: Residual function of explanted pulse generators. AAMI 1973; 7:203–207.

Parsonnet V, Myers GH, Gilbert L, et al: Prediction of impending pacemaker failure in a pacemaker clinic. Am J Cardiol 1970; 25:311–319.

Pennock RS, Dreifus LS, Morse DP, et al: Cardiac pacemaker function. JAMA 1972; 222: 1379.

Rosenqvist M, Edhag O: Pacemaker dependance in transient high-grade atrioventricular block. PACE 1984; 7:63–70.

Ruben S: Sealed zinc-mercuric oxide cells for implantable cardiac pacemakers. Ann NY Acad Sci 1969; 167:627.

Rubenstein JJ, Laforet EG: Pacemakers runaway following intermittent output failure. PACE 1983; 6:645–647.

Schneider AA, Kulp JW: Lithium-iodine batteries for cardiac pacemakers. Med Electron 1978; 9:50–54.

Shaw GB, Evans A, Brewster GM, et al: Telephone monitoring of patients with pacemakers in the west of Scotland. Br Med J 1981; 283:127–129.

Sholder J, Levine PA, Mann BM, et al: Bidirectional telemetry and interrogation in cardiac pacing. In SS Barold, J Mugica (Eds): The Third Decade of Cardiac Pacing. Futura, Mount Kisco, 1982, pp 145–166.

Smyth NPD, Purdy DL, Sager D, et al: A new multiprogrammable isotopic powered cardiac pacemaker. PACE 1982; 5:761–767.

Smyth NPD, Millette M: The isotopic cardiac pacer: A ten year experience. PACE 1984; 7:82–89.

Steiner RM, Morse D: The radiology of cardiac pacemakers. JAMA 1978; 240:2574–2576.

Stone JM, Bhakta RD, Lutgen J: Dual chamber sequential pacing management of sinus node dysfunction: Advantages over single-chamber pacing. Am Heart J 1982; 104: 1319–1327.

Tyers GF, Foresman RA JR, Brownlee RR, et al: An automated tester for evaluation of pacemaker battery performance and reliability. J Surg Res 1974; 16:262–267.

Tyers GFO, Brownlee RR: The non-hermetically sealed pacemaker myth. Or, Navy-Ribicoff 22,000-FDA-Weinberger. J Thorac Cardiovas Surg 1976; 71:253.

van Gelder LM, El Gamal MI: False inhibition of an atrial demand pacemaker caused by an insulation defect in a polyurethane lead. PACE 1983; 6:834–839.

Venkataraman K, Bilitch M: Clinical experience with a programmable pacemaker. PACE 1980; 3:605–611.

Ward DE, Camm AJ, Spurrell RAJ: Ambulatory monitoring of the electrocardiogram: An important aspect of pacemaker surveillance. Biotelemetry 1977; 4:109–114.

Welti JJ: Pacemaker surveillance "A La Française": An attempt to detect faulty series of permanent pacemakers at an early stage. PACE 1978; 1:342–344.

Chapter 16

TELEMETRY

Seymour Furman

Telemetry is the transmission of data from an implanted pulse generator to an extracorporeal receiver. Unidirectional telemetry, i.e., from the pulse generator to the programmer, is being supplanted by bidirectional telemetry in which commands are transmitted from the programmer to the pulse generator and responses are transmitted from the generator to the programmer. Telemetry may be of great value in routine analysis of pacemaker function, during interpretation of complex electrocardiograms, and especially when troubleshooting a malfunction. Transmission is of two broad varieties: hardware and physiological data. It is broken down further into six categories:

1. hardware identification;
2. the electrogram (EGM);
3. ECG interpretation channels;
4. Memory contents including information placed into memory by the physician and memory of pacemaker (i.e., Holter) function;
5. Programmed settings;
6. Battery impedance and status, lead impedance, and battery drain and pulse generator output in charge per pulse and on a continuing basis.

Combinations of the above (Table I) are common.

It is also important to recognize that not all that is printed from a programmer need be telemetered. Because of the complexity of modern programming, programmers commonly deliver a tape with the programmed details printed out. Some printouts show only what the operator has selected and the programmer transmitted. There is no implication that the signals have been received or that pacemaker function has been changed. In that instance, independent verification, such as on an ECG and an oscilloscope or other instrument, is required to ascertain that programming has, indeed, occurred. In other instances the programmed commands and a telemetered confirmation will be printed. The operator must be aware of which data is a repetition of what has been entered into the programmer and what is actually telemetered from the implanted pacing system (Figure 1) (Table II).

Table I
Pacemaker Telemetry

1. Programmed pacemaker settings
2. Measured pacemaker stimulation parameters
3. Battery and lead status (current flow and impedances)
4. Pulse generator and electrode hardware data
5. Real-time pace sense events (ECG interpretation channel)
6. Electrogram (EGM)
7. Memory contents

```
           PACESETTER SYSTEMS INC.
              Version 1.5  - 1315

DATE:    DEC  6, 1984 11:49 AM

MODEL:  283  SERIAL:    14036

PATIENT: ...............................................

PHYSICIAN: .............................................


---------------- PROGRAMMED PARAMETERS ----------------

MODE  . . . . . . . . . . . . . . . . . . . . . . . DDD
RATE  . . . . . . . . . . . . . . . . . . . . . . .  70 PPM

VENTRICULAR CHANNEL:
  REFRACTORY . . . . . . . . . . . . . . . . . . . 325 MSEC
  PULSE WIDTH . . . . . . . . . . . . . . . . . . . 0.5 MSEC
  PULSE AMPLITUDE . . . . . . . . . . . . . . . . . 5.0 VOLTS
  SENSITIVITY . . . . . . . . . . . . . . . . . . . 3.0 MVOLT

ATRIAL CHANNEL:
  REFRACTORY . . . . . . . . . . . . . . . . . . . 325 MSEC
  PULSE WIDTH . . . . . . . . . . . . . . . . . . . 0.5 MSEC
  PULSE AMPLITUDE . . . . . . . . . . . . . . . . . 5.0 VOLTS
  SENSITIVITY . . . . . . . . . . . . . . . . . . . 1.2 MVOLT

AV INTERVAL . . . . . . . . . . . . . . . . . . . 190 MSEC

MAX. TRACK RATE . . . . . . . . . . . . . . . . . 110 PPM

BLANKING PERIOD . . . . . . . . . . . . . . . . . 38 MSEC

MAGNET:  OFF


------------------- MEASURED DATA -------------------

PACEMAKER RATE . . . . . . . . . . . . . . . . 70.0 PPM

MAGNET RATE . . . . . . . . . . . . . . . . . . 80.0 PPM

CHANNEL MEASUREMENTS:

                VENTRICLE      ATRIUM
  PULSE VOLTAGE    4.7          4.7   VOLTS
  PULSE CURRENT    8.0          9.8   MAMPS
  PULSE ENERGY      19           24   µJOULES
  PULSE CHARGE       4            5   µCOULOMBS
  LEAD IMPEDANCE   588          480   OHMS

BATTERY DATA: ( W.G.8074 - NOM.2.3 AHR )
  IMPEDANCE . . . . . . . . . . . . . . . . . . 1.0 KOHMS
  VOLTAGE . . . . . . . . . . . . . . . . . . . 2.71 VOLTS
  CURRENT . . . . . . . . . . . . . . . . . . . 25 µAMPS
```

Figure 1. *A printout of hardware data from a dual-chamber pacemaker lists the output, sensitivity, and interval settings that have been programmed. These are not actually telemetered, rather they repeat the programmed settings. The telemetered data is indicated as "measured" data.*

Table II
Programmed Pacemaker Settings

---

1. Mode
2. Rate
3. Pulse amplitude, duration voltage
4. Sensitivity
5. Refractory period

6. Hysteresis
7. AV delay
8. Upper and lower rates
9. Sensor function

HARDWARE IDENTIFICATION

Hardware identification may include battery status, battery voltage and impedance and lead impedance, the model and serial number of the pulse generator, date of manufacture, and date of implant (if placed into memory). Hardware that has been identified on x-ray can be identified in more detail, often including setting of mode of operation, output, sensitivity, etc., by subsequent telemetry.

Hardware telemetry can be useful in determining the cause of malfunction. Several manufacturers allow telemetry of lead impedance during analysis of pacemaker function so that diagnosis of lead deterioration or fracture can be supported noninvasively. If records of lead impedance, measured intraoperatively at implant or via telemetry early after implant, are available, then telemetric interpretation of impedance increase, indicating lead fracture, or decrease, indicating insulation disruption, can be determined before revision is undertaken (Figure 2). Battery depletion can be indicated by a decrease in the magnetic pacer rate on ECG or by an increase in the impedance of a lithium battery measured telemetrically (Table III).

Table III
Pulse Generator and Electrode
Hardware Data

---

1. Battery voltage
2. Battery current drain
3. Battery impedance
4. Lead/electrode impedance

```
        QUANTUM                    QUANTUM
     PACING SYSTEM              PACING SYSTEM
    INTERMEDICS, INC.          INTERMEDICS, INC.
 ------------------------    ------------------------
 DATE   10-22-84            DATE   07-31-85
 PATIENT                    PATIENT
     W      , M                 W        W
 PROGRAMMED SETTINGS        PROGRAMMED SETTINGS
    AMPLITUDE                  AMPLITUDE
        2                          2
    PULSE WIDTH                PULSE WIDTH
        2                          2
    SENSITIVITY                SENSITIVITY
        4                          4
    RATE                       RATE
        7                          MAGNET
 ------------------------    ------------------------
 PROGRAMMED TELEMETRY       MAGNET TELEMETRY
 MEASUREMENTS               MEASUREMENTS

 --PACER PARAMETERS-         --PACER PARAMETERS--

    RATE                       RATE
     72.2 PPM                   86.2 PPM

    INTERVAL                   INTERVAL
     830 MSEC                   696 MSEC

    PULSE WIDTH                PULSE WIDTH
     .31 MSEC                   .64 MSEC

    PULSE AMPLITUDE            PULSE AMPLITUDE
     5.47 VOLT                  5.56 VOLT

    OUTPUT CURRENT            OUTPUT CURRENT
     11.4 MILLIAMPS             2.3 MILLIAMPS

 --LEAD PARAMETERS--         --LEAD PARAMETERS--

    LEAD IMPEDANCE            LEAD IMPEDANCE
     454 OHMS                   2360 OHMS

    CHARGE DELIVERED          CHARGE DELIVERED
     3.50 UCOLS                 1.50 UCOULS

    ENERGY DELIVERED          ENERGY DELIVERED
     18.3 UJOULES              8.3 UJOULES

 --BATTERY PARAMETERS--      --BATTERY PARAMETERS--

    BATTERY VOLTAGE           BATTERY VOLTAGE
     2.8 VOLTS                  2.80 VOLTS

    BATTERY CURRENT           BATTERY CURRENT

     14.4 UAMPS                 10.3 UAMPS

    BATTERY IMPEDANCE         BATTERY IMPEDANCE
     1.0 KOHMS                  1.0 KOHMS
```

Figure 2.   *A telemetric diagnosis of lead fracture can be made when the lead impedance increases greatly from its stable value. In this instance, the lead impedance on 10–22–84 was 454 ohms, on 7–31–85 it was 2360 ohms. Lead fracture was confirmed on x-ray. Note that the impedance reduced output current, battery current drain, and the energy delivered. The changes in rate, interval, and pulse width were not relevant.*

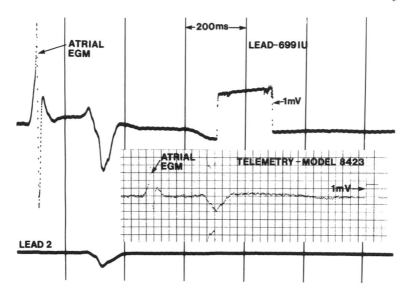

Figure 3.   *The atrial electrogram, telemetered from a single-chamber unipolar pacemaker is illustrated and compared to the electrogram derived directly from the lead at a bandwidth of 0.1-2000 Hz. Despite the restricted telemetry frequency response, the overall quality and timing of the atrial EGM can be determined.*

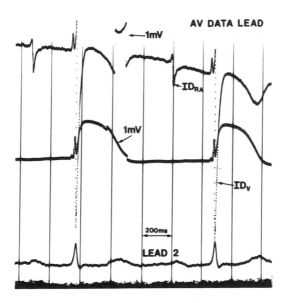

Figure 4.   *An AV data lead has terminals in the ventricle and in the atrium in a single lead and is able to record atrial and ventricular events simultaneously on the same channel. As there is also a ventricular electrode for conventional sensing and stimulation, three electrogram channels are possible.* **ABOVE:** The AV data channel with atrial and ventricular electrograms. **MIDDLE:** The ventricular electrogram from the lead tip. **BELOW:** Lead 2.

ELECTROGRAM

The electrogram is an especially important aspect of data transmission as it indicates the quality of the signal the pacemaker senses. It also determines the software decisions of the generator. The intrinsic deflection may be readily visible and indicates the time of sensing of antegrade and retrograde events and allows a decision concerning the quality of sensing and pacing function (Figure 3). The two major defects of EGM data transmission are the restricted response of the radio frequency link, which is limited to approximately 300 Hz, and the electrocardiograph upon which the data is printed, which may be further limited to 100 Hz (Figure 4). Both limitations reduce data quality. Only a few systems can telemeter atrial and ventricular electrogram channels simultaneously (Figure 5). Often this is accomplished by splitting the frequency response in such a way that the transmission frequency for each channel is no more than 100–150 Hz, which severely limits the quality of the electrogram (Figures 6 and 7). For systems that cannot transmit atrial and ventricular electrograms simultaneously, important relationships between atrial and ventricular function are not readily discernible via telemetry except as a far-field signal on either the atrial or the ventricular telemetered electrogram. ECG interpretation channels, therefore, may have an even greater capacity for troubleshooting, as the activity of both atrial and ventricular channels is indicated, although in a format that indicates pacer and cardiac activity by a variety of coded lines. Unfortunately each ECG interpretation channel presentation is different for each manufacturer so that anyone who uses hardware provided by several different manufacturers will need to learn to read and interpret several different ECG interpretation channels. Even

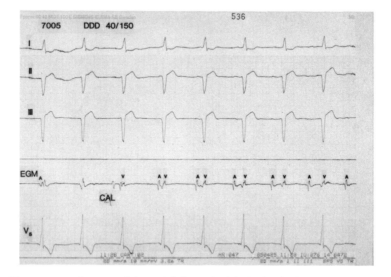

Figure 5.   *Electrogram telemetry of the atrial channel with the far-field ventricular EGM recorded simultaneously. The surface leads give the impression that AV conduction with first-degree AV block is present. The atrial EGM clearly demonstrates the lack of relationship between atrial and ventricular events, i.e., complete AV block.*

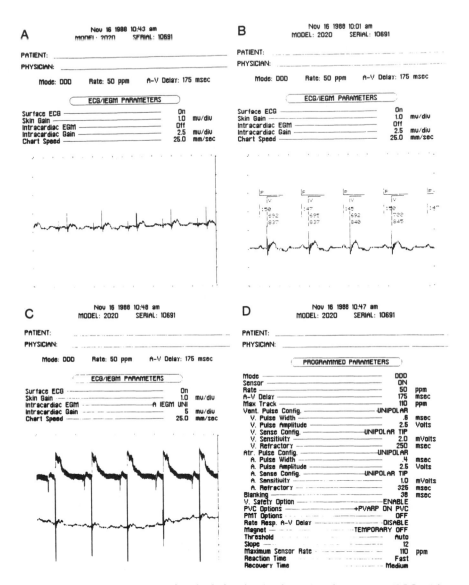

Figure 6. *Four programmer tapes after dual-chamber implantation show: A. An ECG with spontaneous atrial events and ventricular stimulation and response. B. An ECG with timing indications printed on each P-QRS event, with the duration of the AV delay, the VA interval and the VV interval all indicated. C. The atrial EGM during atrial sensing and ventricular pacing. The atrial EGM is about 5 mV in amplitude and is followed by the very large ventricular channel stimulus. D. A final printout of all pacemaker settings.*

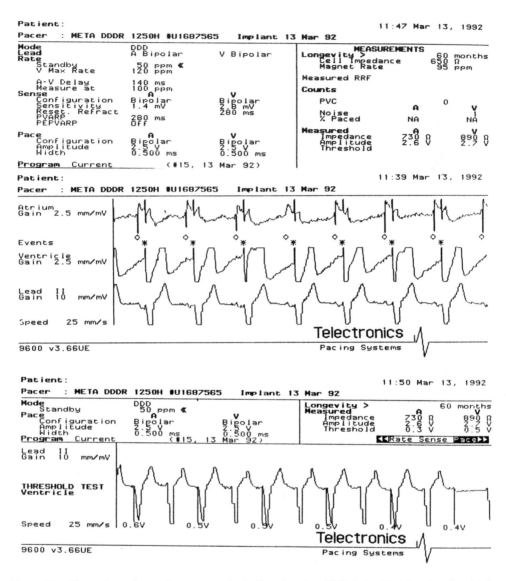

Figure 7. *Three-channel recordings can evaluate the telemetered EGM. In this telemetry the atrial and ventricular channels are inscribed simultaneously with the ECG. Other data such as lead impedance and estimated battery longevity at the output settings (output voltage, pulse duration and stimulation rate) are indicated as well.*

for the same manufacturer some approaches have been introduced, then abandoned, and a new approach begun.

While the transmission of the electrogram is an important capability and will assume greater importance in the future, some telemetric EGM transmissions are more useful than others. (Figures 8A, and 8B). Telemetry of the electrogram may allow calibration and determination of its amplitude. While this may be broadly useful, the bandwidth of pulse generator electrogram telemetry capability may not be the same as that of it's sensing channel so that accurate determination of the sensitivity threshold may not be possible with this mechanism. In usual circumstances this discrepancy may have little importance, but in marginal situations the programming physician or technician should be wary about drawing too careful a correlation between telemetered electrogram amplitude and sensitivity setting.

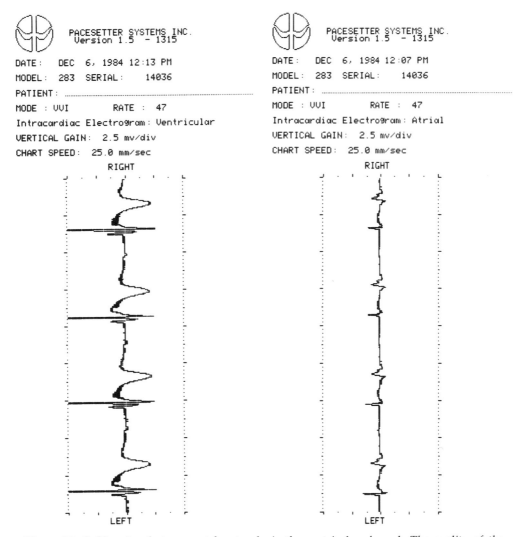

Figure 8A (left). *An electrogram telemetered via the ventricular channel. The quality of the signal can be interpreted as can its amplitude, in this instance about 7.5 mV. The P wave can be discerned as a small distant signal.* **B (right).** *The electrogram telemetered via the atrial channel. The atrial intrinsic deflection is followed by a far-field QRS complex approximately 250 ms later. The amplitude of the atrial electrogram is approximately 2.5 mV.*

Table IV
Real-time Pace and Sense Events
(ECG Interpretation Channel)

1. Sensing
2. Pacing
At atrial and/or ventricular levels

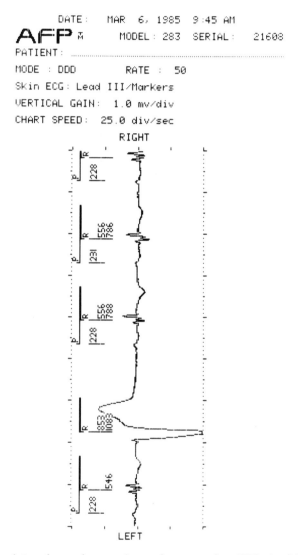

Figure 9. *Timing intervals can be superimposed on a surface ECG, in this instance lead III simultaneously with the various intervals. The first P wave is sensed 228 ms before the QRS complex. The first conducted QRS is sensed near its beginning on the surface, but the VPC is sensed later within the deflection. The escape intervals between events and the refractory intervals are clearly indicated.*

ECG INTERPRETATION CHANNEL

ECG interpretation (Marker Channel™, Main Timing Events, etc.) channels are designed to indicate the pacing and sensing function of single- and dual-chamber pacemakers (Table IV). The instant of sensing or pacing is indicated with associated events, such as the onset of alert and refractory and safety pacing intervals, by a mark on the programmer printout. As sensing occurs at the intrinsic deflection, the mark indicates the timing of those events (Figure 9). ECG interpretation channels (which do not telemeter the electrogram) can indicate the relationship between atrial and ventricular sensing and stimulus emission (Figure 10). As the mark is an artifact of the pacemaker sensing and output circuits, an indicator of pacemaker response to cardiac function exists. In some telemetry, an artifactual ECG will have marks on it giving the impression of an actual ECG. A ladder diagram also exists in conjunction with an ECG, which indicates, much as a conventional ladder, the relationship between atrial and

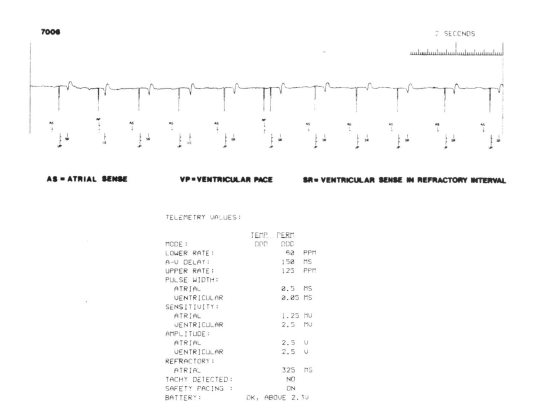

AS = ATRIAL SENSE   VP = VENTRICULAR PACE   SR = VENTRICULAR SENSE IN REFRACTORY INTERVAL

```
TELEMETRY VALUES:

                      TEMP   PERM
MODE :                DDD    DDD
LOWER RATE :                 60    PPM
A-V DELAY :                  150   MS
UPPER RATE :                 125   PPM
PULSE WIDTH:
   ATRIAL                    0.5   MS
   VENTRICULAR               0.05  MS
SENSITIVITY:
   ATRIAL                    1.25  MV
   VENTRICULAR               2.5   MV
AMPLITUDE:
   ATRIAL                    2.5   V
   VENTRICULAR               2.5   V
REFRACTORY:
   ATRIAL                    325   MS
TACHY DETECTED:              NO
SAFETY PACING :              ON
BATTERY:              OK, ABOVE 2.3V
```

Figure 10. *ECG interpretation channels can indicate what the pacemaker senses when pacing occurs and the relationships between the various sensed and paced events. In this illustration, atrial sensing and ventricular sensing are normal, ventricular pulse duration is below threshold of capture. QRS complexes result from conduction following a spontaneous P wave that is normally sensed. The QRS complexes fall into the ventricular refractory period after the ventricular stimulus. They are unsensed and do not begin a timing cycle.*

ventricular events, adding the appropriate alert, refractory, and blanking intervals (Figure 11).

A variety of different ECG interpretation channels, some wholly artifactual, others with telemetered EGMs or ECGs, exist. In each instance it is important to distinguish whether the apparent signal (ECG or EGM) is artifactual or real.

The mark placed on a telemetry printout can indicate a sensed atrial or ventricular event that starts a pacemaker cycle or one that occurs too early or too late in the timing cycle to begin a timing event. It can also indicate a stimulus emission from either ventricular or atrial channel, which, if not reflected on the ECG, can suggest a lead fracture (Figure 12). As sense and pace markers exist for both channels (in the dual-chamber pacemaker), the exact relationship between the two is shown, and in some systems, can be recorded simultaneously with the ECG and clarify the ECG and pacemaker function. ECG interpretation channels clearly indicate which electrocardiographic events are being sensed properly and which start a timing cycle (Figure 13). The mark indicates which events do not begin such a cycle and which are unsensed. The persistence of retrograde conduction can be recognized and quantified, and data used to determine the appropriate duration of a programmed atrial refractory interval. Most of the EGM and ECG interpretation channels print out on programmer paper tape. This defect will be corrected as printers and multichannel electrocardiographs become available that will allow input from the programmers either via a computer link or by direct input. However, even as of this writing (October 1992) such a capability does not exist. In some the electrogram can be printed out on a multichannel recorder, while the ECG interpretation channel can only be printed on programmer tape (Figure 14).

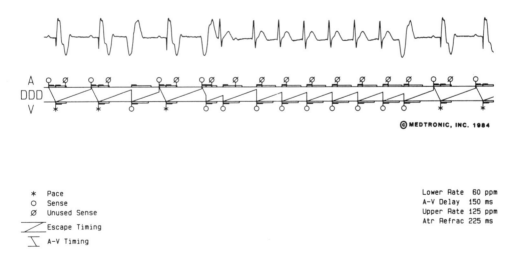

©MEDTRONIC, INC. 1984

*	Pace		Lower Rate	60 ppm
O	Sense		A-V Delay	150 ms
Ø	Unused Sense		Upper Rate	125 ppm
	Escape Timing		Atr Refrac	225 ms
	A-V Timing			

Figure 11. An automatic programmer-drawn ladder diagram is a useful telemetric indication of pacemaker function in which pace and sense events, and atrial and ventricular refractories can be indicated much as in a hand-drawn ladder diagram. This is a simulated ECG and does not represent actual cardiac events. A real ECG must be available to correlate with the ladder diagram findings.

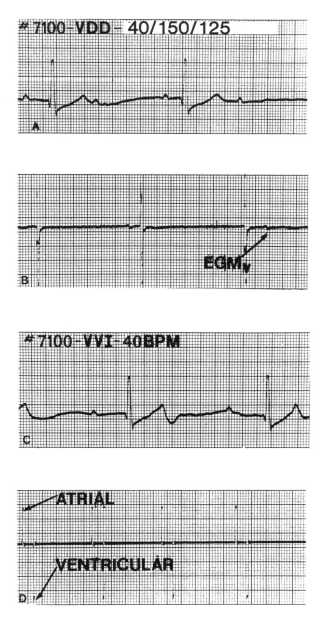

Figure 12. *A patient with complete heart block and an implanted VDD (atrial synchronous, ventricular inhibited) was seen without pacemaker stimuli on the electrocardiogram. A. The ECG is in the VVI mode programmed to a rate of 40 bpm. There is no evidence of pacemaker activity. B. Telemetry of the ventricular EGM shows only a small deflection and ventricular stimuli not seen on the ECG at a rate of 40 bpm. C. Programming the VDD mode with an AV interval of 150 ms, a lower rate limit of 40 bpm, and an upper rate limit of 125 bpm again shows no evidence of pacemaker activity. D. ECG interpretation channel telemetry shows normal sensing of atrial events, the absence of sensing of ventricular events, emission of ventricular stimuli at the programmed AV interval without visibility on the ECG, and the absence of ventricular capture. The most likely fit for these findings was ventricular lead fracture, which was subsequently radiographically confirmed.*

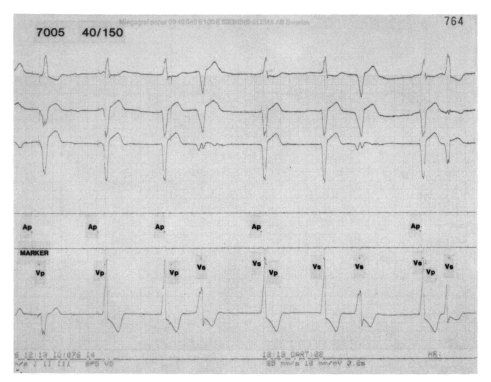

Figure 13. *Intermittent failure of atrial sensing and ineffective atrial stimuli are clearly indicated on the ECG interpretation channel. Three spontaneous ventricular events V_s are properly sensed. Ventricular complexes five and eight are sensed after the atrial stimulus during the safety pacing interval. Two ventricular marks occur, the first V_s for ventricular sensing, the second V_p for the "safety" stimulus. No ventricular stimulus V_p clearly captures the ventricle.*

MEMORY CONTENTS

Memory contents fall into two subcategories: data placed into memory by the physician and that resulting from pacemaker activity. The latter category can be further subdivided into activity generated by stimulation and that of sensed events (Table V).

<table>
<tr><td colspan="2" align="center">Table V
Measured Impulse Stimulation Parameters</td></tr>
<tr><td>1. Interval (rate)</td><td>4. Voltage</td></tr>
<tr><td>2. Duration</td><td>5. Charge and energy</td></tr>
<tr><td>3. Current</td><td></td></tr>
</table>

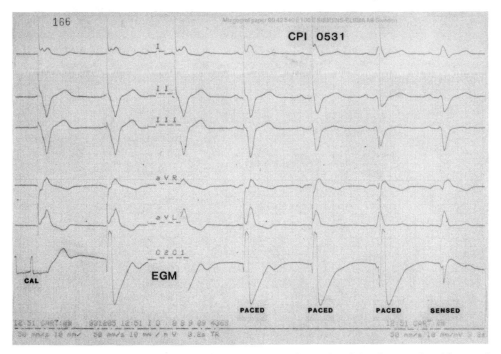

Figure 14. *Telemetry of the single-chamber electrogram is best printed simultaneously with several other electrocardiographic channels. In this display of five surface leads and the electrogram only, the last is an unpaced EGM. The CAL is 5 mV and the spontaneous EGM is, therefore, approximately 5 mV in amplitude and occurs late in the simultaneously recorded surface leads. The preceding EGM is a fusion beat with the stimulus occurring earlier than the intrinsic deflection of the ventricular depolarization.*

Data Placed Into Memory

Several pulse generators have a memory into which coded data can be entered. This data includes lead model and threshold, electrogram amplitude, and pacemaker settings at implant, medications the patient is consuming, and the indication for pacemaker implant. If the system is used, all of this data is entered by a coding arrangement provided by the manufacturer and can be read later from the pulse generator by the programmer. As there is no commonly accepted coding for different conditions, this data may be useful for the physician with the appropriate programmer, but less valuable should the patient visit another physician.

Data Derived During Pacemaker Operation

Several pacemakers can store information concerning pacemaker activity. Categories can consists of: (a) atrial paced beats; (b) ventricular paced beats; (c) atrial and/or ventricular sensed beats; (d) ventricular premature contractions, which are defined as spontaneous ventricular events not preceded by a sensed or paced atrial event, and atrial premature contractions defined as atrial events that are sensed at specific times of the cardiac cycle during which atrial activity is not anticipated (Figure 15) (Table VI).

```
283-01-017019                    AUG 29 '85 09:22 AM   •
    MODE SELECTION                    DDD              I
                                                       II
PACING RATE                            50  PPM         I
PACING INTERVAL                      1200  MSEC        E
VENTRICULAR TRACKING LIMIT            100  PPM         P
FALLBACK RATE                         100  PPM         N
A - V DELAY                           250  MSEC        E
                                                       D
                        ATRIAL   VENTRICULAR           I
POST VENT REFRACTORY      315         200  MSEC        C
PULSE WIDTH               0.45        0.45 MSEC        S
PULSE AMPLITUDE           5.4         5.4  VOLTS
SENSITIVITY               .8          3    MV          I
                                                       II
    •         INQUIRE CONFIRMED                        • •
```

```
283-01-017019                    AUG 29 '85 09:24 AM   •
            COSMOS TELEMETRY DATA                      I
PACING RATE                            50  PPM         II
PACING INTERVAL                      1,200 MSEC        I
AVERAGE CELL VOLTAGE                   2.72 VOLTS      E
CELL IMPEDANCE                         2.97 KOHMS      P
                        ATRIAL   VENTRICULAR           N
SENSITIVITY              0.8          3    MV          E
LEAD IMPEDANCE           333         343  OHMS         D
PULSE AMPLITUDE          5.20        5.29 VOLTS        I
PULSE WIDTH              0.45        0.45 MSEC         C
OUTPUT CURRENT          13.4        13.8  MA           S
ENERGY DELIVERED        27.4        29.8  UJ
CHARGE DELIVERED         6.03        6.21 UC           I
    NOTE: DURING TRANSMISSION, PULSE GENERATOR        II
    REVERTS TO ASYNCHRONOUS PACING AT PROGRAMMED      C
    RATE AND MODE (SINGLE- OR DUAL-CHAMBER).          .
```

```
283-01-017019                    AUG 29 '85 09:22 AM   •
    DIAGNOSTIC DATA ( CARDIAC CYCLES )                 I
                                                       II
EVENT COUNTERS LAST CLEARED.. JUN 26, 03:00 PM         T
NO. OF PREMATURE VENTRICULAR EVENTS.... 15,688         E
NO. OF ATRIAL SENSE EVENTS FOLLOWED                    P
    BY VENTRICULAR SENSE EVENT...... 3,488,825         M
NO. OF ATRIAL SENSE EVENTS FOLLOWED                    E
    BY VENTRICULAR PACE EVENT............. 581         D
NO. OF ATRIAL PACE EVENTS FOLLOWED                     I
    BY VENTRICULAR SENSE EVENT.......... 5,436         C
NO. OF ATRIAL PACE EVENTS FOLLOWED                     S
    BY VENTRICULAR PACE EVENT.......... 1,061
PERCENT PACED - ATRIUM.................... 0%          I
PERCENT PACED - VENTRICLE................. 0%          II
            DISPLAY MISCELLANEOUS EVENTS               C
                                                       •
```

Figure 15. *Printout of telemetry from dual-chamber model 283–01. The top section consists of pacemaker settings determined by the INQUIRE command. The middle section is the telemetered hardware data. The lower section (Diagnostic data) is that of the pacemaker memory contents of data derived during pacer function. As the event counters are CLEARED and reset when read, it is possible to determine the number of events during the interval from the past clearing of the memory registry. In this instance, the pacemaker was largely inhibited, but the atrium was stimulated 5436 times with AV conduction inhibiting ventricular output. Other events are as indicated.*

Table VI
Memory Contents

A. Patient Data:
   1. I.D. number
   2. Indications for pacing
   3. Medication, etc.

B. Pacemaker Data:
   1. Type and location of electrode
   2. Stimulation thresholds
   3. Model and serial number
   4. Date of implant, etc.

C. Processed Data:
   1. Ratio of paced to sensed beats
   2. Absolute number of paced beats

This data can be valuable if implantation is accomplished with less than absolute evidence of AV block or of sinus arrest or if atrial or ventricular ectopic activity occurs. Once the pacemaker is implanted it can be set at a rate sufficiently low so that if a stimulus is emitted, it can be assumed that pacing is necessary. Coupled beats and runs of sensed tachycardia can be counted both as individual events and runs of tachycardia. All of the data recorded for some pulse generators is numeric. P waves and QRS complexes are not recorded individually. The compromises made in diagnosis of various arrhythmias do not allow the recording of the QRS complexes or P waves. This is a major defect as the reading of the actual ECG or EGM is of great value. This Holter capability will be very useful when it exists, but as the digitized ECG consumes very large amounts of computer memory, such Holter recordings are unlikely to be available soon, although the progressive development of high capacity computer memory chips will eventually provide such capability.

Evolution of this variety of telemetry has produced an event counter telemetry that can be displayed graphically and is especially useful for rate modulated pacemakers. For example, a rate modulated pacemaker may be programmed to a presumed satisfactory sensor setting. Holter monitoring of the pacemaker response to a given exercise is useful but costly and may be especially delayed in data availability so that it becomes difficult to make accurate assessments and adjustments. Event memory and telemetry can record a brief period of exercise and provide a graphic display of the sensor response to exercise. As the response is in the pulse generator memory it may be played back and analyzed promptly, in time to reprogram and retest. (See Figure 28, Chapter 11.)

In some pulse generators the sensor may be in the passive mode so that its activity is recorded into memory but it does not actually affect the cardiac rate. Once again such a capability may allow programming of sensor function without altering the actual pacing rate. For example, an excessively sensitive or responsive sensor may be evaluated without causing an excessive pacemaker, and therefore cardiac, rate. A graphic display of sensor activity will thus yield sensor function while allowing control by the spontaneous cardiac rhythm (Figure 16).

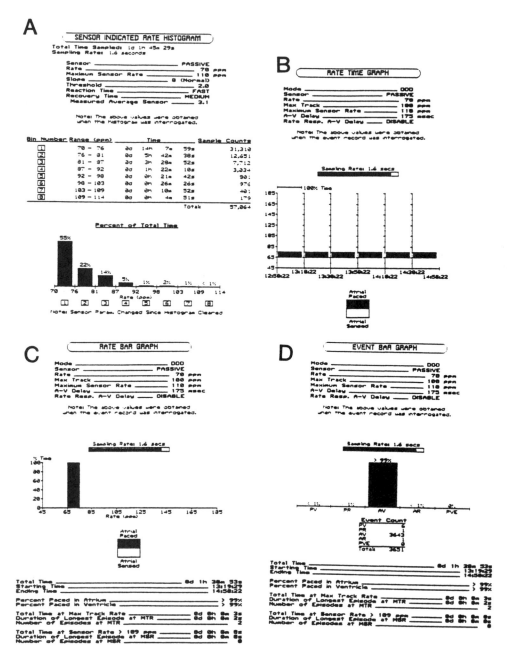

Figure 16. Telemetry of memory of paced events (Holter capability) can become relatively elaborate. These printouts are from a DDDR unit. In this instance the recording was for a period of 1 day, 1 hour, 45 minutes and 29 seconds, at a sampling frequency of 1.6 seconds. A. With the sensor in the passive mode, i.e., not driving pulse generator output, the sensor determined a rate of 70–76 bpm (55% of the time), i.e., in excess of 14 hours and 7 minutes. The sensor-determined rate was between 76–81 bpm 22% of the time. B. Because the sensor was passive and the atrial rate was slower than the lower rate limit, the pacemaker paced the atrium all of the time during the six intervals sampled. C. This bar graph is of the proportion of time the atrium was actually paced at each rate. As the sensor was passive and this recording was made over 1 hour and 38 minutes (between 13:19:29 and 14:58:22) during special observation, all atrial pacing was at a rate of 70 bpm. D. This bar graph indicates the proportion of pacing or sensing both chambers, or pacing one and sensing the other. AV = atrial and ventricular pace; PV = atrial sense/ventricular pace; PR = atrial and ventricular sense; AR = atrial pace/ventricular sense; PVE = premature ventricular event. In this graph an excess of 99% of all beats were atrial and ventricular paced.

UTILITY OF TELEMETRY

Telemetry is useful in four broad categories: (1) derivation of device settings and evidence of lead and battery integrity, including the output settings of the generator and additional data such as lead and battery impedance and battery voltage, indicating remaining longevity of the unit; (2) memory of operational events; (3) definition and interpretation of complex electrocardiograms; and (4) troubleshooting. As a relatively recent addition to pacemaker technology, telemetry capabilities have not been fully explored and innovations can be anticipated as the electronic base of telemetry becomes more sophisticated.

The four functions are partially restrained because of the absence of a means of transmitting, recording, and displaying data. Each manufacturer uses a recording device and unique language. Some are relatively easy to operate, with a recording that is rapid and readily interpretable, while others are arcane. The hard copy printers are often slow and present a barrier to use rather than providing assistance. Still, even single-chamber modern pulse generators are so complex and programmable in so many different ways that automatic transmission of data for record keeping purposes is very useful. When programming a modern six function (a common number of functions for a multiprogrammable model) single-chamber pulse generator, a single printout of the new programmed setting is preferable to a two person team (one to program and the other to transcribe data).

Telemetry of battery impedance and voltage is useful, but the availability of a magnetic rate that is correlated with battery status (a technique widely used for two decades) is almost as good and has the advantages of being well understood and interpreted on an ECG alone, requiring only the use of a magnet, which is more widely available than a programmer. Magnet rate related to battery voltage is universally used and understood so that magnet application represents a variety of universal telemetry. Unfortunately, different pulse generators have different magnet rates indicating normal battery depletion or requiring elective pulse generator replacement so that additional information is required. In practice it is easier to derive magnet rate data via transtelephonic monitoring with a magnet and a pulse generator magnetic rate than with telemetry of data, which must be done in the patient's presence rather than from a remote location. An ECG interpretation channel indicating the instant of sensing and refractory and alert intervals is useful even in a single-chamber pulse generator and much more useful in a dual-chamber generator.

Telemetry of memory function such as the number of times paced and the number of sensed events may be useful, but until there is a clear indication from the generator that a recorded paced event was indeed in response to need, the data will be of limited value. This "Holter" function will await the availability of adequate computer memory to allow the recording of an ECG of reasonable facsimile within the pulse generator and its telemetry to an external recorder. The widespread use of such telemetry will also probably await agreement on interfaces for the production of hard copy.

Printing of programmed settings to allow rapid knowledge of pulse generator function and the use of ECG interpretation channels is important. While useful in single-chamber pulse generators, both are far more useful in dual-chamber pacing. While six programmable functions (and additional rate modulation functions) are common in single-chamber pulse generators, many more functions and modes of operation are needed in dual-chamber generators. The relationship between events on the electrocardiogram and the intervals between atrial and ventricular events, refractory and alert intervals, and upper and lower rate limits can only be recorded in a comprehensible fashion by a hard copy indication of the interplay between the pacemaker and the heart. It is in this area that telemetry of ECG interpretation channels is useful. With increasing complexity of the device, certainly when pacemakers are used more extensively

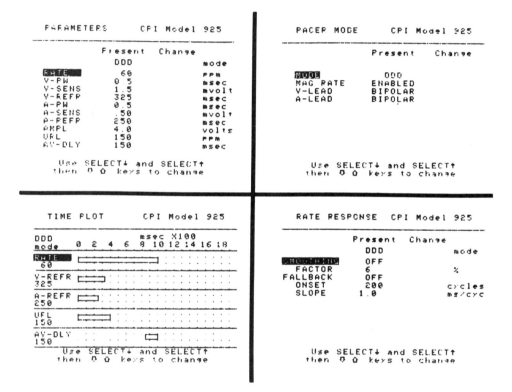

Figure 17. Data available from CPI Model 925 "DELTA" programmer pacemaker printout. The upper left corner of the figure displays the parameters at which the pacemaker is currently programmed. In the upper right corner is a screen indicating whether or not the magnet rate is enabled and if the leads are functioning in a unipolar or bipolar mode. In the lower left corner is a display of the rate, ventricular refractory period, atrial refractory period, upper rate limit, and AV delay plotted in a bar graph to allow the use of a graphic display of the relationship of the various programmed intervals and how a change in one interval affects another programmed change. The lower right corner is the final screen of telemetered information and reflects whether or not smoothing and/or fallback is being utilized.

for tachycardia management, telemetry will be more widely available and more widely used (Figure 17).

SPECIFIC TELEMETRY FINDINGS

1. Physiological findings relevant to the conditions for production of endless loop tachycardia may be determined by ventricular pacing and telemetry of the atrial response (Figure 18).

V-A Retrograde Conduction Evaluation

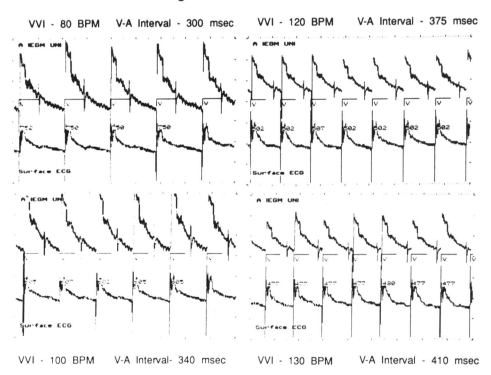

Figure 18. *Evaluation of retrograde conduction after a pacemaker has been implanted can be readily done with adequate telemetry. In this instance telemetry was of the atrial channel EGM during ventricular pacing at rates of 80, 100, 120, and 130 bpm. Each pair is of the ECG below and the atrial EGM above. The large stimulus deflection of each pair is of the ventricular stimulus while the smaller following line is the atrial EGM. The interval between the two is readily determined. Progressive prolongation of the VA interval with increased rate of stimulation occurred, although VA conduction was retained even at a rate of 130 bpm. Annotation of rate and VA interval was added to the telemetry.*

2. Pathological findings associated with rapid and irregular DDD pacemaker response (Figures 19 and 20).

3. Misinterpretations may occur or reversible malfunction may be detected (Figure 21).

4. Lead fracture or insulation deterioration is readily determined with specific telemetry data (Figures 22 and 23).

5. ECG interpretation, difficult on conventional ECG, may be elucidated by an ECG and a simultaneous ECG interpretation channel (Figures 24–27).

6. The proper sensitivity setting to sense atrial events and reject far-field ventricular events may be assisted (Figure 28).

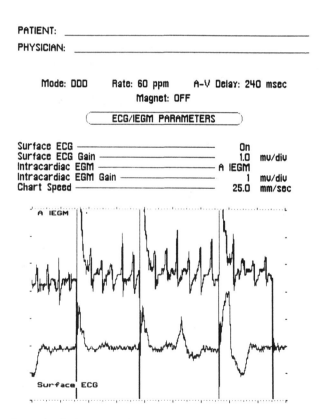

Figure 19. *A patient who had apparently developed atrial fibrillation underwent telemetry to confirm that impression. The ECG is below, the EGM above, the recording at 25 mm/s. Telemetry was of the atrial channel only, although ventricular events are often readily sensed via the atrial channel.*

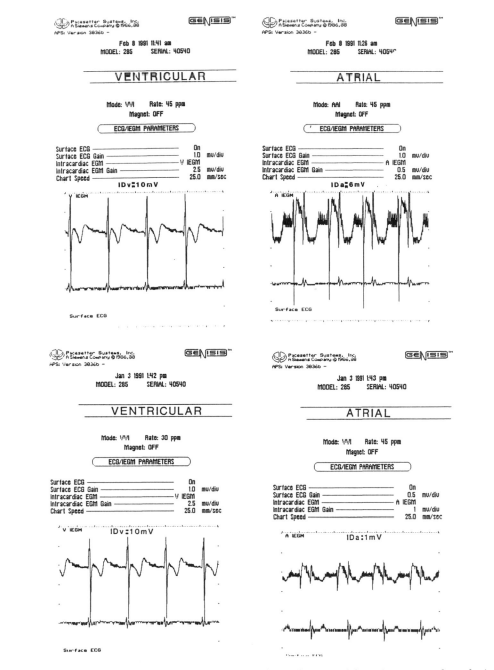

Figure 20. *A patient with a dual-chamber pacemaker and poor atrial sensing was evaluated. A. Ventricular EGM telemetry revealed an amplitude of approximately 10 mV. The atrial EGM was about 1 mV—equal in amplitude to the far-field ventricular EGM. B. After operative revision, in which the atrial lead was repositioned, the untouched ventricular lead telemetered an EGM equal to that preoperatively. The atrial EGM had increased in amplitude to 3 mV, the far-field ventricular EGM remained at 1 mV. The atrial EGM was now satisfactory for consistent atrial sensing.*

```
MODEL 9710A PROGRAMMER/9743 MEMORY MOD
PATIENT: _____
PHYSICIAN: _____
MODEL SELECTED: ELITE 7074
PACER SER. NO.  YE2110807


PRINTER ON AT  TUE 02 XXX 83 01:57:50
TELEMETRY VALUES:


                      TEMP  PERM

MODE:                 VOO   VVI
RATE:                 65    50    PPM
PULSE WIDTH:
   VENTRICULAR              0.42  MS
SENSITIVITY:
   VENTRICULAR              2.5   MV
AMPLITUDE:
   VENTRICULAR              4.2   V
VENTRICULAR BLANKING:      24    MS
SAFETY PACING:             ON
A. SENSE CONFIGURATION:    BIPOLAR
V. SENSE CONFIGURATION:    BIPOLAR
AV PACE CONFIGURATION:     BIPOLAR
PACER SER. NO.:            YE2110807
BATTERY:                   REPLACE PACER
CHECK MAGNET RATE TO CONFIRM EOL.
```

```
PROGRAMMING BATTERY RESET    02:24:00
RESET-PACER-BATT-STATUS CONFIRMED
VALUES JUST PROGRAMMED:
PACER BATT STATUS:    RESET



TELEMETRY VALUES:


                      TEMP  PERM

MODE:                 VOO   VVI
RATE:                 85    100⁻  PPM
PULSE WIDTH:
   VENTRICULAR              0.42  MS
SENSITIVITY:
   VENTRICULAR              3.0   MV
AMPLITUDE:
   VENTRICULAR              5.0   V
VENTRICULAR BLANKING:      24    MS
SAFETY PACING:             ON
A. SENSE CONFIGURATION:    BIPOLAR
V. SENSE CONFIGURATION:    BIPOLAR
AV PACE CONFIGURATION:     BIPOLAR
PACER SER. NO.:            YE2110807
BATTERY:                   OK
```

Figure 21.   *Telemetry data may be misleading unless it can be interpreted properly. The telemetry data shown was derived immediately after implantation while the patient remained on the procedure table. (Left) The telemetry was of low battery voltage (end of life) with the recommendation that the generator be replaced. The unit had been shipped in the cold and had entered the low voltage, battery depletion mode. Once reprogrammed, telemetry indicated normal pacemaker function. This sequence is diagnostic of a cold lithium iodine cell.*

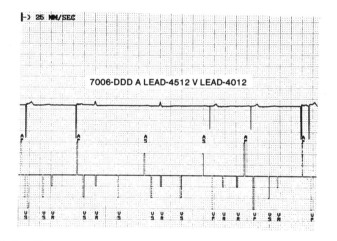

Figure 22.   *Marker Channel™ analysis of electrocardiographic pacemaker malfunction with no x-ray findings. The ECG is above showing satisfactory atrial pacing and sensing via a model 4512 atrial lead. Ventricular lead function, model 4012, is abnormal on the ECG. The Marker Channel™ is below, divided into atrial and ventricular function by the horizontal line. Atrial function above the horizontal is normal with satisfactory sensing (AS) and pacing (AP). Below the line there are three ventricular pace stimuli (VP) that are seemingly properly timed. There are many ventricular sense events (VS) that do not correspond to an event on the ECG, but recycle the pulse generator, and additional ventricular sense events that fall into a ventricular refractory period (VR) and do not recycle the pulse generator. This jumble of events can only be associated with ventricular lead failure, later confirmed at exploration.*

PG 2020–VENTRICULAR LEAD–1016

⟨ MEASURED DATA ⟩		⟨ MEASURED DATA ⟩	
Pacer Rate __4/8/92 – 9:59AM__ 49.7 ppm		Pacer Rate __4/8/92 – 10:15AM__ 49.7 ppm	
Ventricular:		**Ventricular:**	
Pulse Amplitude	3.5 Volts	Pulse Amplitude	.1 Volts
Pulse Current	8.4 mAmperes	Pulse Current	>49.9 mAmperes
Pulse Energy	14 μJoules	Pulse Energy	8 μJoules
Pulse Charge	4 μCoulombs	Pulse Charge	1 μCoulombs
Lead Impedance	416 Ohms	Lead Impedance	<250 Ohms
Atrial:		**Atrial:**	
Pulse Amplitude	3.1 Volts	Pulse Amplitude	3.1 Volts
Pulse Current	5.8 mAmperes	Pulse Current	4.9 mAmperes
Pulse Energy	18 μJoules	Pulse Energy	18 μJoules
Pulse Charge	4 μCoulombs	Pulse Charge	4 μCoulombs
Lead Impedance	618 Ohms	Lead Impedance	628 Ohms
Battery Data: (W.G. 8874 – NOM. 2.3 AHR)		**Battery Data: (W.G. 8874 – NOM. 2.3 AHR)**	
Voltage	2.84 Volts	Voltage	2.82 Volts
Current	37 μAmperes	Current	38 μAmperes
Impedance	<1 KOhms	Impedance	<1 KOhms

Figure 23. *Lead failure may be detected by telemetry data. In this patient, seen because of symptoms consistent with intermittent loss of ventricular capture, initial ECG and telemetry were unremarkable (left). Sixteen minutes later another telemetry transmission provided useful information. Battery drain had increased six times, the pulse amplitude had decreased, and pulse energy and charge had decreased correspondingly. These findings are diagnostic of insulation failure, which was confirmed at exploration. Lead impedance had fallen below 250 ohms (from a previous reading of 416 ohms). Atrial lead data, recorded simultaneously, showed no change.*

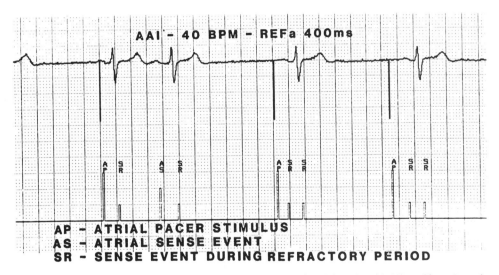

AP – ATRIAL PACER STIMULUS
AS – ATRIAL SENSE EVENT
SR – SENSE EVENT DURING REFRACTORY PERIOD

Figure 24. *Marker Channel™ telemetry in the presence of atrial pacing (AAI) malfunction of a patient with sinus bradycardia can clarify the issue. Atrial stimuli are emitted at appropriate times and on the ECG some seem to capture the atrium. On telemetry it is seen that none capture the atrium, although all P waves are properly sensed. Those that occur during the sensitive portion of the pulse generator cycle (AS, second from left) properly inhibit and recycle the pacemaker. The far-field QRS complexes are also sensed via the atrial lead and are therefore considered atrial events, but fall into atrial refractoriness (SR) and do not recycle the pulse generator. In the third and fourth complexes the atrial stimulus (AP) is ineffective and both spontaneous events, the P wave and the far-field QRS fall during the 400 ms refractory period started by the atrial stimulus (AS). Atrial sensing was determined to be satisfactory, there was no atrial capture.*

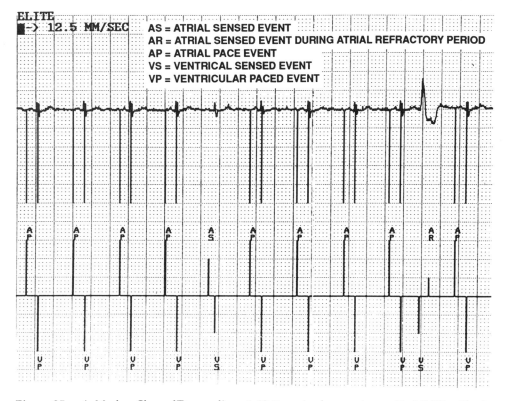

Figure 25.   *A Marker Channel™ recording at 12.5 mm/s shows a transmitted ECG with the pacemaker stimuli emphasized for legibility. The interpretation channel (below) is divided into atrial events above the horizontal line and ventricular events below the line. Each mark is annotated as indicated at the top of the illustration. The first four complexes at the left have paced atrial events (AP) and paced ventricular events (VP). The fifth complex from the left shows a sensed atrial event (AS) with a shorter atrial marker and a sensed ventricular event (VS) with a shorter ventricular marker. The second complex from the right is a premature ventricular beat that inhibits pacemaker output. It is marked as a sensed ventricular event (VS). The atrium depolarizes during the refractory interval, which follows the VPB, and is sensed as an atrial event occurring during a refractory interval (AR).*

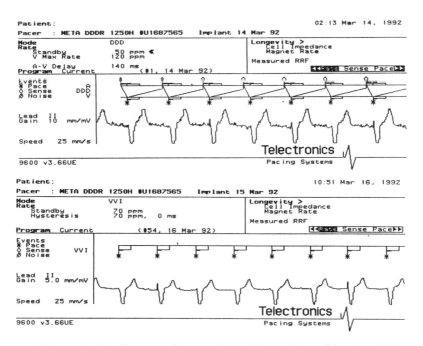

Figure 26. *Elaborate ladder diagram telemetry (Main Timing Events™) assists ECG interpretation. The programmed settings are left above. The ladder diagram of a pacemaker in the DDD mode has the ECG below the ladder. Each event on the ladder is indicated as a "sensed" event, a "paced" event, or as noise. The ladder indicates sensed atrial events followed by paced ventricular events. The small bars on the ladder indicate the duration of blanking, refractory, and AV intervals. The lower strip is of a pacemaker in the VVI mode, indicating the stimuli and the blanking and refractory intervals.*

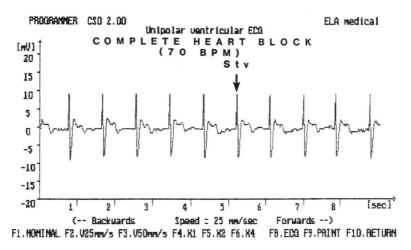

Figure 27. *An EGM derived following a ventricular channel stimulus for management of complete heart block. The stimuli at a coupling interval of 850 ms produce a consistent ventricular response.*

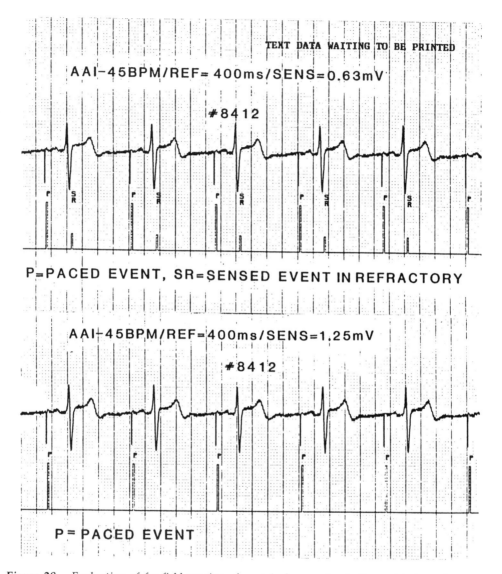

Figure 28. Evaluation of far-field sensing of ventricular events via the atrial channel can be demonstrated via telemetry. In these illustrations continuous atrial pacing was present with the pacemaker in the AAI mode. In each instance the ventricular event was conducted, the refractory period was 400 ms in duration and only the atrial sensitivity was changed. Above is the telemetry ECG with the Marker Channel™ immediately below. At a high sensitivity (0.63 mV) the ventricular event was sensed during the refractory period that followed the atrial channel stimulus. It was sensed (SR) but not used to start a timing cycle. The lower illustration at a lesser sensitivity (1.25 mV) demonstrates that the far-field ventricular events were no longer sensed.

BIBLIOGRAPHY

Barold SS, Falkoff MD, Ong LS, et al: Crosstalk due to activation of atrial sense marker function of DDD pulse generators. PACE 1987; 10:293–301.

Byrd C, Schwartz S, Wellenstein E, et al: Computer aided analysis of pacemaker function Comput Cardiol 1984; 11:147.

Castellanet MJ, Garza J, Shaner SP, et al: Telemetry of programmed and measured data in pacing system evaluation and follow-up. J Electrophys 1987; 1:360–375.

Duffin EG: The marker channel: A telemetric diagnostic aid. PACE 1984; 7:1165–1169.

Gladstone PJ, Duxbury GB, Berman ND: Arrhythmia diagnosis by electrogram telemetry. Involvement of dual chamber pacemaker. Chest 1987; 91:115–116.

Halperin JL, Camunas JL, Stern EH, et al: Myopotential interference with DDD pacemakers: Endocardial electrographic telemetry in the diagnosis of pacemaker-related arrhythmias. Am J Cardiol 1984; 54:97–102.

Hayes DL, Higano S, Eisinger G: Utility of rate histograms in programming and follow-up of a DDDR pacemaker. Mayo Clin Proc 1989; 64:495–502.

Irnich W, Effert S: Telemetric control of pacemaker function. Dtsche Med Wochenschr 1971; 19:811–814.

Kruse I, Markowitz T, Ryden L: Timing markers showing pacemaker behavior to aid in the follow up of a physiological pacemaker. PACE 1983; 6:801–805.

Levine PA: Confirmation of atrial capture and determination of atrial capture thresholds in DDD pacing systems. CPPE 1984; 2:465–473.

Levine PA: The complementary role of electrogram, event marker and measured data telemetry in the assessment of pacing system function. J Electrophys 1987; 1:404–416.

Levine PA, Lindenberg B, Mace R: Analysis of AV universal (DDD) pacemaker rhythms. CPPE 1984; 2:54–73.

Levine PA, Sholder J, Duncan JL: Clinical benefits of telemetered electrograms in assessment of DDD function. PACE 1984; 7:1170–1177.

Lindenberg BS, Hagan CA, Levine PA: Design dependent loss of telemetry: Uplink telemetry hold. PACE 1989; 12:823–826.

Luceri RM, Castellanos A, Thurer RJ: Telemetry of intracardiac electrograms: Applications in spontaneous and induced arrhythmias. J Electrophys 1987; 1:417–424.

Martin D, Venditti F: Use of event markers during exercise testing to optimize morphology criterion programming of implantable defibrillator. PACE 1992; 15:1025–1032.

Olson WH, McConnell MV, Sah RL, et al: Pacemaker diagnostic diagrams. PACE 1985; 8:691–700.

Sarmiento JJ: Clinical utility of telemetered intracardiac electrograms in diagnosing a design dependent lead malfunction. PACE 1990; 13:188–195.

Scheibelhofer W, Kaliman J, Mayr H, et al: Reversible end-of-life indicator leading to erroneous pacemaker implantation. Pitfalls of telemetry. PACE 1984; 7:952–954.

Sholder J, Levine PA, Mann BM, et al: Bidirectional telemetry and interrogation in cardiac pacing. In SS Barold, J Mugica (Eds): The Third Decade Of Cardiac Pacing. Futura, Mount Kisco, 1982, p. 145–166.

Sutton R, Citron P: Electrophysiological and hemodynamic basis for application of new pacemaker technology in sick sinus syndrome and AV block. Br Heart J 1979; 41:600–612.

Sutton R, Perrins EJ, Duffin E: Interpretation of dual chamber pacemaker electrocardiograms. *PACE* 1985; 8:6–16.

Taylor KD: An FM telemetry demodulator for telephone pacemaker clinics. Biomed Eng 1978; 25:87–90.

Uhley HN: An inexpensive receiver for ECG telemetry. Am Heart J 1976; 91:346–348.

Ward DE, Camm AJ, Spurrell RAJ: Ambulatory monitoring of the electrocardiogram: An important aspect of pacemaker surveillance. Biotelemetry 1977; 4:109–114.

Chapter 17

PROGRAMMABILITY

David L. Hayes

Programmability is defined as the ability to make noninvasive, stable, but reversible changes in pacemaker function. The pulse generator contains predetermined circuits from which one or several features or functions can be selected for variation within a restricted range. Using a "pacemaker programmer" many parameters of pacemaker function can be changed or varied. It is not possible to produce a completely new program with available pacemakers. (Although investigational work is being carried out with "software-based" pacemakers in which new programs, not part of the manufacturing process, can be written, there are no such commercially available products at this time.)

The first modern programmable pacemakers were introduced in 1972. In this pacemaker, a magnetic code was introduced from an external programmer to manipulate four levels of output and six rates. Since 1972, numerous changes have evolved in pacemaker programming capabilities. Radiofrequency signals are now exclusively used to communicate between the pacemaker and the programmer. The number of programmable features and the variability of each feature has also expanded greatly.

All pacemakers implanted in the United States are programmable to some degree. The North American Society of Pacing and Electrophysiology/British Pacing and Electrophysiology Group (NASPE/BPG) code designates the degree of programmability and rate modulation in the fourth position. 'O' indicates that none of the parameters of the pacing system can be noninvasively altered. 'P' is simple programmability, one or two parameters can be changed but this code doesn't specify which parameters. 'M' is multiparameter programmability that indicates three or more parameters can be changed. 'C' reflects the ability of the pacemaker to communicate with the programmer, namely it has telemetry. By convention, and in actual operation, it also means that the pacemaker has multiparameter programmability. An 'R' in the fourth position indicates that the pacemaker has a special sensor to control the rate independent of endogenous electrical activity of the heart. Virtually all pacemakers with a sensor also have extensive telemetric and programmable capabilities. There is not sufficient space within the code to indicate which sensor is being utilized. (See Chapter 6, "Pacemaker Codes," Table I.)

The degree of programmability varies widely among pulse generators (Table I). The first and greatest variable is whether the pacemaker paces a single-chamber or has dual-chamber capabilities. The variables in dual-chamber pacemakers are in large part related one to another in maintaining and optimizing AV synchronous performance. Dual-chamber programmable parameters are discussed here, but additional information can be found in Chapter 7, "Comprehension

Table I
Potential Programmable Values

Mode	Ventricular refractory period
Lower rate limit	Pulse width (atrial and/or ventricular)
Maximum pacing rate*[1]	Pulse amplitude (atrial and/or ventricular)
Hysteresis	Sensitivity (atrial and/or ventricular)
AV delay*	Blanking period*
Adaptive AV delay*	Polarity
Atrial refractory period	Rate adaptation (On or Off)[2]
Post-ventricular atrial refractory period*	Rate adaptive sensor variables[3]

* Applicable to dual-chamber pacemakers only; [1] In dual-chamber rate adaptive pacemakers the maximum pacing rate may be a single programmable value or there may be independently programmable maximum P-tracking rate and maximum sensor-driven rate; [2] Rate adaptation may be a function of the programmed mode, i.e., the pacemaker may have DDDR as a programmable option, or rate adapation may require programming "on" in conjunction with the desired pacing mode, i.e., programming the mode to DDD and rate adaptation "on" will delivery DDDR pacing; [3] Rate-adaptive sensor variables are not listed separately because they vary significantly from sensor to sensor.

of Pacemaker Timing Cycles"; Chapter 9, "Pacemaker Electrocardiography"; and Chapter 11, "Rate Modulated Pacing."

MODE PROGRAMMING

Single-Chamber Pacemakers

Most programmable single-chamber pacemakers can be programmed to the inhibited, triggered, or asynchronous mode. The inhibited (AAI, VVI) mode is most commonly used for long-term pacing. The triggered (AAT, VVT) mode is helpful during follow-up to determine normal sensing (Figures 1 and 2). The triggered mode cannot be inhibited (this is only partially true in at least one older pulse generator) and is therefore useful when noncompetitive pacing is associated with EMI. The asynchronous (AOO, VOO) mode rarely is used for long-term pacing because it is potentially competitive with spontaneous conducted or ectopic activity.

If the single-chamber pacemaker is capable of rate adaptation other programmable mode options will include VVIR and VOOR for ventricular application and AAIR and AOOR for atrial application. (Not all single-chamber rate adaptive pacemakers will offer rate adaptation in the asynchronous mode.)

(Reference is sometimes made to the SSI, SSIR, SST, or SOO mode. Manufacturers are also allowed to use "S" in both the first and the second positions of the pacemaker code to indicate that the device is capable of pacing a single cardiac chamber. Once the device is implanted and connected to a lead in either the atrium or the ventricle, "S" should be changed to either an "A" or a "V" in the clinical record to reflect the chamber in which pacing and sensing are occurring.)

Table II
Programmable Pacing Modes

VOO-Ventricular pacing; no sensing	DOO-Dual-chamber pacing; no sensing
VVI-Ventricular pacing; ventricular sensing and inhibition	DVI-Dual-chamber pacing; ventricular sensing and inhibition; no tracking of the atrium
VVT-Ventricular pacing; ventricular sensing and triggering	DVIR-Dual-chamber pacing; ventricular sensing and inhibition; no tracking of the atrium; AV sequential rate modulation
VVIR-Ventricular pacing; ventricular sensing with inhibition; rate modulated pacing	DDI-Dual-chamber pacing; dual-chamber sensing and inhibition; no tracking of the atrium
VOOR-Ventricular pacing; no sensing; rate modulated pacing	DDIR-Dual-chamber pacing; dual-chamber sensing and inhibition; no tracking of the atrium; AV sequential rate modulation
AOO-Atrial pacing; no sensing	VDD-Ventricular pacing; dual-chamber sensing, tracking of atrium with ventricular inhibition
AAI-Atrial pacing; atrial sensing and inhibition	VDDR*-Ventricular pacing; dual-chamber sensing, tracking of atrium with ventricular inhibition and ventricular rate modulation
AAT-Atrial pacing; atrial sensing and triggering	DDD-Dual-chamber pacing; dual-chamber sensing and inhibition; tracking of the atrium
AAIR-Atrial pacing; atrial sensing with inhibition; rate modulated pacing	DDDR-Dual-chamber pacing; dual-chamber sensing and inhibition; tracking of the atrium; AV sequential rate modulation
AOOR-Atrial pacing; no sensing; rate modulation	DOOR-Dual-chamber pacing; insensitive; AV sequential rate modulation
	OOO-Pacemaker is programmed OFF (allows assessment of underlying rhythm)

* VDDR is a misnomer by the NASPE/BPG code for pacing modes. The "R" in this context would generally indicate the capacity of dual-cvhamber sensor-driven pacing. However, VDD by definition excludes atrial pacing. The designation of VDDR is being used by manufacturers as a device that operates in a P-synchronous mode except when sensor-driven during which time pacing may be VVIR or DDDR depending on the specific device.

In dual-chamber pacemakers, multiple single- and dual-chamber modes are usually available. Dual-chamber rate-adaptive pacemakers may have as many as 21 programmable modes: DDD, DDDR, DOO, DOOR, DDI, DDIR, DVI, DVIR, VDD, VDDR, VVI, VVIR, VVT, VOO, VOOR, AAI, AAIR, AAT, AOOR, OOO. (See Table II.)

RATE PROGRAMMABILITY

Rate programmability is the most frequently used programmable feature in single-chamber pacemakers. It is almost always used in routine pacemaker programming. During programming for pacemaker follow-up, if the patient's intrinsic rate is greater than the programmed rate, the imposed rate is increased in order to assess the threshold of stimulation. If the patient is pacing at the programmed lower rate, the rate should be decreased to determine the status of the patient's underlying conduction (Figure 1). It is necessary to know this prior to checking stimulation threshold, i.e., if the patient is pacemaker-dependent and has no reliable ventricular escape rhythm loss of capture during threshold determination could have severe clinical consequences.

The major use of chronic rate programming in a single-chamber pacemaker is to allow a patient to remain in sinus rather than in paced rhythm when sinus bradycardia with intermittent sinus arrest or intermittent AV block exists. Programming a rate of 60 bpm or even as low as 40 to 50 bpm may allow the patient's intrinsic rhythm to exist as much of the time as possible and pacing will occur only in the event of a more profound sinus bradycardia or asystole. In many single-chamber pacemakers the nominal value remains 70 bpm. Slower pacing rates, i.e., slower than nominal, are also helpful in patient's with symptomatic ventriculoatrial (VA) conduction. In these patients pacing rates fast enough to prevent symptomatic bradycardia but slow enough to minimize pacing will minimize symptoms of pacemaker syndrome. (Hysteresis may also be helpful in this regard, see below.)

More rapid pacing rates, i.e., greater than 70 bpm, are used most commonly in pediatric patients and are sometimes useful when faster pacing rates may be

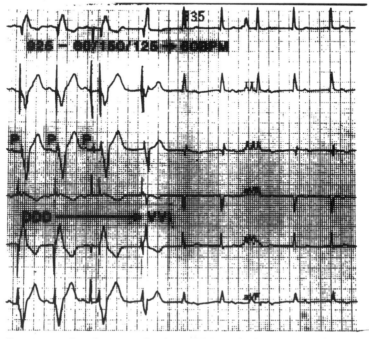

Figure 1. *Reprogramming the pacemaker from DDD mode, lower rate 60 bpm, upper rate 125 bpm, to VVI mode, rate 60 bpm, allows the patient's intrinsic rhythm to predominate. Determination of the status of the underlying ventricular escape rhythm should be done prior to determination of stimulation thresholds.*

necessary to enhance cardiac output, i.e., post-operatively. In a few patients, a faster rate may suppress an atrial or ventricular arrhythmia.

In dual-chamber devices capable of atrial tracking and/or rate adaptation, both a lower and upper rate must be programmed. The programmed lower rate determines the lowest ventricular rate that will be allowed. The lower rate usually is programmed in the 50 to 70 bpm range depending on the individual patient and other factors discussed for determining the lower rate for single-chamber pacemakers.

The upper rate defines the fastest paced ventricular rate that will be allowed. Determining the appropriate upper rate is dependent on the patient's exercise requirements and associated cardiac and other medical problems. Although some dual-chamber pacemakers allow independent programming of the upper rate limit it is the TARP (total atrial refractory period = post-ventricular atrial refractory period + AV interval) that will effectively determine the maximum achievable paced rate. (See Chapter 4, "Comprehension of Pacemaker Timing Cycles.")

In dual-chamber rate adaptive pacemakers, the upper rate limit may be a single programmable value or independent programming of the maximum tracking rate and maximum sensor-driven rate may be required. (See Chapter 9, "Pacemaker Electrocardiography" and Chapter 11, "Rate Modulated Pacing.")

A newer feature for lower rate limit control is that of a circadian response™ (Intermedics, Inc.). This feature allows a lower rate to be programmed for the approximate time during which the patient is sleeping. A separate, potentially faster lower rate limit may then be programmed for waking hours. (For example, the lower rate limit during waking hours may be programmed to 70 bpm and the lower rate limit during sleeping hours may be programmed to 50 bpm.)

HYSTERESIS PROGRAMMING

Programming of hysteresis permits prolongation of the first pacemaker escape interval after a sensed event. A pacemaker programmed at a cycle length of 1000 ms (60 bpm) and a hysteresis of 1200 ms (50 bpm) allows 200 ms more for another sensed QRS complex. Should another QRS complex not be recognized, the pacemaker will stimulate continuously at the programmed rate of 60 bpm, an escape interval of 1000 ms (Figure 2) until a sensed event restarts the

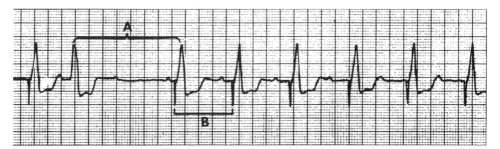

Figure 2. *Hysteresis in a VVI pacemaker programmed to a lower rate of 70 bpm (B) and hysteresis at 40 bpm (A).*

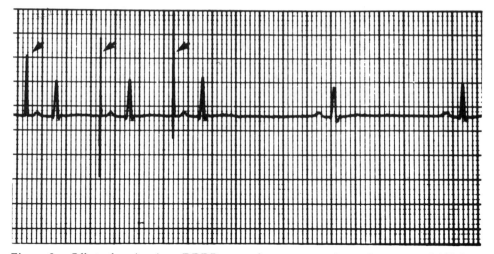

Figure 3. *Offset of pacing in a DDDR pacemaker programmed to a lower rate of 100 bpm, hysteresis at 50 bpm. (Pacing stimuli noted by arrows.) After 256 cycles of pacing at 100 bpm, pacing is suspended for the pacemaker to "search" for the intrinsic lower rate. If the lower rate is greater than the hysteresis rate, 50 bpm in this example, pacing is inhibited until the rate again falls below 50 bpm.*

cycle. The advantage of hysteresis is in the ability to maintain spontaneous AV synchrony as long as possible. This may prevent symptomatic retrograde VA conduction. In most patients with symptomatic VA conduction, hysteresis provides reliable backup pacing and increases the potential for the patient's own rhythm.

Hysteresis is now a programmable option in some dual-chamber pacemakers. Dual-chamber pacing with hysteresis has been advocated for patients with carotid sinus hypersensitivity who require pacing for cardioinhibition but who also have a significant vasodepressor component. "Search" Hysteresis (Intermedics, Inc.) is a modification of conventional hysteresis. In conventional hysteresis, once pacing begins it continues until a spontaneous event such as a premature ventricular beat or sinus rhythm inhibits the pacing sequence. In "Search" Hysteresis, following 256 stimuli at the more rapid rate, the prolonged escape interval is permitted to allow a slower spontaneous rate to begin. If no spontaneous rate occurs, stimulation resumes at the more rapid rate, with cycling at each 256 stimuli (Figure 3).

PROGRAMMING OF OUTPUT
(Pulse Width and Voltage Amplitude)

Output of the pacemaker is probably the most important programmable feature. Programming output can be used to extend pulse generator life by output reduction or to solve the clinical problem of rising stimulation threshold. Presently available pulse generators have programmable output, from a minimum of approximately 1 μJ to a maximum of almost 200 μJ. With good implant technique and newer low-threshold lead designs it is common to program the voltage output to 2.5 V rather than the previously more commonly used 5.0 V. By programming the output at an efficient but safe level, the projected battery life can be increased significantly. A decrease in energy output can also be used to eliminate extracardiac (diaphragmatic or pectoral muscle) stimulation. Conversely, in some patients, increasing thresholds develop after implantation. These high thresholds may be transient or permanent (Figure 4). The threshold may increase to an output requirement of 100 or more microjoules without obvious lead displacement. Output programmability is useful in transient and permanent situations. In patients with a transient elevation, maximal output can be used until thresholds return to a stable chronic level. In patients with chronic high thresholds, the pulse generator can be programmed to higher output to permit reliable pacing (albeit with reduced pulse generator longevity).

The output function to be programmed for the most effective control of a rising threshold depends on actual threshold. Both pulse duration and output voltage (amplitude) are programmable in most pacemakers. Programming the pulse duration to greater than 1 ms approaches rheobase, the lowest voltage threshold at an infinitely long pulse duration. This does not provide much additional pacing margin of safety and causes high current and energy drain. If pulse duration programmability defines a threshold greater than 1 ms in du-

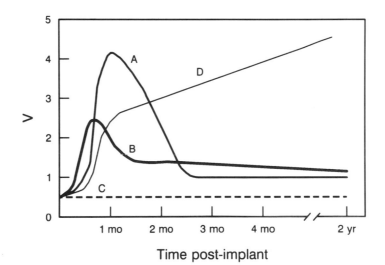

Time post-implant

Figure 4. *At implantation, patients A, B, C, and D have a similar threshold of approximately 0.75 V at 0.5 ms pulse duration. Stimulation threshold evolution for the 4 patients differs significantly. A more marked increase in the early threshold, exceeding 4 V, developed in patient A, but the threshold decreased thereafter to a stable long-term level. Threshold in patient B peaked at approximately 2.5 V two to three weeks after implantation with the chronic threshold approximately twice the acute threshold. Patient C had a steroid (dexamethasone) eluting lead and demonstrated a lower acute threshold of stimulation and during follow-up no significant increase in threshold occurs. Patient D is the least common threshold evolution seen. Initial thresholds are similar to those of patients A and B, but the threshold gradually continues to climb. This response may occur with "exit-block."*

ration, then output voltage increase is the better option. If the threshold is high, the rheobase may be above a specific voltage setting no matter how long the programmed pulse duration. If pulse duration threshold is high, then output voltage is more useful. Conversely, if pulse duration threshold is very low, i.e., in the range of 0.05 to 0.1 ms at a given output voltage, consider a reduction of voltage and a modest prolongation of pulse duration. It is possible to program output based on delivered energy at threshold. The rationale for the various methods of output programming is discussed in Chapter 2, "Basic Concepts." Output programmability should not, at any time, be a substitute for proper lead placement.

Determination of the stimulation threshold is an important consideration in setting pulse generator output and should be a part of routine pacemaker follow-up. The process of determining stimulation threshold can be prolonged, tedious, and, if subthreshold output is reached and not promptly corrected, dangerous. If the patient has a reliable ventricular escape rhythm, ventricular voltage amplitude and/or pulse duration can be decreased until capture is lost. Stimulation threshold should be considered the output settings at which capture is reestablished (Figures 5 and 6).

If the patient is pacemaker-dependent, programming the pacemaker to subthreshold output parameters will result in ventricular asystole. Every pace-

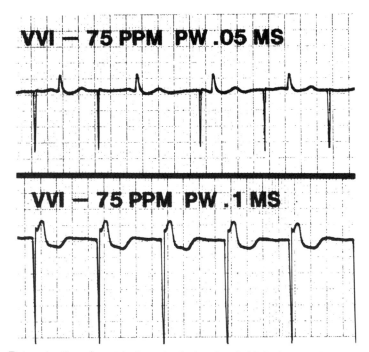

Figure 5. *Determination of ventricular stimulation threshold during routine pacemaker follow-up. The pacemaker is programmed VVI, rate 75 ppm, voltage amplitude 2.5 V, and pulse duration (PW) 0.05 ms in the upper panel and 0.1 ms in the lower panel. Capture is consistently lost at 0.05 ms but restored at 0.1 ms. The stimulation threshold is 2.5 V/0.1 ms.*

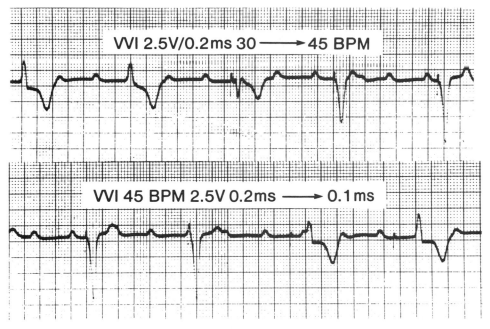

Figure 6. *Determination of ventricular stimulation threshold during routine pacemaker follow-up. Initial portion of the ECG demonstrates an intrinsic rhythm of complete heart block with a ventricular escape rate of approximately 43 bpm. At 2.5 V/0.2 ms pulse duration there is ventricular capture which is seen following reprogramming of the rate to 45 bpm. When the pulse duration is subsequently decreased to 0.1 ms, there is failure of ventricular capture and the ventricular escape rhythm is seen.*

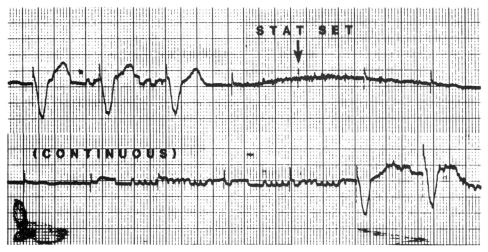

Figure 7. *A continuous ECG recording that begins with a pacemaker being programmed to subthreshold values during determination of stimulation threshold and results in ventricular asystole. The "stat set" was activated immediately upon recognition of failure to capture. However, nominal parameters are not restored for approximately 6 seconds during which time the patient remains asystolic.*

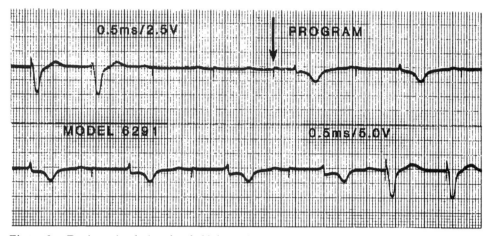

Figure 8. *During stimulation threshold determination, ventricular capture is lost with the pacemaker programmed to 0.5 ms/2.5 V. The pacemaker was reprogrammed at the arrow to 0.5 ms/ 5.0 V, but it takes 8 seconds for effective capture to occur. Fortunately the patient has a slow ventricular escape rhythm.*

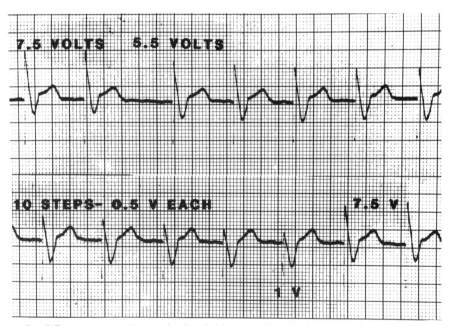

Figure 9. *When programming to the threshold test mode there is a pause longer than the usual escape interval (between stimuli two and three). Thereafter, from the nominal full output of 5.5 V, the output decreases by 0.5 V steps until 1 V is reached. The unit then returns to the programmed output. Should capture be lost, removal of the programmer from the pulse generator returns full output at the next stimulus. Pacing threshold can be readily calculated by counting the number of stimuli.*

maker is equipped with an emergency or "stat set" button that will restore nominal pacing parameters if activated. However, there may be a significant delay between activation of the stat set parameters and actually achieving restoration of nominal pacing parameters (Figures 7 and 8).

Many pacemakers have programmable features that allow automatic threshold testing (Figure 9). This can be done during programming in which the programming sequence reduces pulse duration through each step until the sequence is stopped manually.

Other methods are available that give an exact voltage threshold or an indication of a narrow pacing margin of safety. One manufacturer incorporates a Threshold Margin Test™ with magnet application. With this technique magnet application results in a rate of 100 bpm for 3 beats followed by asynchronous pacing at the programmed rate. The first and second pacing artifacts at a rate of 100 bpm are of normal, i.e., programmed, pulse duration. The third pacing artifact at a rate of 100 bpm is at 75% of the programmed pulse duration. Loss of capture on the third beat indicates a narrow pacing margin of safety (Figure 10). Another approach is a proprietary mode called Vario™. This is a program-

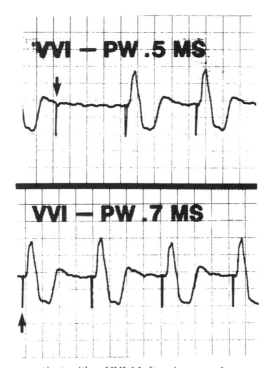

Figure 10. *ECG from a patient with a VVI Medtronic pacemaker programmed to a rate of 70 bpm and 5.0 V. In the upper panel the pulse duration is 0.5 ms. There is failure to capture with the first pacing artifact seen (arrow). This pacing artifact is the third of three asynchronous pulses at 100 bpm that occur with magnet application. As part of the Threshold Margin Test™, the pulse duration of this pacemaker stimulus is 75% of the programmed pulse duration of 0.5 ms. A suprathreshold stimulus is at 0.5 ms, but at 75% of this output duration (equivalent to a pulse duration of 0.375 ms) failure to capture occurs. In the lower panel the programmed pulse duration is 0.7 ms. The first pacing artifact is again the third of the three asynchronous pulses and is therefore at 75% of programmed, or 0.525 ms, and capture is maintained.*

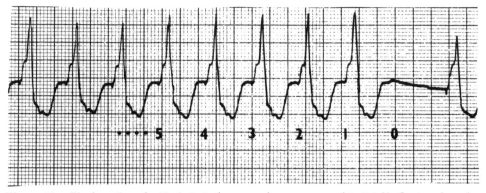

Figure 11. *Final portion of a Vario test of a pacemaker programmed to 5.0 V. Capture is maintained at 0.3 V, indicated here by "1," and appropriately there is no capture when output is 0 V. A paced ventricular event occurs at the programmed lower rate of 60 bpm.*

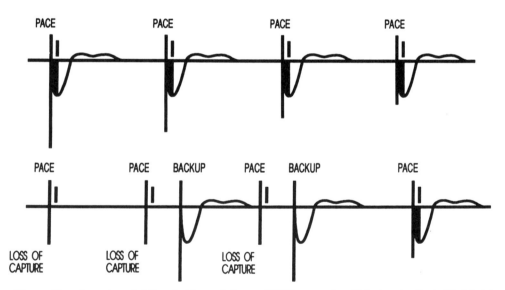

Figure 12. *An automated threshold search from a VVIR pacemaker (Telectronics Sentri™, Model 1210). The threshold search sequence begins with a pacer stimulus of 3.2 V and decrements by 0.1 V on each successive cycle until capture is lost for 3 successive cycles. After the 2nd and 3rd stimuli where there is loss of capture, a backup stimulus at twice the pulse duration is emitted 120 ms after the stimulus where there is loss of capture. Once the stimulation threshold has been determined a safety margin of 0.8 V is added. Feld GK, Love CJ, Camerlo J, et al: A new pacemaker algorithm for continuous capture verification and automatic threshold determination: Elimination of pacemaker afterpotential utilizing a triphasic charge balancing system. PACE 15:174, 1992.*

mable option in multiprogrammable pacemakers from several manufacturers. In the Vario mode, magnet application results in 16 asynchronous beats at the magnet rate of 100 bpm followed by 16 asynchronous beats at a rate of 125 bpm. During the 16 beats at 125 bpm the voltage output is reduced by $\frac{1}{15}$ progressively until zero output is reached (Figure 11). Removal of the magnet returns full output at the next stimulus. The Vario mode can be activated for the test procedure only or programmed "on" permanently.

The feasibility of automatic output regulation has been explored since the early 1970s with prototype devices implanted in humans. Despite the desirability of such a feature, automatic output regulation has never been made available in a clinically released pacemaker. Automatic output regulation has been a programmable option in several pacemakers that have undergone or are undergoing clinical investigation (Figure 12). This feature automatically determines capture threshold and adjusts output accordingly. At least one investigational device has also included capture verification whereby capture is verified after every fourth cycle and if loss of capture is identified, the output is adjusted and capture verification continued on a beat-by-beat basis until capture is regained and a safety margin is added. Because output adjustment is so critical for both extremes, i.e., maintaining an adequate safety margin and for prolonging battery longevity, automatic output regulation will most certainly become a standard feature of future pacemakers.

SENSITIVITY PROGRAMMABILITY

All noncompetitive pulse generators sense and filter the intracardiac electrogram delivered through the electrode(s). For atrial and/or ventricular sensing, the R and P waves must be of significant amplitude (millivolts) and slew rate (dV/dt) for proper sensing to occur. The sensitivity of the pulse generator is the R (or P) wave of the lowest amplitude that the pacemaker will recognize as a ventricular (or atrial) depolarization. The pacemaker definition of whether it is an R or P wave depends on the channel through which it is sensed. Events sensed through the atrial channel will be defined as P waves, those via the ventricular channel as R waves. Nominal ventricular sensitivity is usually in the range of 1.2 to 2.5 mV and nominal atrial sensitivity is usually in the range of 0.5 to 1.2 mV. Although the amplitude of the intracardiac R or P waves may be adequate at the time of implantation, this amplitude may decrease for a variety of reasons, including metabolic and drug effects and lead dislodgment. Each focus of intrinsic activity, be it atrial or ventricular, is not equally sensed, and some foci (conducted or ectopic) may not reach an adequate level of amplitude or slew rate to be sensed. Some extrasystoles may be sensed, while conducted beats may not be sensed and vice versa. Sensitivity programming can be accomplished by an increase in the sensitivity of the amplifier, for example, decreasing the amplitude of the signal required to trigger the unit but maintaining the same frequency spectrum. (The terminology is confusing in that the amplifier is made more sensitive as the number decreases, i.e., 1.25 mV is more sensitive than 2.5 mV.)

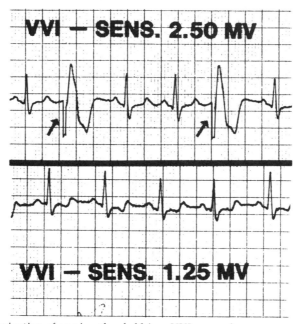

Figure 13. *Determination of sensing threshold in a VVI pacemaker programmed to a rate of 60 bpm. In the upper panel the sensitivity is programmed to 2.5 mV and there is failure to sense (arrows). In the lower panel the sensitivity has been reprogrammed to 1.25 mV and there is normal sensing.*

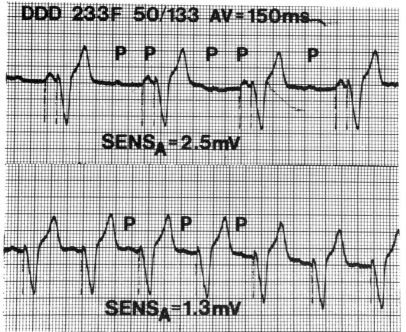

Figure 14. *Atrial sensitivity programming of a dual-chamber (DDD) pacemaker changes atrial sensing and mode of operation. Upper panel: Insensitivity to spontaneous P waves allows an atrial stimulus to produce an atrial contraction followed by a ventricular stimulus, both at the lower rate limit (50 bpm). Lower panel: Increasing atrial sensitivity from 2.5 mV to 1.3 mV allows atrial sensing and the restoration of atrial synchrony.*

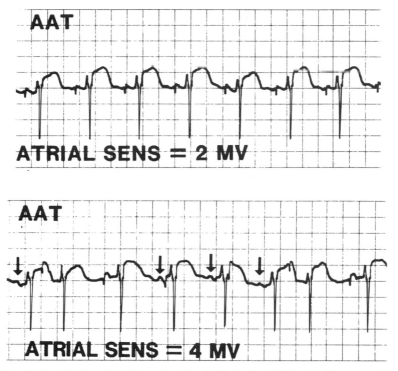

Figure 15. *Determination of atrial sensing thresholds in the AAT mode. Upper panel: the pace-maker has been programmed to AAT, rate 60 bpm, atrial sensitivity of 2 mV. A pacemaker artifact can be seen in each intrinsic P wave, indicating that each P wave is being sensed appropriately. Lower panel: atrial sensitivity has been programmed to 4 mV. Arrows indicate intrinsic P waves that are not sensed because there is no atrial pacing artifact delivered. Other atrial pacing artifacts are delivered inappropriately because of the undersensing.*

Determining the sensing threshold can be determined during routing pace-maker follow-up by programming the pacemaker to less sensitive values until there is failure to sense (Figures 13 and 14). (Sensing thresholds could also be determined by altering sensing values when programmed to a triggered pacing mode, i.e. AAT or VVT.) (Figure 15).

Sensitivity programmability to increase or decrease sensitivity has saved additional operative procedures. Increased sensitivity is especially useful in atrial pacing as the electrograms are usually far smaller than those obtained during ventricular pacing. Decreasing sensitivity is useful in eliminating over-sensing of nonphysiological electromagnetic interference signals (Figure 16) or such physiological signals as pectoral muscle artifacts (Figure 17).

Automatic sensitivity adjustment has received less attention and less in-terest than auto-programming of other features but has nonetheless been in-vestigated. The purpose of automatic sensitivity would be to prevent or mini-mize episodes of both over- and undersensing. This feature has been incorporated in some pacemakers but did not perform as expected. Investiga-tions have demonstrated marked variation in electrogram size that should be a continued impetus to develop an auto-sensing feature.

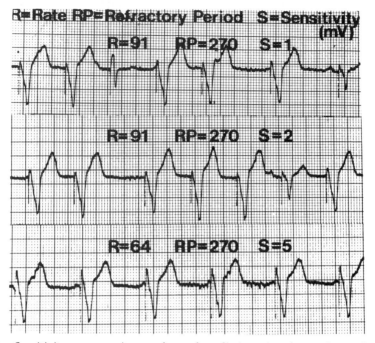

Figure 16. *Sensitivity programming can be used to eliminate interference from a lead fixation mechanism. Because of interfering signals sensed by the pacemaker, the fifth interval is prolonged. At this time, the sensitivity level for ventricular pacing was 1 mV. Reprogramming and reduction of sensitivity to 2 mV did not eliminate artifact sensing, but further reduction to 5 mV produced consistent pacing without false inhibition.*

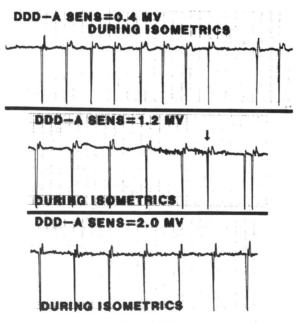

Figure 17.

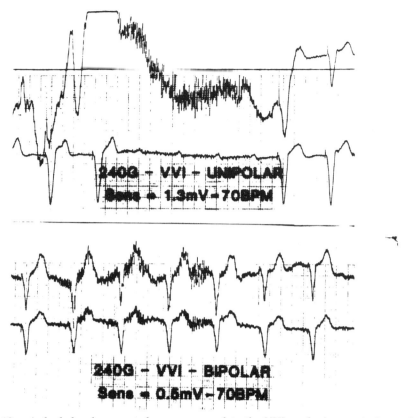

Figure 18.   *A dual-chamber pacemaker programmed to the VVI mode, into unipolar and then bipolar sensing to assess resistance to electromyographic interference. Upper: Programmed to a sensitivity of 1.3 mV, EMI causes inhibition of output and allows ventricular asystole. Lower: In the bipolar mode at a more sensitive value of 0.5 mV, EMI does not inhibit output.*

POLARITY PROGRAMMABILITY

Polarity programmability is now available on many pacemakers. This allows programming from unipolar to bipolar functions. (In some dual-chamber pacemakers the polarity of the atrial and ventricular channels are independently programmable and in others they are not.) This feature is most helpful in patients who have myopotential or electromagnetic inhibition in the unipolar mode but not in the bipolar mode (Figure 18). Unipolar and bipolar electrograms have

Figure 17.   *In P-synchronous pacemakers, VDD or DDD, oversensing of myopotentials on the atrial lead may result in inappropriately fast rates because of ventricular tracking of the false signals. In this example from a patient with a unipolar DDD pacemaker, isometrics were performed at various atrial sensitivity values to determine the potential for tracking of myopotential interference. Top panel: Atrial sensitivity is most sensitive at 0.4 mV and there is irregular rapid ventricular pacing as myopotentials are tracked. Middle panel: Atrial sensitivity at 1.2 mV results in less myopotential interference but it is not completely eliminated (arrow). Lower panel: At an atrial sensitivity of 2.0 mV there is no myopotential interference.*

Bipolar

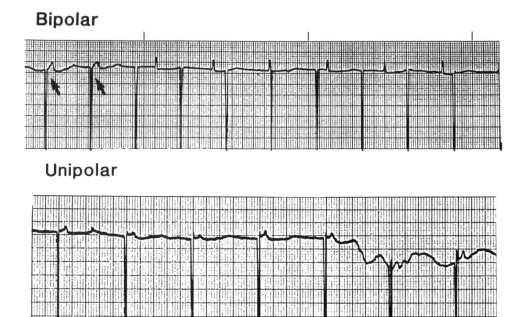

Unipolar

Figure 19. *ECG tracings from a patient with a VVI pacemaker. Upper panel: In the bipolar configuration there is intermittent failure to capture. Capture is demonstrated only with the first two pacing stimuli (arrows). Lower panel: When programmed to the unipolar configuration at the same pulse duration and voltage, there is consistent capture.*

distinctly different characteristics, and programming from one polarity to the other may eliminate the sensing of an unwanted electrogram or interfering signal. It is possible but improbable that there will be superior sensing in one polarity configuration over the other.

Polarity programmability may be helpful in a patient with a lead fracture by converting from the bipolar to the unipolar configuration, i.e., by eliminating the fractured portion of the lead, normal pacing may be restored through the remaining intact pole of the pacing lead (Figure 19). This alternative should usually be considered a temporary measure because whatever force resulted in one fractured conductor may eventually lead to fracture of the second.

REFRACTORY PERIOD

Single-Chamber Pacemakers

Refractory period programming in single-chamber pacing is not commonly required. However, it can be advantageous in some situations. If the refractory period is so long that some ventricular electrograms are not sensed, the subsequent pacemaker stimulus could fall on the T wave of the unsensed beat.

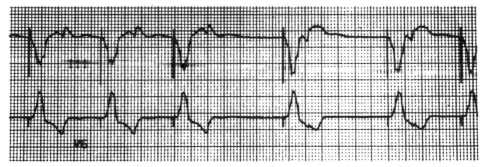

Figure 20. *ECG from a patient with a VVI pacemaker programmed to rate 70 bpm (857 ms), sensitivity 2.5 mV. There are RR cycles that are longer than 857 ms. A portion of the T wave is being sensed and resets the timing cycle. This can be determined by measuring back 857 ms from the 4th QRS complex.*

Conversely, too brief a refractory period can allow sensing of the T wave and inappropriate inhibition of the pulse generator (Figure 20). In older pulse generators there was occasional oversensing of the afterpotential following the pacemaker stimulus. This problem is rarely seen but can be corrected by prolonging the refractory period or reducing the pulse duration if an adequate pacing margin of safety is present.

If a single-chamber pacemaker is used for atrial pacing, a longer refractory period is desirable to avoid sensing of the QRS electrogram, especially if the pacemaker is unipolar (Figure 21).

Dual-Chamber Pacemakers

Refractory periods in dual-chamber dual-sensing units are much more complex than in single-chamber units because the events and timing cycles in one channel impact on the other. When programmed to a dual-chamber sensing

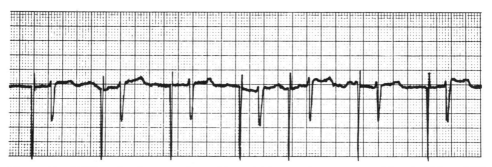

Figure 21. *ECG tracing from a patient with an AAI pacemaker programmed to rate 90 bpm (667 ms). There are AA cycles longer than 667 ms. The only correct interval is between the fourth and fifth atrial pacing artifacts. Measuring back 667 ms from the atrial pacing artifacts following the longer cycles determines that the QRS has been sensed and reset atrial pacing.*

mode (VDD, DDI, DDD), refractory periods exist for each sensing channel. The refractory period for the ventricular channel will behave as for single-chamber sensing. The operation of the refractory period on the atrial channel is quite different. Following an atrial stimulus or a sensed atrial event, the atrial sensing amplifier becomes refractory for the AVI plus the programmed atrial refractory interval after the ventricular event, the post-ventricular atrial refractory period (PVARP). (The total atrial refractory period or TARP is the sum of the AVI and PVARP.) Immediately following a ventricular sensed event, an intrinsic QRS complex, or PVC, the atrial sensing amplifier will become refractory for the programmed refractory period.

Programmable flexibility of the atrial refractory period is especially important because of its role in preventing endless loop tachycardia (ELT) (Figures 22 and 23). Because ELT can occur only when the atrial refractory period is shorter than the retrograde conduction time, this is an especially important interval. Not all patients, however, have intact VA conduction and some have short retrograde conduction times. There are other programmable options to avoid ELT other than a prolonged PVARP. The pacemaker may have a programmable option of "PVARP extension." If this feature is enabled, the PVARP will be

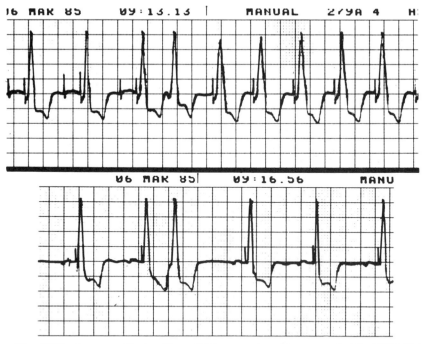

Figure 22. ECGs from a patient with a DDD pacemaker. Upper panel: The PVARP is programmed to 225 ms. The fourth QRS complex is a premature ventricular contraction that produces a retrograde P wave and an ELT at the programmed upper rate of 110 bpm. Lower panel: The PVARP has been lengthened to 325 ms. The third complex is premature, but with a longer PVARP, the retrograde P wave is not sensed and ELT does not occur.

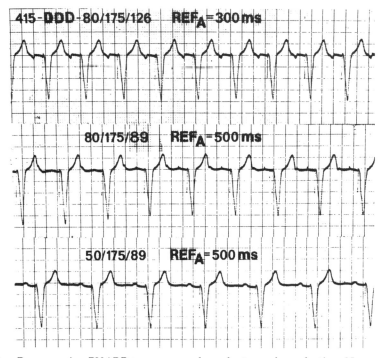

Figure 23. *Programming PVARP to manage prolonged retrograde conduction. Upper panel: The PVARP is briefer than the retrograde conduction time, 300 ms. Retrograde P waves are sensed and an ELT is sustained at a coupling interval of 640 ms (94 bpm) below the pacemaker upper rate limit. Middle panel: The PVARP is prolonged to 500 ms. Retrograde P waves cannot be sensed, and pacing and sensing occur at a coupling interval of 750 ms (80 bpm). The upper rate limit is effectively reduced to an interval of 675 ms (89 bpm). Lower panel: The lower rate has been reduced to an interval of 1200 ms (50 bpm) and atrial sensing is restored.*

lengthened a defined duration if a premature ventricular contraction is sensed. In actuality, the pacemaker cannot distinguish a PVC from any other ventricular beat. The most common mechanism for designating a ventricular depolarization as a PVC is if the pacemaker senses two ventricular events without an intervening atrial event. Should this happen, the PVARP will be extended in an effort to avoid sensing the potential retrograde atrial activation that occurs as a result of the PVC. PVARP extension may result in confusing ECG presentations. If the extended PVARP encompasses the subsequent atrial or ventricular event there will be the appearance of undersensing. This is considered "functional undersensing" because it is a function of the extended PVARP (Figure 24).

Algorithms to detect and interrupt ELT have been incorporated in DDD pacemakers for many years but were not uniformly effective. Some DDD pacemakers utilize algorithms that automatically alter the post-ventricular atrial refractory period (PVARP) and/or the AV interval. Prevention of ELT with newer algorithms has been successful.

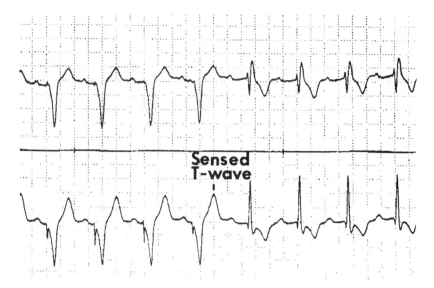

Figure 24. *ECG from a patient with a DDD pacemaker with PVARP extension. The upper and lower ECG tracings occur simultaneously. The T wave that follows the fourth paced ventricular complex is oversensed. Because the pacemaker senses two consecutive events that are thought to represent ventricular activity, the paced QRS complex and the T wave, without sensing an intervening atrial event, the PVARP extension occurs. PVARP is extended to 480 ms. The subsequent P wave falls into the extended PVARP and is therefore not sensed. The next native QRS complex is sensed and because there has been no sensed atrial activity the PVARP extension is continued. This appearance of atrial failure to sense with a first-degree AV block is functional undersensing due to the PVARP extension.*

Automatic regulation of the PVARP is a newer programmable feature. With shorter RR or VV cycles that may occur with atrial tracking or with sensor-driven pacemakers it would seem logical for the PVARP to shorten proportionately to the entire cycle length. Automatic regulation of the PVARP has been introduced in DDDR pacemakers to prevent tracking of pathological atrial rhythms. If a P wave falls in the PVARP (the PVARP automatically decrements as the sensor-driven interval decreases), the next atrial stimulus is omitted, and if the next P wave occurs before the subsequent ventricular output, it will not initiate an AV delay. It is in effect operating in the VVIR mode. This will continue until the P to P interval is longer than the adapted PVARP. When P waves no longer fall within the adapted PVARP, AV synchrony is restored. The early experience with this ability to distinguish between and react to physiological versus pathological atrial rhythms appears to be successful.

ATRIOVENTRICULAR INTERVAL (AVI)

In dual-chamber pacemakers an AVI must be programmed. Optimal programming of the AVI is discussed in Chapter 5, "Hemodynamics of Cardiac

Pacing." The AVI is no longer a single programmable value in many dual-chamber pacemakers. The AVI and it's programmable variations are described and illustrated in Chapter 9, "Pacemaker Electrocardiography."

BLANKING PERIOD

The blanking period is the time during and after a pacemaker stimulus when the opposite channel of a dual-channel pacemaker is insensitive. The intent is to avoid sensing the electronic event of one channel in the opposite channel. The blanking period usually is programmable. It may be desirable to prolong the blanking period to prevent crosstalk (Figure 25). It may be necessary to

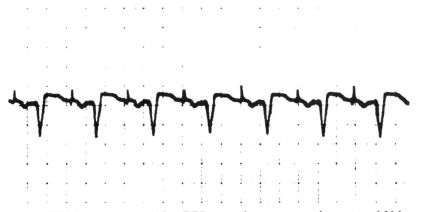

Figure 25A. *ECG from a patient with a DDI pacemaker programmed to a rate of 86 bpm, AVI of 165 ms, and a blanking period of 13 ms. The interval from the atrial pacing stimulus to the intrinsic QRS complex is actually 220 ms. This abnormality occurs because the atrial output is sensed on the ventricular sensing circuit and inhibits ventricular output. There is intact AV nodal conduction with a first-degree AV block.*

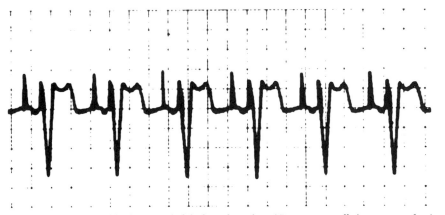

Figure 25B. *When the blanking period is lengthened to 35 ms, crosstalk is prevented. A ventricular pacing stimulus occurs 165 ms after the atrial pacing stimulus, i.e., at the programmed AVI.*

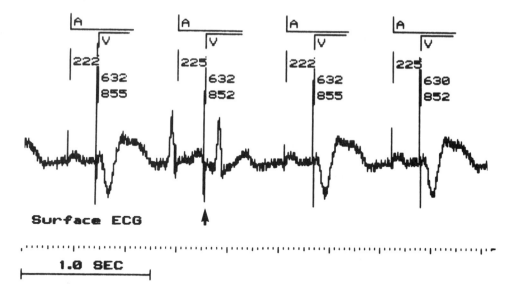

Figure 26. *Surface ECG obtained telemetrically from a DDD pacemaker. The pacemaker is pro-grammed DDD, lower rate 60 bpm, AVI 225 ms, blanking period 51 ms. An intrinsic QRS occurs simultaneously with an atrial pacing stimulus. (The atrial pacing stimulus is masked by the QRS complex but it's presence is verified by the "A" marker above.) The intrinsic deflection of the QRS complex occurs within the blanking period and is not sensed. Therefore, a ventricular pacing stim-ulus is delivered at the programmed AVI and occurs in the T wave (arrow). The ventricle is still refractory and the pacing stimulus is ineffective. However, it is closely followed by another intrinsic QRS complex.*

shorten the blanking period if ventricular extrasystoles are sensed during the blanking period. This could potentially result in pacing during the early portion of ventricular repolarization (Figure 26). Shortening the blanking period should diminish the likelihood of the QRS occurring within the blanking period.

PROGRAMMING RATE ADAPTIVE VARIABLES

Parameters that determine rate adaptation in a sensor-driven pacemaker vary considerably depending upon the sensor incorporated. Programming rate adaptive parameters is discussed in Chapter 11, "Rate Modulated Pacing."

PHANTOM PROGRAMMING

Several categories of phantom or false programming have been defined, including misprogramming from faulty program emission signals, dysprogram-ming from anomalous sources, and, most commonly, purposeful programming by a health-care provider who fails to inform the patient or record the repro-gramming for future reference. Faulty program emission signals were more com-mon when programming was accomplished via magnetic reed switch program-

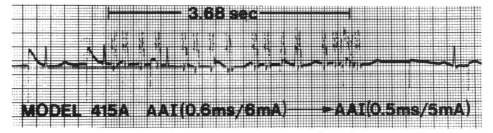

Figure 27. *Magnetic reed switch programming used in several older pacemakers required a prolonged transmission time. Programming this dual-chamber pulse generator in the AAI mode from one output to another uses a pulse code 3.68 seconds in duration. If the programmer is decoupled, i.e., moved away from proper position in relation to the implanted pacemaker during code transmission, a false code can be transmitted or programming will be unsuccessful.*

ming (Figures 27 and 28). With radiofrequency transmission of programming signals, phantom programming is uncommon.

There are several sources of phantom programming that occur or are detected in a hospital setting. The first is exposure to cold. The pulse generator may be exposed to severe cold in the cargo hold of an aircraft or the trunk of an automobile during delivery. New microprocessor-based pulse generators will revert, following exposure to severe cold, to a back-up mode which is different for each pacemaker. A special programming sequence usually is necessary to restore normal operation. Reversion to the back-up mode could also be caused

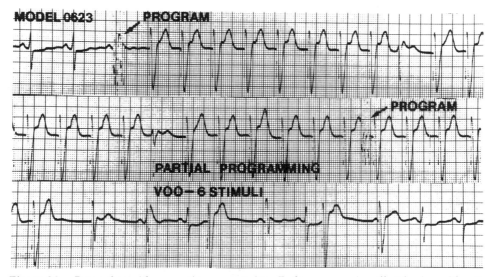

Figure 28. *Pacemaker with magnetic programming. Each programming effort begins with a 5-stimulus sequence at a coupling interval of 600 ms (100 bpm). Thereafter, six asynchronous stimuli are emitted at the newly programmed coupling interval. Inhibited pacing is then resumed. A programming attempt caused the 100 bpm rate, but because only partial programming had occurred, the newly programmed rate of 60 bpm did not begin until reprogramming (middle) completed the programming process.*

by cardioversion or electrocautery. If the possibility of such reversion is not anticipated in each of these instances, pacemaker malfunction may be thought to be present.

When phantom programming occurs outside of the hospital setting, a detailed analysis of possible sources of reprogramming should be discussed with the patient in an attempt to determine and avoid the cause and ascertain that pacemaker malfunction does not exist. With the EMI shielding provided in current pacemakers, false programming as a result of exposure to EMI is seen infrequently. When a patient presents with the pacemaker programmed to parameters other than those on record, the following causes should be considered:

1. Reprogramming by another physician without notification of the pacemaker center;
2. Medical equipment/hospital environment, i.e., electrocautery and magnetic resonance imaging;
3. Exposure to large internal combustion engines;
4. Exposure to welding equipment;
5. Home appliances (rarely) (Figure 29).

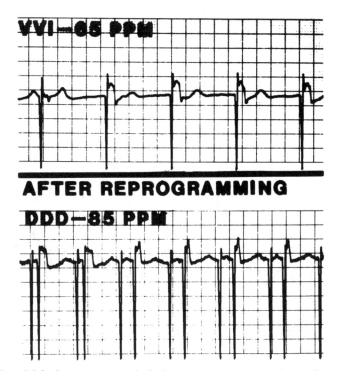

Figure 29. *Two ECGs from a patient who had experienced reprogramming of an implanted pacemaker by a faulty kitchen appliance. The upper tracing was obtained during transtelephonic monitoring and shows the pacemaker in the VVI mode at a rate of 65 bpm, the fallback mode for this pacemaker. The patient had been previously programmed to the DDD mode. After reprogramming, the bottom tracing reflects magnet application to the pacemaker that results in AV sequential pacing at 85 bpm.*

PROGRAMMING DURING ROUTINE FOLLOW-UP

The importance and utility of noninvasive programmability during routine follow-up and troubleshooting cannot be overstated. To be certain that the pacemaker is thoroughly evaluated and to optimize pacemaker function, a definite approach to programming should be adopted. The following programming sequence for a rate adaptive dual-chamber pacemaker (DDDR) can be adapted for other pacing modes.

1. *Assess magnet response.*
2. *Determine status of underlying rhythm.* If the patient is pacing, program the rate of the pacemaker to the lowest programmable value, i.e., 30 or 40 bpm.
3. *Determine ventricular stimulation threshold.* Program the pacemaker to VVI mode. Decrease voltage amplitude to lowest programmable value. If capture is maintained, decrease pulse duration until capture is lost. Increase pulse duration as needed to restore capture and record the voltage/pulse duration threshold parameters. If the patient has no ventricular escape rhythm determination of ventricular stimulation threshold poses some risk to the patient and should only be attempted by experienced personnel.
4. *Determine atrial stimulation threshold.* If the patient has intact AV nodal conduction program to AAI mode. Proceed as described for ventricular stimulation threshold by decreasing voltage and then pulse duration until loss of capture occurs. Regain atrial capture and record threshold parameters. If AV nodal conduction is not intact, program to DVI or DDD at a rate fast enough to override intrinsic atrial rate.
5. *Determine sensing thresholds.* Beginning with ventricular sensing, program to VVI and decrease sensitivity until there is failure to sense and record the value where sensing was last maintained. Alternatively program to VVT and do the same. In the AAI, DVI or DDD modes, depending on status of AV nodal conduction, determine atrial sensing thresholds. AAT mode can also be used and is often helpful because intrinsic P waves may be very difficult to appreciate on a single lead monitoring system.
6. *Determine appropriate upper rate limit.* Taking into consideration patient's age, physical requirements and associated medical conditions, set the upper rate limit accordingly.
7. *Consider PVARP.* Knowing the underlying conduction disturbance requiring pacing will provide some clue as to whether the patient will have intact VA (retrograde) conduction. For example, with sinus node dysfunction only, VA conduction is likely intact. With AV nodal disease there is less likelihood that there is VA conduction, but even with complete antegrade block, retrograde conduction is still possible. Review programmable options for prevention of endless loop tachycardia.
8. *Consider AVI.* There is controversy regarding the most appropriate way to program the AVI. If there is no conduction through the native AV nodal pathway then an AVI of 100 to 150 ms at the lower rate is probably most appropriate. If there is intact AV nodal conduction a longer AVI will allow conduction through the native pathway. If differential AVI and/or rate adaptive AV intervals are programmable options, consider potential advantages of turning then "on."
9. *Program rate adaptive parameters.* Exercise assessment, either formal or informal, is necessary if the pacemaker is to be programmed to a rate adaptive pacing mode. (See Chapter 11, "Rate Modulated Pacing.")

BIBLIOGRAPHY

Barold SS, Falkoff MD, Ong LS, et al: Oversensing by single-chamber pacemakers: Mechanisms, diagnosis, and treatment. Cardiol Clin 1985; 3:565–585.

Barold SS, Falkoff MD, Ong LS, et al: Programmability in DDD pacing. PACE 1984; 7:1159–1164.

Begemann MJS, Boute W: Automatic refractory period. PACE 1988; 11:1684–1692.

Belott PH, Sands S, Warren J: Resetting of DDD pacemakers due to EMI. PACE 1984; 7:169–172.

Berman ND: T wave sensing with a programmable pacemaker. PACE 1980; 3:656–659.

Billhardt RA, Rosenbush SW, Hauser RG: Successful management of pacing system malfunction without surgery: The role of programmable pulse generators. PACE 1982 5:675–682.

Erkkila KI, Singh JB: Reversion mode activation by myopotential sensing in a ventricular inhibited demand pacemaker. PACE 1985; 8:50–51.

Feld GK, Love CJ, Camerlo J, et al: A new pacemaker algorithm for continuous capture verification and automatic threshold determination: Elimination of pacemaker afterpotential utilizing a triphasic charge balancing system. PACE 1992; 15:171–178.

Fieldman A, Dobrow RJ: Phantom pacemaker programming. PACE 1978; 1:166–171.

Furman S: Spurious pacemaker programming. PACE 1980; 3:517–518.

Furman S, Pannizzo F: Output programmability and reduction of secondary intervention after pacemaker implantation. J Thorac Cardiovasc Surg 1981; 81:713–717.

Gabry MD, Behrens M, Andrews C, et al: Comparison of myopotential interference in unipolar-bipolar programmable DDD pacemakers. PACE 1987; 10:1322–1330.

Griffin JC, Schuenemeyer TD, Hess KR, et al: Pacemaker follow-up: Its role in the detection and correction of pacemaker system malfunction. PACE 1986; 9:387–391.

Harper GR, Pina IL, Kutalek SP: Intrinsic conduction maximizes cardiopulmonary performance in patients with dual chamber pacemakers. PACE 1991; 14(11 part 2):1787–1791.

Harthorne JW: Programmable pacemakers: Technical features and clinical applications. Cardiovasc Clin 1983; 14:135–147.

Hauser RG, Susmano A: After-potential oversensing by a programmable pulse generator. PACE 1981; 4:391–395.

Hayes DL: Endless Loop Tachycardia—The problem has been solved? In SS Barold, J Mugica (eds.) New Perspectives in Cardiac Pacing. Mount Kisco, New York. Futura Publishing Co., 1988,pp. 375–386.

Ilvento J, Fee JA, Shewmaker S: Automatic mode switching from DDDR to VVIR. A management algorithm for atrial arrhythmias in patients with dual chamber pacemakers. (abstract) PACE 1990; 13:1199.

Jocheim R, Lutzmann A, Bisler H, et al: Comparison of sensing behaviour of unipolar and bipolar electrodes. Herz Kreisl 1991; 23:113–118.

Jung W, Manz M, Luderitz B: Which programmable pacemaker features are available and what is their clinical relevance. Herz 1991; 16:158–170.

Lamaison D, Girodo S, Limousin M: A new algorithm for a high level of protection against pacemaker mediated tachycardia. PACE 1988; 11:1715–1721.

Lee MT, Baker R: Circadian rate variation in rate-adaptive pacing systems. PACE 1990; 13:1797–1801.

Levine PA: Proceedings of the policy conference of the North American Society of Pacing and Electrophysiology on programmability and pacemaker follow-up programs. Clin Prog Pacing Electrophysiol 1984; 2:145–191.

Luceri RM, Hayes DL: Follow-up of DDD pacemakers. PACE 1984; 7:1187–1194.

Marketwitz A, Hemmer W, Weinhold C: Complications in dual chamber pacing: A six-year experience. PACE 1986; 9:1014–1018.

Mond HG: Unipolar versus bipolar pacing—Poles apart. PACE 1991; 14:1411–1424.

Nalos PC, Nyitray W: Benefits of intracardiac electrograms and programmable sensing polarity in preventing pacemaker inhibition due to spurious screw-in lead signals. PACE 1990; 13:1101–1104.

Nitzsche R, Gueunoun M, Lamaison D, et al: Endless-loop tachycardias: Description and first clinical results of a new fully automatic protection algorithm. PACE 1990; 13: 1711–1718.

O'Keefe JH Jr, Hayes DL, Holmes DR Jr, et al: Importance and long-term utility of a multiparameter programmable pulse generator. Mayo Clin Proc 1984; 59:239–242.

Pless P, Simonsen E, Arnsbo P, et al: Superiority of multiprogrammable to nonprogrammable VVI pacing: A comparative study with special reference to management of pacing system malfunctions. PACE 1986; 9:739–744.

Rosenqvist M, Vallin HO, Edhag KO: Rate hysteresis pacing: How valuable is it? A comparison of the stimulation rates of 70 and 50 beats per minute and rate hysteresis in patients with sinus node disease. PACE 1984; 7:332–340.

Sinnaeve A, Piret J, Stroobandt R: Potential causes of spurious programming: Report of a case. PACE 1980; 3:541–547.

Smyth NPD, Sager D: A multiprogrammable pacemaker with unipolar or bipolar option. Am Heart J 1983; 106:412–414.

Sulke AN, Chambers JB, Sowton E: The effect of atrio-ventricular delay programming in patients with DDDR pacemakers. Eur Heart J 1992; 13:464–472.

Sweesy MW, Batey RL, Forney RC: Activation times for "emergency back-up" programs. PACE 1990; 13:1224–1227.

Toivonen L, Valjus J, Hongisto M, et al: The influence of elevated 50 Hz electric and magnetic fields on implanted cardiac pacemakers: The role of the lead configuration and programming of the sensitivity. PACE 1991; 14:2114–2122.

Chapter 18

ELECTROMAGNETIC INTERFERENCE, DRUG-DEVICE INTERACTIONS, AND OTHER PRACTICAL CONSIDERATIONS

David L. Hayes

Electromagnetic interference (EMI) can be defined as electrical signals of nonphysiological origin that affect pacemaker function. EMI can be broadly classified as galvanic, electromagnetic, or magnetic. Galvanic interference requires direct contact with electrical current, i.e., defibrillation/cardioversion, cautery, and diathermy. Electromagnetic or electrically coupled interference does not require direct contact, i.e., arc welding, Ham radios, electrical appliances, metal detectors. Magnetic interference occurs when a patient comes in close contact with an intense magnetic field, i.e., nuclear magnetic resonance imaging.

The pacemaker is designed to filter out EMI but not all interference is avoided. The pacemaker circuitry is designed to attenuate (decrease) any interference outside the normal range of a cardiac electrogram (10 Hz—100 Hz). This is accomplished via the bandpass filter(s) incorporated in the pacemaker. EMI is most commonly a problem for the pacemaker patient within the hospital environment. Outside the hospital there are potential sources of EMI but they less frequently create a clinical problem.

The response of the pacemaker to EMI is dependent upon the EMI source, pacing mode, and pacing polarity. Regardless of the source, EMI is of more concern for the pacemaker-dependent patient in whom inhibition of the pacemaker by EMI may render the patient asystolic. Although there are many potential sources of EMI (Table I), there are a limited number of EMI sources that more commonly create clinical problems. The following sources of EMI will be considered: individually:

Electrocautery/cardioversion/defibrillation
Magnetic resonance imaging (MRI)
Extracorporeal shock wave lithotripsy (ESWL)
Transcutaneous nerve stimulation
Diathermy
Therapeutic radiation
Radiofrequency ablation
Electroshock therapy
Nonmedical equipment

ELECTROCAUTERY/CARDIOVERSION/DEFIBRILLATION

Interference with pacemaker function by electrocautery, cardioversion, defibrillation, or electroconvulsive or electroshock therapy is possible and should be considered before the procedure. Prior to any procedure involving any electrical device it is important to know how the pacemaker is programmed so that correct programmed parameters can be restored should the device be reprogrammed by the procedure.

In all instances, the electrocautery or paddles for cardioversion/defibrillation should ideally be kept at least 4–6 inches away from the pacemaker itself. For cardioversion, the pads should optimally be placed in an anteroposterior position rather than to the left and right of the anterior portion of the chest. This positioning minimizes the chance of placing the paddle over the pulse generator or having the current path go directly to the lead system.

After any electrical intervention, i.e., electrocautery during surgery, cardioversion, or electric shock therapy, the pacemaker should be interrogated because the pacing function may have been changed. Potential effects of electrocautery follow.

The most common problem encountered with electrocautery is pacemaker inhibition (Figure 1). As long as the electrical intervention is only brief, it is not of concern in most patients. If prolonged electrocauterization occurs, the pacemaker may revert to the noise mode and pace the heart asynchronously, a change that rarely leads to difficulty (Figure 2 and 3). If the patient is to undergo a surgical procedure in which electrocauterization could be fairly constant, the anesthesiologist should be consulted, and consideration given to reprogramming the pacemaker to an asynchronous mode to avoid intermittent inhibition or, in nonprogrammable pacemakers, to taping a magnet over the unit to convert it to an asynchronous mode. This course of action should be definitely considered in patients who are pacemaker-dependent. The cautery electrode should ideally be kept about 4–6 inches away from the pacemaker because damage to the pacemaker circuitry is possible if used in close proximity. Cautery will interfere with electrocardiographic monitoring so it is desirable to have some other means of monitoring such as an audible finger pulse or intra-arterial line.

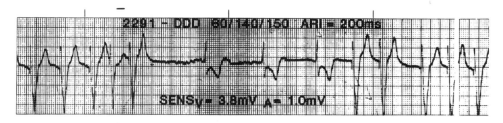

Figure 1. *DDD pacing with P-synchronous pacing at the beginning and end of the example. EMI results in inhibition of the ventricular channel of the pacemaker with 3 ventricular escape beats occurring at a rate less than the programmed lower rate of 60 bpm.*

EFFECTS OF ELECTROCAUTERY

1. Reprogramming.
2. Permanent damage to the pulse generator.
3. Inhibition of the pulse generator.
4. Reversion to a fall-back mode,* noise reversion mode, or electrical reset. (*The characteristics of the fall-back mode should be known so that its presence is not confused with malfunction or end-of-life.)
5. Myocardial thermal damage secondary to transmission of electrical discharge to the heart via the lead(s) (resulting in myocardial infarction or ventricular fibrillation or both)

The pacemaker could also be programmed to its "backup" mode of operation (Figure 4). Electrocautery is a sufficiently powerful electrical interference that the implanted generator may be reprogrammed rather than only inhibited. For example, if a patient with a DDD pacemaker is operating in the asynchronous single-chamber mode (VOO) after EMI, the most likely occurrence has been reprogramming to its protected (backup) mode. The pacemaker can be readily reprogrammed to its former function. Other pacemakers may require access to special codes before the device can be programmed out of "backup."

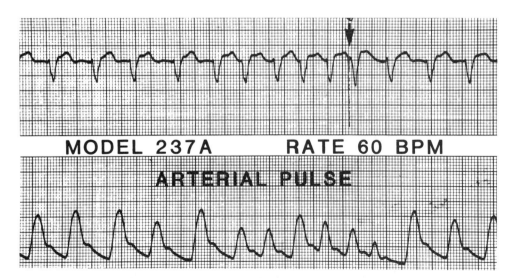

MODEL 237A   RATE 60 BPM

ARTERIAL PULSE

Figure 2. *A VVI pacemaker is in place which at a rate of 60 bpm is inhibited by a more rapid spontaneous rate. After the fifth regularly timed spontaneous beat an irregular series of beats occur. They end with the emission of a pacemaker stimuli (arrow). The second beat preceding the pacemaker stimulus had started a timing cycle. The next beat fell into a noise-sampling portion of the cycle, forcing the next stimulus. This ECG had previously been mistaken as ventricular undersensing.*

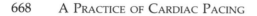

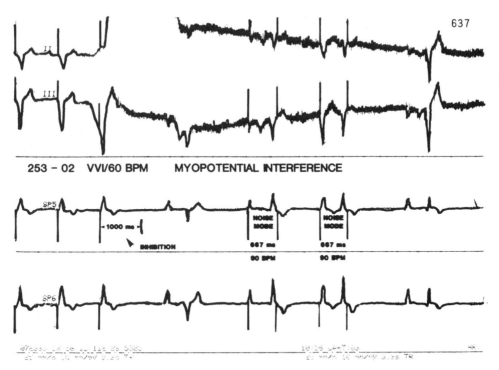

Figure 3. ECG tracings from a unipolar VVI pacemaker programmed to 60 bpm. Standard leads II and III are shown above, and simultaneous special function leads positioned to reduce interference on the ECG, SP5 and SP6, are shown below. Myopotential interference begins with the third pacing artifact. This initially causes inhibition of the pacemaker as evidence by intervals greater than 1000 ms or 60 bpm lower rate limit. In the presence of continued myopotential interference, the pacemaker reverts to the "noise mode" as evidenced by pacing at a rate of 90 bpm, 667 ms intervals.

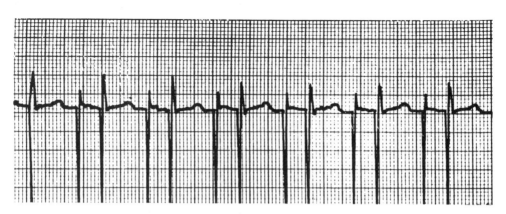

Figure 4A. Pre-operative ECG tracing from a pacemaker programmed to DDD, lower rate 80 bpm, AVI 150 ms. Consistent AV sequential pacing is seen.

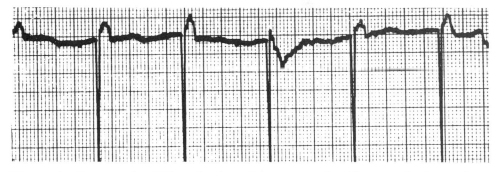

Figure 4B. *Post-operative ECG tracing from the same pacemaker. The pacemaker is now functioning VVI at 65 bpm. These are back-up parameters for this pacemaker indicating that the pacemaker was reprogrammed during the surgical procedure.*

If cardioversion is performed, the pads should be kept 4–6 inches away from the pacemaker to minimize the chance of damage to the device. Cases have been reported in which, despite adherence to these guidelines, the angle of the electrical shock to the lead or pacemaker was sufficient to cause pacemaker damage. The pacemaker should always be interrogated after an electrical intervention to ascertain that it is still programmed correctly and functioning normally.

The potential effect at the electrode-myocardial interface should also be considered. Although rare, an electrical impulse delivered at the appropriate angle to the pacemaker lead can be transmitted through the electrode directly to the endocardium or myocardium where it can produce arrhythmias or local endocardial necrosis with high threshold and poor sensing.

MAGNETIC RESONANCE IMAGING

Magnetic resonance imaging (MRI) is a commonly used and important diagnostic tool. The MRI system, with its powerful static, time-varying magnetic and radiofrequency fields, can affect normal pacemaker operation and function. At the very least, exposure to MRI causes all pacemakers to revert to an asynchronous mode because of reed switch closure. This effect can be avoided only in pacemakers in which the magnet response can be programmed "off." Investigations of MRI and pulse generator interaction have shown that MRI does not permanently damage the reed switch or other pulse generator components. The radiofrequency artifacts do not alter the acutely programmed variables, change the normal magnet rate, or induce pacing in most pacemakers tested. Certain single- and dual-chamber pacemakers implanted in animals and exposed to MRI can pace at the radiofrequency pulse period used during radiofrequency scanning. Because the radiofrequency pulse period may be set at extremely short intervals for some diagnostic procedures (available range of 20 to 2000 ms), patients with susceptible pacemakers could theoretically be paced at rates as high as 3000 bpm.

No generalizations can be made concerning which pacemaker patients can be exposed safely to magnetic resonance scanning, and, in general, MRI should be avoided in a patient with an implanted pacemaker. In pacemaker patients in whom MRI scanning is needed and no alternative procedure can provide the necessary diagnostic information, several approaches have been used. In non-pacemaker-dependent patients, if the patient can be programmed to an output where there is consistent failure to capture, MRI may be attempted. In this case, even if the pacemaker were susceptible to rapid pacing via the radiofrequency signals, the patient should be protected from effective rapid pacing rates. If the pacemaker can be programmed to the OOO mode, or "off," the nonpacemaker-dependent patient probably can be scanned safely. Alternatively, the pacemaker may be explanted for the duration of the MRI, but again, this is only applicable to the nonpacemaker-dependent patient and is not without risk. Even with strict sterile technique the patient would be exposed to some increased risk of infection. It must be remembered that if the area of the body that is to be imaged is in close proximity to the pacemaker site, if MRI is undertaken, the pacemaker-induced artifact may obscure the images. Because MRI is generally felt to be contraindicated in patients with permanent pacemakers, the patient must be thoroughly aware of the risks if MRI is performed even with any of the above cautions.

EXTRACORPOREAL SHOCK WAVE LITHOTRIPSY

Extracorporeal shock wave lithotripsy is used frequently for the treatment of nephrolithiasis and less frequently for the treatment of cholelithiasis. This method can potentially cause problems with permanent pacemakers. The shock waves produced by the lithotripsy device usually are synchronized to the patient's ventricular depolarization or to the output stimulus of the pacemaker. Testing of pacemakers in vitro and limited in vivo experience has shown that lithotripsy does not interfere with fixed rate VVI pacing as long as the focal point of the lithotriptor is at least 6 inches from the pacemaker. In patients with dual-chamber pacemakers, synchronization of the lithotriptor with the atrial output can result in inhibition of ventricular output. Therefore, the pacemaker should be reprogrammed to the VVI or VOO mode for the duration of the treatment. In patients with an activity-sensing, rate adaptive pacemaker sensing of the shock waves can result in increased pacing rates and damage to the piezoelectric crystal if placed near the focal point of the lithotriptor.

GUIDELINES FOR LITHOTRIPSY IN PACED PATIENTS

1. Program the pacemaker to the VVI or VOO mode.
2. Keep the focal point of the lithotriptor no closer than 6 inches from the pacemaker.
3. Cardiac monitoring throughout the procedure.

TRANSCUTANEOUS NERVE STIMULATION

Transcutaneous nerve stimulation (TENS) is used frequently for a number of neurological and musculoskeletal problems. It appears to be safe in most patients with a permanent pacemaker and rarely causes inhibition, interference, or reprogramming, although an occasional patient with interference with pacemaker function has been observed (Figure 5). It is not known how close to the pacemaker the transcutaneous nerve stimulator can be placed, and it is best to avoid applying the stimulator to a vector or path that would be parallel to the pacing lead. Pacemaker-dependent patients should be monitored during initial transcutaneous nerve stimulation to be certain no inhibition occurs. Most of the information regarding transcutaneous nerve stimulation in patients with permanent pacemakers has been obtained with relatively modern pacemakers. It is possible that some older pacemakers with less sophisticated filtering capabilities may be more susceptible to interference.

In patients with VDD or DDD pacemakers TENS can potentially result in an increase in ventricular rate. If the noise created by the TENS were sensed as atrial activity, the pacemaker could track the noise and increase the ventricular rate.

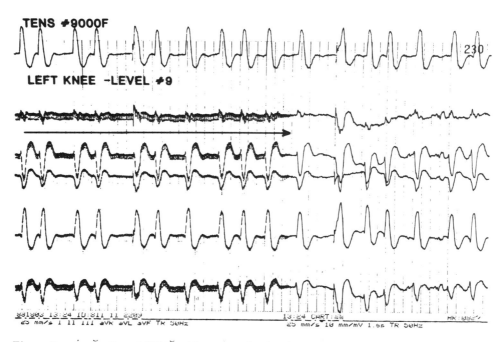

Figure 5. *Application of TENS with a pacemaker in place. The pacemaker is programmed VVI, 70 bpm. While interference with the ECG is visible, no interference with pacemaker function has occurred.*

DIATHERMY

Some types of diathermy equipment can cause pacemaker inhibition. Patients who are to receive such therapy should be alerted to notify the treating physician. Diathermy placed directly over the pulse generator may heat components sufficiently to destroy its function.

THERAPEUTIC RADIATION

Diagnostic x-ray does not interfere with pacemaker function. Therapeutic radiation levels can have a damaging effect on pacemaker function. Modern pacemakers contain complementary metal oxide semiconductors (CMOS) for their integrated circuits, while older generators had discrete components. CMOS circuits are damaged more readily by lower levels of radiation than were discrete components. Specifically, when the metal oxide semiconductor is exposed to ionizing radiation, damage occurs to the silicone and silicone oxide insulators within the semiconductors. Therapeutic radiation may be of sufficient intensity to result in complete failure or random damage to circuit components. Sudden output failure or runaway may occur. As the damage to the circuit is random and the radiation dose cumulative, from one therapeutic exposure to the next, no specific prediction relative to dose can be made. There have been some reports of pacemaker damage in CMOS devices from as small a radiation dose as 1000 rads, while in others, 3000–15000 rads have been reported to cause damage.

This effect is of particular importance in patients undergoing radiation for thoracic or chest wall malignancies. In patients in whom the pacemaker is within

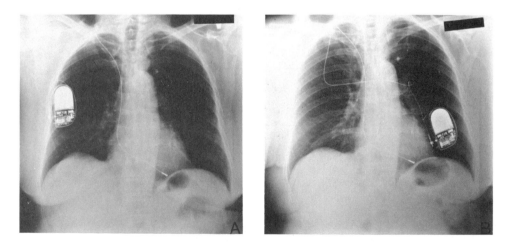

Figure 6A.   *A permanent pacemaker in the right pectoral position and the lead entering the right external jugular vein.* ***B.*** *Carcinoma of the right breast developed and because the pacemaker would have been in the field of therapeutic radiation, the pacemaker was moved to the left chest wall. The lead was temporarily disconnected and tunneled subcutaneously to the left side of the chest where it was reconnected to the pulse generator.*

the field of radiation, for example, those with carcinoma of the breast, moving the pulse generator to another site may be required (Figures 6A and 6B). If the pulse generator is not in the field of radiation it should still be shielded to prevent damage.

RADIOFREQUENCY ABLATION

There has been increasing use of radiofrequency ablation for the treatment of tachyarrhythmias. Precautions are necessary if radiofrequency ablation is performed in the patient with a permanent pacemaker since the pacemaker could potentially be inhibited or reprogrammed with radiofrequency exposure. To insure correct programming the pacemaker should be interrogated following the radiofrequency procedure. The possibility of a "runaway" pacemaker is theoretically possible but unlikely. The appropriate pacemaker programmer should be available during the procedure.

ELECTROSHOCK THERAPY

Electroshock or electroconvulsive therapy for the treatment of depression in the patient with a permanent pacemaker usually will not result in any pacemaker problems. It is theoretically possible that the electrical therapy could reprogram the pacemaker, and for this reason the pacemaker should be interrogated following the electroshock therapy to determine that the pacemaker is still programmed correctly.

NONMEDICAL EQUIPMENT AND DEVICES

Permanent damage to implanted pacemakers by electrical equipment normally encountered at home or at work has not been reported and is unlikely. The most frequent occurrence is temporary interference with pacemaker activity while the patient is in the presence of sustained electrical interference. Interpreted by the pacemaker as cardiac electrical activity, this electrical interference may inhibit pacemaker function episodically but will not damage the pacemaker.

There are potentially significant restrictions for occasional patients. Each circumstance is different and involves the individual decision of the implanting physician and the patient. In patients who work in environments with equipment capable of causing significant electromagnetic interference, i.e., close proximity to heavy motors, such as internal combustion engines, or arc welding, temporary interference with pacemaker activity can result in pacemaker inhibition. In these situations, patients may be required to change occupations or at least avoid specific equipment. If the potential for such EMI is known before implant, the use of bipolar leads can minimize or eliminate the problem. When the patient's livelihood involves the use of equipment that may cause EMI it is helpful to have the patient return to the workplace, with another adult, while wearing an ambulatory electrocardiographic monitor. Brief exposure to the potentially problematic equipment at close proximity with simultaneous electrocardiographic recording will help to determine whether a real problem exists. If the patient has a pacemaker with the capability of storing event records, examination of the stored records after exposure to the usual work environment may help to determine whether the EMI is of concern. On occasion it may be necessary to request an engineer from the pacemaker company to visit the patient's workplace and determine potential EMI exposure (Figure 7).

Patients invariably inquire whether a microwave oven or radar detectors of the type used in airports interfere with pacemaker function. With present-day pulse generators, microwaves should not cause any problem. Metal detectors could theoretically cause inhibition of a single beat but should not result in any significant clinical sequelae.

Table I provides a summary of commonly encountered EMI sources and the pacemaker response. Some of the sources in the table do not cause EMI but have been included because of questions commonly asked by patients.

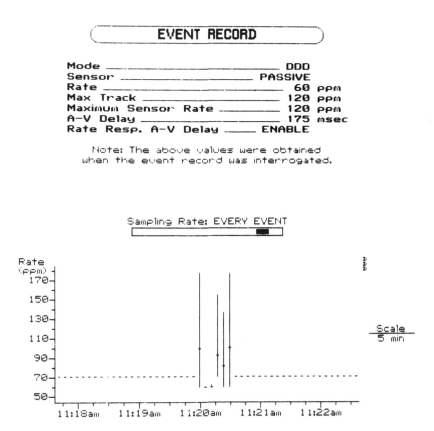

Figure 7. Event records obtained during in vitro testing of the work environment of a pacemaker patient that contained a large degaussing coil. **(A)** Telemetry on a 5-minute scale representing 4 minutes of paced activity with stable pacing at a rate of 70 bpm as noted by the dashed line with the exception of approximately 30 seconds at 11:20 AM when the degaussing coil is turned on.

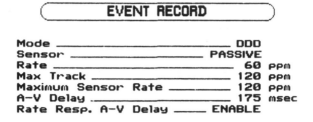

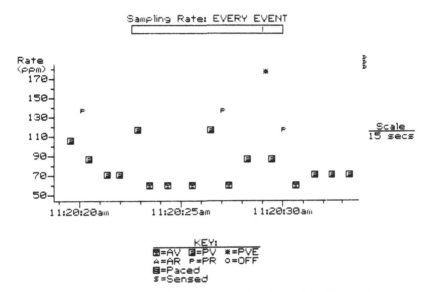

Figure 7B. *Telemetry on a 15-second scale representing the period when pacing was not stable (previously identified in A). Erratic pacemaker activity is demonstrated by events greater than and less than 70 bpm. Because the rate should have been strictly controlled at 70 bpm in this in vitro testing system, the events at rates other than 70 bpm represent oversensing in both the atrium and ventricle and asynchronous pacing due to noise reversion. Stable P-synchronous pacing returned when the coil was turned off.*

Table I

Source	Pacer Damage	Total Inhibition	1-beat Inhibition	Asynch/ noise	Rate Increase	Uni/Bi
Ablation	Y	Y	N	N	Y	U & B
Acupuncture	N	Y	Y	Y	N	U & B
Airport detector	N	N	Y	N	N	U
Antitheft device	N	N	Y	N	N	U
Arc welder	N	Y	Y	Y	N	U & B
Cardioversion	Y	N	N	N	N	U & B
Cautery/coag	Y	Y	Y	Y	Y1	U & B
CB radio	N	N	Y	N	N	U
CT Scanner	N	N	N	N	N	
Defibrillation	Y	N	N	N	N	U & B
Diathermy	Y	Y	Y	Y	Y	U & B
Drill, electric	N	N	Y*	N	N	U
ECT/EST	N	Y	Y	Y	Y3	U
Electric blanket	N	N	Y*	N	N	U
Electric shaver	N	N	Y*	N	N	U
Electric switch	N	N	Y*	N	N	U
Electrolysis	N	N	Y	Y	N	U
Electrotome	N	N	Y*	N	N	U
Ham radio	N	N	Y	N	N	U
Heating pad	N	N	N	Y	N	U
Lithotripsy	Y3	Y*	Y*	Y*	Y2	U & B
Metal detector	N	N	Y*	N	N	U
Microwave	N	N	N	N	N	
MRI	Y	N	Y	Y	Y	U & B
PET scanner	Y	N	N	N	N	U & B
Powerline	N	N	N	Y	N	U & B
Radar	N	N	Y*	N	N	U
Radiation, Dx	N	N	N	N	N	
Radiation, Rx	Y	N	N	N	Y	U & B
TENS	N	Y	N	Y	Y2	U
TV remote	N	N	N	N	N	
TV transmitter	N	Y*	Y*	Y*	N	U
Ultrasound, Dx	N	N	N	N	N	
Ultrasound, Rx	Y3	N	N	N	N	U
Arc Welder	N	N	Y	Y	N	U & B

[1] Modified from Telectronics: Electromagnetic interference and the pacemaker patient. Technical Notes. May 1991, No 110.

1 = Impedance-based pulse generators; 2 = DDD mode only; 3 = Piezoelectric crystal-based pulse generators; * = Remote potential for interference.

EMI AND IMPLANTABLE CARDIOVERTER DEFIBRILLATORS (ICD)

The effects of EMI on ICDs are somewhat more complex and are discussed in Chapter 12, "Implantable Cardioverter Defibrillators."

EFFECT OF DRUGS ON CARDIAC PACEMAKERS

When a new drug is prescribed for a patient already taking medications, consideration must be given to potential drug interactions. The same considerations must be given to the patient with a permanent pacemaker. Drug effect on pacemaker performance usually is thought of in terms of an increase or decrease in pacing (capture) threshold. With rate adaptive pacemakers there are considerations that must be given to the potential effects of some drugs on sensor function.

Numerous drugs have been implicated in pacemaker malfunction, usually as an increase in pacing thresholds and less commonly as a change in sensing thresholds. While there are undoubtedly many instances where a specific drug has complicated pacing therapy, there are few drugs that consistently result in pacing problems.

Class IA agents, i.e., quinidine, procainamide, and disopyramide, have been shown to have mixed effects on pacing thresholds. Procainamide has resulted in failure to capture in a patient with toxic levels of the drug but has not convincingly been shown to increase pacing thresholds at therapeutic levels in humans. Quinidine-induced increases in pacing thresholds have not been shown in humans. Disopyramide at toxic levels has been reported to cause failure to capture, but again there has been no significant problem with pacing thresholds when the drug is at therapeutic levels.

Class IB agents, i.e., lidocaine, tocainide, and mexilitene, are not generally recognized as having a clinically significant effect on pacing thresholds. There are individual studies describing an effect of each of these agents in humans and/or animals, but from a practical standpoint the use of these drugs in paced patients is safe.

At the present time the greatest concern is with Class IC antiarrhythmics. Flecainide, encainide, and propafenone have been shown to raise pacing thresholds. One study found flecainide to raise pacing thresholds by as much as 200%. These drugs are probably best avoided in pacemaker-dependent patients. If there is no alternative drug therapy for such patients, the patient must be carefully observed to be certain that the rise in pacing threshold does not exceed the output capability of the pacemaker. (It is in such a patient that automatic output regulation would be particularly useful. If this option were available and programmed "on," intermittent automatic pacing threshold determinations would detect a rise in pacing threshold and automatically increase the pacemaker output to avoid loss of capture.)

Beta blockers do not usually have any significant effect on pacing thresholds, although there is controversy in the literature. It is well documented that sympathetic stimulation usually lowers pacing thresholds. It has been suggested that beta blockade would raise pacing thresholds, but study results have been inconsistent. Clinically this class of drugs has not been problematic in terms of any significant rise in pacing threshold. Calcium channel blockers have not been convincingly shown to have any significant effect on chronic pacing thresholds in humans. Amiodarone has been shown to affect defibrillation thresholds but there is no convincing evidence that amiodarone significantly affects pacing thresholds.

From a practical standpoint, Class IC drugs must be used cautiously in pacemaker patients, especially in those who are pacemaker-dependent. It is unlikely that any of the other antiarrhythmic drugs discussed would create clinical problems when the drug is at therapeutic levels. However, the possibility of a rise in threshold should always be considered in pacemaker-dependent patients, and the pacemaker output should be programmed to allow an adequate pacing margin of safety.

It is also important to consider drugs that may lower the pacing threshold. Corticosteroids are the most important of these. In the 1960s it was reported that systemic steroids could transiently result in lower pacing thresholds for patients with failure to pace because of rising thresholds or exit block. However, systemic therapy with steroids not only caused the usual side effects associated with steroid use but the lower thresholds are almost never sustained after the steroid is discontinued. In recent years steroid-eluting leads have been developed to allow the local effect of the steroid at the electrode/myocardial interface without any systemic side effects. The drug is slowly eluted, and it is estimated from canine studies that a low concentration of steroid will be maintained in the area of the electrode tip for the lifetime of a patient. Human studies have shown that the steroid-eluting lead prevents the usual rise in pacing threshold in the first 4 to 6 weeks after implantation and that pacing thresholds remain flat during long-term follow-up. Patients with documented exit block and high chronic pacing thresholds have also shown low, stable thresholds with a steroid-eluting lead.

Sympathomimetic agents usually lower pacing thresholds as will any activity that results in increased sympathetic tone. Epinephrine, ephedrine, and isoproterenol have been reported to decrease pacing thresholds but are rarely used clinically for this purpose.

Hyperkalemia is well documented to result in an increase in pacing thresholds. The level of hyperkalemia at which threshold changes occur will vary from patient to patient. When serum potassium levels exceed 7.0 mEq/L there will almost always be an increase in pacing threshold. When this occurs, the treatment of choice is obviously to correct the electrolyte disturbance, but in the interim, programming the pacemaker to a higher output may restore pacing.

Sensing thresholds are much less commonly recognized as being affected by cardioactive drugs, and significant clinical sensing problems have not been recognized with any of the drugs discussed in relation to pacing thresholds.

DRUG/PACEMAKER SENSOR INTERACTION

It is becoming apparent that the function of sensors used for rate adaptive pacing can be altered by concomitant drug therapy. This can necessitate changing the drug or the dosage of the drug or reprogramming the pacemaker to maintain optimal rate modulation. To date there have been only a few such interactions reported, but there will undoubtedly be more given the increasing use of pacemakers capable of rate modulation. The most widely used sensor is an activity or motion sensing device. This is accomplished by incorporating a piezoelectric crystal into the pacemaker. With the patient resting, little or no activity would be sensed and the pacing rate would remain at or near the programmed lower rate limit. Cyclosporine-induced tremors in a cardiac transplant patient have been reported to result in rapid resting heart rates because of pacemaker sensing of the patient's involuntary movements. Theoretically, any drug that results in tremors or involuntary motion could cause an activity sensing device to pace at faster rates. This would require discontinuation of the drug, or in the case where no alternative drug is acceptable, e.g., drugs used in the treatment of a transplant patient, the sensor parameters would have to be programmed to a less sensitive level to minimize inappropriate sensor activation.

Any sensor whose operation is dependent on intracardiac measurements could potentially be affected by antiarrhythmic drugs or any drug that might alter cardiac depolarization or repolarization. Sensors that modulate pacing rate based on measurements of the QT interval, paced depolarization interval, dP/dt and stroke volume/pre-ejection interval all measure a parameter dependent upon ventricular function and/or depolarization/repolarization. Any drug that can alter either of these could theoretically alter sensor function. This concern is more theoretical than proven at present.

PRACTICAL CONSIDERATIONS

Patients with an implanted device have practical concerns that are related to activity, environmental effects on the pacemaker, effects of the surgical procedure, and responsibilities of long-term care of the device. Some concerns about the environmental effect on a pacemaker stem from experience with early-generation pacemakers and electrical equipment and are no longer valid. They still must be addressed, and the anxieties of the patient allayed.

The optimal time for patient instruction is before hospital discharge after pacemaker or defibrillator implantation. Patients can be instructed in postoperative care of the incision, restrictions, techniques of taking and interpreting the pulse, basic principles and techniques of cardiac pacing and/or cardioversion defibrillation, and details of device follow-up.

PHYSICIAN-PATIENT INTERACTION

Some patients become psychologically dependent on the implanted pacemaker. They date many life, other cardiac, and certainly medical events to the implant and existence of the pacemaker. Some even presume that the existence of the pacemaker cures a variety of unrelated cardiac conditions. The physician should attempt to emphasize that the pacemaker effectively manages a specific cardiac condition that does not cure all illnesses.

The patient must be encouraged to adopt the attitude that an illness is being managed and that cooperation in its management is required. The patient should recognize that prudent steps should be taken to protect the device and to maintain its correct function. The patient should also recognize that health may deteriorate, and the device may undergo progressive, routine, or, albeit rare, even sudden failure. A prudent attitude devoid of apprehension and denial of disease is helpful.

Physician

A physician who implants a pacemaker or one who is responsible for follow-up of a patient with an implanted pacemaker should recognize the prolonged responsibility entailed. Electrical, electronic, or physiological malfunctions may occur, and the lead system of the pulse generator may malfunction or be recalled.

Communications may be received from the manufacturer about a particular problem with a pulse generator or lead and it may be necessary to notify the patient about the potential problem. The physician should keep accurate records of the patient's location and if the patient moves from the physician's area of responsibility, he or she should insist that pacemaker follow-up be continued elsewhere.

The physician should recognize, as should the patient, that the existence of a pacemaker does not protect against illnesses or problems unrelated to the rhythm disturbance for which the device was implanted. The physician should not blame each unrelated ache or pain on the implanted device. Pain in the shoulder adjacent to a pacemaker may be pacemaker-related or it may be due to a bursitis or some other rheumatologic problem; precordial distress may be pacemaker syndrome but it may also be angina pectoris, esophageal reflux, or musculoskeletal pain. Only careful evaluation can make the distinction.

Patients invariably inquire whether household appliances and other commonly encountered electrical activity will interfere with pacemaker function. With present-day pulse generators, most patients will not encounter electrical devices that will cause significant interference.

ILLNESS, SURGERY, AND PREGNANCY

The patient with a cardiac pacemaker is subject to other illnesses and medical conditions. Tolerance to the stress of illness, surgery, and pregnancy is a function of the patient's intrinsic cardiac reserve. A limiting factor of varying significance is the lessened ability of a patient with a non-rate adaptive pacemaker to increase the cardiac output in response to fever or stress. Nevertheless, the patient with a non-rate adaptive pacemaker and preserved left ventricular function can increase stroke volume and thus maintain cardiac output. If left ventricular function is poor and cardiac output is rate-dependent, the patient will do less well.

Care and attention to the device and its interaction with the host is a lifelong responsibility, but it need not be especially burdensome. Modern devices function for long periods, usually without any intervention. While some become troublesome, this is the exception rather than the rule. Understanding of what the device can accomplish, how it is to be observed, and how to protect it and the patient from harm will lead to prolonged satisfactory function. The personal physician should have some broad knowledge of pacemaker function and where to seek consultation. The patient should not fix all illnesses on the pacemaker and equally should not assume that its presence is a guard against all cardiac disease.

COMMON QUESTIONS

Travel

Patients who have cardiac pacemakers should carry a personal identification card that lists the type of pacemaker, type of lead system, and the patient's physician. Providing the patient with a list of physicians in the city they are traveling to who are knowledgeable in pacemaker care may be helpful. Travel should not be limited. The only requirement is that the patient carry the transmitter necessary for transtelephonic analysis and be in a part of the world where reliable telephone service exists and responsible medical attention is available.

Neither commercial air travel nor the metal detectors used in airports is a problem for pacemaker patients. A pacemaker may activate the metal detector, but having the identification card available should avoid any confusion.

WORK

A patient should be able to return to their previous occupation and recreational activity with few exceptions (See "Nonmedical Equipment and Devices," this chapter). All patients, especially those who are pacemaker-dependent, should be warned to refrain from driving for 2 to 3 weeks after pacemaker implantation to be certain to avoid problems related to lead dislodgment.

SPORTS

Contact sports must be restricted. There should be no limitations on other activities. For patients who insist on being involved in contact sports, it should be made clear that direct trauma can result in damage to the pacemaker itself or fracture of the lead. Contact sports in which there is little risk of direct trauma to the placement site are reasonable if the patient wears a protective garment or dressing over the pacemaker.

Patients frequently inquire about several specific activities. One is golfing, which is not restricted after the first 2 to 3 weeks after implantation. Patients also ask about the use of a rifle or shotgun. This should be discussed before implantation. If this activity is important to the patient, the pacemaker should be placed on the side opposite the shooting arm to avoid damage due to recoil. Patients also often ask about swimming. Swimming can be done after the incision has healed. Patients should be reassured that there is no danger of water causing problems with the pacemaker circuit.

SEXUAL ACTIVITY

Sexual activity is permitted as tolerated and is limited only by the cardiac reserve. Patients tend to be reluctant to ask questions about sexual activity. This topic is included in the literature and audiovisual material provided for the patient's instruction.

CLOTHING

Clothing usually has little impact on the pacemaker. Patients with epicardial implants who have the pulse generator in the abdominal position should not wear a tight belt crossing the lead system because the belt can become a fulcrum about which the leads may bend or break. A woman may ask whether her brassiere will affect the pacemaker or lead. A brassiere will not damage the pacemaker lead, but the very thin patient or the patient in whom the pacemaker is poorly positioned may have some discomfort. A soft sponge or rubber pad may alleviate pressure on the leads or pulse generator. In some patients, a brassiere may support the breast and decrease discomfort related to the pacemaker itself. In occasional patients with pendulous breasts, a brassiere may be worn at night to minimize discomfort.

Patients also ask whether seat belts, especially shoulder straps, cause any problems with the pacemaker. They should be reassured that with transvenous systems in which the pacemaker has been placed in the anterior chest wall, there is no problem with seat belts or shoulder restraints. Patients who have epicardial systems should follow the same precautions as those noted above for wearing a tight belt.

BIBLIOGRAPHY

Adamec R, Haefliger JM, Killisch JP, et al: Damaging effect of therapeutic radiation on programmable pacemakers. PACE 1982; 5:146–150.
Barold SS, Falkoff MD, Ong LS, et al: Resetting of DDD pulse generators due to cold exposure. PACE 1988; 11:736–743.

Belott P, Sands S, Warren J: Resetting of DDD pacemakers due to EMI. PACE 1984; 7: 169–172.

Bianconi L, Boccadamo R, Toscano S, et al: Effects of oral propafenone therapy on chronic myocardial pacing threshold. PACE 1992; 15:148–154.

Blacher RS, Basch SH: Psychological aspects of pacemaker implantation. Arch Gen Psychiat 1970; 22:319–323.

Catipovic-Veselica K, Skrinjaric S, Mrdenovic S, et al: Emotion profiles and quality-of-life of paced patients. PACE 1990; 13:399–404.

Chen D, Philip M, Philip PA, et al: Cardiac pacemaker inhibition by transcutaneous electrical nerve stimulation [published erratum appears in Arch Phys Med Rehabil 1990; 71(6):388]. Arch Phys Med Rehabil 1990; 71:27–30.

Cooper D, Wilkoff B, Masterson M, et al: Effects of extracorporeal shock wave lithotripsy on cardiac pacemakers and its safety in patients with implanted cardiac pacemakers. PACE 1988; 11:1607–1616.

Dohrmann ML, Goldschlager NF: Myocardial stimulation threshold in patients with cardiac pacemakers: Effect of physiologic variables, pharmacologic agents, and lead electrodes. Cardiol Clin 1985; 3:527–537.

Erdman S, Levinsky L, Strasberg B, et al: Use of the new Shaw Scalpel in pacemaker operations. J Thorac Cardiovasc Surg 1985; 89:304–307.

Erkkila KI, Singh JB: Reversion mode activation by myopotential sensing in a ventricular inhibited demand pacemaker. PACE 1985; 8:50–51.

Fetter J, Aram G, Holmes DR Jr, et al: The effects of nuclear magnetic resonance imagers on external and implantable pulse generators. PACE 1984; 7:720–727.

Fetter J, Patterson D, Aram G, et al: Effects of extracorporeal shock wave lithotripsy on single chamber rate response and dual-chamber pacemakers. PACE 1989; 12:1494–1501.

Frohlig G, Dyckmans J, Doenecke P, et al: Noise reversion of a dual-chamber pacemaker without noise. PACE 1986; 9:690–696.

Furman S: Radiation effects on implanted pacemakers. PACE 1982; 5:145.

Gabry MD, Behrens M, Andrews C, et al: Comparison of myopotential interference in unipolar-bipolar programmable DDD pacemakers. PACE 1987; 10:1322–1330.

Gay RJ, Brown DF: Pacemaker failure due to procainamide toxicity. Am J Cardiol 1974; 34:728–732.

Gettes LS, Shabetai R, Downs TA, et al: Effect of changes in potassium and calcium concentration on diastolic threshold and strength-interval relationships of the human heart. Ann NY Acad Sci 1969; 167:693–705.

Hayes DL: Effects of drugs and devices on permanent pacemakers. Cardiology 1991; 1: 70–75.

Hayes DL, Holmes DR Jr, Gray JE: Effect of 1.5 tesla nuclear magnetic resonance imaging scanner on implanted permanent pacemakers. J Am Coll Cardiol 1987; 10:782–786.

Hayes DL, Trusty J, Christiansen J, et al: A prospective study of electrocautery's effect on pacemaker function. (abstract) PACE 1987; 10:442.

Hellestrand KJ, Burnett PJ, Milne JR: Effect of the antiarrhythmic agent flecainide acetate on acute and chronic pacing thresholds. PACE 1983; 6:892–899.

Holmes DR Jr, Hayes DL, Gray JE, et al: The effects of magnetic resonance imaging on implantable pulse generators. PACE 1986; 9:360–370.

Irnich W: Interference in pacemakers. PACE 1984; 7:1021–1048.

Irnich W, Barold SS: Inteference protection in cardiac pacemakers. In SS Barold (ed.): Modern Cardiac Pacing. Mount Kisco, NY, Futura Publishing Company, 1985, pp. 839–855.

Kaye GC, Butrous GS, Allen A, et al: The effect of 50 Hz external electrical interference on implanted cardiac pacemakers. PACE 1988; 11:999–1008.

Kruse IM: Long-term performance of endocardial leads with steroid-eluting electrodes. PACE 1986; 9:1217–1219.

Langberg J, Abber J, Thuroff JW, et al: The effects of extracorporeal shock wave lithotripsy on pacemaker function. PACE 1987; 10:1142–1146.

Lau CP, Linker NJ, Butrous GS, et al: Myopotential interference in unipolar rate responsive pacemakers. PACE 1989; 12:1324–1330.

LaBan MM, Petty D, Hauser AM, et al: Peripheral nerve conduction stimulation: Its effect on cardiac pacemakers. Arch Phys Med Rehabil 1988; 69:358–362.

LeVick CE, Mizgala HF, Kerr CR: Failure to pace following high dose antiarrhythmic therapy—reversal with isoproterenol. PACE 1984; 7:252–256.

Levine PA, Barold SS, Fletcher RD, et al: Adverse, acute and chronic effects of electrical defibrillation and cardioversion on implanted unipolar cardiac pacing systems. J Am Coll Cardiol 1983; 1:1413–1422.

Manwaring M: What patients need to know about pacemakers. Am J Nurs 1977; 77:825–828.

Mickley H, Petersen J, Nielsen BL: Subjective consequences of permanent pacemaker therapy in patients under the age of retirement. PACE 1989; 12:401–405.

Mohan JC, Kaul U, Bhatia ML: Acute effects of antiarrhythmic drugs on cardiac pacing thresholds. Acta Cardiol 1984; 39:191–201.

Montefoschi N, Boccadamo R: Propafenone induced acute variation of chronic atrial pacing threshold: A case report. PACE 1990; 13: 480–483.

Preston TA, Fletcher RD, Lucchesi BR, et al: Changes in myocardial threshold. Physiologic and pharmacologic factors in patients with implanted pacemakers. Am Heart J 74:235, 1967.

Rasmussen MJ, Hayes DL, Vlietstra RE, et al: Can transcutaneous electrical nerve stimulation be safely used in patients with permanent cardiac pacemakers? Mayo Clin Proc 1988; 63:443–445.

Reiffel JA, Coromilas J, Zimmerman JM, et al: Drug-device interactions: Clinical considerations. PACE 1985; 8:369–373.

Rodriguez F, Filimonov A, Henning A, et al: Radiation-induced effects in multiprogrammable pacemakers and implantable defibrillators. PACE 1991; 14:2143–2153.

Sager DP: Current facts on pacemaker electromagnetic interference and their application to clinical care. Heart Lung 1987; 16:211–221.

Salel AF, Seagren SC, Pool PE: Effects of encainide on the function of implanted pacemakers. PACE 1989; 12:1439–1444.

Singer I, Guarnieri T, Kupersmith J: Implanted automatic defibrillators: Effects of drugs and pacemakers. PACE 1988; 11:2250–2262.

Surawicz B, Chlebus H, Reeves JT, et al: Increase of ventricular excitability threshold by hyperpotassemia-possible cause of internal pacemaker failure. J Am Med Assoc 1965; 191:71–76.

Telectronics: Electromagnetic interference and the pacemaker patient. Technical Notes, May 1991, No. 110.

Toivonen L, Valjus J, Hongisto M, et al: The influence of elevated 50 Hz electric and magnetic fields on implanted cardiac pacemakers: The role of the lead configuration and programming of the sensitivity. PACE 1991; 14:2114–2122.

Venselaar JLM: The effects of ionizing radiation on eight cardiac pacemakers and the influence of electromagnetic interference from two linear accelerators. Radiother Oncol 1985; 3:81–87.

Warnowicz MA: The pacemaker patient and the electromagnetic environment. Clin Prog Pacing Electrophys 1983; 1:166–176.

Zullo MA: Function of ventricular pacemakers during resuscitation. PACE 1990; 13:736–744.

Chapter 19

TROUBLESHOOTING

Seymour Furman

Implantable pacemakers will have occasional deficiencies with pacing and/or sensing, and pacemaker patients require periodic management of pacing defects. Complex modern devices must be analyzed carefully to understand the significance of pacing defects. Analysis must be undertaken in a logical and rational manner. Troubleshooting can occur during two different circumstances: nonoperatively (or preoperatively) and intraoperatively. During preoperative (or nonoperative) evaluation, direct access to the generator does not exist. Modern pulse generators have both programmability and telemetry that, added to x-ray and ECG findings, can often determine the nature of a specific malfunction. This chapter will deal with pacemaker hardware rather than physiological malfunction. Data from each of the other chapters, especially electrocardiography and radiology, has a bearing on this chapter and should be reviewed as this text is read.

Noninvasive evaluation will often allow management of difficulties by nonoperative change of pacemaker function. If nonoperative correction of pacemaker malfunction is impossible, then operative intervention will be required and will follow a second set of procedures to be described later. As in every medical discipline, preoperative diagnosis is preferable to intraoperative diagnosis. Management of problems must be undertaken in a rational and sequential manner (Table I).

Table I
Management of Complications of Pacing

I. A. Knowledge of Hardware Function
   B. Careful Records
   C. Knowledge of Possible Difficulties
      1. Surgical
      2. Physiological
      3. Specific hardware
      4. Interference or radiation damage
II. Careful Preoperative Analysis
III. Careful Intraoperative Analysis
IV. Rational Repair

Identify the Symptomatic Nature of the Malfunction

Unless infection or local pain exist, malfunction usually will be manifest by return of symptoms that required pacemaker implant initially, i.e., fatigue, syncope, or mental confusion. Malfunction may be noted by palpitations resulting from coupled beats, episodes of tachycardia, or pounding in the neck and chest, which are associated with pacemaker syndrome. A careful history to define the nature of the malfunction may be less necessary if syncope recurs, although it must be remembered that syncope, especially in the elderly, may be caused by bradycardia, tachycardia, or events unrelated to an implanted pacemaker or cardiac rate and rhythm. Alternatively, approximately one-third of patients will have significant but asymptomatic pacemaker malfunction.

Electrocardiographic Determination of Malfunction

A number of findings on ECG should be sought (Table II):

a. Is capture satisfactory in the sensitive period of the cardiac cycle for atrium, ventricle, or both?
b. Is sensing normal?
c. Is there any evidence of pacemaker function. If so, is it at a "normal" rate, is it very slow, is it rapid, or is it so rapid that it is impossible or unlikely that any pacemaker during normal operation could function in that manner; is it at a runaway rate, i.e., faster than 140 stimuli per minute; does cardiac capture occur at any rate?
d. Runaway pacemaker: rapid pacing rates that result from electronic malfunction have been referred to as "pacemaker runaway." Runaway has been the most lethal variety of pacemaker malfunction because of the rapid rates that can occur and because of instability of the pacemaker circuit. Runaway almost always occurs without warning of any other preliminary malfunction. In some, stimulation rates were sufficiently slow so that a patient with a relatively healthy myocardium could survive a short episode of ventricular pacing runaway.

Table II
Troubleshooting DDD Pacemakers—I

Free-Running ECG

1. Is the pacing rate as programmed?	5. Are the pulse durations as programmed?
2. Is the AV delay as programmed?	6. Are both channels operating:
3. Is the atrium:	a. individually?
a. sensed properly?	b. together?
b. paced properly?	
4. Is the ventricle:	
a. sensed properly?	
b. paced properly?	

In others, the rapid rate was coupled with a decrease in pacemaker output for each stimulus, occasionally below pacing threshold. Few, if any pacemakers capable of high-rate runaway remain in service. Modern pacemakers are carefully designed to reduce the possibility of stimulation rates in excess of about 140 bpm. Many are also designed to reduce the incidence of runaway by requiring two separate and unrelated electronic failures before runaway can occur. Although it is still possible for more rapid rates to occur, pacemaker runaway has become extremely unusual. If runaway rate is seen, the pacemaker should be removed as an emergency under sterile conditions if time permits, or if necessary, in the emergency department under unsterile conditions. If sterile, a new generator can be attached to the lead system immediately; if unsterile, the implanted lead can be used for temporary pacing. The pulse generator that has demonstrated runaway should not be left in situ for observation. Normal function may alternate with runaway at a lethal level without warning. Once runaway has occurred, the unit must be deemed unreliable and potentially disastrous, even if it appears to return to normal function (Figure 1).

A distinction between runaway and a ventricular or atrial triggered (VVT/AAT) pacemaker tracking a native tachycardia must be made. Magnet application with cessation of sensing of spontaneous cardiac activity will assist in the distinction. Magnet application will, almost always, have no effect on a generator during runaway.

e. No output: Sudden "no output" is a common mode of electronic failure. (Although electronic failure of modern pace generators is, itself, uncommon, much less common than in former discrete component generators.) In this instance, no pacemaker activity will be found either during free running or magnet application. Despite the impression that the sudden absence of pacemaker function leaves the patient unprotected and that pacemaker-dependent patients will suffer severely even with recurrent syncope, this situation is less dangerous than runaway. Possibly 30% of patients are sufficiently pacemaker-dependent as to have 5 seconds or more of asystole following sudden pacemaker failure.

f. Is the pacemaker single- or dual-chamber? If dual-chamber, is there evidence of atrial and ventricular pacing? Does all recycle occur from ventricular sen-

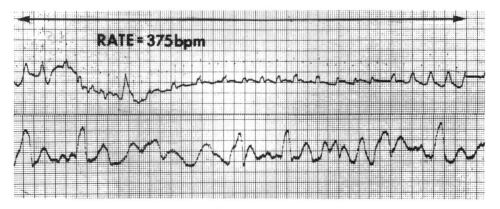

Figure 1.   *Runaway pacemaker, the most potentially lethal of all pacemaker complications, still occurs. This runaway, seen during March 1985 in an external pacemaker, stimulated the ventricle at about 350 beats per minute and caused ventricular fibrillation and death.*

Table III
Troubleshooting DDD Pacemakers—II

Magnet ECG

1. Is the pacing rate as programmed?
2. Is the AV delay as programmed?
3. Are the outputs as in the magnet mode?
4. Have the timing cycles become those of the magnet mode?

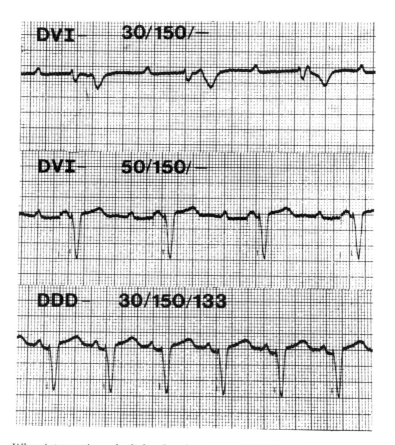

Figure 2.   *When interpreting a dual-chamber electrogram (ECG) it is important to recognize which chamber(s) are sensed and which are paced. Timing cycles are started and ended by sensed and paced events. Top: The DVI mode senses only ventricular activity. The unsensed atrial event does not initiate a timing cycle. As the ventricular rate is more rapid than the automatic pacemaker rate of 30 bpm, both atrial and ventricular channels are inhibited. Middle: The spontaneous ventricular rate is slower than the pacemaker rate so that continuous ventricular pacing occurs, always preceded by an atrial stimulus, in this instance competitive with unsensed atrial activity. Below: In the DDD mode, atrial sensing exists, and each sensed event starts an AV interval—in this instance, of 150 ms duration. Each sensed P wave is thus followed by a ventricular stimulus.*

sing only? Does escape after a sinus pause occur via an atrial escape, i.e., is the pacemaker DVI, DDI, or DDD, or does escape occur only by a ventricular stimulus, i.e., VDD? Is each P wave tracked with a ventricular stimulus following each P wave? The answer to each of these questions will assist in determining the mode of pacemaker operation and whether operation is normal (Table III) (Figure 2).

Identify the Pacemaker

All pacemaker function is defined by the design of the individual pacing device, and unusual function may appear to be present when, in fact, it is normal operation of an unexpected variety. One possibility is the unusual atrial and ventricular recycle during normal function of a committed AV sequential pacemaker.

X-Ray the Pacing System

All pulse generators can be radiographically identified. Some are clear with a manufacturer's logo and model number while others have a letter designation. Most can be identified by the x-ray configuration of the battery and circuit. All manufacturers provide tables and charts of identifying material, and a number of pacing books tabulate the data under one cover. Computer programs and compendia of pacemaker (pulse generator and leads) data allow ready identification of a pulse generator x-ray so that the pulse generator can be identified. Once the generator has been identified its mode of function should be known and if it is one for which the physician has the appropriate programming hardware, s/he should proceed with diagnosing the malfunction. If not, the manufacturer can be asked to provide the appropriate programmer and technical consultation. The lead system can be identified as unipolar or bipolar, whether a bifurcated bipolar lead has been unipolarized and whether the electrode tip is in the atrium or ventricle, or whether leads are in both atrium and ventricle for a dual-chamber system. Modern bipolar leads have an inline connector so that the former distinction between unipolar and bifurcated bipolar can no longer be made. But, a bipolar lead has two electrodes at its tip so that distinction remains. As many modern pulse generators, either single or dual chamber, can be programmed between unipolar and bipolar, the identification of a bipolar lead does not guarantee that the pacing system is in the bipolar mode. Of course, a unipolar system cannot be programmed to bipolar. X-ray can identify fracture, lead displacement, or inadequate connection and consequent intermittent pacing (Figure 3). Unfortunately insulation deterioration (a relatively common means of failure during the past decade) cannot be identified by x-ray.

X-ray and ECG are the two basic approaches for evaluating a pacing system. In many modern pacemakers, telemetry of pacemaker function is an important addition (Table IV).

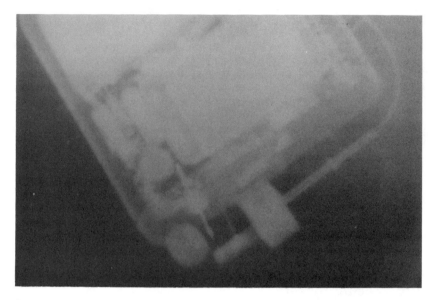

Figure 3. *Intermittent sensing and pacing were caused by inadequate placement of the lead pin connector into the receptacle of the pulse generator. Contact between the generator and the lead was, therefore, intermittent. Correction was by resetting the pin and the set screw. The defect is readily visible on x-ray.*

Table IV
Troubleshooting DDD Pacemakers—III

Chest X-ray—PA and Lateral

Is the atrial lead in RA appendage?
Is the ventricular lead in RV apex?
Is either lead fractured?
Are connections to the PG secure?

LEAD DESTRUCTION

Pacemaker implantation is commonly and widely achieved via subclavian puncture. To accomplish safe introduction of the needle and introducer, the vein that is entered traverses the costoclavicular space, as do the leads. Medial subclavian puncture is recommended as it is less likely that the subclavian artery or the pleural space will be entered. This approach traverses the costoclavicular ligament and provides an additional point of stress. The costoclavicular space may be narrow so that one and, especially, two leads already stressed by the costoclavicular ligament may bind further and be subjected to continual pressure and local friction and pressure. In the event of continual pressure and friction,

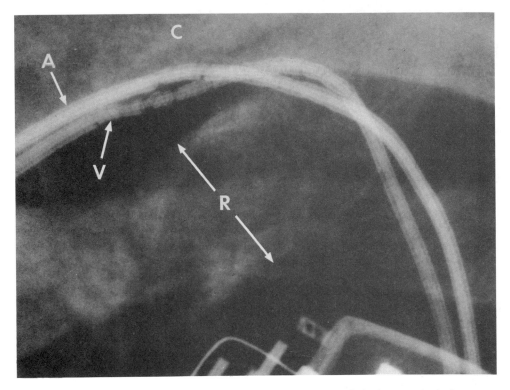

Figure 4. *Pressure caused destruction of atrial and ventricular leads in the costoclavicular space. The insulation of both leads is extensively notched with the conductor exposed. No ligatures have been placed in this region. A = atrial lead; V = ventricular lead; C = clavicle, R = first rib. (Courtesy of F. Earl Fyke, III, M.D.)*

insulation deterioration, especially of a polyurethane lead, will be rapid. Early failure of leads after such implantation can be detected radiologically, and as in other polyurethane deterioration, will be initially manifest by oversensing and possibly pacemaker inhibition (Figure 4). Telemetry of lead impedance and of the electrogram or other ECG interpretation channel may be especially useful in diagnosing insulation deterioration. Reduction of lead impedance is an indication of loss of insulation, while increase in impedance will indicate beginning loss of the metal conductor. The ECG interpretation channel will show the false signals generated by make and break metal contacts in an electrolyte solution that produce small electrical transients which are adequate to trigger and recycle a pulse generator.

PULSE GENERATOR MANIPULATION

Pulse generators should lie in the subcutaneous tissue, usually in the right or left pectoral region. The well-sited pulse generator will be well medial of the anterior axillary fold, and will be sufficiently inferior to the clavicle so that body movement, especially of the arm, will not cause the generator to impinge on the axilla or the clavicle. The pulse generator should be comfortable while the patient is at rest and pain free during body and, especially, arm movement. The skin overlying the generator should be nontender, of normal color, and without local heat. The pulse generator should not be adherent to the skin, subcutaneous tissue, or the underlying fascia. If any of these circumstances exist, the unit may be malpositioned or infected.

Other possibilities exist: One is that the pocket may be too small and the skin may have been pulled too tightly over the implanted generator. Excessively tight skin will be continually painful and skin necrosis (decubitus) with exposure of the pulse generator may occur. A generator placed too laterally will impinge on the anterior axillary fold and be uncomfortable whenever the arm is moved. The pulse generator may not be implanted in the subcutaneous plane, rather in the subcuticular plane so that the subcutaneous fat is deep to the pulse generator and the skin is superficial. Even a small generator will then protrude and will be clearly visible even in a heavy patient. The site will be continuously exquisitely painful, even if it is not touched, but more so even if the overlying skin is lightly touched. This finding is pathognomonic. Only replacement of the pulse generator in the subcutaneous space will relieve this distress. The generator may also have been placed immediately inferior to the clavicle. Then, with each movement of the arm it will ride superiorly and rub against the clavicle causing local distress. If even closer to the clavicle, arm movement may cause the generator to move superiorly and visibly push against and raise the skin. In all these instances the generator must be operatively replaced in the subcutaneous tissue or placed more inferiorly or more medially. Nonoperative management will be unsuccessful.

A lead fracture, the rare fracture of the header (connector) on the pulse generator, or a loose set screw holding the lead may be demonstrated by manipulating the pulse generator and lead. With the ECG running, the pulse generator is grasped through the skin and moved superiorly, inferiorly, medially, and laterally. A lead fracture may be detected by distraction of the fragments. With the patient in the standing position, holding a weight in the arm on the side of the pacemaker is also useful to distract lead fragments. X-ray with a weight can also be helpful in demonstrating fracture.

If infection of the pacemaker site is suspected because of local erythema, swelling, fluid collection, pain, or adherence of the pulse generator to surrounding tissue, wound culture is wise. As bacteria can be introduced, extreme care to avoid contamination should be exercised. The pulse generator site should be carefully shaved (if necessary) and washed as if for an operative procedure. It should then be painted with antiseptic solution and draped with sterile towels. The person performing the wound culture should wear sterile gloves and a sterile gown over clothing. Anesthetic solution and saline for intravenous use or for irrigation should be available as should sterile syringes and aerobic and anaerobic culture media. Saline for parenteral injection often contains an antibacterial preservative, and cultures diluted with it will be sterilized. An antibiotic solution for subsequent irrigation is useful. If the site appears to be infected it can be irrigated after the culture is taken, as that will provide short-term symptomatic relief while awaiting culture growth and determining the future course.

A dependent portion of the wound is infiltrated with local anesthetic. A #14 or #16 angiocath can then be introduced through the anesthetized site. This relatively large needle size is useful as purulent fluid is thicker and more viscous than either serous fluid or liquefied blood, and a larger lumen will be useful in its aspiration. The needle is directed toward the device and should strike it. The sensation of hitting a hard metallic object is unmistakable. As much fluid as possible should be withdrawn from the space around the pulse generator. If the fluid is too viscid or if little has accumulated, sterile saline (for intravenous use, not for injection) can be introduced and then aspirated. The fluid removed is sent for culture. As much as possible of the accumulated fluid is removed. Antibiotic solution then can be instilled and removed several times until the return is relatively clear. If the wound culture eventually demonstrates infection this process may provide brief symptomatic relief, but should not be confused as being curative.

RADIATION DAMAGE

Implanted pulse generators are not damaged by diagnostic levels of radiation. However, the thousands of RADs that are used for therapeutic radiation can damage and destroy an implanted generator. Older generators, which were constructed with discrete resistors, condensers, and transistors, were far less sensitive to radiation damage than are newer generators with complementary metal oxide semiconductor (CMOS) circuits. The difference between the two pacemaker designs is striking and older concepts of pacemaker resistance are not relevant to modern multiprogrammable single- or dual-chamber pulse generators.

If radiation therapy is required, the generator should not be in the radiation field and should be carefully shielded from scatter. If shielding is impossible, for example, in the case of breast or lung cancer in which the pulse generator lies directly in or adjacent to the radiation field, the generator should be moved to another site. A radiation dose is cumulative and the eventual mode of generator failure is random. The generator may lose sensing or output, suddenly stop, or suddenly runaway. Leads can be radiated without risk.

SUPERFAST RECHARGE

An occasional patient with a unipolar dual-chamber pulse generator model 7005 implanted will complain of episodic or continuous local muscle stimulation at the site of the pulse generator. Evaluation will demonstrate that such local stimulation occurs only when the atrium is being stimulated and not during ventricular stimulation alone or with atrial sensing and ventricular stimulation. Analysis of the atrial stimulus artifact will show it to be normal. Other evidence of lead insulation failure, the most common cause of local pectoral muscle stimulation, will be absent. Muscle stimulation during atrial pacing is likely to persist despite reduction in atrial channel output, even if it is below the stimulation capture threshold.

The event occurs because of a superfast recharge circuit placed into the atrial channel output and is intended to reduce the necessary duration of the ventricular blanking period, which begins with the atrial stimulus. Reduction in duration of the recharge time allows a shorter blanking period, but produces a greater amplitude recharge stimulus, though of shorter duration. This stimulus may, in a few patients, be a suprathreshold for stimulation of the local (pectoral) musculature.

As there is no certain means of stimulating the atrium and avoiding local musculature stimulation, the best means of management is the reduction of the incidence of atrial pacing. Model 7005 has no VDD mode, i.e., with atrial sensing but without pacing. Should atrial pacing be required to maintain synchrony, then local muscle stimulation may be unavoidable. If atrial activity is normal, then the lower rate limit should be reduced below the anticipated slowest atrial rate (this may be a problem for sleeping atrial rates), so that only sensing will occur. As atrial stimulation may occur during upper rate operation, especially should fixed ratio AV block occur, it is wise to increase the upper rate limit as high as is reasonable.

Should all other means of management fail, pulse generator replacement may be required. As this mechanism is part of normal operation of model 7005, replacement of one unit by another of the same model is not likely to help. Another model pulse generator will be required. The number of 7005 pulse generators implanted is decreasing as patients die and other units become depleted. Successor models have modified the rapid recharge circuit so that local muscle stimulation will not occur. Few model 7005 units now remain in service.

PULSE GENERATOR INSULATION DEFECT

Insulation defect, which is known to exist and be extremely troublesome in lead systems, can also exist on a pulse generator. Unipolar pulse generators (and bipolar generators that are programmable unipolar-bipolar) are insulated on one side, generally that opposite to the side engraved with the pulse generator identification. The insulated side should be placed toward the muscle, and the uninsulated side toward the subcutaneous tissue. The insulation material can be removed or rubbed from the pulse generator. Should that occur, two circumstances may follow. The first is that electromyographic interference (EMI) may occur and inappropriately inhibit the pulse generator. Alternatively, a small area of defect may shunt a relatively high current density to the muscle, causing a local twitch with each stimulus. This is especially true in the case of the atrial stimulus in a pulse generator with a superfast recharge circuit (see above). It may not then be possible to program an atrial channel output sufficiently low to avoid local muscle stimulation. This may be especially true in a patient with chronotropic incompetence who requires continued atrial stimulation.

If the pacemaker can operate in the effective VDD mode, in which there is no atrial stimulation, the effect may be avoided. If there is no possibility of ending atrial channel stimulation, operative intervention will be required. Once the insulation defect is found, an accessory silicone rubber boot may be placed on the generator. Alternatively, the pulse generator may be replaced. This condition is unusual, but has been seen by the author on several occasions. It should be suspected when local muscle stimulation occurs in model 7005, in the absence of atrial stimulation. It may occur with other pulse generators as well. No detectable defect may be present during routine, postoperative evaluation, as the current leak is extremely close to that which occurs during normal unipolar DDD pulse generator function.

PACING SYSTEM ANALYZER

The pacing system analyzer (PSA) is the basic device for determination of threshold of pacing and sensing. Equally important, it allows testing the function of an implanted pulse generator and lead system during pacemaker implant and during intraoperative analysis of pacemaker malfunction. As with any other device, knowledge of its proper operation is essential to derivation of useful data. This is especially true for the PSA, as these devices are not universally compatible with all implanted pacemaking systems, either for the lead system or for the pulse generator. For this reason, it is a wise policy to use the same make PSA as the generator to be tested and implanted. As each PSA operates somewhat differently, its manual should be carefully read and understood. There are two major differences that affect the method of interpretation of data derived from a PSA.

Measurement of Output Voltage

Constant voltage output is used in all present-day implantable pulse generators. One major manufacturer had used a constant current circuit, but it no longer provides the product. Some constant current pulse generators remain implanted, although all will have been removed in the near future. In a constant voltage output, the actual current flow is largely determined (within limits) by the impedance of the lead system. If the output voltage is 5 V and the impedance is the relative standard of 500 ohms, the current flow will be 10 mA. If however, a short circuit exists, and the impedance is only 250 ohms, then the current flow may be 20 mA and rapidly deplete the pulse generator battery. A PSA that measures constant voltage output will read both voltage outputs similarly and calculate current output at the higher level. (See Chapter 2, Basic Concepts.)

The sensing circuits of different pacing system analyzers use different criteria. Each manufacturer's standard differs from a natural intrinsic deflection depolarization; all are artificial. The sensing circuit of a pulse generator may test differently on each PSA and therefore, the specific response of each generator must be known for each specific PSA. As the volume of detail involved will probably exceed the management capability of most laboratories, and as manufacturers are unwilling to provide data concerning test results of generators not of their manufacture, it is best to use the PSA provided by the manufacturer of the pulse generator being tested. Electrogram (EGM) telemetry may differ from the measurement of an electrogram measured directly on a PSA so that data derived from telemetry may differ from that derived during direct measurement by a PSA.

At the conclusion of noninvasive pacemaker function evaluation, the nature of the malfunction is usually known. If unknown, it is likely that all possible diagnostic modalities have not been exhausted.

DIAGNOSTIC MODALITIES

1. Passive ECG
2. X-ray
3. ECG-free running and in the magnet mode
4. Ambulatory ECG (Holter monitoring)
5. Programming
6. Manipulation of the pulse generator (to accentuate lead fracture or insulation defect)
7. Telemetry

Most often, these maneuvers will give sufficient information to allow preoperative diagnosis of pacemaker malfunction. It is as important to begin surgical intervention well informed (concerning pacemaker malfunction) as in any other surgical approach. Because of the limited causes of malfunction, the cause usually can be ascertained preoperatively. Each approach, preoperative evaluation and operative assessment, offers the possibility of diagnostic procedures unavailable to the other; each should be used. For example, a hairline lead fracture may be visible on x-ray, but invisible to the unaided eye following exposure of the pacemaker hardware but, once again, present as a high impedance on telemetry or at operation. A summary of the procedure for troubleshooting dual-chamber pacemakers is contained in Tables II, III, IV, and V.

Table V
Programmability for Lead Malfunction

Operative Repair	*Increase Sensitivity*
1. Fracture	1. Poor electrogram
Decrease Output	*Reduce Sensitivity*
1. Diaphragmatic stimulation	1. Electromagnetic interference
2. Phrenic nerve stimulation	2. Electromyographic interference
Increase Output	*Change Mode*
1. Insulation failure	1. Electromagnetic interference
2. Poor position	2. Electromyographic interference
3. Displacement	3. "Noisy lead"
4. High threshold	
5. Threshold evolution	

TELEMETRY

Telemetric data transmission that includes hardware, stimulation, physiology, and electrogram data is becoming increasingly more available and important in troubleshooting pacemaker defects and analyzing the intricacies of normal pacemaker function. (See Chapter 16, Telemetry.) Recording of the telemetric data of lead impedance will be valuable in determining lead insulation failure, which will be indicated by a reduction of impedance. Unfortunately, lead impedance measurement that has been available from one major manufacturer for about half a decade (written in 1992) is only now becoming more widely available. Lead impedance telemetry is becoming more widely available and will soon be a functional component of most pulse generators from all manufacturers. A very low telemetered impedance, i.e., 200 ohms, or a very high impedance, i.e., 2000 ohms seems to provide diagnostic information. More moderate impedance changes may be nonspecific or result from measurement errors and have no clear meaning. Both low and high impedance resulting from structural damage are likely to be associated with more dramatic findings.

OPERATIVE ASSESSMENT OF PACEMAKER MALFUNCTION

If noninvasive assessment of pacemaker malfunction has been unsuccessful in determining the nature of the problem or if the programmability available has not been adequate for resolution of the problem, then operative intervention is undertaken (Table V).

The Incision

If it has been determined with a reasonable degree of certainty that the pulse generator only is at fault, then it alone should be approached. The incision can be made over the center of the implanted generator, which can then be lifted from the subcutaneous or submuscular pocket detached from the lead(s), which can then be tested for contact with the chamber of placement and for electrical and mechanical integrity. This is usually the case if pulse generator battery depletion has occurred.

If the leads have been determined preoperatively to require replacement or reposition, then the incision should be made via the original implant incision that had been placed to approach the venous system. If the leads need not be manipulated, an incision over them risks damage as they are difficult to palpate in the subcutaneous tissue and can readily be cut scalpel or scissors. If the revision does not require dissection of leads, they should not be approached.

The Wound

When the wound is opened it should be inspected and reviewed for infection. An infected wound should be abandoned (see Infection, Chapter 14). A clean wound is free of purulence, erythema, and tenderness. Upon opening the wound, if the lining of the pacer site is reddened or purulent or there is other than a small volume (1–2 cc) of clear light yellow fluid, then the wound should be cultured and not reused as a pacer site. Malposition of the pulse generator, which may be high, lateral, superficial, or any combination, will cause continuing, unrelenting patient discomfort until surgically relieved (see above).

Pulse Generator and Leads

The Leads are Exposed

Measurement should be made of the impedance of each lead separately. If the lead is bipolar, then the impedance measurement should be of the bipolar pair. Measurement should be with any of the pacing system analyzers commercially available. The impedance is a measurement determined at a specific pulse duration and at a specific output, usually 10 mA (constant current) or 5 V (constant voltage). Lead impedance is very important data and varies with the method of measurement; it is, therefore, important that measurement be undertaken so that readings at the time of implant and later, at secondary intervention, are comparable.

Low Impedance

Late evolution of impedance after implantation is modest, i.e., several years after implantation, impedance will not be more than 20% greater than the impedance at the time of implantation (again measured by similar techniques). Virtually all electrode impedances will approximate 500 ohms, as all are designed to that general specification. Some will be as low as 400 ohms and others will be as high as 950 ohms. Any significant deviation outside of these limits should suggest strongly the possibility of electrode defect.

If the impedance is lower than the given range, an insulation defect can be anticipated with current leak into the tissue before reaching the electrode. In the presence of a bipolar lead system, the possibility exists that the short circuit is between the two conductors. If low impedance is present, current is escaping either to the surrounding tissue (local muscle stimulation may occur) in a unipolar or bipolar lead system, or between the two conductors in a bipolar system (Figure 5). If insulation damage is visible (in a unipolar system) in the exposed tissue it can probably be repaired. If it is at the connector, repair is readily possible with equipment provided by all manufacturers. If the insulation is deteriorated the lead cannot be salvaged. If the disruption is somewhere within the venous system, repair will be difficult or practically impossible. If one limb of a bipolar system is intact, the resolution may be by unipolarization of the lead system but only if the lead to the tip is intact, not the lead to the electrode ring (Figure 6). While programming from bipolar to unipolar may be accomplished with an inline bipolar lead and a unipolar-bipolar programmable pulse generator, conductor fracture in one conductor may cause early fracture in the

SHORT CIRCUIT

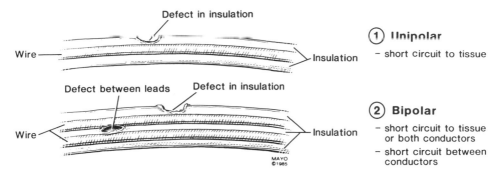

Figure 5. *Short circuit of a pacer lead follows insulation deterioration. In the unipolar system, short circuit allows escape of current to the surrounding tissue. In the bipolar lead, the defect may be to the surrounding tissue of one conductor, both conductors, or between the two.*

other. Once again the programming revision can be done only if the conductor to the tip remains intact. If insulation deterioration has occurred, rather than a traumatic insulation loss, deterioration will continue and the lead must be taken out of service. The lead may be removed, although this may be very difficult, or the lead may be abandoned in place.

While a lead fracture protects an implanted pacemaker from depletion, an insulation disruption can cause rapid depletion. A constant voltage pacemaker

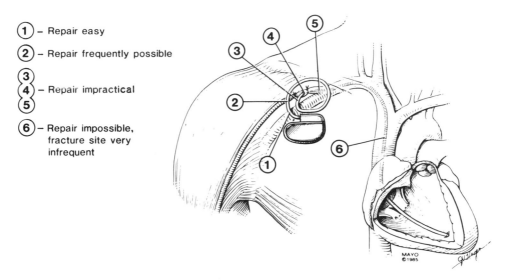

Figure 6. *Lead fracture still occurs as a constant, ongoing phenomenon following implant. For a unipolar lead, attempt at repair depends on the site of fracture. If fracture is well beyond (i.e., outside) entry to the vein, repair may be easy; if adjacent to entry to the vein, it is impractical; and if within the vein, the fracture site is unapproachable.*

will deliver a current at short circuit that will be limited only by the low internal resistance of the output circuit. Consequently, a constant voltage unit can deliver large currents and deplete itself rapidly. If revision is undertaken for lead insulation failure, the generator should be investigated carefully for evidence of depletion before it is reused. This is especially true for insulation defects of polyurethane leads in which the defect is commonly associated with short circuit to the subcutaneous tissue or between the two conductors of a bipolar lead. Consideration to replacing the pulse generator should be given even if it has been implanted only for a short time and tests satisfactorily. Generators do not provide an indication of substantial depletion until end of service life has occurred. One further clue may be telemetry (if it exists) of cell impedance that for the lithium iodine cell increases progressively with its depletion. An impedance well over 1000 ohms indicates substantial depletion and the pulse generator should be replaced.

High Impedance

If lead impedance is high it is important to check the measurement. Calibrate the PSA. If the PSA is satisfactory, short circuit the test cables used to measure the lead impedance, one to the other. The impedance on the PSA should now approximate zero or the minimum reading of the PSA. Separate the two clips, the impedance should be infinite. If these findings are consistent, the PSA is probably operating satisfactorily and the cables are intact. Most PSA impedance measurements allow a range of 250–2000 ohms, so these will be the measurement limits. If the impedance exceeds the presumed upper limit or if it is higher by 50% or more than that at implant, lead fracture or conductor deterioration has probably occurred. Such a fracture may not be visible on x-ray. Negative x-ray findings do not eliminate the possibility of fracture. Elevated lead impedance is a more sensitive indicator of fracture than x-ray. If the impedance reading is above 1000 ohms, fracture is almost certain; if it is above 2000 ohms, i.e., reading at infinity, lead fracture is certain. If the break is outside the venous system and in the subcutaneous tissue, repair depends on whether an adequate length is present to repair without stress. If repair cannot be accomplished either with low or high impedance conditions, the connector pin should be insulated or removed and the lead abandoned or removed.

A lead that is clean (uninfected) and has been chronically in place may be difficult to remove. If it is fractured within the venous system, i.e., distal to the point at which it can be grasped it may not be possible to remove it without an invasive procedure. Abandonment of an uninfected lead may be preferable to an attempt at removal. Occasionally, total removal of a lead will be unsuccessful leaving fragments of the lead in situ. Such fragments may cause more difficulty than an intact, inactive lead. Removal of an inactive lead should be performed only after carefully considering the consequences of leaving the lead in place or removing it destructively. If the high impedance is felt to be caused by lead failure, several options exist: abandonment, partial removal, or complete removal.

Threshold of Pacing

Each lead should be tested for pacing threshold and whether the threshold is within the output capability of the pulse generator. If the threshold is low (compared to the output capability of the pulse generator), then all is well. If the threshold is in the general middle range of output, the generator can be programmed to accommodate threshold. If threshold is near or above maximum pulse generator output, the lead requires revision. The distinction between high threshold and lead defect lies in the impedance. High or low impedance associated with lack of capture indicates lead defect. Normal impedance with high threshold implies defect of the electrode myocardial interface.

It is generally easy to decide when threshold is well within the output capability of the pulse generator intended for implant. It is equally easy to determine when threshold is excessively high. The major difficulty occurs when threshold is high but margin still exists. The following rules may be useful:

1. Determine that the lead impedance is normal, i.e., that high threshold is not a result of a lead defect;
2. Determine that the voltage and current thresholds are proportional. If the voltage threshold is high, the current threshold should be proportionally high. High voltage threshold and low current threshold indicate high impedance and lead fracture. Low voltage threshold and high current threshold indicate short circuit or lead defect. For virtually all pacing system analyzers the voltage is measured directly, just as the impedance, and the current flow is derived, i.e., calculated from the two. It should be recognized that voltage threshold and impedance are measured values, current is derived.
3. A stable, sharply defined threshold that is high may be useful. If threshold is high and varies as it is tested, it is unreliable and should not be used. High pulse generator output consumes the battery rapidly, and all estimates of prolonged pacemaker longevity are based on "normal" levels of output. If "normal" output cannot accommodate pacing and an adequate safety margin, lead revision or replacement should be undertaken. Special circumstances may, of course, dictate that prolonged longevity is less important than immediate and short-term restoration of pacing. "Normal" output can be considered to be a maximum output voltage of 5 V and a pulse duration of 0.5–1.0 ms. However, the most modern pacemakers will have an abbreviated longevity even at 5 V and 0.5 ms, and their longevity is based on a continuing output at 2.5 V, a far more efficient setting.
4. 7.5–10 V outputs consume the battery rapidly. Such outputs should be used sparingly and only for good reason in special circumstances.

Once pulse duration threshold has been determined at 2.5 V, output should be set at 2.5 V and at least triple the pulse duration threshold. This situation will work well if threshold pulse duration is briefer than 1.0 ms. If threshold pulse duration is determined at 2.5 V, output should be set at least three times the threshold pulse duration if that pulse duration does not exceed 1.2 ms. If pulse duration threshold at 2.55 V output is 0.5 ms or greater, a 5 V setting should be used for an adequate safety margin, recognizing the abbreviated longevity that will result.

Sensing Threshold

As with the pacing threshold, the amplitude of the electrogram should be measured either directly on a physiological recorder or with a PSA. If the electrogram is of amplitude and slew rate (frequency content) adequate to be readily sensed, no revision is required. If not, the lead may require repositioning. The display of the electrogram on a physiological recorder has the additional virtue, not available on the PSA, of identifying the chamber in which the lead lies. Since erroneous placement of an atrial appendage lead in the outflow tract of the right ventricle can occur, display of the atrial EGM is especially valuable and will definitively identify the site of the lead; simple electrogram amplitude will not (Figure 7). If the signal (i.e., the EGM) is too small to be sensed by the maximum sensitivity of the pulse generator, lead revision is required. If the signal is adequate, attention can be turned to the pulse generator.

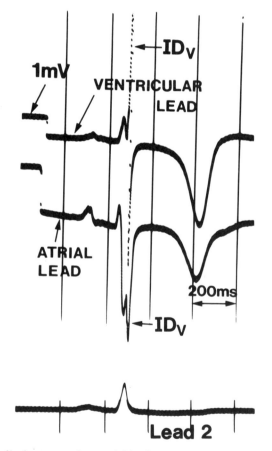

Figure 7. *Following displacement of an atrial lead to the right ventricular outflow tract, x-ray was reported as normal. Simultaneous electrogram recording from the atrial and ventricular leads demonstrated ventricular electrograms from both leads simultaneous with the QRS complex on the surface.*

Electrogram

One of the best tests for lead integrity and placement is determination of the electrogram via the implanted lead. In a number of generators, the electrogram can be telemetered noninvasively and indicate by its quality whether the lead is intact. If this capability does not exist or if there is any doubt at all, the electrogram derived from the implanted lead should be displayed during pacemaker revision. The appearance of the implanted lead electrogram should be similar to that shown elsewhere in this text (Chapter 3, Sensing and Timing the Cardiac Electrogram). A carefully done electrogram using cables now provided by various manufacturers and displayed on a physiological recorder should be recorded at 0.1–2000 Hz and will be clean and well defined. An electrogram recorded on an electrocardiograph will be frequency-limited but will be readily recognizable and interpretable (Figures 8 and 9). Possible defects include:

1. Artifacts on the EGM indicating the reason for "false recycle" (Figure 10);
2. 60-Hz interference, indicating a loss of lead continuity;
3. Intermittent loss of signal, i.e., intermittent lead contact;
4. Small EGM, below the level of sensing capability (Figure 11).

In each instance it is important to be certain that the connecting cables are intact as defects in the cables can mimic each of these problems.

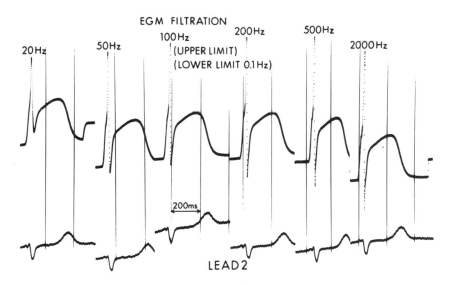

Figure 8. *The quality of the electrogram (EGM) depends on the frequency response of the recorder. In each of these tracings, the lower frequency response is 0.1 Hz, the upper is as listed. Since much of the electrogram amplitude is at higher frequency levels, recording at a lower frequency limits the amplitude of the recording. The recording at 100 Hz will approximate that on an electrocardiograph. It is best to record the EGM at an upper frequency cutoff of 500 or more Hz.*

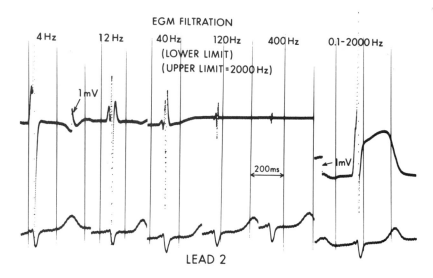

Figure 9. *The quality of the electrogram (EGM) depends on the frequency response of the recorder. In each of these tracings, the upper frequency response is 2000 Hz, the lower is as listed. Since much of the electrogram amplitude is also at lower frequency levels, recording at a higher frequency only limits the amplitude of the recording. It is best to record the electrogram at a lower frequency response of 0.1 Hz and an upper limit of at least 500 Hz.*

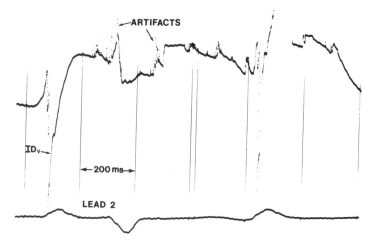

Figure 10. *An electrogram recorded with superimposed random artifacts. These artifacts may result from a poor connection between test lead and pacing lead, or lead fracture. The persistence of these artifacts after careful attention to the various connections is an indication of conductor deterioration even if no fracture is visible on x-ray.*

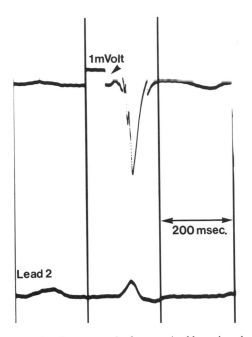

Figure 11. *A good ventricular electrogram is characterized by a sharply defined intrinsic deflection of adequate amplitude, with an intrinsic deflection that has minimal visible slope. A poor electrogram is characterized by visible slope, poor amplitude (in this instance no more than ³/₄ mV), and occasionally, a reversal of the intrinsic deflection, which makes each component too small to be sensed.*

RETAINED LEAD

Occasionally, a lead will be damaged or will have deteriorated so that it no longer can be in use. When such a lead is found to be present because of high threshold, uncorrectable sensing, or impending insulation deterioration or lead fracture, the lead should not be reused. Two additional circumstances exist: the lead may be infected or it may be clean. If it is infected it must be removed, otherwise cure of the infection and sterilization of the blood will be virtually impossible. While occasional reports of infection relief without removal of hardware have appeared, these should be regarded with suspicion. The only certain means of clearing the infection is lead removal with subsequent antibiotic management.

If the lead is clean it may be abandoned in situ. The connector pin should be insulated with a cap provided for that purpose. The lead should be carefully attached to the subcutaneous tissue with nonabsorbable ligature so that it cannot migrate.

LEAD REMOVAL

If the lead is infected it must be removed. The lead must be carefully mobilized, and a secure portion of the lead in the subcutaneous tissue grasped.

Gentle traction under fluoroscopy should be exerted while watching the lead move from the right ventricular apex into the superior vena cava and out, via the site of insertion. If implantation is via thoracotomy, then repeat thoracotomy will be necessary. The incision is made to approach the electrode at the myo- cardial level. Once the electrode is carefully removed from the myocardium by unscrewing or by cutting the ligatures holding it, the electrode is cut from the lead and removed. The lead can then be removed by traction as it moves through the tract in the subcutaneous tissue. Removal of the electrode at the myocardial level is usually easily accomplished if infection is present, as it has already been lifted from the heart by the infectious process (Figure 12).

If the transvenous lead cannot be removed by gentle manual traction, weighted traction can be used. The lead is exposed, and a hemostat grasps the exposed end. A weight over a pulley at the end of the operating table or the bed then applies continuous traction until the lead falls from the heart. The process may occupy several hours. Once the pulley is in place, water is added to a plastic bag to serve as the weight until several ventricular premature con- tractions (VPC) are seen. Approximately 350 mL will be required to start. Water is then continually added until VPCs occur as the traction removes the lead from the myocardium. This process contaminates the lead, which must be removed eventually, once this process has started (Figure 13).

Atrial leads can also be removed, but since the atrium is fragile it may be lacerated by the procedures listed above. Only a few successful removals of a retained atrial lead have been reported, and the risk of removal of an atrial lead by traction is uncertain. If traction is deemed too risky, then thoracotomy may be used with amputation of the atrial appendage.

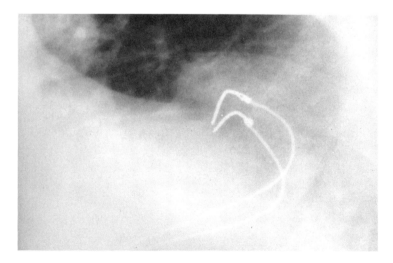

Figure 12.   *An infectious mass surrounds the two electrodes implanted by thoracotomy, which are no longer capable of stimulating the heart. At exploration, the electrodes lay free in a gelatinous infected mass.*

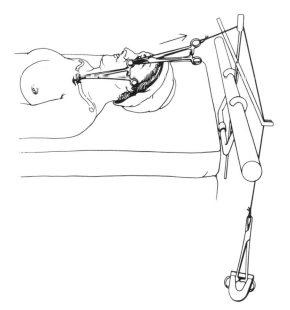

Figure 13. *Removal of a chronically implanted ventricular lead can usually be accomplished by slow, progressive, and gentle traction. The lead must be surgically mobilized and then attached to a Buck's traction on which progressive weights are placed. The weight is increased progressively to the level at which an occasional ventricular premature contraction (VPC) occurs. As the lead moves from the ventricle, the weight can be increased.*

Locking Guide Wire Technique

During the past few years a technique has been developed that has been successful in removal of endocardial atrial and ventricular leads. The level of success is such that while infected leads must be removed, some workers now routinely remove uninfected leads to rid the venous system and right ventricle of unnecessary hardware. The approach is highly successful, with few complications of disruption of the ventricle or, rarely, but more commonly the atrium. Should laceration of atrium or ventricle occur, emergency evacuation of the pericardium will be required, most likely by an open chest approach.

The technique involves an approach external to the lead and another within the coil. Therefore it is suitable only for leads in which the conductor has a lumen, i.e., all transvenous leads, but not epicardial leads. The hardware consists of locking guide wires that are introduced into a lead lumen, hard plastic tubes that are introduced over the lead, sizers that ascertain the size of the locking guide wire to be used, and a tool to dilate the lead lumen to accept the locking stylet (Figure 14). The lead is exposed in the subcutaneous tissue and detached from the pulse generator. Any ligatures or a sleeve which may hold the lead in place is removed so that the lead is fully mobilized. The connector is cut from the lead with a sharp tool so that the coil is not crushed. The lumen dilating tool is inserted for 1–2 cm. The sizers are then gently inserted about 2–3 cm to determine the size of the lumen so that the properly sized locking

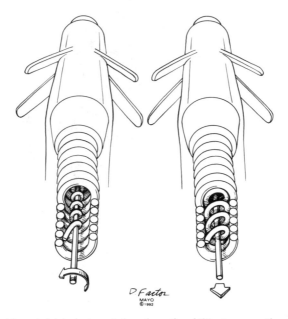

Figure 14. *The locking stylet technique is based on the ability to grasp the coil (the inner coil of a bipolar lead) with a locking guide wire so that inflexible traction can be applied to the tip of the lead. Left: The locking guide is inserted and rotated counterclockwise. The locking whisker is insinuated and grasps the coil. Rotation can then be relaxed and traction applied.*

guide wire can be introduced. The locking guide wire should fit as snugly as possible while still moving freely. Once the lumen is dilated and the proper sized locking guide wire selected, the guide wire is removed from its sheath and a fine wire "whisker" at the distal end of the wire is drawn from a position against the wire to one standing apart from the wire at a 45° angle.

The wire is gently introduced under fluoroscopic control and with continual rotation to the end of the lead to be removed. Once it is in this position the rotation is reversed and the guide wire "locked." With this maneuver the lead, which is normally flexible and can be elongated by traction, is now locked to the guide wire which cannot be elongated. Traction on the guide wire will now be transferred to the lead. Traction forcefully applied to the locked guide wire will now begin to pull the lead from its position in the atrium or the ventricle. If the lead can be fully removed that ends the procedure and a second lead, if present, may be approached. If the lead is adherent to the ventricular apex or if it appears to be adherent to the venous system, the external plastic tubes are placed over the now taut lead. The guide wire has a loop at its proximal end that is grasped by an additional metal wire that allows the tube of appropriate size to be placed over the lead. It is insinuated along the lead with continual rotation to break adhesions to the venous system. If this completes the freeing of the lead it can be removed. If the lead remains adherent to the apex of the ventricle, the tube is advanced to the point of ventricular attachment where traction on the lead and countertraction with the plastic tube will exert sufficient force to free the lead (Figure 15).

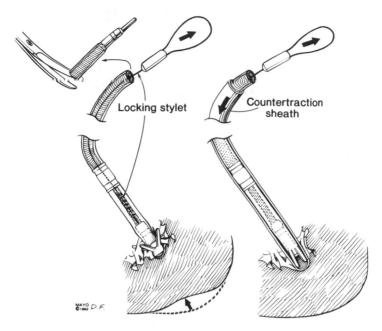

Figure 15. *The entire process is described as follows: The connector is cut from the lead. The locking stylet is then insinuated into the lead (see Figure 13). Traction is applied to the lead which may pull it from the heart. Right: If additional traction is required, the plastic sheath is placed over the lead and pushed against the myocardium to provide countertraction, while the locking guide pulls on the lead.*

Equipment specifically designed to remove retained leads by a femoral approach is also commercially available. The technique, while modified specifically for the purpose of lead removal, is similar to that described above for endocardial lead removal via the femoral route, described below. The details are in the manufacturer's literature.

Lead Removal—Femoral Route

A chronically implanted lead can often be removed if tension can be applied to the lead near its tip. The technique used at the Mayo Clinic is as follows. If the tip of the lead cannot be removed by traction, a pigtail catheter is passed into the heart via the femoral vein. The pigtail portion of the catheter is positioned around the permanent pacing lead as near the tip as possible (Figure 16). Twisting the pigtail catheter multiple times in a clockwise direction will entwine the pacing lead in the pigtail catheter (Figure 17). Traction is then applied to the pigtail catheter. Traction applied to the pacing lead near its point of endocardial attachment will frequently free the lead (Figure 18A). If the lead tip is dislodged from the endocardial surface, continued traction is placed on the pigtail catheter and the lead is pulled into the inferior vena cava. Because the entwined pacing lead and pigtail catheter are bulky and with traction the pigtail

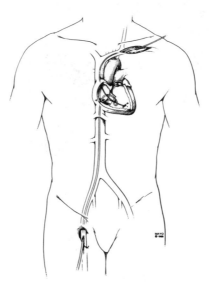

Figure 16.   *A pigtail catheter is passed via the right femoral vein into the right ventricle. The pigtail portion of the catheter is positioned around the permanent pacing lead as near to the tip of the lead as possible.*

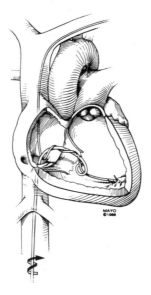

Figure 17.   *The pigtail catheter is then twisted in a clockwise fashion. This effectively entwines the pigtail catheter and the permanent pacing lead.*

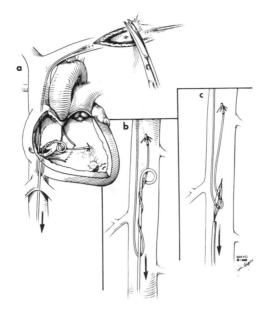

Figure 18. *(A) With the pigtail catheter and the permanent pacing lead firmly entwined, traction is applied on the pigtail catheter in an attempt to free the lead tip from the endocardial surface. (B) If traction is successful in freeing the tip of the lead, the lead is pulled into the inferior vena cava. The pigtail catheter is rotated in a counterclockwise direction to free the pigtail catheter and is removed via the femoral vein. (C) The pigtail catheter is replaced with a Dotter retriever. The wire basket is extended, and under fluoroscopy, it's positioned so that a portion of the pacing lead is within the wire basket. The wire basket is then retracted around a portion of the pacing lead so that the pacing lead is firmly caught in the Dotter retriever. Traction is then applied to the Dotter retriever in an attempt to extract the whole lead via the femoral vein. The most proximal portion of the pacing lead (the lead connector) should be transected prior to extraction.*

catheter may slip off the free end of the pacing lead, the pigtail catheter is removed in a counterclockwise direction (Figure 18B). Once the pigtail catheter is removed, a Dotter retriever is passed into the inferior vena cava via the femoral vein. The Dotter retriever consists of a retractable wire basket that is passed within a sheath. When the wire basket is extended beyond the sheath, the basket opens, and the operator attempts to catch a portion of the pacing lead in the wire basket. When the retractor is then pulled back, the pacing lead will be firmly entrapped in the Dotter retriever. Applying traction on the Dotter retriever, the lead then can be extracted via the femoral vein. Prior to attempting extraction, the connector portion at the proximal end of the pacing lead must be transected (Figure 18C).

If initial traction on the entwined pigtail catheter fails to dislodge the tip of the pacing lead, any redundancy in the lead is pulled into the inferior vena cava in an effort to form a small loop of pacing lead that can subsequently be grasped by the Dotter retriever (Figure 19A). Again, by turning the pigtail catheter in a counterclockwise direction, the pigtail catheter is freed from the pacing lead and removed. The Dotter retriever is then passed into the inferior vena cava and with the basket extended, an attempt is made to capture the loop of pacing lead

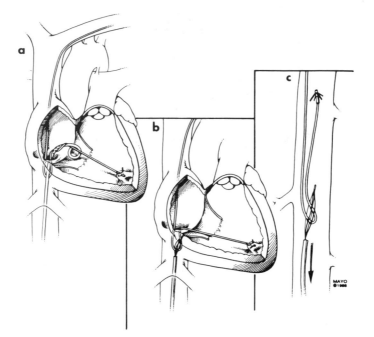

Figure 19.   (A) With the pigtail catheter firmly entwined with the permanent pacing lead, traction is applied, but the lead tip cannot be dislodged from the endocardial surface. Traction is applied on the pigtail catheter and the still attached lead in an effort to position a small loop of the pacing catheter within the inferior vena cava. The pigtail catheter is then rotated in a counterclockwise direction in an effort to separate the pigtail catheter from the pacing lead. The pigtail catheter is then removed. (B) The Dotter retriever is passed into the inferior vena cava. With the Dotter retriever extended, an attempt is made to snare the loop of the pacing lead in the Dotter retriever. Once this is accomplished, the basket portion of the Dotter retriever is retracted, firmly securing a portion of the pacing lead in the Dotter retriever. Traction is then applied on the Dotter retriever to free the tip of the pacing lead from the endocardial surface. (C) If the tip of the pacing lead is successfully dislodged from the endocardial surface, the lead is extracted via the femoral vein.

within the inferior vena cava in the Dotter retriever. Once the pacing lead has been entrapped in the wire basket, the retractor is pulled back and with the pacing lead firmly snared, traction is placed on the Dotter retriever in an effort to dislodge the tip of the lead (Figure 19B). The Dotter retriever is sometimes successful in dislodging the lead tip when the pigtail catheter has failed, because better traction can be applied with the pacing lead securely snared in the Dotter retriever. If the lead tip is successfully dislodged, continued traction is placed on the Dotter retriever, and the lead is extracted by the femoral vein (Figure 19C). Extracting the lead via the femoral vein, while it is still entangled in the Dotter retriever can potentially damage the femoral vein because of the bulk of the catheters being extracted. In our experience, no significant hematomas have resulted from the extraction, nor has venous repair ever been required. A pressure dressing should be placed over the puncture site, and the site must be carefully observed.

LEAD REMOVAL BY OPEN HEART SURGERY

If all other approaches for removal of an infected lead(s) have failed, removal is still mandatory if cure of endocarditis is to occur. If the lead cannot be safely removed, and this may be especially so for atrial leads, a direct approach by thoracotomy must be made.

If a ventricular lead has been removed and only the atrial lead remains, it may be attached at the atrial appendage. With median sternotomy, the superior and inferior vena cava are dissected and looped with tapes and the azygos vein is also occluded. The attachment of the atrial lead to the atrial appendage can be palpated, and with inflow occlusion the tip of the atrial appendage can be amputated, freeing the lead. The amputated atrium is then reclosed with a partially occluding clamp and repaired. Separately, the site of insertion of the lead, probably at the pectoral area, is opened, and the lead mobilized and withdrawn from the venous system. This approach does not involve cardiopulmonary bypass and can be accomplished briefly (with 1 to 2 minutes of inflow occlusion, or none at all).

If the atrial lead cannot be removed, as above, a ventricular lead is adherent to the ventricular apex, or a lead has deteriorated and traction only causes it to unravel, leaving portions of the lead within the ventricle, open heart surgical approach is required for its removal. The chest is opened via median sternotomy and cardiopulmonary bypass is established. The right atrium is opened and the ventricular lead is grasped as it traverses the tricuspid valve. The lead is detached from the valve, and the traction on it pulls the point of ventricular attachment to the tricuspid valve. The site of attachment may be encased in infected thrombus, which can now be removed along with tricuspid valve vegetations. As much infected tissue as possible should be debrided. The fibrous tissue holding the lead in place can be readily identified and cut with a scalpel. The lead can then be readily removed from the ventricle. The fibrous mass should be debrided, but need not be entirely resected.

Having freed the lead from within the heart, the site of attachment to the pulse generator in the pectoral region can be approached, and the lead withdrawn. A chronically implanted lead may have become adherent to the subclavian vein, which may be lacerated by traction. Bleeding may then be virtually uncontrollable.

Once the lead and vegetations have been removed from the heart, the atriotomy can be reclosed in routine fashion and cardiopulmonary bypass ended. If the patient has been on prolonged antibiotic management, and the blood stream has been sterilized, thoracotomy implantation of new myocardial leads may be accomplished at this time. Antibiotic administration should be continued for the full course of management of bacterial endocarditis.

At Montefiore Medical Center 12 patients have undergone open heart surgical removal of infected leads with the first on July 27, 1973. Ten have been long-term cures with uninfected survival as long as 17 years. One 89-year-old patient is alive and well and free of infection 15 months (as of March 1993) after open heart removal of an infected lead. We do not consider a cure to have been achieved until the patient has been absolutely well for 1 year. One patient died postoperatively with a retained infected lead fragment in the vascular system, but not in the heart.

The Pulse Generator

The pulse generator should be tested to determine whether it is operating properly. Most of the available PSA systems will allow the determination of pulse generator output, sensitivity, and pulse duration. The pulse generator should be programmed to several of its capabilities and then checked with the PSA. If the generator has been programmed to the outputs displayed on the programmer, then it is probably functioning normally and may be reused. Sterile programming heads and cables are readily available. If the pulse generator is contaminated during testing, it should not be returned to the original pacer site but be resterilized with ethylene oxide and reused in the same patient. Directions for resterilization with ethylene oxide are beyond the capability of this text; temperature limits should not be exceeded. If ethylene oxide sterilization is used, the device should be allowed to aerate for several days, and should be adequately washed with saline to remove residual gas before reimplantation. The generator should be carefully inspected for mechanical defects, especially at the connector. If the unit is sterile and intact mechanically and electrically, it can be reused, but most warranties will be voided. Each manufacturer may have a different policy and this should be checked. If in doubt, use a new generator suitable for the patient.

Pulse Generator Reuse

Reuse of a previously implanted pulse generator is an issue fraught with legal and ethical problems. In the United States a unit from one patient cannot be refurbished by a manufacturere or other commercial organization and implanted in another patient. Reuse of a generator that has been removed and is to be reimplanted during the same procedure into the same patient is commonly performed and is appropriate. Reuse of a pulse generator removed from a patient, then cleansed, sterilized, and reused in the same patient at a later date is appropriate. Nevertheless, subjecting the pulse generator to that process will usually void the manufacturer's warranty and if incorrectly done, may destroy the generator (see above). The U.S. Food and Drug Administration stated in Compliance and Policy Guide 7124.12 dated October 1, 1980 the policy that "Pacemaker Reuse is an objectionable practice."

Pulse Generator Eccentricity

Pacemaker eccentricity is an apparent deviation from presumed normal function, but is normal function for that model. Eccentricities should be distinguished from unexpected function, which has been designed to be normal pulse generator function. There are many such eccentricities of both single- and dual-chamber pulse generators. All represent normal rather than abnormal function and when found, should not lead to a conclusion of malfunction.

Single-chamber pulse generator eccentricities include:

1. Prolonged periods of asystole during programming of models 5984/5. Depending on the rate from which the device is programmed to the rate at which it is programmed, a period of almost 4 seconds of asystole may occur (Figure 20). (This unit is no longer manufactured but many remain in service.)
2. Partial programming during programming of devices using magnetic reed switch manipulation. Partial rate programming may result in an intermediate rate. For example, the 0505 generator rate moves during rate programming from the previous rate of 100 bpm, and finally to the new rate. It may remain at 100 bpm and can be returned to the normal function by repeating the programming sequence (Figure 21). (This unit is no longer manufactured but many remain in service.)
3. Several models of unipolar dual-chamber pacemakers can use the opposite leads (atrial and ventricular) as the ground for sensing and pacing. A unipolar pacemaker requires the pacemaker case in contact with the tissue to complete the circuit. In this instance, the pulse generator can be lifted from the wound and continue to pace and sense well.
4. Several models of dual-chamber pacemakers will stimulate the ventricle if the threshold is in the low normal range during pacing in the AAI mode due to current leak within the circuit. This effect (cross stimulation) is not subject to correction by reduction of ventricular output, but only by reduction of atrial output.
5. Crosstalk is the sensing of the atrial stimulus in the ventricular channel with consequent inhibition of output in that channel. It occurs more often during high atrial output, and reduction of output can often reduce or eliminate crosstalk. Other methods of management include increase of the duration of the ventricular blanking period, programming to the triggered mode in the ventricular channel, and reducing ventricular sensitivity.
6. The single-chamber pacemaker may sense the repolarization effect following

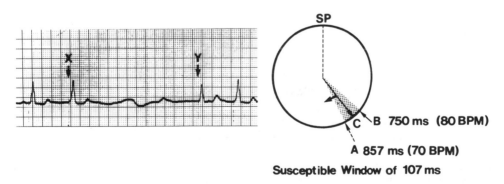

SP

B 750 ms (80 BPM)

A 857 ms (70 BPM)

Susceptible Window of 107 ms

Figure 20. *Asystole can occur during programming from a lower to a higher rate in one make of multiprogrammable pacemaker. The timing "clock" has a 2000 ms cycle (lowest rate 30 bpm) starting from "SP". The programmed rate acts as a release point (A). When the moving cursor (the diagrammatic arrow C) reaches A the stimulus is released. If, after the cycle has started and the cursor (C) has passed the higher rate (which it reaches first) but not reached the lower rate, the lower rate stop (A) can be moved (by rate programming) behind the advancing cursor. No "stop" exists, and no stimulus is emitted until that stop is reached. Depending on the rates programmed, the maximum duration of asystole can be almost 4 seconds.*

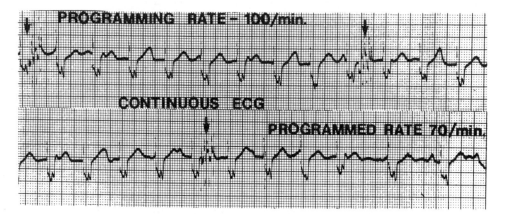

Figure 21. *Partial programming can occur, especially in pulse generators that are programmed by magnetic reed "dithering" and that move through an intermediate step before reaching the programmed value. In this unit, model 0505, the intermediate rate during rate or output programming is 100 bpm for four stimuli. Each programming episode is indicated by an arrow. Only the last completes the programming cycle. Partial programming results from incomplete transmission of the signal caused either by distance from the pulse generator or by removing the programming head before the programming transmission has been completed. Note that the programming signal is about 0.3 seconds in duration. Thousands of these generators remain in service.*

a high output stimulus. Reduction of stimulus amplitude or increase in duration of the ventricular refractory period may resolve the problem.

Many other eccentricities will be manifest as devices proliferate and become more complex. It is most important that these be distinguished from truly abnormal function.

INTERPRETATION OF DATA

The interpretation of data is of utmost importance in the decision concerning the kind of revision to be undertaken. The PSA can only provide numerical data for such interpretation. In the end, all interpretations are made because of the operator's knowledge of pacing hardware and physiology. Some guides are valuable, including the following useful measurements:

1. voltage threshold;
2. current threshold;
3. impedance;
4. electrogram.

Based on intraoperative data derived from these four factors, diagnosis and resolution can be made (Table VI). Troubleshooting of implanted hardware problems may be extremely difficult or relatively simple as the number of problems and resolutions are limited.

Table VI
Lead and Electrode Test Data

	Fracture	Insulation Failure	Displace-ment	High Threshold	Poor Sensing	Poor Position
Voltage	High	Low	High	High	Normal	High
Current	Variable May be normal	High	High	High	Normal	High
Impedance	High	Low	Normal	Normal	Normal	Normal
Electrogram	Variable	Variable	Low	May be normal	Low	Low
Resolution	Repair	Repair	Reposition	Higher output or reposition	High sensitivity	Reposition

DIAGNOSIS OF MALFUNCTION

The failure of different components of the pacing system should be analyzed to assist in making a rational choice concerning revision. There are characteristic deficiencies that lead to the conclusion that the electrode, lead, pulse generator circuit, or power source is at fault.

The prevalence of polyurethane leads at risk, models 6972, 6990U, 6991U, 4002, and 4012 implanted in over 200,000 patients, makes it likely that defects

---

DIAGNOSIS OF MALFUNCTION

POWER SOURCE
1. Rate decline in the magnet mode;
2. Loss of capture in a high threshold lead system;
3. Loss of sensing as a late manifestation;
4. Erratic stimulation rate as a late manifestation.

CIRCUIT
1. Erratic stimulation rate and erratic magnet rate;
2. Erratic or absent sensing of cardiac signals and absent sensing of chest wall stimuli;
3. Programming defect;
4. Telemetry defect;
5. Absent or erratic magnetic mode;
6. Sudden "no output" lead intact on x-ray

ELECTRODE
1. High threshold, apparently normal pulse generator function;
2. Poor sensing, apparently normal pulse generator function;
3. High threshold with poor sensing;

4. Oversensing, i.e., false recycle from inapparent events is frequently electrode/lead in origin.

LEAD
1. Absent sensing and pacing usually is caused by a lead fracture;
2. False sensing may result from insulation defect;
3. Polyurethane lead deterioration causes the following complex:
   a) low lead impedance;
   b) early battery depletion (caused by large output drain in a constant voltage pacemaker);
   c) false sensing and recycle from artifacts;
   d) high threshold;
   e) stimulation of the pectoral musculature caused by subcutaneous insulation defect;
   f) stimulation of the right phrenic nerve caused by local insulation defect;
   g) undersensing of spontaneous cardiac activity.

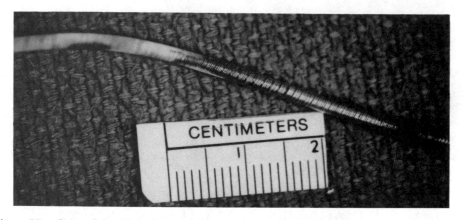

Figure 22.   *Some of the original polyurethane leads underwent spontaneous deterioration during contact with body fluids. Pressure of a ligature could also destroy the underlying polyurethane. Milky opacification of the clear polyurethane, cracking, and insulation loss with short circuit all occurred.*

will be widely seen. Failure rates of up to 20% occur and as the failures are time-dependent, more are likely to be seen. If unusual pacemaker failure circumstances are observed with one of these urethane leads, the possibility of lead failure should be considered promptly (Figure 22).

REVISION AND REPAIR

High threshold electrode: Program to high pacemaker output but if the threshold persists, operatively revise the electrode position. *Malposition of the lead:* Revise the position by operative intervention.

Ventricular lead perforation: Withdraw the lead into the main right ventricular cavity. Although it is rare, one should check to make sure there is no pericardial bleeding.

Lead fracture: (a) repair if the fracture site is accessible, and a new connector can be placed without repair of the lead itself; (b) abandon the lead if the fracture is intravascular or if the stump remaining in the subcutaneous tissue is too short to repair securely; (c) remove the lead if it is infected.

Insulation failure: (a) repair if accessible, but not if the insulation failure is caused by general deterioration of the material; (b) if a recalled urethane lead or one known to be subject to in situ deterioration, remove or abandon; (c) abandon and insulate the connector.

Pulse generator depletion: replace the generator.

Pulse generator electronic failure: replace the generator if failure is of the pulse-forming or sensing circuits. Other circuits such as telemetry can malfunction without affecting vital pacemaker function. Consult the manufacturer, as many malfunctions are generic to a design rather than unique to a single unit, and the manufacturer may be willing to provide valuable advice concerning function expectation.

SUMMARY

Troubleshooting of implanted cardiac pacemakers involves knowledge of the hemodynamics, electrophysiology, radiography, and electrocardiography of pacing. If the findings on x-ray or ECG are clear-cut and straightforward, then diagnosis of the problem and its resolution may be straightforward. If the findings are subtle or confusing, the diagnosis and consequent resolution can be very difficult. Diagnosis can, in the end, be made from the perspective of maximum information concerning pacemaker function and interaction with the patient.

BIBLIOGRAPHY

Alicandri C, Fouad FM, Tarazi RC, et al: Three cases of hypotension and syncope with ventricular pacing: Possible role of atrial reflexes. Am J Cardiol 1978; 42:137–142.

Aulenbacher CE: Hydrothorax from subclavian vein catheterization. J Am Med Assoc 1970; 214:372 (letter to editor).

Ausubel K, Furman S: The pacemaker syndrome. Ann Int Med 1985; 103:420–429.

Ausubel K, Gabry MD, Klementowicz PT, Furman S: Pacemaker-mediated endless loop tachycardia at rates below the upper rate limit. Am J Cardiol 1988; 61:465–467.

Barber K, Amikam S, Furman S: Atrial lead malposition in a dual chamber (DDD,M) pacemaker. Chest 1984; 84:766.

Barold SS, Falkoff MD, Ong LS, et al: Hyperkalemia-induced failure of atrial capture during dual-chamber cardiac pacing. J Am Coll Cardiol 1987; 10:467–469.

Barold SS, Gaidula JJ: Failure of demand pacemaker from low-voltage bipolar ventricular electrograms. J Am Med Assoc 1971; 215:923.

Barold SS, Levine PA: Autointerference of demand pulse generators. PACE 1981; 4:274–280.

Bernard RW, Stahl WM: Mediastinal hematoma: Complication of subclavian vein catheterization. NY State J Med 1974; 74:83–84.

Calfee RF: Therapeutic radiation and pacemakers. PACE 1982; 5:160–161.

Campo I, Garfield GJ, Escher DJW, et al: Complications of pacing by pervenous subclavian semifloating electrodes including two extra-luminal insertions. Am J Cardiol 1970; 26:627.

Carter R, Dickerson SC, Berry R: Axillary-subclavian vein thrombosis as a complication of permanent transvenous cardiac pacing. VA Med 1978; 105:515–518.

Chatterjee K, Sutton R, Davies JG: Low intracardiac potentials in myocardial infarction as a cause of failure of inhibition of demand pacemakers. Lancet 1968; 1:511.

Chauvin M, Brechenmacher C: Muscle stimulation caused by a pacemaker current leakage: The role of the insulation failure of a polyurethane coating. J Electrophysiol 1987; 1:326–29.

Christensen KH, Nerstrom B, Baden H: Complications of percutaneous catheterization of subclavian vein in 129 cases. Acta Chir Scand 1967; 133:615–620.

Collins DWK, Black JL, Sinclair IN: Predicted early failure of cardiac pacemakers. PACE 1985; 8:544–548.

Coumel P, Mugica J, Barold SS: Demand pacemaker arrhythmias caused by intermittent incomplete electrode fracture. Diagnosis with testing magnet. Am J Cardiol 1975; 36:105–109.

Crook, BRM, Gishen P, Robinson CR, et al: Occlusion of the subclavian vein pacemaker electrodes. Br J Surg 1977; 64:329–331.

Daly JE, Whitte AA: Non-invasive analysis of simulated pacemaker failure available in multiprogrammable pulse generators. PACE 1982; 5:4–9.

Danielson GK, Shabetai R, Bryant LR: Failure of endocardial pacemaker due to late myo-
    cardial perforation. Successful restoration of cardiac pacing by conversion to an epi-
    cardial system. J Thorac Cardiovasc Surg 1967; 54:42–48.
Davies JG, Siddons H: The detection of impending failure in implanted pacemakers.
    Thorax 1969; 24:74–77.
Dekker E, Buller J, Schuilenburg RM: Aids to electrical diagnosis for pacemaker failure.
    Am Heart J 1965; 70:739.
Epstein E, Quereshi MSA, Wright JS: Diaphragmatic paralysis after supraclavicular punc-
    ture of subclavian vein. Br Med J 1976; 1:693–694.
Falkoff M, Ong LS, Heinle RA, et al: The noise sampling period: A new cause of apparent
    sensing malfunction of demand pacemakers. PACE 1978; 1:250–253.
Farhat K, Nakhjavan FK, Cope C, et al: Iatrogenic arteriovenous fistula: A complication
    of percutaneous subclavian vein puncture. Chest 1975; 67:480.
Fisher JD, Furman S, Parker B, et al: Pacemaker failures characterized by continuous
    direct current leakage. Am J Cardiol 1976; 37:1019–1023.
Flanagan JP, Gradisar IA, Gross RJ, et al: Air embolus: A lethal complication of subclavian
    venipuncture. N Engl J Med 1969; 281:488–489.
Frick MH: Efficiency of a pacemaker clinic to prevent sudden pacing failures. Br Heart
    J 1973; 35:1280–1284.
Frumin H, Furman S: Endless loop tachycardia started by an atrial premature complex
    in a patient with a dual chamber pacemaker. J Am Coll Cardiol 1985; 5:707–710.
Fulkerson PK, Leier CV, Vasko JS, et al: Use of chest wall stimulation to localize and
    treat pacemaker sensing failure. J Electrocardiol 1980; 13:283–284.
Furman S, Escher DJW, Lister J, et al: A comprehensive scheme for management of
    pacemaker malfunction. Ann Surg 1966; 163:611.
Furman S, Escher DJW, Parker B, et al: Electronic analysis for pacemaker failure. Ann
    Thorac Surg 1969; 8:57.
Fyke FE III: Simultaneous insulation deterioration associated with side-by-side subclavian
    placement of two polyurethane leads. PACE 1988; 11:1571–1574.
Gabry MD, Behrens M, Andrews C, et al: Comparison of myopotential interference in
    unipolar-bipolar programmable DDD pacemakers. PACE 1987; 10:1322–1330.
Gerst PH, Bowman FO, Fleming WH, et al: An evaluation of function and failure of
    cardiac pacemakers. J Thorac Cardiovasc Surg 1967; 54:92–102.
Giedwoyn JO: Pacemaker failure following external defribrillation. Circulation 1971; 44:
    293.
Goldman BS, MacGregor D: Management of infected pacemaker systems. CPPE 1984; 2:
    220–235.
Goldman BS, Noble EJ, MacGregor DC: Pacemaker panic. Am J Cardiol 1972; 30:705 (letter
    to editor).
Goldman LI, Mailer WP, Drezner AD, et al: Another complication of subclavian puncture:
    Arterial laceration. J Am Med Assoc 1971; 217:78.
Gould L, Maghazeh P, Reddy CVR: Subclavian vein thrombosis following cardiac pace-
    maker implantation. Vasc Surg 1978; 12:262–268.
Gould L, Patel C, Betzu R, et al: Pacemaker failure following electrocautery. CPEP 1986;
    4:53–55.
Gould L, Patel S, Gomes GI, et al: Pacemaker failure following external defibrillation.
    PACE 1981; 4:575–577.
Griepp RB, Daily PO, Shumway NE: Subclavian-axillary vein thrombosis following im-
    plantation of a pacemaker catheter in the internal jugular vein. J Thorac Cardiovasc
    Surg 1970; 60:889.
Gschnitzer F: Thrombose der Vena subclavia and axillaris nach Herzschrittmacher Im-
    plantation. Wien Klin Wschr 1972; 84:393.
Haas JM, Strait GB: Pacemaker-induced cardiovascular failure hemodynamic and angi-
    ographic observations. Am J Cardiol 1974; 33:295–299.
Hanson J: Sixteen failures in a single model of bipolar polyurethane-insulated ventricular
    pacing lead. PACE 1984; 7:389–394.

Hauser RG: Bipolar leads for cardiac pacing in the 1980's: A reappraisal provoked by skeletal muscle interference. PACE 1982; 5:34–37.

Hauser RG, Edwards LM, Giuffre VW: Limitations of pacemaker system analyzers for the evaluation of implantable pulse generators. PACE 1981; 4:650–657.

Hauser RG, Giuffre VW: Clinical assessment of cardiac pacemaker performance. J Cont Ed Cardiol 1979; 14:19–35.

Hayes D, Holmes D Jr, Merideth J, et al: Apparent pacemaker failure due to reversion circuitry within the programming device. PACE 1984; 7:237–239.

Hearne SF, Maloney JD: Pacemaker system failure secondary to air entrapment within the pulse generator pocket. A complication of subclavian venipuncture for lead placement. Chest 1982; 82:651.

Heilbrunn A: Fatal subdural hematoma: An unusual complication of pacemaker failure. Chest 1970; 57:283–285.

Hepburn F: Discriminating between types of pacemaker lead failure. J Med Eng Tech 1978; 2:130–135.

Janosik D, Stratmann HG, Walter KE, et al: Torsades de pointes: A rare complication of temporary pacing for permanent ventricular pacemaker failure. PACE 1985; 8:558–561.

Katzenberg CA, Marcus FI, Heusinkveld RS, et al: Pacemaker failure due to radiation therapy. PACE 1982; 5:156–159.

Klein B, Mittelman M, Katz R, et al: Osteomyelitis of both clavicles as a complication of subclavian venipuncture. Chest 1983; 83:143.

Kohler F, Schmitt CG, Ellringmann U: Extraction of tricuspid valve tissue and myocardium, as a complication of transvenous cardiac pacing. Thoraxchirurgie 1977; 25:97–100.

Kukral JC: Transvenous pacemaker failure due to anomalous venous return to the heart. Chest 1971; 59:458–461.

Lasky II: Pacemaker failure from automobile accident. J Am Med Assoc 1970; 211:1700 (letter to editor).

Levick C, Mizgala H, Kerr C: Failure to pace following high dose antiarrhythmic therapy—reversal with isoproterenol. PACE 1984; 7:252–256.

Levine PA: Confirmation of atrial capture and determination of atrial capture thresholds in DDD pacing systems. CPPE 1984; 2:465–73.

Levine PA: Pacemaker pseudomalfunction. PACE 1981; 4:563–565.

Levine PA, Barold SS, Fletcher RD, et al: Adverse, acute and chronic effects of electrical defibrillation and cardioversion on implanted unipolar cardiac pacing systems. J Am Coll Cardiol 1983; 1:1413–1422.

Levine PA, Klein MD: Myopotential inhibition of unipolar pacemakers: A disease of technologic progress. Ann Int Med 1983; 98:101–103 (editorial).

Levine PA, Seltzer JP: Magnet rates and recommended replacement time indicators of lithium pacemakers. (Part 2). CPPE 1983; 1:287–292.

Lewin AA, Serago CF, Schwade JG, et al: Radiation induced failures of complementary metal oxide semiconductor containing pacemakers: A potentially lethal complication. Int J Radiat Oncol Biol Phys 1984; 10:1967–69.

Lister JW, Escher DJW, Furman S, et al: Heart block: A method for rapid determination of causes of pacing failure in artificial pacemaker systems. Am J Cardiol 1966; 18:64–72.

Lister JW, Furman S, Stein E, et al: A rapid determination of pacemaking defects in patients with artificial pacemakers. Bull NY Acad Med 1964; 40:982.

MacGregor DC, Noble EJ, Morrow JD, et al: Management of a pacemaker recall. J Thorac Cardiovasc Surg 1977; 74:657.

Martin CM, Klein JJ: Pseudofusion beats masquerading as pacemaker failure. J Electrocardiol 1974; 7:179.

McGrath LB, Gonzalez-Lavin L, Morse DP, et al: Pacemaker system failure and other events in children with surgically induced heart block. PACE 1988; 11:1182–1187.

McGuire LB, Breit RA, Steinberg S, et al: Reflections on an epidemic of premature pacemaker failures. PACE 1981; 4:335–338 (editorial).

McGuire LB, Nolan ST: The care of patients at increased risk of premature pacemaker failure. J Am Med Assoc 1979; 24:701–703.

McWilliams E, Buchalter M, O'Neill C: An unusual form of pacemaker failure. PACE 1984; 7:765–766.

Misaki T, Iwa T, Mastunaga Y: Atrial amplitude mapping to avoid P wave sensing failure. (abstract) PACE 1983; 6:A–3.

Mond HG, Sloman JG: The malfunctioning pacemaker system. Part I. PACE 1981; 4:49–60.

Mond HG, Sloman JG: The malfunctioning pacemaker system. Part II. PACE 1981; 4:168–181.

Mond HG, Sloman JG: The malfunctioning pacemaker system. Part III. PACE 1981; 4:304–308.

Nagatomo Y, Ogawa T, Kumagae H, et al: Pacing failure due to markedly increased stimulation threshold 2 years after implantation: Successful management with oral prednisolone: A case report. PACE 1989; 12:1034–1037.

Nathan DA, Lister JW, Keller JW, et al: Percutaneous access to implanted electrodes. Am J Cardiol 1971; 27:397.

Nevins MA, Landau S, Lyon LJ: Failure of demand pacemaker sensing due to electrode fracture. Chest 1971; 59:110–113.

Obel IWP: Transient phrenic nerve paralysis following subclavian venipuncture. Anaesthesiology 1970; 33:369–370.

Ong LS, Barold SS, Craver WL, et al: Partial avulsion of the tricuspid valve by tined pacing electrode. Am Heart J 1981; 102:798–799.

O'Reilly MV, Murnaghan DP, Williams MB: Transvenous pacemaker failure induced by hyperkalemia. J Am Med Assoc 1974; 228:336–337.

Oseran D, Ausubel K, Klementowicz PT, et al: Spontaneous endless loop tachycardia. PACE 1986; 9:379–386.

Pappas G, Shoultz Ch A Jr, Blount SG Jr: Fractured intracardiac transvenous pacemaker catheter. An unusual case of pacemaker failure. Am Heart J 1969; 78:807.

Parsonnet V, Myers GH, Manhardt M: A pacemaker follow up clinic: An analysis of detection of signs of impending pacemaker failure. In P Samet, N El-Sherif (eds): Cardiac Pacing. Grune & Stratton, New York, 1980, p. 257.

Parsonnet V, Myers GH, Gilbert L, et al: Prediction of impending pacemaker failure in a pacemaker clinic. Am J Cardiol 1970; 25:311–319.

Phillips R, Frey M, Martin RO: Long-term performance of polyurethane pacing leads: Mechanisms of design-related failures. PACE 1986; 9:1166–1172.

Pourhamidi AH: Radiation effect on implanted pacemakers. Chest 1983; 84:499–500.

Preston TA, Fletcher RD, Lucchesi BR, et al: Changes in myocardial threshold. Physiological and pharmacologic factors in patients with implanted pacemakers. Am Heart J 1967; 74:235–242.

Quertermonus T, Megahy SM, DasGupta DS, et al: Pacemaker failure resulting from radiation damage. Radiology 1983; 148:257–258.

Raymond R, Nanian K: Insulation failure with bipolar polyurethane leads. PACE 1984; 7:378–380.

Reinhart S, McAnulty JH, Dobbs J: Type and timing of permanent pacemaker failure. Chest 1982, 82:433–435.

Rockland R, Parsonnet V, Myers GH: Failure modes of American pacemakers: In vitro analysis. Am Heart J 1972; 83:481.

Rowley BA: Electrolysis: A factor in cardiac pacemaker electrode failure. IEEE Trans Biomed Eng 1963; 10:176.

Rubenstein JJ, Laforet EG: Pacemaker runaway following intermittent output failure. PACE 1983; 6:645–647.

Rubin IL, Arbeit SR, Gross H: The electrocardiographic recognition of pacemaker failure and function. Ann Intern Med 1969; 71:603.

Ryden L, Hedstrom P, Leijonhufvud S: A new apparatus for detection of impending pacemaker failure in patients treated with implanted pacemakers. Cardiovasc Res 1970; 4:242.

Seltzer JP, Levine P: Magnet rates and recommended replacement time indicators of the available implanted pulse generators in North America (part I). CPPE 1983; 1:81–84.

Seltzer JP, Levine PA, Watson WS: Patient-initiated autonomous pacemaker tachycardia. PACE 1984; 7:961–969.

Sheridan DJ, Reid DS, Williams DO, et al: Mechanical failure causing leakage with unipolar pacemakers. Significance and detection. Eur J Cardiol 1978; 8:1–8.

Slepian M, Levine JH, Watkins L Jr, et al: Automatic implantable cardioverter defibrillator/permanent pacemaker interaction: Loss of pacemaker capture following AICD discharge. PACE 1987; 10:1194–1197.

Smith SA, Weissberg PL, Tan L: Permanent pacemaker failure due to surgical emphysema. Br Heart J 1985; 54:220–221.

Sowton E: Detection of impending pacemaker failure. Isr J Med Sci 1967; 3:260.

Stanford W, Coyle FL, Dooley BN, et al: Transvenous pacemaker failure; migration of catheter lead by patient manipulation. Ann Thorac Surg 1968; 5:162.

Stroobandt R, Willems R, Depuydt P, et al: The superfast atrial recharge pulse: A cause of pectoral muscle stimulation in patients equipped with a unipolar DDD pacemaker. PACE 1989; 12:451–455.

Sudduth B, Goldschlager N: Retrograde ventricule atrial conduction and atrial refractoriness: A cause of apparent failure of atrial capture. CPEP 1986; 4:56–59.

Tegtmeyer CJ, Bezirdjian DR, Irani FA, et al: Cardiac pacemaker failure: A complication of trauma. South Med J 1981; 74:378–379.

Tulgan H: Electrocardiographic misrepresentation of impending pacemaker failure. Ann Intern Med 1970; 72:251.

Van Beek GJ, den Dulk K, Lindemans FW, Wellens HJJ: Detection of insulation failure by gradual reduction in noninvasively measured electrogram amplitudes. PACE 1986; 9:772–775.

van Mechelen R, Hart C'T, de Boer H: Failure to sense P waves during DDD pacing. PACE 1986; 9:498–502.

Walker PR, Papouchado M, James MA, et al: Pacing failure due to flecainide acetate. PACE 1985; 8:900–902.

Warnowicz MA, Goldschlager N: Apparent failure to sense (undersensing) caused by oversensing: Diagnostic use of noninvasively obtained intracardiac electrogram. PACE 1983; 6:1341–1343.

Weinman J: Comments. Electrolysis. A factor in cardiac pacemaker electrode failure. IEEE Trans Biomed Eng 1964; 11:114–115.

Yarnoz MD, Attai LA, Furman S: Infection of pacemaker electrode and removal with cardiopulmonary bypass. J Thorac Cardiovasc Surg 1974; 68:43–46.

Yatteau RF: Medical Intelligence: Brief recordings. Radar-induced failure of a demand pacemaker. N Engl J Med 1970; 283:1447–1448.

GLOSSARY

ALERT PERIOD: That part of the ventricular or atrial cycle during which the pacemaker is sensitive, i.e., "alert" to incoming signals.

AMPERE (A):   The basic unit of electrical current. Pacemaker systems require small amounts of current, measured in thousandths of an ampere (milliampere, abbreviated mA) or in the millionths of an ampere (microampere, abbreviated (μA). The fluid equivalent is a measure of flow, i.e., quarts or gallons of water/sec.

AMPERE HOUR: The basic unit of battery capacity. All batteries are rated in ampere-hours and output voltage. The voltage is specific for any one battery, the overall capacity depends on the size of the cell, i.e., greater or lesser ampere-hour capacity. The implication is that under standardized conditions the battery will deliver a given number of amperes for a stated number of hours. The equivalent might be the capacity to deliver a specific number of gallons of water for a specific number of hours.

ANODE: The positive terminal of a pacemaker or electrode. In a battery, the terminal that receives electrons.

ASYNCHRONOUS: A mode of operation in which the pacemaker is insensitive to incoming signals from the chamber being paced. The antonym of asynchronous in pacing terms is not synchronous, rather it is responsive.

AV BLOCK: The mode of approach to the upper rate interval by maintaining the AV interval constant until a P wave is unsensed or blocked.

AV CONDUCTION: A description of the conduction of atrial impulses from the atrium through the AV node and the His-Purkinje system to the ventricle. The term in also applied to the conduction of paced beats from the atrium to the ventricle via the pacemaker.

AV INTERVAL: (Atrioventricular interval, AV delay) The interval between the sensed or paced atrial event and the next sensed or paced ventricular event.

AV SYNCHRONY: The relationship between atrial and ventricular systole. This relationship is lost in patients with AV block. AV synchrony is maintained with P synchrony pacing and at times, but not always, with AV sequential pacing.

AUTOMATICITY: An electrophysiological mechanism of arrhythmia in which there is abnormal impulse formation. Automatic arrhythmias can usually not be reliably induced or terminated by electrical stimulation.

AUTONOMOUS PACEMAKER TACHYCARDIA (APT):   A tachycardia of a dual-chamber pacemaker in which the arrhythmia is begun by a combination of pacemaker and sensed cardiac events, but once begun is sustained without regard to cardiac interaction. No electronic malfunction exists.

BATTERY: The power source of the pulse generator. Strictly speaking, a battery consists of more than one cell. Each cell of a battery is of a specific chemistry and develops a specific voltage. In a cell or battery of cells power is evolved from a chemical reaction.

BEGINNING OF LIFE (BOL):   The electronic characteristics of a pulse generator when it has been freshly manufactured. These are usually maintained until the approach of end of life. This term relates to the operation of the pulse generator battery.

BIPOLAR: Both pacemaker electrical terminals, anode and cathode, are in contact with stimulatable tissue.

BLANKING PERIOD: The time during and after a pacemaker stimulus during which the opposite channel of a dual channel pacemaker is insensitive. The intent is to avoid sensing the electronic event of one channel in the opposite channel.

CAPACITOR (Condenser):   A device that can store an electrical charge. It is made of two conductors separated by an insulator, or by an electrolyte or air.

CARDIAC OUTPUT: The volume of blood ejected per unit of time, measured in liters per minute. This may be adjusted to account for body surface to yield the cardiac index, i.e., liters per minute per meter^2.

CAROTID SINUS SYNCOPE (CSS):   Attacks of syncope and related symptoms that usually occur with the patient in the upright position and that can be reproduced regularly by means of mechanical stimulation of the carotid sinus.

CATHODE: The negative terminal of a pacemaker or electrode. In a battery, the terminal that emits electrons.

CELL: See Battery.

CHRONAXIE TIME: See Strength-Duration Curve.

COMMITTED: A dual-chamber pacemaker in which the delivery of an atrial stimulus forces the delivery of a ventricular stimulus. Either both stimuli are emitted or neither.

COMPLEMENTARY METAL OXIDE SEMICONDUCTOR (CMOS):   Low power semiconductor.

CONDUCTOR: A material that allows the passage of electrical current. As all materials will allow the passage of current at a sufficiently high voltage, a conductor is one which will allow the passage of current at a low voltage.

CONNECTOR: The mechanism that connects the output of the pulse generator to the lead. There are two parts, one on the generator, the other on the lead.

CONSTANT CURRENT: A pacemaker that maintains its constancy of current output over a wide range of impedance. The output voltage is as required to maintain the current output constant.

COULOMB (C): The measure of charge. It is equivalent to the term gallons. As pacemaker outputs are small, the common measurement would be in the micro terms, i.e., 1/1,000,000 of a coulomb (μC).

CROSSTALK: Sensing of electronic events generated in one channel in the other channel. Sensing an atrial stimulus in ventricular channel with consequent recycle is an example.

CYCLE LENGTH: The interval in milliseconds from one event to the next. The term is used in measuring cardiac rate or a pacemaker stimulation rate.

DEFIBRILLATION THRESHOLD (DFT): The energy in Joules that consistently terminates ventricular fibrillation.

DEMAND (Standby): A noncompetitive pacemaker, i.e., in a VVI pacemaker, a ventricular output is on "standby" and released only in the absence of an intrinsic ventricular event within a defined interval.

DISCRIMINANT P WAVE SENSING: The ability of the pacemaker to discriminate between an antegrade and a retrograde P wave. Such discrimination could be helpful in preventing endless loop tachycardia.

dP/dt: An abbreviation denoting the change in pressure that occurs over a given amount of time. When applied to cardiac hemodynamics, this refers to contractility. dP/dt measurements have been used as a biological sensor for rate modulation.

dV/dt: See slew rate.

DUAL-CHAMBER: A pulse generator that can stimulate and/or sense atrium and/or ventricle.

ECCENTRICITY: An apparent deviation from presumed normal function but which is normal function for that model.

EJECTION FRACTION: The relationship between the volume of blood ejected and the end-systolic (ES) and end-diastolic (ED) volume. ED volume— ES volume/ED volume.

ELECTROCARDIOGRAM (ECG, EKG): The electrical signal emitted by active cardiac tissue recorded from the body surface.

ELECTRODE: The interface with living tissue across which the stimulus is transmitted. It is usually metal or carbon.

ELECTROGRAM (EGM): The electrical signal emitted by active cardiac tissue recorded from within or upon the heart.

ELECTROMAGNETIC INTERFERENCE (EMI): Electrical signals of non-physiological origin that affect pacemaker function.

ELECTROMYOGRAPHIC INTERFERENCE (EMI): Electrical signals of muscular origin that affect pacemaker function.

ELECTROPHYSIOLOGICAL TESTING: An invasive study with placement of a variable number of catheters in the heart for stimulation and recording. During this study the basic properties of conduction and refractoriness are assessed. The mechanism of tachycardia is assessed by analyzing conduction and termination sequences.

ENDLESS LOOP TACHYCARDIA (ELT):   (Pacemaker-Mediated Tachycardia; Pacemaker-Mediated Re-entry Tachycardia; Pacemaker Circus Movement Tachycardia). A re-entry arrhythmia in which the dual-chamber pacemaker acts as the antegrade limb of the tachycardia and the natural pathway as the retrograde limb.

END OF LIFE (EOL):   The electronic characteristics of a pulse generator when it should be electively removed from service. This term relates to the operation of the pulse generator battery.

EPICARDIAL LEAD: A lead stimulating the heart by onlay upon the epicardial surface of the atrium or ventricle.

EPIMYOCARDIAL LEAD: A lead placed into the myocardium from the epicardial surface of the heart. All modern leads implanted by thoracotomy are myocardial, colloquially referred to as "epimyocardial."

ESCAPE INTERVAL: The interval between a sensed or paced event to the next paced event (see hysteresis).

EVOKED RESPONSE: The response of the myocardium to a pacemaker stimulus. The response may be modified by the activity state of the cardiac tissue and is used as a biological sensor for rate adaptive pacing.

FIXATION: The means of attachment of an endocardial electrode to the endocardium once it is introduced. Two modes exist:
Active: The electrode actively grasps the endocardium via fine metal pins, a jawlike device, or a screw.
Passive: The lead proximal to the electrode is irregular with a conical "shoulder" fins or tines. Local tissue reaction places enough fibrous tissue about the lead irregularity to hold it in place.

FUSION BEAT: A ventricular or atrial depolarization which starts from two foci (one spontaneous, the other, a pacemaker stimulus) and has characteristics of each.

HEADER: The portion of a pulse generator that contains the receptacle(s), which receive the lead connector pins.

HERMETIC: The ability to seal a device so that neither water vapor nor any other gas can enter or leave the "hermetic seal." The standard measurement technique is in leakage of helium molecules.

HERTZ (Hz):   Frequency of a signal in cycles per second.

HYSTERESIS: A difference in the duration of the pacemaker escape interval depending on whether it is started by a sensed or paced event. The interval may be shorter or longer than the escape interval and will be referred to as "positive or negative," although in the context, the terms are undefined.

IMPEDANCE: The total impediment to the flow of electrical current in a conductor. It is a more complex function than resistance alone and accounts for all impediments to the flow of current.

IMPLANTABLE CARDIOVERTER DEFIBRILLATOR (ICD): A permanently implanted device with the function of sensing ventricular tachycardia and/or ventricular fibrillation and delivering an electrical shock when such a rhythm has been detected.

INHIBITED (INHIBITORY): A pacemaker response in which a stimulus is withheld in response to a sensed event.

INTERVAL: The elapsed time between pacemaker and/or cardiac events. A more useful concept than rate.

INTRINSIC DEFLECTION: The portion of the electrogram that represents the depolarization wave moving past the sensing electrode. It is the part of the electrogram that is sensed because of adequate amplitude and slew rate (frequency content).

JOULE (J): The unit of energy. It is the product of current volts and time. In pacemakers, microJoules (μJ) would be used; in defibrillators, Joules would be used.

LEAD: The insulated wire that connects the output of the pulse generator to the electrode.

LOWER RATE INTERVAL: Also referred to as the "lower rate limit," etc. It is the maximum interval the pacemaker will allow between two pacemaker ventricular stimuli or between a sensed ventricular event and the next ventricular paced event.

MAGNET MODE: The response of a pacemaker to the closure of its magnetic switch. Many different magnetic modes exist so that the mode of operation for a specific pacemaker must be known.

MAXIMUM SENSOR RATE: The programmed value for a rate modulated pacemaker that determines the maximum rate that can be achieved with the artificial sensor. In a rate modulated dual-chamber pacemaker the maximum sensor rate may be the same, higher, or lower than the maximum atrial trigger (tracking) rate.

MAXIMUM TRACKING RATE: The maximum rate (or minimum coupling interval) at which an atrial sensing pacemaker will respond to atrial events. In a rate modulated dual-chamber pacemaker the maximum tracking rate may be the same, higher, or lower than the maximum sensor rate.

MINUTE VENTILATION: Respiratory rate × tidal volume = minute ventilation. This parameter is used as a biological indicator for rate modulated pacing.

MYOCARDIAL ELECTRODE: An electrode that penetrates the myocardium and is held in place by a suture, or by a plastic, fabric, or rubber plate.

NOISE MODE: The pacemaker operation when it receives signals defined as being electrical noise. For example, the asynchronous (VOO) operation of a ventricular inhibited pacemaker during sensing of 60 Hz current.

NONCOMPETITIVE: A pacemaker that senses cardiac function and avoids a stimulus during the sensitive portion of a spontaneous depolarization.

OVERDRIVE PACING: Pacing at a more rapid rate than a tachycardia in order to interrupt and terminate a re-entrant arrhythmia.

OVERVOLTAGE: A reverse voltage developed by a reactive metal in a biological solution, i.e., a non-noble metal electrode, e.g., Elgiloy (a steel alloy) in contact with myocardium. The more noble (i.e., nonreactive) the metal, the lower the overvoltage. Overvoltage is part of the impedance measurement.

PACEMAKER: The entire cardiac stimulating system, it includes power source (battery) and circuit, which are always one package, lead, and electrode.

PACEMAKER-INDUCED ARRHYTHMIA (PIA):   An arrhythmia caused by a pacemaker stimulus or stimuli that once begun continues without further pacemaker function, e.g., ventricular fibrillation.

PACEMAKER-MEDIATED ARRHYTHMIA (PMA):   An arrhythmia that requires a pacemaker to start and be sustained, e.g., atrial fibrillation or flutter sensed by the pacemaker to drive the ventricle, endless loop tachycardia.

PACEMAKER SENSOR: A sensor incorporated into an implantable pulse generator for the purpose of detecting a physiological or nonphysiological function in order to modulate its rate, and possibly, other characteristics.
Closed Loop: A pacemaker sensor that responds to a physiological stimulus such as dP/dt, O_2 saturation, or evoked response.
Open Loop: A pacemaker sensor that responds to a nonphysiological stimulus such as motion or activity.

PACEMAKER SYNDROME: A syndrome of pounding in the chest and neck and waves of weakness during cardiac pacing that results from loss of AV synchrony and retrograde activation of the atrium. Other causes include restricted cardiac output, because of the absence of rate increase with exercise.

POLARIZATION: Resistance to the flow of current because of the accumulation of electrons about an electrode. These act as an insulator until diffused. Polarization is measured as part of the impedance.

POST VENTRICULAR ATRIAL REFRACTORY PERIOD (PVARP):   Interval following a ventricular event in a DDD^R, VDD, or DDI^R pacemaker during which the actual sensing channel is refractory.

PRE-EJECTION INTERVAL: The interval from the beginning of ventricular depolarization to the beginning of ventricular ejection. The pre-ejection interval is made up of the electrical mechanical interval plus the isovolumetric contraction time. When used as an indicator for rate modulation, timing starts with a pacemaker stimulus.

PROBABILITY DENSITY FUNCTION: A technique that determines the diagnosis of ventricular fibrillation by the time the electrogram spends at the isoelectric line, more during sinus or ventricular tachycardia, and less with ventricular fibrillation.

PROGRAMMING: The ability to alter a pacemaker setting noninvasively. A variety of selections exist each with its own designation. If inadvertent or undetected, it is phantom programming.

PSEUDOFUSION BEAT: A spontaneous cardiac depolarization with a superimposed stimulus. The depolarization is of unpaced origin only.

PULSE DURATION: The duration of the pacemaker stimulus from its beginning to the return to the zero line. Some pulse shapes require measurement from the beginning to some other point. This is specified by the manufacturer.

PULSE GENERATOR: The metal enclosed power source and electronic circuit with its attached lead connector. The pulse generator is often mistakenly referred to as the pacemaker.

RATE: The reciprocal of the sustained pacemaker stimulation interval. The number of beats per minute, spontaneous or paced.

RATE MODULATED: A pacemaker that is able to adjust its stimulation interval (rate) based on input from a biological sensor. It is considered synonymous with rate responsive, rate adaptive, and sensor driven.

RATE RESPONSIVE: The change in pacemaker stimulation interval caused by sensing a physiological function other than the intrinsic atrial rhythm. The physiological functions sensed may be stimulus-T interval, activity, right ventricular temperature, minute ventilation, etc.

RATE SMOOTHING: Capability to avoid marked RR cycle variations by placing limits on how much a subsequent RR cycle length can vary from the preceding cycle length. In general, this is programmable in values of percent, i.e., 3, 6, 12 percent. When rate smoothing is utilized in a DDD device, it will result in AV dissociation.

REED SWITCH: A magnetically activated switch sealed (usually in glass) and contained within a pulse generator. Open (electricity does not flow), the generator functions in one way, closed (current flows) by placement of a magnet, in another manner, referred to as the magnet mode. Unless a magnet is placed, the resting position of the switch is ''open.''

REENTRY: The most common mechanism of tachycardia. It requires two pathways with differential conduction and unidirectional block. Reentrant arrhythmias can usually be induced and terminated by electrical stimulation.

REFRACTORINESS: A measure of the recovery of excitability of the cardiac tissue under electrophysiological investigation.

REFRACTORY PERIOD: A time after a sensed or paced event during which the pacemaker is insensitive.

REFRACTORY PERIOD (ATRIAL):   The time after a sensed or paced event during which the atrial pacemaker or channel of a dual-chamber pacemaker is insensitive. The intent is to avoid sensing a physiological event.

REFRACTORY PERIOD (VENTRICULAR):   The time after a sensed or paced event during which the ventricular pacemaker or channel of a dual-chamber pacemaker is insensitive. The intent is to avoid sensing a physiological event.

RESISTANCE: The impediment to the flow of electrical current in a conductor. All conductors present some degree of resistance to the flow of current. It is the ratio of the voltage to current of an electrical circuit connected to a direct current source. The measurement of resistance is in ohms.

RESISTANCE, INTERNAL: The resistance to the flow of current within a battery. This limits the ability to deliver current flow. A high internal resistance battery may have the overall capacity to deliver a large amount of electrical capacity, but only at a slow rate. The lithium iodine battery fails by increase of internal resistance rather than depletion of the iodine or the lithium. At a sufficiently high internal resistance (approximately 50,000 ohms), the ability of current to flow out of the battery is reduced below the needs of the pulse generator circuit.

RHEOBASE: See Strength-Duration Curve

SAFETY PACING: A mechanism in which an event sensed during a defined interval after the end of the ventricular blanking period causes emission of a ventricular stimulus. It is designed to eliminate crosstalk or EMI inhibition of the ventricular channel.

SCANNING PACEMAKER: An underdrive pacemaker which progressively scans diastole in an attempt to stimulate during the critical time window during which tachycardia can be terminated.

SENSOR DRIVEN: A pacemaker that is capable of rate modulation via a sensor. Sensor driven may be used as a synonym for rate modulation, rate adaptive, and rate responsive pacemakers.

SINGLE-CHAMBER: A pulse generator that can stimulate and sense one cardiac chamber only. Often the same generator can be used for either atrium or ventricle.

SLEW RATE: The rate of movement of an electrical field, measured in volts/second. It is characteristic of a biological signal such as an electrogram. By a complex mathematical process known as the Fourier transform it can be converted into a series of signals of different frequencies.

STANDBY (DEMAND):   A noncompetitive pacemaker.

STRENGTH-DURATION CURVE: The quantity of charge, current, voltage, or energy required to stimulate the heart at a series of pulse durations. The *RHEOBASE* is the lowest point on such a curve at an infinitely long pulse duration. *CHRONAXIE TIME* is the pulse duration twice the rheobase value.

STROKE VOLUME: The volume of blood ejected per heart beat. It equals end-diastolic volume minus end-systolic volume.

STYLET: The thin flexible wire that can be shaped and inserted in the lumen of the pacing lead to allow its manipulation.

SUTURELESS LEAD: A myocardial lead in which the means of its introduction is the means of its fastening. One example is the "corkscrew-" like electrode, which once screwed into the myocardium is fixed in position and stimulates the heart.

SYNCHRONIZED: A stimulus emitted simultaneously with a sensed atrial or ventricular event so that the pacemaker stimulus falls into the absolute refractory interval of spontaneous depolarization.

SYNCHRONOUS: A pacemaker stimulus that is emitted in response to a sensed event after an appropriate delay, as in atrial synchronous.

TACHYCARDIA: A ventricular rate more rapid than 100 bpm. It may be entirely normal as in sinus tachycardia, a response to exercise, emotion, fever, etc.
Malignant: A tachycardia that accelerates and may result in ventricular fibrillation.
Monomorphic: A tachycardia that originates from one ventricular focus.
Polymorphic: A tachycardia that originates from more than one ventricular focus.
Supraventricular: A tachycardia that originates above the ventricle, i.e., sinus, atrial fibrillation, or flutter, etc.

THRESHOLD: The threshold of cardiac stimulation is the least cathodal electrical stimulus which, when delivered in diastole after the absolute, relative refractory and the hypersensitive periods, is able to maintain consistent capture of the heart.
Acute: The threshold immediately after implantation of the lead-electrode system.
Chronic: The threshold after stability has been reached.

TIME WINDOW: Range of critical coupling intervals during which extrastimuli can initiate and terminate tachycardia.

TOTAL ATRIAL REFRACTORY PERIOD (TARP):   The time in which the atrial pacemaker channel is insensitive. It usually consists of the AV interval and the atrial refractory interval after the ventricular event.

TRIGGERED: (See Synchronized.) A pacemaker response in which a stimulus is emitted in response to a sensed event.

UNDERDRIVE PACING: Pacing at a slower rate than a tachycardia which can interrupt and terminate a re-entrant arrhythmia.

UNIPOLAR: All pacemaker systems have two electrical terminals for each channel, one anodal, the other cathodal. If one (always the cathode) is in contact with sensitive tissue while the other is remote, i.e., away from the heart, the system is termed unipolar.

UPPER RATE INTERVAL: Also referred to as the "upper rate limit," "maximum tracking rate," etc. It is the minimum interval of response of the pacemaker ventricular channel to signals received via the atrial channel. It is the shortest interval the pacer will allow between two ventricular stimuli, or between a sensed ventricular event and a ventricular stimulus. The concept of interval is much more useful than that of rate.

VA CONDUCTION (ventriculoatrial):   The conduction of a ventricular impulse retrograde to the atrium via the AV node.

VA INTERVAL (ventriculoatrial):   The interval between the sensed or paced ventricular event and the next sensed or paced atrial event.

VOLT (V):   The force with which current is driven. The proper term is electromotive force which is measured in volts. Pacemaker output is indicated in volts. Biological signals, such as electrogram amplitudes, are indicated in millivolts (mV).

VULNERABLE PERIOD: That portion of the electrical complex, either atrial or ventricular, during which stimulation may induce arrhythmia.

WENCKEBACH: AV conduction at progressively greater intervals until one P wave is unsensed. The cycle then restarts.

WENCKEBACH UPPER RATE LIMIT: A mode of approach to the upper rate interval by automatically prolonging the interval between the sensed or paced ventricular event. This is also referred to as pseudo-Wenckebach behavior.

INDEX